A tailored education experience —

Sherpath book-organized collections

Sherpath is the digital teaching and learning technology designed specifically for healthcare education.

Sherpath book-organized collections offer:

Objective-based, digital lessons, mapped chapter-by-chapter to the textbook, that make it easy to find applicable digital assignment content.

Adaptive quizzing with personalized questions that correlate directly to textbook content.

Teaching materials that align to the text and are organized by chapter for quick and easy access to invaluable class activities and resources.

Elsevier ebooks that provide convenient access to textbook content, even offline.

INTERPERSONAL RELATIONSHIPS

Professional Communication Skills for Nurses

9th
EDITION

Kathleen Underman Boggs, PhD, FNP-CS

Family Nurse Practitioner, Associate Professor Emeritus College of Health and Human Services
University of North Carolina Charlotte, Charlotte, North Carolina

ELSEVIER

Elsevier
3251 Riverport Lane
St. Louis, Missouri 63043

Notice

Practitioners and researchers must always rely on their own experience and knowledge in evaluating and
using any information, methods, compounds or experiments described herein. Because of rapid advances
in the medical sciences, in particular, independent verification of diagnoses and drug dosages should be
made. To the fullest extent of the law, no responsibility is assumed by Elsevier, authors, editors or contributors for any injury and/or damage to persons or property as a matter of products liability, negligence or
otherwise, or from any use or operation of any methods, products, instructions, or ideas contained in the
material herein.

Previous editions copyrighted 2020, 2016, 2011, 2007, 2003, 1999, 1995, and 1989.

Content Strategist: Yvonne Alexopoulos
Senior Content Development Specialist: Rae Robertson
Publishing Services Manager: Deepthi Unni
Project Manager: Thoufiq Mohammed
Design Direction: Ryan Cook

Printed in India

Last digit is the print number: 9 8 7 6 5 4 3 2 1

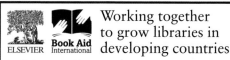

To Michael, the love of my life, granddaughters Sydney and Taya, and all of you choosing nursing.
Kathleen Underman Boggs

REVIEWERS AND CONTRIBUTORS

REVIEWERS

Roseann Colosimo, PhD, RN
Associate Professor
University of Nevada, Las Vegas
Las Vegas Nevada

Ruth Ozug, WHNP-BC
Assistant Professor of Nursing
Marian University
Indianapolis, Indiana

CONTRIBUTORS

Saretha Rebecca Lavarnway, MS
Educational Consultant and Faculty
Board of Education
Charleston, South Carolina

PREFACE

The ninth edition is designed as a key interactive communication skill reference for nursing students and professional nurses. It has been updated and expanded to include new understandings of patient-centered communication and the support for self-management strategies needed in contemporary healthcare environments. Simulation exercises with reflective analysis discussions allow students to process the pros and cons of various approaches and modern practice issues across clinical settings. Patient-centered relationships, self-management of chronic disorders, collaborative interprofessional communication, and team-based approaches remain the primary focus.

Our healthcare system is undergoing rapid change. New healthcare delivery models reflect greater emphasis on care delivery in the community, with patients assuming more responsibility for self-management of chronic conditions. It is anticipated that more than 50% of nursing positions will be community based rather than within the acute care hospital setting. The nation's population is more culturally diverse at many different levels—psychosocial, educational, with multiple resource availability, requiring individualized communication strategies. There are explanatory models for the same illness and varied underlying principles about treatment. Nurses are educationally prepared to function at a higher level than ever before. They are expected to master communication skills so as to play a key role in promoting and supporting patients to make healthy behavior changes.

ABOUT THE CONTENT

Interpersonal Relationships: Professional Communication Skills for Nurses consists of 27 chapters. The ninth edition reflects lessons learned during the COVID-19 pandemic with a new chapter emphasizing the need for self-care. Nurses are strongly encouraged to use intrapersonal communication strategies to help them manage the stress inherent in their nursing practice. The ninth edition continues to emphasize the therapeutic role of nurse–patient communication in a range of healthcare applications, including preventive health applications. Nurses follow patients through the life cycle so they need to master communication throughout the life cycle of our patients, including end-of-life communication. Content supports healthcare applications across a broad service continuum of care that includes hospitals, long-term care, ambulatory and public health, rehabilitation, and palliative and home care.

Chapter topics in the ninth edition mirror the nation's shift from a healthcare system structured around medical disease to one based on an integrated holistic health approach to healthcare that begins with the patient's perception, values, concerns, and preferences. Contemporary healthcare relationships consider every health experience as a holistic *human experience*, which requires a fresh, new perspective and level of patient and family involvement. This belief is reflected throughout the text in the types of communication strategies presented.

Although the text continues to draw evidence-based principles from nursing, medical science, technology, psychology, public health, and systems-based communication, the new contemporary healthcare landscape emphasizes a more personalized level of care, which honors the personal dignity, values, and preferences of patients in making significant health decisions and in implementing meaningful care choices in care. Patients are expected to actively engage in their own care and, in partnership with their care providers, to make meaningful care decisions related to achievement of mutually determined health goals. Communication skills, combined with patient-centered applications, create the therapeutic partnership that patients nowadays need to have to successfully self-manage long-term chronic disorders.

Emphasis on safety in healthcare is stressed throughout this book and in a full chapter devoted to the importance of communication in making healthcare a quality, safe environment, through nursing practice.

Computer technology has introduced new dimensions to health communication, allowing patients and clinical providers an immediate, transparent access to personal clinical records and secure portals for immediate discussion with providers. Chapter 25 has expanded content related to biomedical technologies documenting improved assessment, medication adherence, patient satisfaction, and sound decision-making. Applications of use of technology at point of care are also discussed. Concepts about the use of electronic records in examination of "Big Data" to analyze documented outcomes of sound clinical nursing practice further emphasize the usefulness of nursing evidence to support safer, more effective clinical judgment and interventions.

CHAPTER FORMAT

Every chapter follows the same format, presenting objectives, basic concepts with related supportive theories, and a clinical application section, connected by a relevant research study or metaanalysis of several studies relevant to the chapter topic.

Next-Generation NCLEX® Examination-Style Case Studies help students prepare for the upcoming 2023 NCLEX® Examination. These new case studies have been added in select chapters throughout the new edition. These are designed to test students on their clinical judgment and decision-making skills and better prepare them for practice. An answer key for the case studies is provided in an appendix at the end of this text.

Developing an Evidence-Based Practice boxes in each chapter offer a summary of research findings related to the chapter subject. This feature is intended to strengthen awareness of the link between research and practice.

Simulation Exercises with critical analysis questions offer an interactive component to the student's study of text materials. This offers opportunities for reflective analysis and offers students an opportunity to practice, observe, and critically evaluate professional communication skills from a practice perspective in a safe learning environment. Experiential practice with relationship-based communication principles facilitates development of confidence and skill in engaging in patient-centered communication across clinical settings. While simulation exercises can be done outside the classroom, in-class discussions are essential to consolidate learning. The shared comments and reflections of other students provide a wider, enriching perspective about the person-centered implications of communication in clinical practice.

Ethical Dilemma boxes are an exemplar related to real-life *ethical dilemmas* faced by direct care nurses and are presented at the end of each chapter. These are intended to stimulate thoughtful analysis and application.

The chapters in this edition can be used as individual teaching modules. The text can also be used as a primary text or as a communication resource, integrated across the curriculum. Chapter text boxes and tables highlight important ideas in each chapter.

This edition presents an updated synthesis of relationships in nursing and team-based health communication, with an emphasis on an integrated collaborative approach to patient- and family-centered professional relationships. Discussion questions for student reflective analysis are placed at the end of each chapter.

This ninth edition continues to give voice to the centrality of patient-centered relational communication strategies as the basis for ensuring quality and safety in professional healthcare delivery. Healthcare has changed dramatically, with the expectation that patients will be actively involved in their care. As the single most consistent healthcare provider in many patients' lives, nurses have an awesome responsibility to provide communication that is professional, honest, empathetic, and knowledgeable in individual and group relationships. As nurses, we are answerable to our patients, our profession, and ourselves to communicate with all those involved with a patient's care in an authentic therapeutic manner and to advocate for the patient's health, care, and well-being within the larger sociopolitical community.

The opportunity to contribute to the evolving development of communication as a central tenet of professional nursing practice has been a privilege as well as a responsibility to our profession.

Kathleen Underman Boggs

ACKNOWLEDGMENTS

We acknowledge our heartfelt appreciation for the contributions of the many professional nurses, students, and other practitioners as well as patients and their families who helped deepen and clarify our evolving thinking and understanding of communication over the past years. Thanks also to the many contributors to communication content over the years.

A resounding acknowledgment is given to the Elsevier editorial staff, particularly Yvonne Alexopoulos, Senior Content Strategist, and Rae L. Robertson, Senior Content Development Specialist. Their expertise, guidance, tangible support, and suggestions were invaluable in the content development of this ninth edition.

The author wishes to acknowledge Dr. Elizabeth Arnold's extensive contributions to the previous editions of this book. Although this 9th edition has been extensively revised, content is based substantially on contributions made by Dr. Arnold and other contributors. Her extensive teaching and clinical expertise informs much of the content, and her excellent writing skills helped make this book a success over the past 25 years.

Kathleen Underman Boggs

1

Communication Theories and Nursing Concepts

OBJECTIVES

At the end of the chapter, the reader will be able to:

1. Describe one-way communication theory is used by nurses to provide safe, quality care.
2. Compare and contrast linear and transactional models of communication.
3. Describe the four core components of nursing's metaparadigm.
4. Analyze one evidence-based practice applicable to nurse–patient communication.

You communicate every day to make your needs known, to convey information or to offer assistance. Socially, you communicate orally, digitally, and in writing. However, professional nurse–patient communication is different, requiring you learn new skills. This introductory chapter lays the groundwork for understanding professional nurse communication competencies. Accurate, effective, timely communication is a key aspect for providing safe and effective patient-centered healthcare. Our basic goal in team communication is to exchange information so we can understand one another as we work together to give care. As students, we learn about, practice, and implement appropriate communication skills. As beginning professional nurses, we are expected to have mastered an understanding of the communication process. The study of communication theory and skills is a complex issue complicated by the fact that knowledge is evolving. While nursing research is at an early developmental stage, applying evidence-based communication practices is a crucial component of care. We use "best practices" to promote wellness and care for those who

are ill. We need to communicate openly, transparently, and frequently (Auriemma et al., 2021).

BASIC CONCEPTS

Definition of Communication

Derived from the Latin word for "sharing," communication is the sending and receiving of information to help people understand one another and their environment. Communication is a social process that connects people and ideas through words, nonverbal behaviors, and actions. It is the method by which we build relationships. Because it is a mutual process, it continually changes over the time of the relationship. Examples of *verbal communication* are words chosen to convey a message. Examples of *nonverbal communication* are use of body language such as facial expressions, making eye contact, or nodding our head to show attentiveness. To be effective, both verbal and nonverbal messages need to be congruent. The vast majority of communication is nonverbal. There is also *written communication*. Consider the case with Laura Cox.

CASE STUDY: Laura Cox, RN

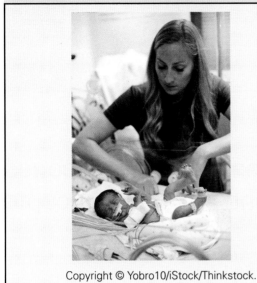

Copyright © Yobro10/iStock/Thinkstock.

Laura Cox is a 21-year-old new graduate nurse who has been working in a neonatal intensive care unit (NICU) for 6 months. Today she cares for Sammy Moe who was admitted at 26 weeks' gestation. He startles at every loud sound. Laura speaks to Sammy in a gentle tone and uses gentle touch to communicate comfort.

Contrast this communication with the following scenario:

Gen West is a very nervous first-year student nurse assigned to Mr Lopez who is recovering from surgery. Gen tells him she wants to care for him and will bathe him. She grimaces while washing his arm, apologizes for the cold water temperature but does not warm it, chats about her boyfriend, and hurries to finish before her instructor comes. Mr Lopez seems not to understand her but senses her anxiety.

1. Is there congruency between verbal and nonverbal behaviors?
2. What messages did these two patients receive?

Communication Theoretical Concepts

Communication theories are derived from multiple fields of study such as psychology, sociology, cultural anthropology, engineering, and management, among others. Communication theories explain the process of information exchange both intrapersonally (internal) and interpersonally (among people). The term communication derives from the Latin "communicare," meaning to share. Communication connects people and ideas through words, nonverbal behaviors, and the written word. People communicate as a key means to share information, ask questions, and seek assistance. Words are used to persuade others, to take a position, or to create an understandable story.

Communication between healthcare providers and patients impacts the way care is delivered. Outcomes of effective interpersonal communication in healthcare relate to higher patient satisfaction and more optimal health status or palliative support at the end of life. Patients are more likely to understand their health condition through meaningful communication and to alert providers when problems arise.

Interpersonal Communication

Interpersonal communication is a continual social process in which at least two people exchange ideas with the intent to influence the behavior or actions of the other. This is true even if the messages are exchanged online (West & Turner, 2018). For the communication to succeed, the sender has to have an idea, encode it with selected words, and send the message. The receiver has to receive it, decode it, and process its meaning. Ideally, the receiver then responds by giving feedback to the sender, sort of signaling "Yes, I hear you" (Munn, 2019).

Message Barriers

It is crucial to the process that the sender validate that both people share the correct message meaning. Conflict arises when the message that is received is not what the sender has intended to send. Sometimes the encoding or decoding gets skewed. Context and environment can also interfere with correct message transmission. Communication is a complex undertaking!

Process

Nurse–patient communication is dynamic, continually changing. The words we choose to use in our effort to communicate are message symbols. Their meaning is central to the way a message is interpreted. It is crucial to create shared meaning. Can you think of a word that might mean one thing to you but holds a very different meaning for an older person or one from another culture? We explain, repeat, summarize, and seek feedback to determine if we have true shared meaning. The environmental context affects message transmission. For example, a noisy television can interfere with our patient's focus.

Components Common to Communication Theories

Process

Communication is a process that is dynamic, changing as the mutual exchange of ideas flows. We use all five of our senses during conversation but primarily rely on vision and hearing for message transfer.

Message

Most **messages** are a factual transfer of information with initial data predominantly being sought by the care provider. Studies show that initial intake interviews are mostly about the nurse getting background information such as presenting the health problem and reason for this visit, as well as other basic facts such as duration of symptoms. To begin to develop a therapeutic nurse–patient relationship, opportunities should be given for the patient to express concerns and ask questions. As the relationship progresses, communication skills are used to convey caring and respect for patient concerns. We can then begin to develop a mutual plan of care to reach desired treatment goals. Educating our patient is another goal for communication.

Sender

A message begins with the words chosen by the sender to convey a specific message. Words may mean different things to different people. Does "cool" mean a factual temperature or is it an affective feeling?

Symbols

Words are used as concrete symbols representing a fact or they can be abstract symbols representing thoughts. Is there a shared meaning for both the nurse and the patient? Are the words chosen appropriate to the purpose of the message and to the setting? Do they advance the purpose of this professional relationship?

Transmission

Most messages are verbal spoken ideas accompanied by nonverbal cues, such as attentive posture, eye contact, and nodding to indicate interest in what is being said.

Meaning

Past experiences and current circumstances influence interpretation of the **meaning** of the message to the receiver. Accurate communication requires that both the sender and the receiver understand the word symbols used and the tone of voice. Meaning is affected by the nonverbal cues the sender is conveying; for example, fidgeting, avoiding eye contact, glancing frequently at a clock convey "I am not really interested in what you have to say."

Receiver

The message is heard by the receiver who then has a cognitive response decoding the factual part of the message. They also interpret the nonverbal message about feelings conveyed.

Feedback

The receiver is expected to acknowledge receipt of the message by signaling understanding about its meaning (**feedback**), giving verification to the sender. Any type of response can alter the content, perhaps modifying what the sender has to say.

Environment

Conversations occur within specific **environments**. Interpretation of the message can be affected by situational variables such as background noise or lack of privacy. The environment is also the context in which the communication takes place. Environment includes time and place, historical context, cultural background, or prior experiences the patient has had with healthcare workers. Glance at Fig. 1.1 for a graphic depiction of these communication theory components.

Systems Theory

Components of systems theory have been adapted to communication among human patients, families, healthcare providers, and organizations. The message sender and environment could be conceptualized as giving output to the receiver, who processes the message (input), interprets the meaning of the message (throughput), then responds, perhaps changing behavior (output), and gives back information to the sender validating what the message means (feedback).

Self-Disclosure

Social penetration theory tells us that conveying some personal information about yourself can be a method of deepening a relationship. While this is true social relationship, there are boundaries that need to be adhered to in a professional nurse–patient relationship limiting what is appropriate to reveal. Generally, nurses do not reveal information about their personal lives or opinions.

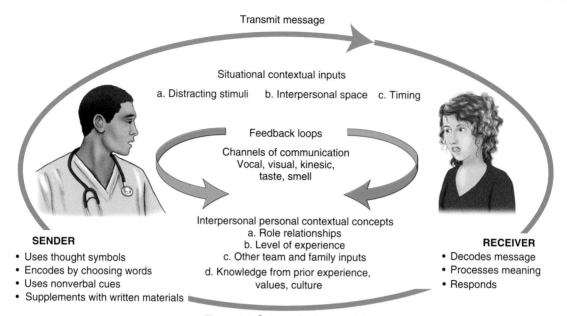

Figure 1.1 Communications model.

Models of Communication

Linear Models

Linear communication models focus only on the sending and receiving of the message. Their components include the sender, receiver, communication channels, and context. They do not describe the development of cocreated meanings. As an example, linear communication is useful in an emergency situation when time is of the essence to convey information.

Transactional Models

Transactional communication models describe interpersonal communication as a reciprocal interaction in which both sender and receiver influence each other's messages and responses as they converse. Each person constructs a mental picture of the other during the conversation, including perceptions about the other's attitudes and potential reactions to the message. The Joint Commission (TJC, 2010) says that effective communication is a two-way process in which messages are negotiated until both parties correctly understand. Communication is influenced by learned patterns of behavior, cultural expectations, personal beliefs, and prior experiences, as well as by the environmental context. Simulation Exercise 1.1 helps you identify differences between linear and transactional formats.

The Healthcare System

Our healthcare system is rapidly evolving. The patient is considered to be at the center of a team of healthcare workers across a variety of organizations (AHRQ, 2017). Nurses usually work for agencies as part of a team of professionals. To do so requires skillful communication not just with a patient but also with management and with colleagues on the healthcare team. As depicted in Fig. 1.2, healthcare is delivered by organizations whose primary mission is to promote, maintain, or restore health.

At the organizational level, communication focuses on the interrelationships across agencies. While part of the goal is to deliver quality healthcare, organizations such as hospitals or home health agencies are businesses. For example, financial solvency is another goal of importance to management. Up to 90% of a manager's time is spent communicating. For example, part of their role is convincing employees to align with corporate goals.

Patient-Centered Care

The practice of competently providing healthcare to a patient and family with their active participation in planning care and making decisions is termed patient-centered care. Concepts such as respect are communicated clearly. Support is provided to help patients attain goals. Ideally,

SIMULATION EXERCISE 1.1   The Meaning of Health as a Nursing Concept

Purpose
To help students understand the dimensions of health as a nursing concept.

Procedure
1. Think of a person whom you think is healthy. In a short report (one to two paragraphs), identify characteristics that led you to your choice of this person.
2. In small groups of three or four, read your stories to each other. As you listen to other students' stories, write down themes that you note.
3. Compare themes, paying attention to similarities and differences, and developing a group definition of health derived from the stories.

4. In a larger group, share your definitions of health and defining characteristics of a healthy person.

Reflective Discussion Analysis
1. Were you surprised by any of your thoughts about being healthy?
2. Did your peers define health in similar ways?
3. Based on the themes that emerged, how is health determined?
4. Is illness the opposite of being healthy?
5. In what ways, if any, did you find concepts of health to be culture or gender bound?
6. In what specific ways can you as a healthcare provider support the health of your patient?

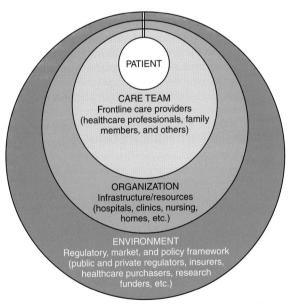

Figure 1.2 Conceptual drawing of a four-level healthcare system, with patient as its core concept. (From National Academy of Engineering, Institute of Medicine, Committee on Engineering and the Health Care System; Reid, P. P., Compton, W. D., Grossman, J. H., et al. (Eds). (2005). *Building a better delivery system: a new engineering/health care partnership* (p. 20). Washington, DC: National Academies Press. Retrieved from http://www.nap.edu/catalog/11378.html.)

care is easily accessed and coordinated, and continuity is ensured. Research identifies practices that are conducive to a positive patient experience as illustrated in Box 1.1 based on Picker Institute principles of patient-centered care.

BOX 1.1   Picker's Eight Principles of Patient-Centered Care

1. Communicates to foster continuity and safe care transition
2. Coordinates care across departments and agencies
3. Informs and educates
4. Provides physical comfort
5. Involves family and provides support
6. Respects patient preferences and makes them partners in planning care
7. Communicates accurately, frequently, and in a timely manner
8. Advocates for access to care

Data from Picker Institute Europe, Oxford, UK.

Nursing

Nursing encompasses both autonomous and collaborative care functions. Nurses focus on promotion of health, prevention of illness, and care of ill patients. Caring is the concept that is viewed as one of the main tenets of the nursing role.

Nursing's Metaparadigm

Nursing's metaparadigm represents the most abstract form of nursing knowledge (Black, 2017). Four core constructs make up professional nursing's **metaparadigm**: *person, environment, health,* and *nursing.* Each of these four conceptual constructs has an internal consistency related to the knowledge structure of nursing, which is described in different ways across theoretical frameworks.

CONCEPT OF PERSON

Knowledge of the "patient as a person" is the starting point in contemporary healthcare delivery. *Person* is defined as the recipient of nursing care. The term "person" is applied to individuals, family units, the community, and selected target populations—for example, infants, elderly, and the mentally ill. For all individuals, mental, physical, and social health are vital strands of life that are closely interwoven and deeply interdependent. Examples include gender, lifestyle, coping styles, habits, and cultural values, which are identified as "person" attributes.

Nurses have a legal responsibility to protect each patient's integrity and health rights to self-determination in healthcare. It is also an *ethical* professional responsibility, whether the person is a contributing member of society, a critically ill newborn, a comatose patient, or a seriously mentally ill individual.

CONCEPT OF ENVIRONMENT

Environment describes the *context* in which health relationships take place. To consider the concept of "person" without considering the environmental factors acting as barriers or supports to healthcare participation is impracticable. Socioenvironmental factors represent the context that directly and indirectly influences a person's health perceptions and health behaviors. At the community level, poverty, education, religious and spiritual beliefs, type of community (rural or urban), family strengths and challenges, level of social support, health resource availability, and ease of care access are significant environmental determinants of health. Contextual factors are important in health promotion, disease prevention, and the capacity of individuals with chronic conditions to take major responsibility for self-management strategies. The importance of environment is underscored in a new American Nurses Association (ANA) Scope and Standard of Nursing Practice (#17): "The registered nurse integrates the principles of environmental health for nursing in all areas of practice" (ANA, 2015).

CONCEPT OF HEALTH

The word **health** derives from the word *whole*. Health is a relative term, subject to personal interpretation. Culture, religious beliefs, and previous life experiences influence how a person perceives and interprets health and illness. For example, in some cultures, where poverty is a significant factor, having a robust body size is considered a sign of a healthy lifestyle. In a different culture, a similar body size would be considered a sign of an unhealthy lifestyle (Schiavo, 2014).

The WHO definition developed in 1948 describes *health* as "a state of complete physical, mental and social well-being, and not merely the absence of disease or infirmity." Present-day health concepts describe health on a continuum as stretching from birth to death. Better nutrition, an emphasis on hygiene, and advances in diagnosis and treatment have reduced the incidence of acute diseases.

People are living much longer, but the incidence of chronic disorders associated with aging has also increased. The Centers for Disease Control and Prevention (CDC) reports that almost half the adult population has one or more *chronic* health conditions. Chronic diseases have overtaken acute disorders as a major cause of death and disability worldwide, accounting for the majority of disease globally.

Contemporary health initiatives reflect an increasing shift in focus to healthy lifestyle promotion, disease prevention, reducing health disparities, early risk assessments, and chronic disease self-care management strategies. **Quality of life** includes both health and well-being. The term refers to an individual's subjective assessment of well-being. At the opposite end of well-being is the human experience of suffering and anguish, in large part, associated with health. A healthy person is the one who is able to productively strive toward *his* or *her* vital goals. For example, an active 80-year-old woman can consider herself quite healthy, despite having osteoporosis and a controlled heart condition.

Paradigm Shift in Healthcare Delivery

We are seeing dramatic changes in how professional nursing is practiced, and where healthcare is delivered. Until recent decades, care was delivered in acute care settings, based on a disease-focused medical model. Many acute disorders that shortened people's lives have been eradicated or are now viewed as manageable chronic conditions. Better diagnostic tools and effective treatments have given rise to improved medical outcomes and longevity. According to the CDC, nearly half of all adults suffer from one or more chronic disorders. Patients are charged with becoming active participants in partnership with their healthcare providers.

There has been a shift to emphasize healthcare initiatives that advance the quality and safety of comprehensive healthcare. The Chronic Care Model is an integrated form of healthcare services, designed to provide safe quality healthcare across designated clinical settings. The model includes proactive health promotion and disease prevention care initiatives. Contemporary healthcare emphasizes health promotion and disease prevention, early intervention for chronic disorders, continuity of care, and activated patient participation as part of the healthcare team. Nurses play an important role in helping people of all ages engage in various health promotion and disease prevention activities needed to promote maximum personal health and well-being. Try Simulation Exercise 1.1, *The Meaning of Health*, which provides an opportunity to explore the multidimensional meaning of health.

PROFESSIONAL NURSING

Nurses represent the largest group of healthcare professionals in the United States with over 3 million registered nurses. Many organizations, including the Pew Commission on Health Professionals, have identified competencies needed for professional nursing practice in the 21st century. In 2012, the IOM charged professional nursing to take a leadership role in shaping a transformed healthcare system. Effective communication links with each competency identified.

Nursing: a Practice Discipline

The science of nursing (theory based, research, clinical guidelines) provides an essential focus and knowledge basis for professional nursing. Evidence-based nursing actions help patients achieve identified health goals through services ranging from health promotion, preventive care, and health education, to include direct care, rehabilitation, palliative care, research, and health teaching. *The patient is at the center of the model, as its core concept.*

Professional nursing represents a practice discipline. Donaldson and Crowley (1978) characterized the nursing discipline as having a specialized perspective.

Professional nursing practice incorporates empirical concepts from the natural and biological sciences, while drawing from the social sciences of psychology, phenomenology, and sociology. Contemporary nurses are expected to integrate evidence-based care principles into practice assessments, and to base their clinical judgments and care decisions on them. Professional nursing combines specialized knowledge and skills with prudent clinical judgment to meet patient, family, and community healthcare needs. Some differentiate between the science and art of nursing, stating that knowledge represents the science of nursing, and caring represents the art of nursing. Both are needed to support the safety and quality of skilled care.

Nursing: an Art

Professional nursing and healthcare practices are grounded in human interactions and relationships. The "art of nursing" references a blending of each nurse's intuitive thinking processes about the nature of health incident from the patient's perspective. The nurse's focus is on developing an individualized understanding of each patient as a unique human being. Perceptions are influenced by the nurse's life knowledge and professional experiences with other patients. Using these data takes into account the interactive factors that nurses must consider to blend their knowledge and skills with scientific understandings to provide safe, quality care. Try Simulation Exercise 1.2 to identify your philosophy of what professional nursing is.

Caring as a Core Value of Professional Nursing

Caring is considered an *essential* functional construct in professional nursing practice, which defines the patient-centered relationship. Caring is an essential element in the development of interpersonal relationships in clinical settings. Think about your most important relationship in healthcare. What made it meaningful to you?

SIMULATION EXERCISE 1.2 What Is Professional Nursing?

Purpose
To help students develop an understanding of professional nursing.

Procedure
1. Interview a professional nurse who has been in practice for more than 12 months. Ask for descriptions of what he or she considers professional nursing to be today, in what ways he or she thinks nurses make a difference, and how the nurse feels the role might evolve within the next 10 years.
2. In small groups of three to five students, discuss and compare your findings.
3. Develop a group definition of professional nursing.

Reflective Discussion Analysis
1. What does nursing mean to you?
2. In what ways, if any, have your ideas about nursing changed now that you are actively involved in patient care as a nurse?
3. Is your understanding of nursing different from those of the nurse(s) you interviewed?
4. As a new nurse, how would you want to present yourself?

Professional caring is about the involvement of the nurse and patient in the encounter, and its meaning to the people involved. Caring does not involve specific tasks. Instead, it involves the creation of a sustained relationship with the other. There are many forms of caring in clinical practice, some visible, others private and personal, known only to the persons experiencing feeling cared for. In a qualitative study, when graduate student nurses were asked to describe a professional caring incident in their practice, they identified the attributes of caring as (1) giving of self, (2) involved presence, (3) intuitive knowing and empathy, (4) supporting the patient's integrity, and (5) professional competence (Arnold, 1997).

FUNCTIONS OF COMMUNICATION WITHIN HEALTHCARE SYSTEMS

More than any other variable, effective interpersonal communication supports the safety and quality in healthcare delivery (see Chapter 2). Communication connects people and ideas through words, nonverbal behaviors, and actions. People communicate as a key means to share information, to ask questions, and to seek assistance. Words are used to persuade others, to take a position, and to create an understandable story. In fact, communication represents the very essence of the human condition. Human communication is unique. Only human beings have complex vocabularies and are capable of learning and using multiple language symbols to convey meaning.

Outcomes of Effective Communication

Communication between healthcare providers and patients impacts the way care is delivered; it is as important as the care itself. Outcomes of effective interpersonal communication in healthcare relate to higher patient satisfaction and productive health changes. Patients are more likely to understand their health conditions through meaningful communication and to alert providers when something is not working. Other specific ways that interpersonal health communication impacts service quality are through

- development of a workable treatment partnership with mutual goals;
- understanding illness from our patient's perspective;
- more effective diagnosis and earlier recognition of health changes;
- better understanding of the patient's condition;
- improved personalized compliance with therapeutic regimes;
- more efficient utilization of health services; and
- stronger, longer lasting positive outcomes.

Two-way communication provides the opportunity to share information, to be heard, and to be validated. Having

the opportunity to provide input empowers patients and families to take a stronger position in contributing to their healthcare.

DEVELOPING AN EVIDENCE-BASED PRACTICE

Evidence-based professional nursing practice serves as a critical foundation for nursing practice. The International Council of Nursing (ICN 2021) defines *evidence-based nursing practice* as a problem-solving approach to clinical decision-making that incorporates a search for the best and latest evidence, clinical expertise and assessment, *and* patient preference values.

Integrating individual clinical expertise and judgment with objective evidence and collaborative interprofessional consultations is recognized as being critical to safe, quality professional nursing care. It is a way of practicing owned by all nurses. Fueled by professional communication, a strong evidence base represents a blending of the nurse's expertise with research findings and best practices guidelines. Nurses partner with patients to merge these data with patient preferences, value beliefs, and personal capacity to cope into jointly constructed action plans to resolve health issues. Ideally, professional nurses integrate their professional clinical expertise with "patterns of knowing" about their patients to customize research-based findings and clinical guidelines in providing skilled, patient-centered care. In each chapter, there is a sample discussion of research studies with suggestions for application to your clinical practice. The *American Journal of Nursing* has run a series of articles in 2020 and 2021 describing this issue. For purposes of this book, the author graded each EPB sample in terms of the strength of the research presented. Is it sufficiently strong to support a change in our practice? Grades are as follows:

- High level of confidence that reported results are true and can be replicated in other studies. There are no discernible problem deficiencies in methodology.
- Moderate. Findings are close to true, but there may be some doubts about methodology. There is moderate confidence that future studies will replicate the same results.
- Low. Only limited confidence in strength of results. More research is needed before applying results to your practice.
- Insufficient. Not enough data were provided about methodology to judge the strength of research. Generally, findings from many studies are needed before changing our practice interventions. A meta-analysis of several studies gives greater confidence.

INTERPROFESSIONAL EDUCATION AND PRACTICE

The IOM Reports advocated health team collaborative care as a key means of delivering complex care, particularly for management of chronic illness. Each health discipline has different vocabularies, training, agendas, and priorities, which must be integrated to achieve coordinated optimal health outcomes using healthcare team concepts. Examples of vocabulary meanings have various meanings among the different disciplines. Principles of team-based healthcare include the following:

- Sharing goals
- Clear roles
- Mutual trust
- Effective communication
- Measurable processes and outcomes

How health providers use collaborative and networking skills to achieve clinical outcomes becomes a measure of system-based team competence.

DEVELOPING AN EVIDENCE-BASED PRACTICE
Sample: Communication Education

Patients with cancer tend to have a high stress level that can be minimized with effective use of communication skills and support. For the Cochrane Database, Moore and colleagues conducted a metaanalysis of 10 studies on effects of use staff training communication programs on patient and family care.

Results
Following communications training, healthcare professionals demonstrated more empathy and improved their use of communication skills such as asking open-ended questions. Findings were supported by Allenbaugh's 2019 study that also found an increase in use of communication skills. However, effects of communication on improving patient health outcomes were not supported. Two studies reported greater patient trust and decreased anxiety.
Strength of Research: Moderate.

Application to Your Clinical Practice
1. Communication skill training can improve direct care communication.
2. Use of effective communication skills can lead to increased empathy some of the time.
3. Effective communication can decrease anxiety in some patients.

References
Allenbaugh, J., Corbell, J., Rack, L., Rubio, D., & Spagnoletti, C. (2019). A brief communication curriculum improves resident and nurse communication skills and patient satisfaction. *J Gen Intern Med. 34*(7), 1167–1173.
Moore, P. M., Rivera, S., Bravo-Soto, G. A., Olivares, C., & Lawrie, T. A. (2018). Communication skills training for healthcare professionals working with people who have cancer. *Cochrane Database Syst Rev. 7*(7), CD003751.

APPLICATIONS

Trends in Healthcare Delivery

For the purposes of this introductory chapter, we highlight some of the major paradigm shifts in healthcare applications that impact care delivery. Healthcare delivery has moved from a "one-professional: one patient" care model to a "many professionals: one patient" model, with reimbursement for quality care rather than quantity of care given. The contemporary practice of healthcare is system based, with the locus of control for decision-making and clinical management of symptoms team shared with the patient and other members of the healthcare team. Healthcare thus becomes a *shared* reality. Recognizing the healthcare team as a microsystem composed of skilled interdependent team members, each representing a relevant discipline involved in the patient's care, creates a different work design and different communication needs.

Care processes are conceptualized as participatory management applications of self-management strategies aimed at controlling the symptoms of chronic disorders. At the center of this care paradigm is the patient. Instead of caring *for* their patients, nurses are charged with working *with* their patients to develop and implement action plans that acknowledge the reality of the patient's health condition, while working to achieve desired clinical outcomes and personal well-being, for everyone—healthcare professionals, patients and their families, researchers, payers, planners, and educators—to make the changes that will lead to better patient outcomes. Specific communication and interprofessional collaborative concepts related to community-based continuity of care initiatives will be presented throughout subsequent chapters in this text.

Management of chronic health problems is linked to, but it is characteristically different from, care delivery for acute health problems. People with chronic health conditions will experience acute health episodes requiring prompt critical treatment. But many chronic problems are preventable, controllable, or resolvable with proactive health promotion actions, and self-managed disease prevention strategies. This paradigm shift from an emphasis on individual disease conditions to population-level disease prevention and wellness promotion reflects the reality of contemporary healthcare demands, including the multiple causes of illness and socioeconomic factors.

Patient Focus

Core components of today's healthcare system include an activated patient and the dual concepts of patient centeredness and patient empowerment. This broader shift in orientation has been strengthened through a decade of IOM reports calling for a transformed healthcare system, in which care is patient driven, and delivered within an interprofessional collaborative care framework.

Team Care

The complexity of patient conditions has given impetus to the use of team models for care as the most efficient means to deliver accessible, high-quality, patient-centered healthcare that addresses wellness and prevention of illness and adverse events, self-management of chronic illness, and interdependent clinical applications. *Interdependence* is a key element in a systems approach that underscores the ways in which various components interact with each other. As providers from different professional health disciplines share responsibility with each other and selected patients, within and across clinical settings, the potential for fragmented or duplicative care is effectively diminished. Interprofessional collaboration is essential to the implementation of safe, quality care in a transformed healthcare system.

Nursing Care Communication Competencies

Multiple professional organizations have established core communication competencies for entry level nurses. These include the following:

- Communicates with patients to determine their preferences, care plan, and preferred goals.
- Communicates openly and clearly, verifying patient understanding.
- Adapts to patient's communication style.
- Communicates responsibly to provide safe care, using tools to improve communication especially at times of "handing over" care responsibility to another nurse.
- Uses informatics to aid in communication with team members and assist in decision-making.

Use of Evidence-Based Practice

We actively seek to use "best practices" in delivering nursing care (QSEN, 2020). Evidence-based practice (EBP) is defined as a problem-solving approach to clinical judgment, which also includes the expertise of clinicians. The goal of EBP is to apply research results to enhance the quality of care and improve patient outcomes. EBP has been shown to improve patient outcome, reduce hospital costs, improve quality, and empower practitioners (Camargo et al., 2018; Edward et al., 2020; Gigli et al., 2020; Melnyk & Fineout-Overholt, 2019). It is slowly being implemented with studies suggesting that some practicing nurses are not knowledgeable. Some agencies have not yet created a culture supportive of EBP use (Yoo et al., 2019). ANA Magnet designated hospitals use EPB as a benchmark of excellent practice. According to Skela-Savie et al. (2020), all European nursing programs integrate EBP use into their curricula. Do all American programs do so? Key steps to EBP use are listed in Table 1.1.

TABLE 1.1 Key Steps to Integrating Evidence-Based Practice Concepts in Patient Care	
Knowledge, Attitude, Skill	**Application to Clinical Practice**
Develop an inquiring attitude, identify clinical problems.	Have an open mind. Be open to changes in "usual" practice; search EBP databases for solutions.
Be accountable.	Use information technology to examine intervention outcomes on your unit, in your agency. Be aware of big data analyses that support specific EBP interventions.
Seek to cultivate organizational support.	Enlist administrators who will support a change in the care culture.
Value EBP as a method to improve quality of care outcomes.	Systematically search for answers to clinical care problems. Seek research to validate new types of interventions. Enlist healthcare team cooperation.
Analyze strength of research and propose changes or develop alternative interventions with colleagues.	Integrate best practice recommendations into care protocols.
Evaluate effectiveness.	Measure, evaluate, and document outcomes.
Be an innovator.	Seek different solutions to rapid changes in environmental conditions.
Disseminate findings.	Share at professional meetings, conferences. Use technology such as blogs to ask questions and present solutions.

SUMMARY

This chapter describes theoretical concepts from communication theories that are useful in nursing and provide foundation for future chapters. This chapter describes core concepts of nursing's metaparadigm to help nurses integrate and apply relational knowledge to benefit patients and families in clinical settings. The nurse as member of a healthcare team was introduced and will be expanded in later chapters. Contemporary professionalism supports team-based processes of multiple professions working together with cross-disciplinary responsibilities and accountability for achieving improved clinical outcomes. The application of evidence-based practice was introduced, and sample research boxes in all subsequent chapters provide opportunities to consider applications to your nursing practice.

> **ETHICAL DILEMMA: What Would You Do?**
> Craig Montegue is a difficult patient to care for. As his nurse, you find his constant arguments, poor hygiene, and the way he treats his family very upsetting. It is difficult for you to provide him with anything but the most basic care, and you just want to leave his room as quickly as possible. How could you use a patient-centered approach to understanding Craig? What are the ethical elements in this situation, and how would you address them in implementing care for Craig?

DISCUSSION QUESTIONS

1. In what ways can you envision communication skills as being as important as your technical skills?
2. In what ways would you envision applying evidence as a nurse to enhance your ability to deliver safe, quality care at the bedside?

REFERENCES

Agency for Healthcare Research and Quality (AHRQ). (2017). *TeamSTEPPS® instructor manual.* Rockville, MD: AHRQ. Available at: https://www.ahrq.gov/teamstepps/ instructor/tools.html. [Accessed 5 May 2021].

American Nurses Association (ANA). (2015). *Scope and standards of nursing* (ed 3). Silver Spring, MD: ANA.

Arnold, E. (1997). Caring from the graduate student perspective. *International Journal for Human Caring, 1*(3), 32–42.

Auriemma, C. L., O'Harhay, M. O., Haines, K. J., Barg, F. K., Halpern, S. D., & Lyon, S. M. (2021). What matters to patients and their families during and after critical illness: A qualitative study. *American Journal of Critical Care, 30*(1), 11–20.

Black, B. (2017). *Professional nursing: Concepts and challenges* (ed 8). St. Louis, MO: Elsevier.

Camargo, F. C., Iwamoto, H. H., Galvao, C. M., Pereira, G., Andrade, R. B., & Masso, G. C. (2018). Competencies and barriers for the evidence-based practice in nursing: An integrative review. *Revista Brasileira de Enfermagem, 71*(4), 2030–2038.

Donaldson, S. K., & Crowley, D. M. (1978). The discipline of nursing. *Nursing Outlook, 26,* 113–120.

Edward, K. L., Galletti, A., & Huynh, M. (2020). Enhancing communication with family members in the intensive care unit: A mixed-methods study. *Critical Care Nurse, 40*(6), 23–32.

Gigli, K. H., Davis, B. S., Ervin, J., & Kahn, J. M. (2020). Factors associated with nurses' knowledge of and perceived values in evidence-based practice. *American Journal of Critical Care, 29*(1), e1–e8.

International Council of Nurses (ICN). (2021). *Nursing definitions.* Geneva, Switzerland: ICN. Available at: http://www.icn.ch/nursing-policy/nursing-definitions/. [Accessed 5 May 2021].

Melnyk, B. M., & Fineout-Overholt, E. (2019). *Evidence-based practice in nursing* (ed 4). Philadelphia: Wolters-Kluwer.

Munn, J. (2019). *Life skills: Communication.* Columbia, SC: self-published.

Quality and Safety Education for Nurses (QSEN) Institute. (2020). *QSEN competencies (Pre-licensure KSAs).* Cleveland, OH: QSEN Institute. Available at: https://qsen.org/ competencies/pre-licensure-ksas/. [Accessed 5 May 2021].

Schiavo, R. (2014). *Health communication: From theory to practice* (ed 2). San Francisco, CA: Jossey-Bass.

Skela-Savie, B., Gotlieb, J., Panczyk, M., et al. (2020). Teaching evidence-based practice (EBP) in nursing curricula in six European countries: A descriptive study. *Nurse Education Today, 94,* 104561.

The Joint Commission (TJC). (2010). *Advancing effective communication, cultural competence, and patient and family-centered care. A roadmap for hospitals.* Oakbrook Terrace, IL: TJC. Available at: www.jointcommission.org/ assets/1/6/aroadmapforHospitalsfinalversion727.pdf. [Accessed 5 May 2021].

West, R. L., & Turner, L. H. (2018). *Introducing communications theory: Analysis and application* (ed 6). New York: McGraw-Hill.

Yoo, J. Y., Kim, J. H., Kim, H. L., & Ki, J. S. (2019). Clinical nurses beliefs, knowledge, organizational readiness and level of implementation of evidence based practice: First step to creating an EBP culture. *PLoS One, 14*(12), 1–2.

SUGGESTED READING

Institute of Medicine (IOM). (2012). The future of nursing: Accomplishments a year after the landmark report (Editorial). *Journal of Nursing Scholarship, 44*(1), 1.

2

Clarity and Safety in Communication

OBJECTIVES

At the end of the chapter, the reader will be able to:

1. Discuss the role communication plays in creating a "culture of safety."
2. Describe why patient safety is a complex system issue and an individual function.
3. Analyze the relationship between open communication, error reporting, and a culture of safety.
4. Create simulations to demonstrate use of standardized tools for clear communication affecting patient care, such as using situation, background, assessment, recommendation (SBAR) in a simulated conversation with a physician.

Communication is the key to safe healthcare. When healthcare workers communicate effectively, fewer errors occur and people are more satisfied. The majority of errors in healthcare are linked to a lack of proper communication. Miscommunication can be between nurses; among interdisciplinary teams (including physicians, physical and occupational therapists, dietitians, and pharmacists); or between nurse and patient. The causes of unsafe events are complex, but patients report communication breakdowns as a major contributing factor (Giardina et al., 2020).

Globally, nurses need to make safety a core priority (ICN, 2020). In the United States, the ability to give safe and effective care is identified by the Quality and Safety Education for Nurses (QSEN) guidelines as an essential competency (www.qsen.org/). According to The Joint Commission (TJC), 60%–70% of reported cases of errors were the result of miscommunication. Some examples of errors are incomplete patient information at time of transition, hospital-acquired infections, incorrect labeling

of lab specimens, patient falls, and, most common of all, medication errors (AHRQ, 2020a). This chapter discusses communication strategies designed to promote a safe environment and focuses on commonly used **standardized communication tools** for clear communication. The tools for clear communication range from effective communication between nurses and physicians, such as using situation, background, assessment, recommendation (SBAR), to simple template checklists used when nurses finish the shift and "handoff" to the next nurse or transfer a patient to another unit or agency. The aim of improving communication is to reduce patient mortality, decrease medical errors, and promote effective healthcare teamwork. A number of agencies and professional organizations are developing and updating guidelines for levels of communication that prevent errors and adverse patient outcomes. Nurses and nursing students must be aware of error prevention and communication strategies to reduce potential threats to safe care at multiple levels in the care system. Consider the Ryte case.

CASE STUDY: **Glen Ryte and Postoperative Complications**

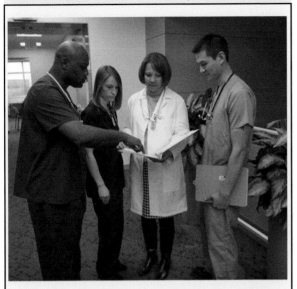

Glen Ryte, age 24, is transferred onto your surgical unit from Recovery Room 1 hour after his appendectomy. You are a staff nurse in the middle of change of shift rounds. Since Mr. Ryte's vital signs are within normal limits, his intravenous (IV) drip flowing well, and his dressing dry and intact, you postpone visiting him until completion of rounds. The recovery room nurse failed to tell you he had a brief episode of falling blood pressure which she handled by increasing his IV rate. By the time you see him, Mr. Ryte's blood pressure has fallen and he looks pale. His abdomen is rigid, possible due to intraabdominal bleeding.

1. What lack of vital communication led to this problem?
2. According to AHRQ (2020b), the nurse's role includes immediate detection and intervention when the patient's condition changes. What would you have done?

BASIC CONCEPTS

Safety Definition

Multiple healthcare organizations have issued definitions of safety. *Safety* is defined by the Institute of Medicine (IOM) as "prevention of harm to the patient." The World Health Organization states that "**patient safety** is the prevention of errors and adverse effects to patients associated with health care" (www.euro.who.int/en/health-topics/Health-systems/patient-safety).

The nursing profession has always had safe practice as a major goal, as identified in the American Nurses Association (ANA) Code of Ethics for Nurses. QSEN and the American Association of Colleges of Nursing offer a broader definition: safety is the minimization of risk for harm to patients and to providers through both system effectiveness and individual performance (Cronenwett et al., 2007).

Safety Incidences

Most errors are preventable. Globally, the World Health Organization (WHO) reports 1 in 10 patients are harmed while receiving healthcare (Lee & Dahinten, 2020). In the United States, 1 in 4 hospitalized patients suffers some level of harm. This is over half a million patients. Approximately 1000 patients die each day due to a preventable hospital error (The Leapfrog Group, 2013). Up to 70% of reported errors have been found to be due to communication problems (TJC, 2020). Hospitals with higher satisfaction scores for physician–nurse communication on average have fewer safety events. Almost as many errors are likely to occur in physicians' offices (Sharma et al., 2020). When asked to identify which profession was responsible for patient safety, 90%–96% of all professional disciplines surveyed said the nurse was responsible! According to TJC, half of nursing errors occur during patient "handoffs." Why haven't we improved?

Goal

Improved safety climate is associated with decreased incidents of patient harm and mortality (Berry et al., 2020). Better communication can lead to safer care. Globally, nurses and their employing agencies are working to create a culture of safety in healthcare organizations at all levels (ICN, 2020). Reflect on the Lakesha Smith case.

Case Study: Student Nurse Lakesha Smith and Medications

After morning rounds, Student Nurse Lakesha says to the staff nurse: "I am assigned to give the meds today. I'll be giving them with my instructor." However, she meant all the oral meds for the team, since her instructor assigned these to her, but not the intravenous (IV) medications. Fortunately, her instructor was there to clarify the message. This is an excellent example of inadequate communication potentially doing harm to the patient. If the IV medications were not given for 8 h, there could have been serious consequences. When policy says to report near misses along with errors, does your agency track near misses by students?

Errors Are Usually System Problems

Since the most common cause of error is incomplete communication during the up to eight daily "handoffs," use of a consistent blueprint, or handoff sheet or tool, is an excellent way to ensure comprehensive and safer handoffs. Just like the use of checklists for central line insertion decreases infections, the use of a consistent handoff tool prevents errors of omission and optimizes nursing care. Errors have a high financial cost, in addition to the human cost, exceeding $29 billion per year just in the United States (AHRQ, 2020b).

GENERAL SAFETY COMMUNICATION GUIDELINES FOR ORGANIZATIONS

Error Databases

Unlike other countries such as Great Britain, in the United States, there is no one national database for reporting unsafe care, making data less readily accessible. The Centers for Medicare and Medicaid Services (CMS) does require reporting for patients who have Medicare.

Improved Communication

US government agencies (e.g., Agency for Healthcare Research and Quality [AHRQ]) and professional nursing groups (e.g., AACN, ANA, QSEN) have made recommendations for clear communication strategies to provide safer care that affect your communication both with other nurses and with other health team members. The AACN recommends using research- and evidence-based safety communication strategies as a basis for your clinical practice. The Leapfrog group has been consistently rating hospital safety through standard indicators, and the report shows some improvement in indicators, such as a 21% decline in hospital infections (The Leapfrog Group, 2013).

BARRIERS TO SAFE, EFFECTIVE COMMUNICATION IN THE HEALTHCARE SYSTEM

Lack of Patient Identifier Number

Nationally, we lack a unique identifier number for each patient. Often agencies use a patient's Social Security number. But not all patients have one. This makes gathering information across agencies difficult and may omit crucial data (Butler, 2020; Shah & Prabhutendolkar, 2020).

Fragmentation

The structure of healthcare organizations is complex. Such systems can be large multistate entities. Merging agencies can hold differing philosophies. Fragmentation of systems can impede communications and become a communication barrier. Although most hospitals have a policy on error reporting, they may lack organizational structure for documenting errors or near misses.

Handoffs or Transfers of Patient Care

Miscommunication errors most often occur during a **handoff** procedure, when one staff member transfers responsibility for care to another staff member. More than half of all incidences of reported serious miscommunications occurred during patient handoff and transfer, when those assuming responsibility for the patient (coming on duty) are given a verbal, face-to-face synopsis of the patient's current condition by those who had been caring for the patient and are now going off duty.

Patient care responsibility is transitioned or handed off to the next shift of nurses or when the patient is transferred to another unit. Transition times are high risk for incomplete communication and consequently result in more errors. This has been attributed to frequent interruptions, inconsistent report format, and omission of key information. Some agencies have adopted standardized handoff communication tools, including the use of checklists on handheld devices. The most ideal clinical handoff is between two nurses in the patient's room with access to the electronic health record (EHR). Discussing the care of the patient with the patient's input is ideal. The use of simple summary aids, like a whiteboard with critical information, like "patient likes to be called Emma" and "ALLERGIC TO SULFA is helpful." The most important part of the handoff is taking the time to adhere to the essential elements, including a thorough review of the assessment and planning of the patient's care.

Underreporting of Errors in a Punitive Climate

Many healthcare providers express concern about reporting errors or near-miss incidents. If we are to create a culture of safety, the system needs to be redesigned to be nonpunitive. A culture of safety is characterized by installing a strong, nonpunitive reporting system; supporting care providers after adverse events; and developing a method to inform and compensate patients who are harmed. Other disciplines have better models for safety. One example is aviation's successful crew resource management (CRM) practice model, which has been used as a template. One necessary step is to require the reporting of near misses so new, safer protocols can be created. Each time an error or near miss occurs, the team members get together and discuss in a nonjudgmental way to determine improved processes to help decrease future errors. *We need to establish a nonpunitive climate. We need to create this new climate of safety in which agencies, policies, and employees maintain a vigilant, proactive attitude toward adverse events.* Recognizing that human error occurs, everyone's focus needs to be on correcting system flaws to avoid future adverse events, rather than finding the one to blame.

INDIVIDUALS AND FACTORS THAT RESULT IN ERRORS

Fatigue

Errors are more likely to occur during long shifts with little rest or nutrition. The risk of error nearly doubles when nurses work more than 12 consecutive hours. Specifically, the last 2 hours of the shift are when nurses are the most fatigued. When a nurse neglects to take a break or refuel with water and a snack, productivity and safety suffer. The effect of fatigue in the final hours of a 12-hour shift is important for all nurses to recognize, so structures can be created to minimize fatigue.

INNOVATIONS THAT FOSTER SAFETY

Communication problems and communication solution strategies identified as "best practices" for creating a culture of safety are summarized in Table 2.1. Beyond individual changes to create safer climates for our patients, we need to advocate for organizational system changes. Leadership is needed to incorporate the 3 C's that promote safer clinical practice:

1. Communication clarity
2. Collaboration
3. Cooperation

Create a Culture of Safety

Agencies are working toward promoting a culture of safety in many ways (AHRQ, 2019a). A major focus is to improve the clarity of communication. This occurs through the use of standardized communication tools and team training. This is evidenced by more than 6000 recent articles and the assessment and intervention tools available from AHRQ's PSNet (http://psnet.ahrq.gov/).

Reducing Risk Factors

Factors that offer protection from risk include teamwork, staffing, handoffs, nurse education level, knowledge of standards, and knowledge of risks to patients. In addition, a lower risk to the patient is present when the nurse is an expert in the use of informatics, including the electronic health record (EHR), medication reconciliation, and having access to all patient records. When viewing the concept of safety and effective nursing care, such a model provides a quick glimpse of the multiple factors to consider. Communication is the thread that is part of the multiple factors. For example, teamwork needs to be led by excellent communicators. EHRs are only useful if those who document communicate well in written form.

Leadership is essential to change to a just culture model, in which the organization creates a balance between accountability of individuals and the institutional system. Establishment of an organizational culture of safety requires us to acknowledge the complexity of any healthcare system. Strong leaders can change the focus to safety practices as a shared value. Creating a safe environment requires us to communicate openly, to be vigilant, to be willing to speak up, and to be held accountable.

Create a Team Culture of Collaboration and Cooperation

Creating effective health teams means getting all team members to value teamwork more than individual autonomy. Team collaborative communication strategies involve shared responsibility for maintaining open communication and engaging in mutual problem-solving, decision-making, and coordination of care. Teamwork failures, including poor communication and failures in physician supervision, have been implicated in two-thirds of harmful errors to patients. Creating a safe environment requires all team members to communicate openly, to be vigilant and accountable, and to express concerns and alert team members to unsafe situations.

Create a Nonpunitive Culture

Establishing a **just culture** system creates expectations of a work environment in which staff can speak up and express concerns and alert team members to unsafe situations. A just culture does not mean eliminating individual accountability, but rather puts greater emphasis on an analysis of the problems that contribute to adverse events in a system.

Establishing open communication about errors is an important aspect of just culture. Most state boards of nursing require nurses to report unsafe practice by coworkers, but many nurses have mixed feelings about reporting a colleague, especially to a state agency. Physicians also have reservations about reporting problems. Barriers to reporting include fear, threat to self-esteem, threat to professional livelihood, and lack of timely feedback and support.

TABLE 2.1   Safe Communication: Problems and Recommended Best Practices

Communication Problem	Best Practice Communication Solution
Healthcare system complexity	Agency establishes safety as a priority. Agency policies adopt procedures to promote transparency and accountability.
Hierarchical status difference with decreased willingness to communicate	Team training such as TeamSTEPPS. Clarify duties of each team member.
Distraction or preoccupation	Policy that isolates you from interruptions (signal to others not to interrupt, such as wearing vest when administering meds). Team members maintain safety awareness as a priority. Control high levels of ambient noise/alarm fatigue. Establish policy to limit interruptions during crucial times.
Heavy workload	Held accountable for evidence-based practice. Support from administration and colleagues. Team members share common safety goals, which each person sees as his or her responsibility.
Stress and practice pressures due to lack of time, leading to use of shortcuts and poor communication	Adherence to safety protocols, especially in med administration. Team huddles, meetings, bedside rounds.
Staff fail to say what they mean; fail to speak up about safety concerns (lack of assertiveness)	All staff receive continuing education that emphasizes safety promotion, communication, and assertiveness training. Use of time-outs.
Attitude of not believing in usefulness of practice guidelines	Ease of access and increased availability of evidence-based practice guidelines specifically relevant to your patient. Value electronic decision-support apps. Participate in team meetings, conference calls, and opportunities to share successes.
Education silos in which each discipline has own jargon and assumptions	Use of standardized communication tools. Team training. Each team member is encouraged to give input.
Cultural differences or language issues	Cultural sensitivity education, especially relevant to adapting communication strategies.
Miscommunication	Adapt communication, and verify receipt of message. Use standardized communication. Participate in simulations and critical event training scenarios to foster clear, efficient communication. Read back and record verbal orders immediately. With patients, use teach-backs or "show me" techniques. Solicit questions.
Avoidance of confrontation and communication with the conflict person	Use conflict resolution skills. Practices open communication. Be assertive in confronting the problem.
Cognitive difficulty obtaining, processing, or understanding Lack of training	Continuing education units about effective communication skills. Avoidance of factors interfering with decision-making, such as fatigue. Seek continuing education units, in-service.
Resistance from patient or family to following guidelines for safe, effective care	Team recognizes that safe outcomes require work and communicates that this must involve patient and family. Bedside rounds, briefings, and involving patient in daily care plan goal setting.

TeamSTEPPS, Team Strategies and Tools to Enhance Performance and Patient Safety.
Data from Leonard, M., Graham, S., & Bonacum, D. (2004). The human factor: The critical importance of effective teamwork and communication in providing safe care. *Quality and Safety in Health Care, 13*(Suppl 1), i85–i90.

Ethical incentives to reporting are protection of the patient and professional protection.

In a nonpunitive reporting environment, staff are encouraged to report errors, mistakes, and near misses. They work in a climate in which they feel comfortable making such reports. In safety literature, compiling a database that includes near-miss situations that could have resulted in injury is important information in preventing future errors. A complete error-reporting process should include timely feedback to the person reporting. Administrators should assume errors will occur and put in place a plan for "recovery" that has well-rehearsed procedures for responding to adverse events.

Best Practice: Communicating Clearly for Quality Care

AHRQ, medical and nursing organizations, and healthcare delivery organizations have undertaken initiatives designed to foster **"best practice"** safer patient care by designing evidence-based protocols for care. *Use "best practices" by increasing use of evidence-based "best practice" versus "usual practice."* The Agency for Healthcare Research and Quality (AHRQ) funds research to identify the most effective methods of promoting clear communication among health team members and agencies and the most effective treatments. This information is used to develop and distribute protocols for best practice, including formats of standard communication techniques. We need more studies of interventions to promote best communication between nurses and physicians with documented outcomes for patients.

Developing an evidence-based best practice requires closing the gap between best evidence and the way communication occurs in your current practice. Apply information from evidence-based best practice databanks for safe practice. The process for development of practice guidelines, protocols, situation checklists, and so on is not transparent or easy. Solutions include gathering more evidence on which to base our practice. When is the "evidence" sufficiently strong to warrant adoption of a standardized form of communication about care? Many best practice protocols are available on free websites, such as AHRQ's (www.ahrq.gov), or proprietary sites, such as Elsevier's ClinicalKey for Nursing.

EHRs improve the safety of patient care and empower providers to have better quality care delivery and more accountability for preventive care and compliance with standard care protocols. EHRs aid in decision support, for example, providing data for the physician about the number of patients who need mammograms. EHRs are discussed in Chapter 25.

Standardized Communication as an Initiative for Safer Care

We are restructuring our healthcare system to make patient care safer. The consensus is that this requires improving communication. Good nurse–physician collaborative communication has empirically been associated with a lower risk for negative patient outcomes and greater satisfaction. The renewed focus on improving patient safety is resulting in the standardization of many healthcare practices. Standardization of communication is an effective tool to avoid incomplete or misleading messages. Standardization needs to be institutionalized at the system level and implemented consistently at the staff level. Safe communication about patient care needs to be clear, unambiguous, timely, accurate, complete, open, and understood by the recipient to reduce errors.

Patient Safety Outcomes

Standardized tools for clear communication prevent harm to patients. Standardization is the best practice. Regulatory agencies have begun mandating the use of standardized communication tools in certain areas of practice. The more consistent the language that is used, the more optimal the outcome.

Nurse-Specific Initiatives

Nurses are often the "last line of defense" against error. Nurses are in a position to prevent, intercept, or correct errors. Nurses do save lives! To prevent errors, nurses need to be clearly communicating to other members of the health team. Your clarity of communication can prevent safety risks, such as medication errors, patient injuries from falls, clinical outcomes related to patient nonadherence to the treatment plan, and high rehospitalization rates. Poor communication can compromise patient safety. One sample is described in the case of Nurse Kay.

Case Study: Ms Jo Kay

Ms Kay, RN, a newly hired staff nurse, has eight patients assigned to her on a surgical unit. She calls the resident for additional pain medication for a patient. Dr Andrews, a first-year resident on a 3-month thoracic surgery rotation, has responsibility for more than 80 patients this weekend when he is on call. Many of these he has never seen. In the phone call, Ms Kay uses nursing diagnoses to describe the patient and is irritated when Dr Andrews does not seem to recognize the patient, nor understand her. What could Kay do to improve the situation?

Decrease Interruptions

Interruptions interfere with a nurse's ability to perform a task safely, yet interruptions have become an almost continual occurrence. These interruptions are tied to an increased risk of errors (AHRQ, 2021). Nonverbal strategies to signal others to avoid distracting communication have been suggested, such as wearing an orange vest when preparing and administering medications.

Improve the Medication Process

A particular focus for error reduction is during the entire medication process, ranging from ordering to administration. The definition of *an adverse medication event* is harm to a patient as a result of exposure to a drug, which occurs in at least 5% of all hospitalized patients (AHRQ, 2019b). We have expanded the definition to include near misses. For example, a nurse prepares an ordered med but recognizes that the ordered dose far exceeds safe parameters. While some medication errors stem from lack of knowledge about the drug, side effects, incompatibility, and other factors involved in ordering or compounding, the majority of errors occur during the nurse's actions in administering the medication. TJC (2007) concluded that drug errors occur when communication is unclear or when a nurse fails to follow the rules for verification: right med, right patient, right dose, and right time.

DEVELOPING AN EVIDENCE-BASED PRACTICE

Globally, studies have examined nurse and safety culture awareness levels as well as current safety practices. Most study methods were descriptive, using focus groups or surveys. Other studies were quasi-experimental, measuring the effects of a safety intervention.

Results

Findings were mixed. Kim's 2020 study of 425 Korean nurses reported only a modest level of safety awareness, while Kaczorowski's 2020 study reported somewhat higher levels of safety awareness in Australian nurses. AHRQ's analysis of 47 American studies found increased safety awareness after implementation of a safety program as compared with a control group. Similarly, several studies including Usher's 2018 study showed increased safety awareness after adoption of handoff checklists or bedside rounds.

Strength of Research: Moderate. Cross-comparison data were not examined, nor was longitudinal effect measured.

Application to Your Clinical Practice

1. Nurses need to increase their awareness of safety threats.
2. Introduction of standardized tools such as checklists that implement safety protocols can increase a culture of safety.
3. Walking to each patient's bedside for change of shift report can impact safety.

References

Agency for Healthcare Research and Quality (AHRQ). (2020). *Making Healthcare Safer III: A Critical Analysis of Existing and Emerging Patient Safety Practices.* Rockville, MD: AHRQ. Available at: www.ahrq.gov/. Accessed May 6, 2021.

Kaczorowski, K. M., Drayton, N. A., & Grimston, M. R. (2020). Gaining perspective into the term "safety culture"; how emergency nurses view its meaning in their everyday practice: A focus group study in an Australian setting. *Australas Emerg Care, 23*(1), 1–5.

Kim, J. H., Lee, J. L., & Kim, E. M. (2020). Patient safety culture and handoff evaluation of nurses in small and medium-sized hospitals. *International Journal of Nursing Sciences, 8*(1), 58–64.

Usher, R., Cronin, S. N., & York, N. L. (2018). Evaluating the influence of a standardized bedside handoff process in a medical-surgical unit. *Journal of Continuing Education in Nursing, 49*(4), 157–163.

APPLICATIONS

Safe Care Climate

A discussion of the **standardized communication tools** used to promote safe interdisciplinary and nursing communication will be the main focus of this application section. Quality and safety education competencies have been developed for all nurses by national nurse leaders, which emphasize safety. The mantra for safe communication should be "simplify, clarify, verify."

Attitude

The NAS (National Academy of Sciences, formerly IOM) has urged organizations to create an environment in which safety is a top priority. Strive to develop an attitude in which safety is always a priority. Our prime goal is to improve communication about a patient's condition among all the people providing care to that patient. Errors occur when we assume someone else has addressed a situation.

Patient Safety Outcome

Once nurses understand the use of clinical guidelines and evidence-based practice procedures and become comfortable accessing this information, they see that they are providing a higher quality of care, improving their decision-making skills, and avoiding errors, resulting in safer care for their patients. They have fewer error incident reports, fewer patient falls, fewer medication events, less delay in treatment for patients, and fewer wound infections, among other outcomes.

Skills Acquisition Through Simulation

Skill acquisition is described as a gradual transition from rigid adherence to rules, to an intuitive mode of reasoning that relies heavily on deep tacit understanding. Communication and practice skills are developed and refined through clinical situation simulations. The students learn in a safe low-stakes simulation lab. The simulations can be low fidelity with model patients or high fidelity with computerized human patient simulators. The students can practice their communication, critical thinking, and clinical judgment skills. Since the instructor is present with several students in the lab, there is a more dynamic experience than the one-on-one in clinical settings. Students should feel free to attempt assessments, get feedback, and improve over time.

Ideally, the simulations should have an interdisciplinary cast of characters. The simulation allows practice without the risk of potentially devastating outcomes in an actual patient care situation.

Simulation laboratories are integrated into most nursing programs and hospitals. You can view sample scenarios on the Internet (even on sites such as YouTube). Practicing clinical assessments and interventions can help build the students' confidence and increase their communication and clinical decision-making skills. In summary, simulations are designed to increase cognitive decision-making skills, increase technical proficiency, and enhance teamwork, including efficient communication skills.

Patient Safety Outcome

More research is needed about the impact of practice simulations on nursing communications that affect actual patient safety. Jeong and Kim (2020) found improved communication in a simulation with SBAR trained groups of student nurses. Certainly, strong evidence shows increased skill proficiency increases patient safety.

INTRODUCTION TO USE OF STANDARDIZED COMMUNICATION TOOLS

Use of Checklists

A checklist is defined as a specific, structured list of actions to be performed in a specific clinical setting whose contents are based on evidence (AHRQ, 2019c). The user's goal is to follow each step in the process. Following a checklist ensures that key steps will not be omitted or important information missed due to *fatigue, pressure, distraction,* or other factors. A checklist is a cognitive guide to accurate task completion or to complete the communication of information. If every step on the list is completed, the possibility of miscommunication or slips leading to error are greatly reduced. Some examples include the WHO's *Surgical Safety Checklist.* Since it was introduced in 2008, use of the WHO checklist has nearly doubled the adherence to surgical standards of care. Another example is the Association of Perioperative Registered Nurses' (AORN) *Comprehensive Surgical Checklist.* This list combines WHO suggestions and TJC guidelines to produce a color-coded list.

Surgical suites and emergent care sites are places that use time-out checklists; these stop everyone in their tasks to verify correctness. Staff verbally review completion of the list to avoid wrong patient, wrong procedure/surgery, and wrong site. TJC, with its universal protocol, does not mandate a specific checklist and just requires that one be used. In 2012, CMS issued requirements to use checklists. AORN has advocated use of a preoperative checklist for years.

Unit checklists are used when, for example, the floor nurse uses a preoperative checklist to verify that everything has been completed before sending the patient to the surgical suite, but then this list is again checked when the patient arrives, but before the actual surgery. Such system redundancies are used to prevent errors. But they have limited and specific uses and do not address underlying communication problems. No standardized protocol exists for checklist development, so use of expert panels with multiple pilot testing is recommended. One example found in most agency preoperative areas is a checklist where standard items are marked as having been done and available in the patient's record or chart. For example, laboratory results are documented regarding blood type, clotting time, and so forth. Adoption of assertion checklists empowers any team member to speak up when they become aware of missing information.

Patient Safety Outcomes

Evidence shows that the use of checklists improves communication and patient safety, especially in areas managing rapid change, such as preoperative areas, emergency departments, and anesthesiology.

Use of Two-Challenge Rule

Communication interventions shown to improve safe communication are listed in Table 2.1. These are best practices. For example, when there is conflicting information or a concern about a potential safety breach, nurses use the "two-challenge rule." The nurse states his or her concern

TABLE 2.2   SBAR Structured Communication Format

S	Situation	Identify yourself; identify the patient and the problem. In 10 s, state what is going on. This may include patient's date of birth, hospital ID number, verification that consent forms are present, etc.
B	Background	State relevant context and brief history. Review the chart if possible before speaking or telephoning the physician. Relate the patient's background, including patient's diagnosis, problem list, allergies, relevant vital signs, medications that have been administered, and laboratory results, etc.
A	Assessment	State your conclusion, what you think is wrong. List your opinion about the patient's current status. Examples would be patient's level of pain, medical complications, level of consciousness, problem with intake and output, or your estimate of blood loss, etc.
R	Recommendation or request	State your informed suggestion for the continued care of this patient. Propose an action. What do you need? In what time frame does it need to be completed? Always include an opportunity for questions. Some sources recommend that any new verbal orders now be repeated for feedback clarity. If no decision is forthcoming, reassert your request.

Data from personal interviews: Bonacum, D., CSP, CPHQ, CPHRM, Vice President, Safety Management, Kaiser Foundation Health Plan, Inc., February 25, 2009; Fleischmann, J.A., Medical vice president of Franciscan Skemp. La Crosse, WI: Mayo HealthCare System, 2008.

twice. This is theoretically enough cause to stop the action for a reassessment.

Use of Situation, Background, Assessment, Recommendation

The **SBAR** method uses a standardized verbal communication tool with a structured format to create a common language between nurses and physicians and others on the health team. It is especially useful when brief, clear communication is needed in acute situations, such as emergent declines in patient status or during handoffs. See Table 2.2 for the SBAR format.

SBAR is designed to convey only the most critical information by eliminating excessive language. It eliminates the authority gradient, flattening the traditional physician-to-nurse hierarchy, making it possible for staff to say what they think is going on. This improves communication and creates collaboration. This concise format has gained wide adoption in the United States and Great Britain. SBAR is used as a situational briefing, so the team is "on the same page." It is used across all types of agencies, groups, and even in e-mails. SBAR simplifies verbal communication between nurses and physicians because content is presented in an expected format. Some hospitals use laminated SBAR guidelines at the telephones for nurses to use when calling physicians about changes in patient status and requests for new orders. Documenting the new order is the only part of SBAR that gets recorded. Refer to Box 2.1 for an example. Then practice your use of SBAR format in Simulation Exercises 2.1–2.3.

BOX 2.1   Situation, Background, Assessment, Recommendation Example

Clinical Example of Use of SBAR Format for Communicating With Patient's Physician

S Situation "Dr. Preston, this is Wendy Obi, evening nurse on 4G at St. Simeon Hospital, calling about Mr. Lakewood, who's having trouble breathing."

B Background "Kyle Lakewood, DOB 7/1/60, a 53-year-old man with chronic lung disease, admitted 12/25, who has been sliding downhill × 2 h. Now he's acutely worse: his vital signs are heart rate 92 bpm, respiratory rate 40 breaths/min with gasping, blood pressure 138/94 mm Hg, oxygenation down to 72%."

A Assessment "I don't hear any breath sounds in his right chest. I think he has a pneumothorax."

R Recommendation "I need you to see him right now. I think he needs a chest tube."

From Leonard, M., Graham, S., & Bonacum, D. (2004). The human factor: The critical importance of effective teamwork and communication in providing safe care. *Quality and Safety in Health Care, 13*(Suppl 1), i85–i90.

Patient Safety Outcomes

Evidence-based reports show that patient adverse events have decreased through the use of SBAR, including decreases in unexpected deaths. Practicing the use of standardized communication formats by student nurses has been found to improve their ability to effectively communicate with physicians about emergent changes in a patient's

SIMULATION EXERCISE 2.1 Using Standardized Communication Formats

Purpose
To practice the situation, background, assessment, recommendation (SBAR) technique.

Case Study
Mrs Robin, date of birth January 5, 1970, is a preoperative patient of Dr Hu's. She is scheduled for an abdominal hysterectomy at 9 a.m. She has been NPO (fasting) since midnight. She is allergic to penicillin. The night nurse reported that she got little sleep and expressed a great deal of anxiety about this surgery immediately after her surgeon and anesthesiologist examined her at the time of admission. Preoperative medication consisting of atropine was administered at 8:40 instead of 8:30 as per order. Abdominal skin was scrubbed with Betadine per order, and an intravenous (IV) drip of 1 L 0.45 saline was started at 7 a.m. in her left forearm. She has a history of chronic obstructive pulmonary disease, controlled with an albuterol inhaler, but has not used this since admission yesterday.

Directions
In triads, organize this information into the SBAR format. Student no. 1 is giving the report. Student no. 2 role-plays the nurse receiving the report. Student no. 3 acts as the observer and evaluates the accuracy of the report.

SIMULATION EXERCISE 2.2 Telephone Conversation Between Nurse and Physician About a Critically Ill Patient

Purpose
To increase your telephone communication technique using structured formats.

Procedure
Read the case, and then simulate making a phone call to the physician on call. It is midnight.

Case
Ms Babs Pointer, date of birth January 14, 1942, is 6-h post-op for knee reconstruction, complaining of pain and thirst. Her leg swelling has increased 4 cm in circumference, and lower leg has notable ecchymosis spreading rapidly. Temperature is 99°F; respiratory rate is 20 breaths/min; pedal pulse is absent.

Reflective Discussion Analysis
Record your conversation for later analysis. In your analysis, write up an evaluation of this communication for accurate use of situation, background, assessment, recommendation (SBAR) format, effectiveness, and clarity.

SIMULATION EXERCISE 2.3 Situation, Background, Assessment, Recommendation for Change of Shift

Purpose
To practice use of situation, background, assessment, recommendation (SBAR) procedure.

Procedure
In postconference, have Student A be the day-shift nurse reporting to Student B, who is acting as the evening nurse. Practice reporting on their assigned patients' conditions, or simulate four or five postoperative patients' status. Use the SBAR format.

Reflective Discussion Analysis
Have the entire postconference group of students critique the advantages and disadvantages of using this type of communication.

condition, and its use has been shown to help develop a mental schema that facilitates rapid decision-making by nurses. This format sets expectation about what will be communicated to other members of the healthcare team.

TJC, the Institute for Health Care Improvement, and AACN all support the use of SBAR as a desirable structured communication format. (TJC requires hospitals to develop a standardized handoff format.) Thus, we consider the SBAR tool as a best practice protocol. In addition to using SBAR when there is a change in a patient's health status, this communication format is used at shift change between nurse colleagues and between nurses and physicians during rounds, transfers, and handoffs from one care setting or unit to another. Some suggest that agencies conduct annual SBAR competency validations.

A distinct advantage of using SBAR or other standardized communication tools between physicians and nurses is that it decreases professional differences in communication styles. In a study by Compton et al. (2012), 78% of physicians surveyed stated they receive enough information to make clinical decisions. Several authors speculate that use of SBAR leads to creation of cognitive schemata in staff. Use of this structured format enables less-experienced nurses to give as complete a report as experienced nurses.

Use of the electronic SBAR format when transferring patients to another unit or during change of shift report has been shown to enhance the amount, consistency, and comprehensiveness of information conveyed, yet to not take any longer than a traditional shift report.

Crew Resource Management-Based Tools

CRM is another communication tool similar to SBAR, which was adapted from the field of aviation. This tool provides rules of conduct for communication, especially during handoff care transitions. Just prior to an event, such as surgery, all members of the team stop and summarize what is happening. Each team member has an obligation to voice safety concerns.

Briefing

In team situations, such as in the operating room, the team may use another sort of standardized format: a **briefing**. The leader (the surgeon, in this case) presents a brief overview of the procedure about to happen, identifies roles and responsibilities, plans for the unexpected, and increases each team member's awareness of the situation. The leader asks anyone who sees a potential problem to speak up. In this manner, the leader "gives permission" for every team member to speak up. This can include the patient also, as many patients will not speak unless specifically invited to do so. A debriefing is usually led by someone other than the leader. It occurs toward the end of a procedure and is a recap or summary as to what went well or what might be changed. This is similar to the feedback nurses ask patients to do after they have presented some educational health teaching, which verifies that the patient understood the material.

Debriefing

Debriefing occurs after a surgery or critical incident. It is a callback or review meeting during which each team member has an opportunity to voice problems that arose, to identify what went well, and to suggest changes that can be made.

Patient Safety Outcomes

Mortality rates have decreased using this tool in the surgical area. Staff identify adverse events that were avoided due to the information communicated during the briefing.

TEAM TRAINING MODELS

Teamwork is described in Chapters 23 and 24 with emphasis on continuity of the physician–nurse communication.

The majority of reported errors have been found to stem from poor teamwork and poor communication. An effective team has clear, accurate communication understood by all. All team members work together to promote a climate of patient safety. To improve interdisciplinary health team collaboration and communication, it is recommended that physicians and nurses jointly share communication training and team-building sessions to develop an "us" rather than "them" work philosophy. When clashes occur, differences need to be settled. Specific conflict resolution techniques are discussed in Chapter 23.

Ideally, the healthcare team would provide the patient with more resources, allow for greater flexibility, promote a "learning from each other" climate, and promote collective creativity in problem-solving. Use of standardized communication tools fosters collaborative practice by creating shared communication expectations. Obstacles to effective teamwork include a lack of time, a culture of autonomy, heavy workloads, and the different terminologies and communication styles held by each discipline. Building in redundancy cuts errors but takes extra time, which can be irritating.

TeamSTEPPS Model

One prominent safety model is Team Strategies and Tools to Enhance Performance and Patient Safety (TeamSTEPPS). This program emphasizes improving patient outcomes by improving communication using evidence-based techniques. Communication skills include briefing and debriefing, conveying respect, clarifying team leadership, cross-monitoring, situational monitoring feedback, assertion in a climate valuing everyone's input, and use of standard communication formats, such as SBAR and the Comprehensive Unit-based Safety Program (CUSP) (the CUSP toolkit is available from AHRQ, 2020a). Creating a team culture means each member is committed to

- open communication with frequent, timely feedback;
- protecting others from work overload; and
- asking for and offering assistance.

AHRQ's CUSP was designed to implement teamwork and communication. It is a multifaceted strategy to help create a culture of safety; urging healthcare workers to use communication tools. CUSP incorporates team training with strategies to translate research into staff's evidence-based practice.

TeamSTEPPS With "I PASS the BATON"

Regarding handoffs, AHRQ's TeamSTEPPS program recommends that all team members use the "I PASS the BATON" mnemonic during any transition by staff in patient care. Table 2.3 explains this communication strategy.

TABLE 2.3	**PASS the BATON**	
I	Introduction	Introduce yourself and your role
P	Patient	State patient's name, identifiers, age, sex, location
A	Assessment	Present chief complaint, vital signs, symptoms, diagnosis
S	Situation	Current status, level of certainty, recent changes, response to treatment
S	Safety concerns	Critical laboratory reports, allergies, alerts (e.g., falls)
B	Background	Comorbidities, previous episodes, current medications, family history
A	Actions	State what actions were taken and why
T	Timing	Level of urgency, explicit timing and priorities
O	Ownership	State who is responsible
N	Next	State the plan: what will happen next, any anticipated changes

Modified from the U.S. Department of Defense. (2005). *Department of Defense Patient Safety Program. Healthcare communications toolkit to improve transitions in care.* Falls Church, VA: TRICARE Management Activity.

Veterans Administration Clinical Team Training Program

The Department of Veterans Affairs has developed a multidisciplinary program for building teams. Based on principles from aviation's CRM, it is an entire program infused with techniques and standardized care strategies to improve open communication. One example is the concept of "assertive inquiry," modeled on aviation CRM, under which any member of the crew is empowered to speak up if they have a safety concern.

PATIENT SAFETY OUTCOMES OF TEAM TRAINING PROGRAMS

Multiple studies tend to demonstrate increased satisfaction, primarily from nurses, when team communication strategies are implemented.

Nursing Teamwork
Care Transitions
The traditional patient report from one nurse handing over care to another nurse (**care transition**) needs to be accurate, specific, and clear and allow time for questions

---

BOX 2.2 Tips to Improve Communication During Handoffs/Transitions

1. Use checklist or standardized sheet during handoff report. Can be electronic list or laminated sheet.
2. Communicate concerns in a timely manner, escalating tone until others listen.
3. Make bedside rounds during change of shift, allowing patient to participate.
4. Follow standardized protocols such as SHARE or SBAR.
5. Engage all staff to value safe communication in transitions.

---

to foster a culture of patient safety. Walking to the bedside and use of a checklist are some recommendations given to foster a more complete report. Using the SBAR format or any other standardized communication format for reports results in a safer environment for your patients, includes patients as active team members, and has been shown not to increase report duration. Consider tips in Box 2.2 that are designed to improve communication during handoffs.

Interdisciplinary Rounds and Team Meetings
Team training is one tool used to increase collaboration between physicians and nurses. The use of teams is a concept that has been around for years within the medical and nursing professions. For example, medicine has used medical rounds to share information among physicians. Contemporary healthcare teams use "interdisciplinary rounds" to increase communication among the whole team—physicians, pharmacists, therapists, nurses, and dieticians. This strategy may increase communication and positively affect patient outcome. For example, daily discharge multidisciplinary rounds have been correlated with decreased length of hospital stay. Some Magnet hospitals use hourly rounding by the nurse and nurse assistant to ensure patient status is assessed.

Interdisciplinary "team" meetings can be held daily or weekly to explore common goals, concerns, and options; smooth problems before they escalate into conflicts; or provide support. There are also *clinical teaching rounds,* where once a week, a physician teaches nurses, with the goal of encouraging physician communication with the nursing staff.

A **huddle** is a brief, informal gathering of the team to decide on a course of action. Huddles reinforce the existing plan of care or inform team members of changes to the plan. A team huddle can be called by any team member.

Callouts and **timeouts** allow staff to stop and review. As mentioned earlier, TJC mandates that staff working in surgery have a time-out in which all team members review the details of the surgery about to take place to prevent wrong patient, wrong site surgeries.

The SHARE Standardized Handoff Tool

Many formats are available to foster complete, organized transfer of information, including electronic handoff checklists. In addition to the checklists already described, TJC released SHARE, a targeted solutions tool (TJC, 2021).

S = Standardize crucial content: give patient's history, key current data

H = Hardwire your system: develop or use standardized tools, checklists

A = Allow opportunities for questions: use critical thinking, share data with entire team

R = Reinforce: common goal, member accountability

E = Educate: team training on use of standardized handoffs with real-time feedback

Patient Safety Outcomes

Strategies to improve interdisciplinary communication break down barriers, increase staff satisfaction, decrease night pager calls to residents, and hopefully help to improve the quality of care.

Technology-Oriented Solutions Create a Climate of Patient Safety

Health information technologies (HITs) are a key tool for increasing safety and a means to decrease healthcare costs and increase quality of care. HITs, text messaging, and dedicated smart phones are some of the technological innovations discussed in Chapters 25 and 26, as are clinical decision support systems, electronic clinical pathways and care plans, and computerized registries or national databanks that monitor treatment.

Electronic transmission of prescriptions involves sending medication orders directly to the patient's pharmacy in the community. This can help decrease errors caused by misinterpretation of handwritten scripts.

Radiofrequency identification (RFID), which puts a computer chip in identity cards or even into some people, is an emerging technology that allows you to locate a certain nurse, identify a patient, or even locate an individual medication. RFID may be able to be incorporated into the nurse's handheld computer.

Prevention of misidentification of the patient is an obvious error prevention strategy. Before administering medication, the nurse needs to verify patient allergies, use another nurse to verify accuracy for certain stock medications, and reverify the patient's identity. TJC's best practice recommendation is to check the patient's name band and then ask the patient to verbally confirm his or her name and give a second identifier, such as date of birth.

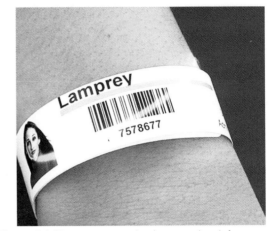

Figure 2.1 Nurse scans patient's name band for accurate identification.

Use of technology, such as *barcoded name bands,* offers protection against misidentification. Some barcoded name bands include the patient's picture, along with the patient's name, date of birth, and barcode for verification of patient identity (Fig. 2.1).

Whiteboards have long been used at the central nursing station to list the census and the staff assigned to care, in delivery suites to list labor status, and in surgical suites to track procedures and staff. Now we have electronic whiteboards, and patients are invited to add to the information displayed on them.

Patient Safety Outcomes

Many agencies, including the Veterans Administration (VA) hospital system, have used barcodes for years. When a new medication is ordered by a physician, it is transmitted to the pharmacy, where it is labeled with the same barcode as is on the patient's name band. The nurse administering that medication verifies both codes by scanning with the battery-operated barcode reader, just as a grocery store employee scans merchandise. Barcode scanning for medication administration has reduced medication administration errors significantly. In a similar fashion, barcoded labels on laboratory specimens prevent mix-ups.

OTHER SPECIFIC NURSING EFFORTS

Following Safety Policies

Implementing unit-based safety programs and following policy helps decrease errors and improve the efficiency of care. Measures to improve efficiency may also increase the time you have for communication with patients. Examples of safety redundant processes are using two identifiers before administering a procedure or medicine.

Work-arounds are shortcuts. Nurses under pressure of time constraints have sometimes developed shortcuts commonly known as work-arounds. These are nonapproved methods to expedite one's work. An example is printing an extra set of barcodes for all your patients who are scheduled to receive medication at 10 a.m. and scanning them all at once rather than scanning each patient's barcode name band in his or her room. High patient to staff ratios and heavy workloads are implicated as main factors. In van der Veen et al. (2020) study, workarounds in medication administrations were observed 62.7% of the time.

Patient Safety Outcomes

Deviating from safety protocols inherently introduces risks. While in the short term, some time may be saved, in the long run, mistakes cost millions of dollars each year, harm patients, and put you at risk for liability or malpractice suits.

Transforming Care at the Bedside

Begun in 2003, Transforming Care at the Bedside (**TCAB;** pronounced *tee-cab*) is an Institute for Healthcare Improvement initiative funded by the Robert Wood Johnson Foundation (RWJF, 2008) to improve patient safety and the quality of hospital bedside care by empowering nurses at the bedside to make system changes.

This program has four core concepts to improve care:
1. Create a climate of safe, reliable patient care. Uses practices, such as brainstorming and retreats for staff nurses, to develop better practice and better communication ideas. One example is that nurses initiate presentation of the patient's status to physicians at morning rounds using a standard format. Another strategy is to empower staff nurses to make decisions.
2. Establish unit-based vital teams. Interdisciplinary, supportive care teams foster a sense of increased professionalism for bedside nurses. This, together with better nurse–physician communication, should positively affect patient outcomes.
3. Develop patient-centered care. This ensures continuity of care and respects family and patient choices.
4. Provide value-added care. This eliminates inefficiencies, for example, by placing high-use supplies in drawers in each patient's room.

Patient Safety Outcomes

Evaluation in more than 60 project hospitals showed that units using this method cut their mortality rate by 25% and reduced nosocomial infections significantly. Nurse–physician collaboration and communication was improved, with both physicians and nurses voicing increased satisfaction.

Patient–Provider Collaborations

Communicating with patients about the need for them to participate in their care planning was the goal set in 2009 by TJC. Goal 13 states, "Encourage patients' active involvement in their own care as a patient safety strategy," which includes having patients and families report their safety concerns. Patients and their families should be specifically invited to be an integral part of the care process. Another strategy is to provide more opportunities for communication.

Emphasize to Patients That They Are Valued Members of the Health Team

Let your patient know he or she is expected to actively participate in his or her care. Safe care is a top goal shared by patient and care provider. Empowering your patient to be a collaborator in his or her own care enhances error prevention. Emphasize this provider–patient partnership, and increase open communication through bedside rounds, bedside change of shift handoffs, and patient access to their own records. In building the relationship, to establish rapport, participants follow the mnemonic PEARLS (*p*artnership; *e*mpathy; *a*pology, such as "sorry you had to wait"; *r*espect; *l*egitimize or validate your patient's feelings and concerns with comments, such as "many people have similar concerns"; *s*upport).

Use Written Materials

In one hospital system, pamphlets are given to patients upon admission, instructing them to become partners in their care. A nurse comes into the patient's room at a certain time each day, sits, and makes eye contact. Together, nurse and patient make a list of today's goals, which are written on a whiteboard in the patient's room. As a part of safety and communication, awareness of language barriers can be signaled to everyone entering the room by posting a logo on the chart, in the room, or on the bed. Use of interpreters and information materials written in the patient's primary language may also reduce safety risks.

Assess Patient's Level of Health Literacy

As mentioned, it is important to make verbal and written information as simple as possible. As a nurse, you need to assess the health literacy level of each patient. Provide privacy to avoid embarrassment. Obtain feedback or teach-backs to determine the patient's understanding of the information you have provided: simplify, clarify, verify!

Patient Safety Outcomes

Data continue to be monitored on safety. Promising trends have been the involvement of patients in monitoring safe care and efforts to promote greater staff engagement, as they mindfully scan their environment for potential hazards (Janes et al., 2021). The evidence does show increases in patient satisfaction after changing to a model of bedside report. AHRQ advises patients to speak up if they have a question or concern, to ask about test results rather than to assume that "no news is good news." Placing information, such as fall prevention posters in the room of an at-risk patient, has been reported by agencies to reduce the number of falls.

SUMMARY

Major efforts to transform the healthcare system are ongoing. We maximize patient safety by minimizing the risk for errors made by all healthcare workers. Because miscommunication has been documented to be one of the most significant factors in error occurrence, this chapter focuses on communication solutions. A number of standardized communications tools are described. Individual and system solution suggestions are offered that should help all nurses practice more safely and effectively.

NEXT-GENERATION NCLEX® EXAMINATION-STYLE CASE STUDY

Addressing Communication Errors During In-Hospital Patient Transfers

A community hospital has provided surgical treatment for 10 patients involved in a multiple-car accident on the interstate. The surgical department's nursing staff has been required to work mandatory overtime to meet the needs of the patients recovering from anesthesia. A nurse preparing to move three patients to the postsurgical unit is asked to delay the transfer process to help admit two new patients from the surgical suite. One of the patients ready for transfer has a chest tube in place to reinflate a collapsed lung. Another patient while now presenting with stable vital signs has a history of congestive heart failure. The third patient with a history of substance abuse is awake and alert with stable vital signs. Due to the current situation, the nurse gives the transfer reports over the telephone to the nurses who will be accepting the patients on the various postsurgical units.

Which issues present risks for incomplete communication between staff during the transfer of these patients from one care site to another? *Select all that apply.*

a. Staff fatigue
b. Frequent interruptions
c. Ineffective staff training
d. Inconsistent report format
e. Omission of key information
f. Lack of relevant safety protocols
g. Poor adherence to established practice guidelines

ETHICAL DILEMMA: What Would You Do?

You are a new nurse working for hospice, providing in-home care for Ms Wendy, a 34-year-old with recurrent spinal cancer. At a multidisciplinary care planning conference 2 months ago, Dr Chi, the oncologist, and Dr Spenski, the family physician, hospice staff, and Ms Wendy agreed to admit her when her condition deteriorated to the point that she would require ventilator assistance. Today, however, when you arrive at her home, she states a desire to forego further hospitalization. Her family physician is a personal friend and agrees to increase her morphine to handle her increased pain, even though you feel that such a large dose will further compromise her respiratory status.

1. What are the possibilities for miscommunication?
2. What steps would you take to get the healthcare team "on the same page"?

DISCUSSION QUESTIONS

1. Give examples you have seen for some of the best-practice communication solutions provided in this chapter.
2. Use the SBAR exercises given. What was the easiest part? Or the hardest? Many schools actually have students' telephone physicians and role-play a scenario. Have you had to do that yet?

REFERENCES

Agency for Healthcare Research and Quality (AHRQ). (2019a). *Patient safety primer: Culture of safety.* PSNet [website]. Rockville, MD: AHRQ.

Agency for Healthcare Research and Quality (AHRQ). (2019b). *Patient safety primer: Handoffs and signouts.* PSNet [website]. Rockville, MD: AHRQ.

Agency for Healthcare Research and Quality (AHRQ). (2019c). *Patient safety primer: Checklists.* PSNet [website]. Rockville, MD: AHRQ.

Agency for Healthcare Research and Quality (AHRQ). (2020a). *AHRQ patient safety tools and resources.* Rockville, MD: AHRQ. Retrieved from https://www.ahrq.gov/patient-safety/resources/pstools/index.html. [Accessed 6 May 2021].

Agency for Healthcare Research and Quality (AHRQ). (2020b). *Making healthcare safer III: A critical analysis of existing and emerging patient safety practices.* Publication #20-0029-EF Rockville, MD: AHRQ. Retrieved from https://www.ncbi.nlm.nih.gov/books/NBK555526/. [Accessed 10 May 2021].

Agency for Healthcare Research and Quality (AHRQ). (2021). *Patient safety primer: Nursing and patient safety.* PSNet [website]. Rockville, MD: AHRQ.

Berry, J. C., Davis, J. T., Bartman, T., et al. (2020). Improved safety culture and teamwork climate are associated with decreases in patient harm and hospital mortality across a hospital system. *Journal of Patient Safety*, 16(2), 130–136.

Butler, M. (2020). COVID-19 magnifies urgent need for patient identification strategies. *Journal of American Health Information Management Association*. Retrieved from https://journal.ahima.org/covid-19-magnifies-urgent-need-for-patient-identification-strategies/. [Accessed 6 May 2021].

Compton, J., Copeland, K., Flanders, S., et al. (2012). Implementing SBAR across a large multihospital health system. *Joint Commission Journal on Quality and Patient Safety*, 38(6), 261–268.

Cronenwett, L., Sherwood, G., Barnsteiner, J., et al. (2007). Quality and safety education for nurses. *Nursing Outlook*, 55(3), 122–131.

Giardina, T. D., Royse, K. E., Khanna, A., et al. (2020). Health care provider factors associated with patient-reported adverse events and harm. *Joint Commission Journal on Quality and Patient Safety*, 46(5), 282–290.

International Council of Nurses (ICN). (2020). *Patient safety*. Geneva, Switzerland: ICN. Retrieved from https://www.icn.ch/nursing-policy/icn-strategic-priorities/patient-safety. [Accessed 6 May 2021].

Janes, G., Mills, T., Budworth, L., Johnson, J., & Lawton, R. (2021). The association between health care staff engagement and patient safety outcomes: Systematic review and meta-analysis. *Journal of Patient Safety*, 17(3), 207–216.

Jeong, J. H., & Kim, E. J. (2020). Development and evaluation of an SBAR-based fall simulation program for nursing students. *Asian Nursing Research*, 14(2), 114–121.

Lee, S. E., & Dahinten, V. S. (2020). The enabling, enacting, and elaborating factors of safety culture associated with patient safety: A multilevel analysis. *Journal of Nursing Scholarship*, 52(5), 544–552.

Robert Wood Johnson Foundation (RWJF). (2008). *The transforming care at the bedside (TCAB) toolkit*. Princeton, NJ: RWJF. Retrieved from http://www.rwjf.org/en/research-publications/find-rwjf-research/2008/06/the-transforming-care-at-the-bedside-tcab-toolkit.html. [Accessed 6 May 2021].

Shah, D., & Prabhutendolkar, S. (2020). Forging ahead with interoperability amid a pandemic. *Journal of American Health Information Management Association*. Retrieved from https://journal.ahima.org/forging-ahead-with-interoperability-amid-a-pandemic/. [Accessed 10 May 2021].

Sharma, A. E., Yang, J., Del Rosario, J. B., et al. (2020). What safety events are reported for ambulatory care? Analysis of incident reports from a patient safety organization. *Joint Commission Journal on Quality and Patient Safety*. Retrieved from https://psnet.ahrq.gov/issue/what-safety-events-are-reported-ambulatory-care-analysis-incident-reports-patient-safety/. [Accessed 6 May 2021].

The Joint Commission (TJC). (2007). Preventing medication errors. In R. A. Porche (Ed.), *Frontline of defense: The role of nurses in preventing sentinel events* (2nd ed.). Oakbrook Terrace, IL: TJC.

The Joint Commission (TJC). (2020). Nursing care center. In *2021 national patient safety goals*. Oakbrook Terrace, IL: TJC.

The Joint Commission (TJC). (2021). *Hand-off communications targeted solutions tool (TST)*. Retrieved from https://www.centerfortransforminghealthcare.org/products-and-services/targeted-solutions-tool/hand-off-communications-tst/. [Accessed 6 May 2021].

The Leapfrog Group. (2013). *Leapfrog Hospital Safety Grade. Latest hospital safety scores show incremental progress in patient safety. New letter grades shift U.S. state rankings*. Retrieved from https://www.hospitalsafetygrade.org/newsroom/display/latest-hospital-safety-scores-show-incremental-progress-in-patient-safety. [Accessed 10 May 2021].

van der Veen, W., Taxis, K., Wouters, H., et al. (2020). Factors associated with workarounds in barcode-assisted medication administration in hospitals. *Journal of Clinical Nursing*, 29(13–14), 2239–2250.

3

Professional Guides for Nursing Communication

OBJECTIVES

At the end of the chapter, the reader will be able to:

1. Discuss nursing communication standards and guidelines for care and communication and expected competencies for beginning professional nurses.
2. Discuss legal and ethical standards in nursing practice relevant to communication, including social media.
3. Construct examples of communications that meet patient privacy legal requirements, such as the American Health Insurance Portability and Accountability Act (HIPAA).
4. Translate empirical knowledge into clinical practice by applying evidence-based practice (EBP) information to construct a case study.

This chapter introduces the student to standards and guidelines that influence nursing care, with the focus on communication in both academia and clinical practice. It provides a brief overview of communication as a component of the nursing process. Globally, standards mandate that nurses provide care with compassion and respect for the inherent dignity, worth, and uniqueness of every individual and are truthful. In addition to these established standards, The National Academy of Sciences has published "Nursing Desired Outcomes (2021)" addressing the nurse's role in promoting health equity.

BASIC CONCEPTS

Standards as Guides to Communication in Clinical Nursing

As nurses, we are guided by standards, policies, ethical codes, and laws. One of the American Association of Critical Care's standards is that nurses need to be as proficient in communication skills as they are in clinical skills (AACN, n.d.). Factors external to the nursing profession, such as technology innovations, research reports, and government mandates, are driving major changes in the way nurses communicate.

In an ideal work environment, we nurses demonstrate professional conduct by using established evidence-based "best practices" to provide safe, high-quality care for our patients. In an ideal work environment, we have excellent communication with our patients, their families, and all members of the interdisciplinary healthcare team. Refer to Box 3.1 for a list of communication characteristics. Effective communication is essential to workplace efficiency and effective delivery of care. A basic tenant is treating all patients with respect. Reflect on the case of Tom Epstein.

BOX 3.1 Characteristics of Safe, Effective Communication

- **Correct**/accurate
- **Clear**/understandable
- **Concise**
- **Concrete**/specific yet complete
- **Confidential**
- **Contemporary**/timely

Advocated, in part, by: Agency for Healthcare Research and Quality (AHRQ); American Nurses Association; American Association of Colleges of Nursing; College of Nurses of Ontario; International Council of Nurses (ICN); Institute of Medicine (IOM), The Joint Commission (TJC); World Health Organization (WHO).

CASE STUDY: **Nurse Conveys Respect to Tom Epstein**

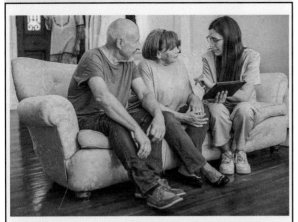

From iStock.com #1255030950; South_agency.

Mr Epstein, age 72, is brought to the hospital for a preadmission visit by his wife. Nurse Barbara McGill greets him, shaking his hand and calling him by his full name. She speaks directly to him, reviewing his history, only asking the wife for information that Mr Epstein is not able to recall. She explains the process for signing papers, getting required lab work and an electrocardiogram.

1. Are seniors sometimes treated as incompetent?
2. How did Barbara communicate respect for Mr Epstein as a unique individual?

BOX 3.2   ANA Standards of Nursing Practice: #10 Communication

- Assesses communication format preferences of healthcare consumers, families, and colleagues.
- Assesses his or her own communication skills in encounters with healthcare consumers, families, and colleagues.
- Seeks continuous improvement of communication and conflict resolution skills.
- Conveys information to healthcare consumers, families, the interprofessional team, and others in communication formats that promote accuracy.
- Questions the rationale supporting decisions when they do not appear to be in the best interest of the patient.
- Discloses observations or concerns related to hazards and errors in care or the practice environment to the appropriate level.
- Maintains communication with other providers to minimize risks associated with transfers and transitions in care delivery.
- Contributes his or her own professional perspective in discussions with the interprofessional team.

Data from American Nurses Association. (2019). *Nursing scope and standards of practice* (4th ed). Silver Spring, MD: ANA.

Effective Communication Concepts

Definition

Effective communication is defined as *a two-way exchange of information* among patients and health providers ensuring that the expectations and responsibilities of all are clearly understood. It is an active process for all involved. Two-way communication provides feedback, which enables understanding by both senders and receivers. It is *timely, accurate, and usable*. Messages are processed by all parties until the information is clearly understood by all and integrated into care. A number of international, national, and professional organizations have issued standards, guidelines, and recommendations impacting the way nurses communicate. Strong emphasis is placed on decreasing miscommunication at high-risk times by using standardized communication tools. Read Box 3.2 for ANA's standards for communication practice.

Difficulties With Communication

Miscommunication problems occur when there are failures in one or more categories: the system, the transmission,

or the reception. The Joint Commission attributes 60% of sentinel events to miscommunication (The Joint Commission, R3 Report, n.d.). The IOM, now the National Academy of Medicine Division of the National Academies of Science, Engineering and Medicine, cites poor communication as a causative factor in 70% of healthcare errors. Current reports continue to show the strong relationship between poor communication and errors (Institute for Healthcare Improvement, 2017).

- **System failures** occur when the necessary channels of communication are absent or not functioning.
- **Transmission failures** occur when the channels exist, but the message is never sent or is not clearly sent.
- **Reception failures** occur when channels exist and necessary information is sent, but the recipient misinterprets the message.

Outcomes

Clarity of communication and truthfulness is stressed in communication guidelines, yet nurses continue to cite this as a problem (Baysal et al., 2019). Why are nurses interested in using communication standards to modify and clarify their own communication? Ideally it is because we are motivated to provide the best, safest possible care.

Outcomes for failure to adhere to established nursing practice and professional performance standards range from harm to patients all the way to professional and legal ramifications, potentially including a negative civil judgment against a professional nurse. Consider the case of Kay Smite, GN.

Case Study: Graduate Nurse Kay Smite and Communication Clarity

Immediately following graduation from her nursing program, Kay Smite, GN, takes an entry position on a busy surgical unit in a small-sized general hospital. With no orientation, she is assigned to work evening shift with one registered nurse and two aides. During her second week when the registered nurse calls in ill, Kay is told by the evening supervisor that she is "charge nurse" this evening, and a float nurse will be sent as soon as possible to help with the workload. A surgeon arrives and rapidly gives verbal instructions to limit his pre-op craniotomy patient's head hair shaving to the incision site only, tomorrow when the preparation procedure is done in the operating suite. As a student, Kay never spoke to a physician. He writes an order stating "patient will be shaved according to head nurse's instructions." He asks Kay to call the operating room to relay these instructions, which she does. Nothing is in the record describing the area to be shaved. When the day shift arrives in the surgical suite, the telephone message from Kay is not passed on. Mr Smith's head is completely shaved, and he threatens a lawsuit.

1. What standards of communication were violated?
2. What do you think is wrong with this entire work environment?
3. What would you change in this unfortunate but true situation?

Professional Standards for Scope of Nursing Practice and Guidelines for Communication

Definition

Scope of practice is defined as the rules, regulations, and boundaries within which a person may practice in a field of healthcare (Benton et al., 2021). Globally, professional practice organizations are issuing practice standards for nursing care that specify clear, comprehensive communication as a requirement.

Regulation

After Benton and associates (2021) completed their analysis of scope of practice for medicine, nursing, and other health professions, they concluded that the model of team collaboration has changed practice roles. Based on their research findings, they advocate a multidisciplinary examination of scope of practice for professionals and the regulatory dimensions governing clinical practice.

- The American Nurses Association (ANA)—The ANA continues to publish "Scope and Standards of Practice" (ANA, 2021). In conjunction with other professional organizations, since the 1990s, they have developed and published standards of practice for many nursing specialized areas of practice. Consult www.nursingworld.org/.
- The Agency for Healthcare Research and Quality (AHRQ)—The Agency **for Healthcare Research and Quality** in the US Department of Health and Human Services has taken a leading role in promoting safer health, funding research to compile evidence and develop "best practices" evidence-based care protocols. For years they operated TeamSTEPPS safety and communication training programs, an operation now continued by the American Hospital Association. An amazing number of resources are available on the Internet (www.ahrq.gov/). Professional standards of practice serve the dual purpose of providing a standardized benchmark for evaluating the quality of their nursing care and offering the consumer a common means of understanding nursing as a professional service relationship. In this way, standards are used to communicate with the public as to what can be expected from professional nurses. The ANA now publishes separate books on standards of practice for each nursing specialty.
- The American Association of Colleges of Nursing—In their guidelines for nursing curricula, they have a specific communication recommendation that students be taught a standard protocol for "handoff" care transition. According to the AACN, student nurses need to master open communication and techniques for interdisciplinary communication including use of technology to communicate (AACN, 2006).
- American Association for Critical Care Nurses—The revised Scope and Standards of Practice states that nurses need to be as proficient in communication skills as they are in clinical skills (Munroe & Hope, 2020). Communication to promote collaboration is also addressed. On their website, this organization has a tool to measure the health of your work environment.
- The International Council of Nurses (ICN)—The ICN published a code of ethics for all nurses globally (ICN, 2012). Code #4 states that we have a responsibility for communicating nursing ethics to other professionals. They identify four fundamental nursing responsibilities: to promote health; prevent illness; restore health;

and alleviate suffering. Each nurse has a responsibility to maintain ethical behavior and sustain respectful collaborative relationships. Among items addressing communication, the code states nurses need to ensure each patient receives accurate, sufficient communication in a timely manner.

- State Boards of Nursing—Each state has a regulatory structure for nursing, organized with a national council (www.NCSBN.org/). Their mission is to ensure a nurse meets professional standards according to the state's nurse practice act. Nurses must comply with the laws and rules to maintain their license. Standards change. For example, students are allowed to count 50% of simulation lab experiences as clinical. During the recent pandemic, hospital-employed students could count work time toward meeting academic requirements. NCSBN developed multistate licensure "Compacts." They advocate for unique identifier numbers for nurses. This would allow lifetime career tracking of nurses signing into Electronic Health Records (NCSBN, 2021).

- The World Health Organization (WHO)—WHO advocates modernization of professional nursing regulations and has made recommendations for nursing workforce policy by 2030. Several national reports also advocate updating nursing regulations to allow for full scope of practice. One example is full prescriptive powers for advanced practice nurses across all states, rather than the hit-and-skip way things are currently done.

- Quality and Safety Education for Nurses (QSEN)—For undergraduates, QSEN identifies six areas of nursing competency as well as the knowledge, skills, and attitudes (KSA) associated with each competency. QSEN's website provides training, resources, and consultants to translate QSEN competencies into teaching strategies. In each of the six competencies, QSEN specifies the *knowledge, skills,* and *attitudes* involved in each:
  - **Patient-centered care.** This competency is defined as empowering the patient/family to be a full partner in providing compassionate, coordinated care. In the KSAs, under "knowledge," you are expected to integrate multiple dimensions of care, including communication, to involve the patient and family. In terms of "skills," you are expected to elicit patient values and preferences during your initial interview and care plan development and to communicate their preferences to other members of the healthcare team. In terms of "attitudes," you are to value expressions of patient values, as well as their expertise regarding their own health status. In meeting the QSEN competency of providing patient-centered care, do you communicate with your patients to engage them in planning care?

  - **Teamwork and collaboration.** With this competency, you are able to function effectively within nursing and on interprofessional teams, to foster open communication, mutual respect, and shared decision-making to achieve quality care. A partial example of expected knowledge objectives for this competency might be that you know the various roles and scope of practice for team members and are able to analyze differences in communication style preferences for patient, family, and other members of the healthcare team. In terms of "skill," you are expected to be able to adapt your own style of communicating and to initiate actions to resolve any conflicts. In terms of "attitudes," your behavior shows that you value teamwork and different styles of communication.

  As you can see in Table 3.1, *communication is a major component* of QSEN's six prelicensure competencies. Effectively working as part of a healthcare team requires open communication, mutual respect, and shared decision-making with the patient and family included.

- Other conceptual models—Several other models are also available that identify core competencies expected of nurses. All of them stress excellent communication, coordination, and collaborative skills. For example, Lenburg's Competency Outcomes Performance Assessment Model includes oral skills, writing skills, and electronic skills.

CODES CONTAINING ETHICAL STANDARDS

Ethical Codes

All legitimate professions have standards of conduct. A Code of Ethics for Nurses provides a broad conceptual framework outlining the principled behaviors and value beliefs expected of professional nurses in delivering healthcare to individuals, families, and communities. Embodied in ethical codes are nursing's core values as illustrated in the CARING diagram in Fig. 3.1. Written codes are found in most nations. An International Code of Ethics was adopted by ICN in 1953 and revised in 2012. This code identifies four fundamental nursing responsibilities as being to promote health, prevent illness, restore health, and alleviate suffering. Moreover, the code says each nurse has the responsibility to maintain a clinical practice that promotes ethical behavior, while sustaining collaborative, respectful relationships with coworkers. Reflect of the ANA's code of Ethics as listed in Box 3.3. Read the Canadian Nurses Association code (CNA, 2017) or the competencies from College of Nurses, Ontario (2018). Among many elements of the code, those addressing communication state we

TABLE 3.1   QSEN's Six Prelicensure Competencies, Definitions, and Selected Communication Examples

Competency	Definition	Partial Examples[a]
1. Patient-centered care (Boggs discussed in every chapter)	Focus on fully partnering with patient to provide care that incorporates his or her values and preferences to give safe, caring, compassionate effective care. To do so requires us to communicate preferences to other health team members.	(K) Integrate understanding of arts, sciences, including communication, to apply nursing process. (S) Use communication skills in intake clinical interview to ask about patient preferences, to develop care plan, to communicate these to others. Use communication tools. (A) Value patient expertise and input.
2. Teamwork and collaboration (Boggs discussed in Chapters 2, 3, 6, 22, 23, and 24)	For teamwork we need mutual respect, open communication, and shared decision-making with all team members.	(K) Know scope of practice. Analyze differences in communication styles. (S) Adapt own style to the needs of the team in the current situation. Communicate openly, share in decision-making, resolve potential conflicts. (A) Respect contributions of every team member.
3. Evidence-based practice (EBP) (Boggs discussed in Chapters 1, 2, 3, and 23, with examples and application to practice in every chapter)	Incorporate the best practices based on newest evidence with our clinical expertise to deliver optimal care.	(K) Identify sources of EBP. Differentiate quality of evidence. (S) Use EBPs, after analyzing research findings and care protocols relevant to our patient's diagnosis; communicate these to others. (A) Value research, appreciate need to seek EBP information.
4. Quality improvement (Boggs discussed in Chapters 2 and 25)	Collect data on common outcome measures of our care to compare with accepted outcomes (benchmarks).	(K) Identify differences between our agency practices and "best practices." (S) Use communication tools to make patient care explicit. (A) Value own and others' contributions.
5. Safety (Boggs incorporated throughout with focused discussion in Chapters 2 and 25)	Minimize risk of harm, analyzing root causes of error, moving from a blame culture to a just culture should increase communication, prevent future problems; result is safer care.	(K) Analyze safety processes in own workplace. (S) Speak up proactively (about potential safety violations) and report near misses. (A) Appreciate how variation from established protocols creates risk.
6. Informatics (Boggs discussed in Chapters 2, 25, and 26)	Use technology to effectively communicate and manage patient care, make decisions, and access evidence-based treatment information.	(K) Contrast benefits and limitations of different communication technologies. (S) Use electronic skills to access available databases to design an effective, evidence-based care plan. (A) Protect confidentiality.

QSEN, Quality and Safety Education for Nurses.
[a]*A,* attitude; *K,* knowledge; *S,* skill.

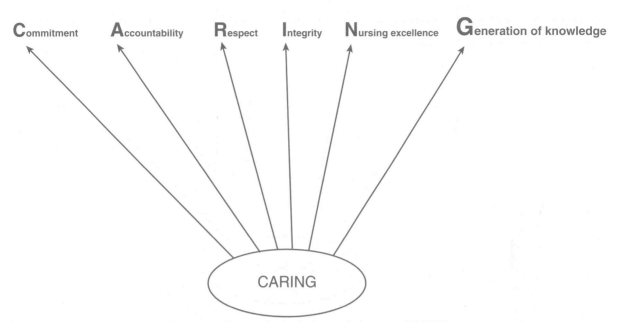

Figure 3.1 Communication in the nursing process (CARING).

BOX 3.3 American Nurses Association Code of Ethics for Nurses

1. The nurse, in all professional relationships, practices with compassion and respect for the inherent dignity, worth, and uniqueness of every individual, unrestricted by considerations of social or economic status, personal attributes, or the nature of health problems.
2. The nurse's primary commitment is to the patient, whether an individual, family, group, or community.
3. The nurse promotes, advocates for, and strives to protect the health, safety, and rights of the patient.
4. The nurse is responsible and accountable for individual nursing practice and determines the appropriate delegation of tasks consistent with the nurse's obligation to provide optimum patient care.
5. The nurse owes the same duties to self as to others, including the responsibility to preserve integrity and safety, to maintain competence, and to continue personal and professional growth.
6. The nurse participates in establishing, maintaining, and improving healthcare environments and conditions of employment conducive to the provision of quality healthcare and consistent with the values of the profession through individual and collective action.
7. The nurse participates in the advancement of the profession through contributions to practice, education, administration, and knowledge development.
8. The nurse collaborates with other health professionals and the public in promoting community, national, and international efforts to meet health needs.
9. The profession of nursing, as represented by associations and their members, is responsible for articulating nursing values, for maintaining the integrity of the profession and its practice, and for shaping social policy.

need to ensure that each patient receives accurate, sufficient communication in a timely manner and to maintain confidentiality.

Professional nurses, regardless of setting, are expected to follow ethical guidelines in their practice. The American Nurses Association Code of Ethics for Nurses with interpretive statements (ANA, 2015) establishes principled guidelines designed to protect the integrity of patients related to their care, health, safety, and rights.

Ethical standards of behavior require a clear understanding of the multidimensional aspects of an ethical dilemma, including intangible human factors that make

---

SIMULATION EXERCISE 3.1   Applying the Code of Ethics for Nurses to Professional and Clinical Situations

Purpose
To help students identify applications of the Code of Ethics for Nurses.

Procedure
Break into small groups of four or five students and role-play the following clinical scenarios:

1. Barbara Kohn is a 75-year-old woman who lives with her son and daughter-in-law. She reveals to you that her daughter-in-law keeps her locked in her room when she has to go out because she does not want her to get in trouble. She asks you not to say anything as that will only get her into trouble.
2. The nursing supervisor asks you to "float" to another unit that will require some types of tasks that you believe you do not have the knowledge or skills to perform. When you explain your problem, she tells you that she understands, but the unit is short staffed and she really needs you to do this.
3. Bill Jackson is an elderly patient who suffered a stroke and is uncommunicative. He is not expected to live.

The healthcare team is considering placement of a feeding tube based on his wife's wishes. Mrs Jackson agrees that he probably will not survive but wants the feeding tube just in case the doctors are wrong.
4. Dr Holle criticizes a nurse in front of a patient, Mrs DiTupper, and her family.

Reflective Discussion Analysis
Share each ethical dilemma with the group and collaboratively come up with a resolution that the group agrees on, using the nurse's code of ethics to work through the situations.

1. Describe some of the challenges your group encountered in resolving different scenarios.
2. Select a situation that offers the most challenge ethically and explain your choice.
3. Justify any problems in which the code of ethics was not helpful.
4. Create a scenario depicting you utilizing the knowledge gained from this exercise in your nursing practice.

---

each situation unique (e.g., personal and cultural values or resources). Chapter 4 discusses nurses and ethics in more depth, while Simulation Exercise 3.1 provides an opportunity to consider the many elements in an ethical nursing dilemma. When an ethical dilemma cannot be resolved through interpersonal negotiation, an ethics committee composed of biomedical experts reviews the case and makes recommendations. Of particular importance to the nurse–patient relationship are ethical directives related to the nurse's primary commitment to the following:

- Patient welfare
- Patient autonomy
- Recognition individual is unique and worthy of respect
- Truth telling and advocacy

LEGAL STANDARDS

Legally nurses are accountable for their own contributions to delivery of high-quality care. As professional nurses, we are legally and morally accountable for both dependent and independent clinical practices (ANA, 2021), accountable for all aspects of the nursing care we provide to patients and families, including documentation and referral. Of special relevance to communication within the nurse–patient relationship are issues of confidentially, informed consent, and professional liability. In one example, Myers

et al. (2020) noted that 47% of legal actions against ICU nurses concerned "failure to monitor" their patient's condition properly.

Classifications of Laws in Healthcare

Statutory Laws
These are legislated laws, drafted and enacted at various government levels. In the United States, Medicare and Medicaid amendments to the Social Security Act are examples of federal statutory laws, while state Nurse Practice Acts are examples of statutory laws.

Civil Laws
These are developed through court decisions, which are created through precedents, rather than written statutes. Most infractions for malpractice and negligence are covered by civil law and are referred to as torts. A tort is defined as a private civil action that causes personal injuries to a private party. Deliberate intent is not present. Four elements are necessary to qualify for a claim of malpractice or negligence.

- The professional duty was owed to patient (professional relationship).
- A breach of duty occurred in which the nurse failed to conform to an accepted standard of care.

- Causality in which a failure to act by professional standards was a proximate cause of the resulting injury.
- Actual damage or injuries resulted from breach of duty.

As nurses, we are legally bound by the principles of civil tort law to provide the care that any reasonably prudent nurse would provide in a similar situation. If taken to court, this standard would be the benchmark against which our actions would be judged.

Criminal Law

These laws are applicable to cases in which there is intentional misconduct or a serious violation of professional standards of care. The most common nurse violation of criminal law is failure to renew a professional nursing license, which means that a nurse is practicing nursing without a license.

Malpractice and Legal Liability in Nurse–Patient Relationships

In the nurse–patient relationship, the nurse is responsible for maintaining the professional conduct of the relationship. Examples of unprofessional conduct or **malpractice** include the following:

- Breaching patient confidentiality
- Verbally or physically abusing a patient
- Assuming nursing responsibility for actions without having sufficient preparation
- Delegating care to unlicensed personnel, which could result in injury
- Following a doctor's order that would result in patient harm
- Failing to assess, report, or document changes in patient health status
- Falsifying records
- Failing to obtain informed consent
- Failing to question a physician's orders, if they are not clear
- Failing to provide required health teaching
- Failing to provide for patient safety (e.g., not putting the side rails up on a patient with a stroke)

Effective and frequent communication with patients and other providers is one of the best ways to avoid or minimize the possibility of harm leading to legal liability.

Documentation as a Legal Record

As described in Chapter 25, nurses are responsible for the accurate and timely documentation of nursing assessments, the care given, and the outcome responses. This documentation represents a permanent record of healthcare experiences. In the eyes of the law, failure to document in written form any of these elements means the actions were not taken.

Communication Affects Application of Standards in Clinical Practice

Communication standards and skills are an integral component of the knowledge, experience, skills, and attitudes encompassed in using the nursing process to deliver care. Discussing case studies and exercises offers opportunities to hone communication skills.

As we emphasized, standards for clear, complete communication are specified in professional codes and guidelines. Nursing students need opportunities to practice effectively communicating before entering the workforce. Throughout this book, emphasis is placed on the importance of guiding your practice through application of both professional standards and evidence in your nursing care. EBP application is a conscious choice to use the most current research to provide "best care" (Brom et al., 2021). Many sources are available to you; for example, guidelines from agencies such as AHRQ or specialty nursing organizations (www.guideline.gov/index.aspx). Repeated study findings show staff nurses are unaware of evidence that could improve their care. Barnsteiner (2017) says that 75% of the time nurses get their information from their experience and only 58% of the time from a policy. Is it true that much of nursing and medicine is not yet based on evidence?

APPLICATION

Nursing Process

The **nursing process** consists of five progressive phases: assessment, problem identification and diagnosis, outcome identification and planning, implementation, and evaluation. As a dynamic, systematic clinical management tool, it functions as a primary means of directing the sequence, planning, implementation, and evaluation of nursing care to achieve specific health goals. Continual and timely communication is a component of each step in the nursing process. Specifically, communication plays a role in the following:

- Establishing and maintaining a therapeutic relationship
- Helping the patient to promote, maintain, or restore health, or to achieve a peaceful death
- Facilitating patient management of difficult healthcare issues through communication
- Providing quality nursing care in a safe and efficient manner

The nursing process is closely aligned with meeting professional nursing standards in providing total care.

DEVELOPING AN EVIDENCE-BASED PRACTICE

Techniques

Acceptance of new care techniques is based on analysis of multiple findings to identify common themes. Froh and colleagues (2021) described the process developed in response to requests from the nursing administration at Children's Hospital of Philadelphia for applying evidence to nursing care during the COVID pandemic. Their process can be used as a template to implement evidence-based clinical practices.

Findings

The process includes the following:

1. Comprehensive review of the literature using standard databases such as Pub Med and CINAHL.
2. Review of international clinical practice guidelines, government and professional medical organizational guidelines, as well as consensus statements.
3. Use of small teams to analyze/digest the evidence and compile tables of evidence in target area.
4. Provide the evidence to staff nurses. This study used "Fast Fact" sheets as handouts to nurses who provide direct care.
5. Use the evidence to support decision-making and to develop policy and procedures for nurses.
6. Increase communication with not only nurses but also other hospital departments.

Strength of research evidence: Strong in the sense that many researchers follow a similar template for discovering evidence that impacts or changes clinical practice.

Application to Your Clinical Practice

Findings support the value of having a nursing research center in hospitals. The process followed by the authors is a template for establishing evidence-based clinical practices. Grady (2021) also supports the need for diverse nurse-led investigative approaches to clinical nursing problems.

References

Froh, E. B., Flood, E. L., Lavenberg, J. G., et al. (2021). Evidence in hand: Optimizing the unique skill set of a hospital-based center for nursing research and evidence-based practice. *Journal of Pediatric Nursing, 56,* 60–63.

Grady, K. L., Rehm, R., & Betz, C. L. (2021). Understanding the phenomenon of health care transition: Theoretical underpinnings, exemplars of nursing contributions, and research implications. *Journal of Pediatric Health Care, 35*(3), 310–316.

Table 3.2 illustrates the relationship. The nursing process begins with your first encounter with a patient and family and ends with discharge or referral. Although there is an ordered sequence of nursing activities, each phase is flexible, flowing into and overlapping with other phases of the nursing process. For example, in providing a designated nursing intervention, you might discover a more complex need than what was originally assessed. This could require a modification in the nursing diagnosis, the identified outcome, the intervention, or the need for a referral. You employ communication skills in each step.

Prioritize

Traditionally, nurses also have used Maslow's Hierarchy of Needs (see Chapter 1) to prioritize goals and objectives. Priority attention should be given to the most immediate, life-threatening problems. Use communication skills to validate these priorities with your patient and health team. Try Simulation Exercise 3.2 to practice considering cultural, age, and gender-related themes when using the nursing process with different types of patients.

Use communication skills to collaborate with health team members and with patient and family members as you implement the nursing process. Your communication skills help you collaborate with your patient to provide safe quality care. After using your communication skills to obtain feedback from your patient, contrasting actual progress with expected outcomes, analyze factors that might have affected goal achievement. Communicate with team members to modify interventions as needed.

ISSUES IN APPLICATION OF ETHICAL AND LEGAL GUIDELINES

Moral Distress

Moral distress is defined as knowing the right thing to do, but outside constraints act to make it nearly impossible to do so. In an AACN survey, 24% of nurses reported experiencing moral distress. ANA (2015) describes their Code of Ethics as "nonnegotiable, encompassing all nursing activities and may supersede specific policies of institutions." If you are unable to provide care, you are obligated to ensure that the patient will have care from

TABLE 3.2 Online Guidelines for Nurses Using Social Media

Principles	Actions
Posts are bound by confidentiality and privacy laws, such as Health Insurance Portability and Accountability Act.	Refrain from posting identifiable patient information. This absolutely applies to photos or videos. It applies even if you do not show their face.
Professional ethical standards need to be followed.	Separate personal from professional information. Use two separate sites? Observe professional boundaries. Do not cross into social friendships.
Social media sites are public forums. Legal liability laws apply. Clicking on "restricted access" does not qualify as a private site.	Any disparaging comments are considered "cyber bullying." Use privacy settings. Understand that colleagues, employers, and even patients may read your posts.
Libel laws and nursing ethical codes apply to online information. Regulatory agencies such as State Boards act on complaints	Social media is permanent and universal. For example, Tweets may be retweeted. Civil, criminal, and professional penalties may apply.

SIMULATION EXERCISE 3.2 Using the Nursing Process as a Framework in Clinical Situations

Purpose
To help develop skills in considering cultural, age, and gender role issues in assessing each patient's situation and developing relevant nursing diagnoses.

Procedure
1. In small groups of three to four students, role-play how you might assess and incorporate differences in patient/family values, knowledge, beliefs, and cultural background in delivery of care for each of the following. Indicate what other types of information you would need to make a complete assessment.
2. Identify and prioritize nursing diagnoses for each to ensure patient-centered care.
   - Michael Sterns was in a skiing accident. He is suffering from multiple internal injuries, including head injury. His parents have been notified and are flying in to be with him.
   - Lo Sun Chen is a young Chinese woman admitted for abdominal surgery. She has been in this country for only 8 weeks and speaks very little English.
   - Maris LaFonte is a 17-year-old unmarried woman admitted for the delivery of her first child. She has had no prenatal care.
   - Stella Watkins is an 85-year-old woman admitted to a nursing home after suffering a broken hip.

Reflective Discussion Analysis
1. The needs of each can be different based on age, gender role, or cultural background. Explain how you account for these differences.
2. Describe any common themes in the types of information each group decided it needed to make a complete assessment.
3. Construct a scenario demonstrating your use of the knowledge gained from this exercise to show how you apply information in your clinical practice.

another well-qualified nurse. ANA supports the rights of patients to self-determination. As a nurse, you have an ethical obligation to support patients' right to make choices. Your professional organization can assist you in lobbying for a healthier work environment, as does the AACN (2020).

Protecting the Patient's Privacy

ANA supports a patient's right to privacy, which is to have control over personal identifiable health information, whereas confidentiality refers to your obligation not to divulge anything said in a nurse–patient relationship. Institutional policies and federal law provide specific

BOX 3.4   Overview of Federal HIPAA Guidelines Protecting Patient Confidentiality

- All medical records and other individually identifiable health information used or disclosed in any form, whether electronically, on paper, or orally, are covered by HIPAA regulations.
- Providers and health plans are required to give patients a clear written explanation of how their health information may be used and disclosed.
- Patients are able to see and get copies of their own records and request amendments.
- Healthcare providers are required to obtain consent before sharing their information for treatment, payment, and healthcare operations. Patients have the right to request restrictions on the uses and disclosures of their information.
- People have the right to file a formal complaint with a covered provider or health plan, or with the US Department of Health and Human Services (DHHS), about violations of Health Insurance Portability and Accountability Act (HIPAA) regulations.

- Health information may not be used for purposes not related to healthcare (e.g., disclosures to employers to make personnel decisions) without explicit authorization.
- Disclosure of information is limited to the minimum necessary for the purpose of the disclosure.
- Written privacy procedures must be in place to cover anyone who has access to protected information related to how information will be used and disclosed.
- Training must be provided to employees about the use of HIPAA privacy procedures.
- Health plans, providers, and clearinghouses that violate these standards will be subject to civil liability, and if knowingly violating patient privacy for personal advantage, can be subject to criminal liability.
- Use and disclosure is permitted for treatment, payment, and healthcare operations activities; for notification; for public health for preventing or controlling disease to lessen an imminent threat; or in cases of abuse, disclosure is permitted to government authorities.

Data from U.S. Department of Health and Human Services (DHHS). (2003). *Summary of the HIPAA privacy rule.* Retrieved from https://www.hhs.gov/sites/default/files/privacysummary.pdf. (Accessed 16 June 2021).

guidelines that all healthcare providers are required to follow. The patient's right to have personal control over personal information is upheld through legal regulations. The ANA Code of Ethics specifically addresses the nurse's responsibility to safeguard the patient's right to privacy.

Health Insurance Portability and Accountability Act Regulatory Compliance

In the United States, federal HIPAA legislation (1996) protects patient privacy (USDHHS, 2003). Key elements are listed in Box 3.4. A nurse is obligated to protect confidential information, unless required by law to disclose that information. Healthcare providers must provide patients with a written notice of their privacy practices and procedures. Agencies are audited for compliance.

HIPAA privacy rules give individuals the right to determine and restrict access to their health information. Patients have the right to access their medical records, request copies, and/or request amendments to health information contained in the record. The Fair Health Information Practices Act of 1997 stipulates civil and criminal penalties for not allowing patients to review their medical records. HIPAA regulations protect the confidentiality, accuracy, and availability of all electronic protected information, whether created, received, or transmitted.

Strict maintenance of written records, including electronic records, is required. Potential issues of privacy involve cell phones, picture taking, use of handheld devices, use of fax machines, Internet user passwords, and the use of electronic monitoring devices.

Healthcare providers must get written authorization before disclosing personal medical information, except in cases of public's health, criminal/legal matters, quality assurance, and aggregate record reviews. Information can be shared among healthcare providers.

The Joint Commission Privacy Regulations

In the United States, TJC requires agencies to have written privacy policies, to orient the staff to these policies, and to demonstrate staff awareness of their privacy policy (The Joint Commission, 2017).

Ethical Responsibility to Protect Patient Privacy in Clinical Situations

Informational privacy is an ethical issue as well as a legal one. Simple strategies that nurses can use to protect the patient's right to privacy in clinical situations include the following:

- Providing privacy for the patient and family when disturbing matters are to be discussed

- Explaining procedures to patients before implementing them
- Entering another person's personal space with warning (e.g., knocking or calling the patient's name) and, preferably, waiting for permission to enter
- Providing an identified space for personal belongings
- Encouraging the inclusion of personal and familiar objects on the nightstand
- Decreasing direct eye contact during hands-on care
- Minimizing body exposure to what is absolutely necessary for care
- Using only the necessary number of people during any procedure
- Using touch appropriately

Confidentiality

Protecting the privacy of patient information and confidentiality are related but separate concepts. **Confidentiality** is defined as providing *only* the information needed to provide care for the patient to other health professionals who are directly involved in their care. The assurance of confidentiality reflects ethical principles such as autonomy and beneficence. Confidential information about the patient cannot be shared with the family or other interested parties without the patient or designated legal surrogate's written permission. Shared confidential information, unrelated to identified healthcare needs, should not be communicated or charted.

Confidentiality within the nurse–patient relationship involves the nurse's legal responsibility to guard against invasion of the patient's privacy related to the following:
- Releasing information to unauthorized parties
- Unwanted visitations in the hospital
- Discussing patient problems in public places or with people not directly involved in their care or on any social media platform
- Taking pictures without consent or using the photographs without the patient's permission
- Performing procedures or tests without permission
- Publishing data about a patient in any way that makes them identifiable without their permission

Professional Sharing of Confidential Information

Nursing reports and interdisciplinary team case conferences are acceptable forums for the discussion of health-related communications shared by patients or families. Other venues include change-of-shift reports, one-on-one conversations with other health professionals about specific care issues, and patient-approved consultations with their families. Select agencies, such as insurance companies, can also access information during audits. Discussion

of patient care should take place in a private room with the door closed. Only relevant information specifically related to assessment or treatment should be shared. Discussing private information casually with other health professionals, such as in the lunch room or on social media, is an abuse of confidentiality. The ethical responsibility to maintain patient confidentiality continues even after discharge.

Mandatory Reporting

Disclosure should be limited. However, under certain circumstances, you are required to report patient personal health information. Certain communicable or sexually transmitted diseases, child and elder abuse, and the potential for serious harm to self or another individual are considered exceptions. The patient should be informed about what information will be disclosed, to whom, and for what reason(s).

Applying Informed Consent

Informed consent is defined as giving care acquiescence knowing the purpose, the extent of the risks and benefits, and the possible alternatives of treatment (AHRQ, 2020). Ethical principles, such as autonomy (self-determination) and beneficence, are the basis for **informed consent.** In today's healthcare market, legal decision-making requires that you educate patients about their care. Informed consent is a patient safety issue and a patient-centered care issue, but primarily it is a legal right protected by common law and case law. It is a focused communication process in which you provide all relevant information related to a procedure or treatment, offering full opportunity for discussion, questions, and expressions of concern, before asking the patient or healthcare agent to sign a legal consent form. Unless there is a life-threatening emergency, all patients have the right to decide about whether to consent. Internationally, part of the ICN Code of Ethics says that nurses ensure that the individual receives accurate, sufficient, and timely information in a culturally appropriate manner on which to base consent for care and related treatment, supporting their right to choose or refuse treatments (ICN, 2012). Box 3.5 lists elements that must be included in an informed consent for it to be legal.

Allowing a patient to sign a consent form without fully understanding the meaning invalidates the legality of consent. Ending the conversation leading to the actual signing of the consent form should always include the question, "Is there anything else that you think might be helpful in making your decision?" Try Simulation Exercise 3.3 to broaden your knowledge of informed consent.

Nurses are accountable for verifying the competency of a patient to give consent. Only legally competent adults

BOX 3.5   Elements of a Legally Valid Informed Consent

- Patient is of legal age.
- Decision is patient-based.
- Consent is signed voluntarily, without coercion.
- Patient has full knowledge of own condition and the treatment purpose, risks, benefits.
- Nurse has verified patient is competent to make decision.
- Patient has knowledge of possible alternative procedures.
- Patient knows they have the right to refuse or discontinue care.
- Patient can convey decision in a meaningful manner.
- If risk is involved, a written consent form is signed (and witnessed) except in emergencies.

SIMULATION EXERCISE 3.3   When Is Informed Consent Legal?

Purpose
To redesign an illegal example of informed consent to comply with legal standards.

Procedure
Read case of Jason Clarence, age 24, who is hospitalized following a motorcycle accident. At a few minutes prior to the 7 a.m. change of shift, nurse Susan Cox rushes into Mr Cox's room, telling him his condition has deteriorated and therefore his surgery has been moved up to 9 a.m. With no further explanation, she asks him to sign the consent for surgery immediately so she can administer pre-op medication before going off duty.

Reflective Discussion Analysis
1. Identify reasons this may be an illegal process.
2. Redesign this case to ensure this is a legal informed consent.

Duration. There is no recommended duration of consent unless it is stipulated in the document, so a form could address repeated procedures. But a new consent form should be signed if the patient's condition changes. Many agencies require that the signature on a consent form be witnessed.

Use of Social Media

Postings on social media platforms are an everyday happening for many. Powerful platforms, such as Facebook, Twitter, LinkedIn, Snapchat, etc., have transformed the way people interact. Consider the case of Cassie Zan, SN.

Case Study: Cassie Zan, SN and Social Media Posts

Cassie is a 17-year-old nursing student who is in her first semester and takes pleasure in the semester-long introduction course assignment to follow care of Clyde, age 4, who has cerebral palsy. She feels this is a great learning experience and that she is contributing to Clyde's progress. Today she uses her smart phone to snap a really cute photo of him enjoying his first ice cream cone and shares it in a post to her friends.

1. What patient rights were violated?

Advances in Communication

Social media is transforming traditional nurse–patient interactions. By allowing us to communicate with hundreds of people simultaneously, we potentially have the power to provide healthcare information and support. We do need to differentiate between general open-to-all social sites, even with privacy settings, and secure restricted sites such as those created by care agencies for internal professional staff use. "A post is forever" is a useful mantra.

Privacy Cautions

TJC has acknowledged instant messaging has a place, but so far they have not given approval for using e-messaging for physician orders, or for conveying other data. Governmental agency privacy regulations apply to you in your off-duty time as well as during clinical time. Students cannot, at any time, reveal private health information. This includes posting any pictures taken in a clinical facility or during a home healthcare visit.

According to the National Council of State Boards of Nursing (NCSBN), nurses breach patient privacy when they post enough to allow recognition of a patient or when they post degrading information (NCSBN, 2012).

can give legal consent; adults who are mentally retarded, developmentally disabled, or cognitively impaired cannot give legal consent. Evaluation of competency is made on an individual basis.

Surrogates. Legislation globally stipulates that a legal guardian or personal healthcare agent (**surrogate**) can provide consent for the medical treatment of adults who lack the capacity to consent on their own behalf. In most cases, legal guardians or parents must give legal consent for minor children, who are defined as those younger than 18, unless the youth is legally considered an emancipated minor.

Consequences for violations can be severe. Student nurses have been dismissed from their schools; state boards have censured, fined, or even revoked the license to practice. Violations of privacy laws also carry a risk of civil lawsuits and sanctions such as fines for the individual. The misuse of electronic communication also has consequences for educational programs, placing in jeopardy the school's relationship with a community agency they rely on for clinical experiences.

BLURRING BETWEEN PROFESSIONAL ROLE AND PERSONAL LIFE

People have become accustomed to posting so much on social media sites that they sometimes do not stop to think about whether a posting violates patient privacy laws or ethical nurse conduct. We need to differentiate between our personal posts and our professional duty to protect patient privacy and confidentially, and to avoid potential harm to patients, coworkers, or employers. Refer to ANA's "Six tips for nurses using Social Media" (ANA, 2011a), part of their "Principles for Social Networking" toolkit (ANA, 2011b). Table 3.2 lists guidelines for social media use.

Simulations

Didactic lectures have been shown to be less effective than experiential exercises, such as applications to clinical cases or scenarios in simulation labs. **Simulations** are used after graduation in continuing education, team training, and systems testing.

SUMMARY

This chapter addresses major factors effecting nursing communication. Standards issued by various agencies and organizations guide nurses in their communications with and about patients. Standards provide a measurement benchmark, used to assess nursing competency as we apply evidence-based practice and clinical guidelines. Ethical and legal aspects of nursing communication, especially HIPAA privacy regulations, have been described. The ANA Standards for Communication and ANA's Code of Ethics for Nurses provide important guides to the choice of communication. The nursing process serves as a clinical management framework, and communication is woven into each of the steps. All phases are patient-centered, where the patient is an active participant and decision-maker. The importance of maintaining the patient's privacy and confidentiality has been stressed, especially with regard to posts on social media platforms.

> **ETHICAL DILEMMA: What Would You Do?**
> As a student nurse, you observe a staff nurse making a medication error, but you are not able to intervene. She is visibly upset by her error. The patient was not actually harmed by the medication error, but the nurse hesitates to report the error. What would you do?

DISCUSSION QUESTIONS

1. Identify three ways to communicate effectively with each member of your patient's healthcare team.
2. Assemble some examples of nurses choosing not to follow written standards for communication, and then critique these examples.

REFERENCES

Agency for Healthcare and Quality (AHRQ). (2020). *AHRQ's making informed consent an informed choice: Training modules for health care leaders and professionals.* Rockville, MD: AHRQ. Retrieved from https://www.ahrq.gov/health-literacy/professional-training/informed-choice.html. [Accessed 16 June 2021].

American Association of Colleges of Nursing (AACN). (2006). Hallmarks of quality and safety: Recommended baccalaureate competencies and curricular guidelines to ensure high-quality and safe patient care. *Journal of Professional Nursing, 22*(6), 329–330.

American Association of Critical Care Nurses (AACN). (2020). *Healthy work environments.* Retrieved from https://www.aacn.org/nursing-excellence/healthy-work-environments. [Accessed 16 June 2021].

American Association of Critical Care Nurses (AACN). (n.d.). Moral distress in nursing: What you need to know. Retrieved from http://www.aacn.org/clinical-resources/moral-distress. [Accessed 21 June 2021].

American Nurses Association (ANA). (2011a). *6 tips for nurses using social media.* Silver Spring, MD: ANA. Retrieved from https://www.nursingworld.org/~4af5ec/globalassets/docs/ana/ethics/6_tips_for_nurses_using_social_media_card_web.pdf. [Accessed 16 June 2021].

American Nurses Association (ANA). (2011b). *ANA's principles for social networking and the nurse: Guidance for registered nurses.* Silver Spring, MD: ANA. Retrieved from https://www.nursingworld.org/~4af4f2/globalassets/docs/ana/ethics/social-networking.pdf. [Accessed 16 June 2021].

American Nurses Association (ANA). (2015). *Code of ethics for nurses.* Silver Spring, MD: ANA.

American Nurses Association (ANA). (2021). *Nursing: Scope and standards of practice* (4th ed.). Silver Spring, MD: ANA.

Barnsteiner, J. (2017). *Opening remarks. Presentation from the QSEN National Conference,* Chicago, IL.

Baysal, E., Sari, D., & Erdem, H. (2019). Ethical decision-making levels of oncology nurses. *Nursing Ethics, 26*(7–8), 2204–2212.

Benton, A. D., Ferguson, S. L., Douglas, J. P., & Benton, D. C. (2021). Contrasting views on scope of practice: A bibliometric analysis of allied health, nursing, and medical literature. *Journal of Nursing Regulation, 12*(1), 4–18.

Brom, H., Carthon, J. M. B., Sloane, D., McHugh, M., & Aiken, L. (2021). Better nurse work environments associated with fewer readmissions and shorter length of stay among adults with ischemic stroke: A cross-sectional analysis of United States hospitals. *Research in Nursing & Health, 44*(3), 525–533.

Canadian Nurses Association. (2017). *Code of ethics for registered nurses.* Ottawa, Canada: CNA. Retrieved from https://www.cna-aiic.ca/-/media/cna/page-content/pdf-en/code-of-ethics-2017-edition-secure-interactive.pdf. [Accessed 16 June 2021].

College of Nurses of Ontario. (2018). *Entryto-practice competencies for registered nurses.* Toronto, Canada: CNO. Retrieved from https://www.cno.org/globalassets/docs/reg/41037-entry-to-practice-competencies-2020.pdf. [Accessed 16 June 2021].

Institute for Healthcare Improvement (IHI). (2017). *New survey looks at patient experiences with medical error.* Retrieved from http://www.ihi.org/about/news/Pages/New-Survey-Looks-at-Patient-Experiences-With-Medical-Error.aspx. [Accessed 16 June 2021].

International Council of Nurses (ICN). (2012). *The ICN code of ethics for nurses, revised.* Geneva, Switzerland: ICN. Retrieved from https://www.icn.ch/sites/default/files/inline-files/2012_ICN_Codeofethicsfornurses_%20eng.pdf. [Accessed 16 June 2021].

Munroe, C. L., & Hope, A. A. (2020). Meeting today's challenges: All in. [editorial]. *American Journal of Critical Care, 29*(5), 334–336.

Myers, L. C., Heard, L., & Mort, E. (2020). Lessons learned from medical malpractice claims involving critical care nurses. *American Journal of Critical Care, 29*(3), 174–181.

National Academies of Sciences, Engineering, and Medicine. (2021). *The future of nursing 2020–2030: Charting a path to achieve health equity.* Washington, DC: The National Academies Press.

National Council of State Boards of Nursing (NCSBN). (2012). www.ncsbn.org/.

The Joint Commission (TJC). (n.d.). *R3 report [online summary briefs].* Oakbrook Terrace, IL: TJC. Retrieved from: https://www.jointcommission.org/standards/r3-report/. [Accessed 16 June 2021].

U.S. Department of Health and Human Services (DHHS). (2003). *Summary of the HIPAA privacy rule.* Retrieved from: https://www.hhs.gov/sites/default/files/privacysummary.pdf. [Accessed 16 June 2021].

SUGGESTED READING

Miller, J. (2020). *Can I do that? Incorporating scope and standards of practice into nursing professional development.* [blog].

National Council of State Boards of Nursing (NCSBN). (2021). *Nurse licensure compact annual report: Fiscal year 2019–2020.* Chicago, IL: NCSBN. Retrieved from https://www.ncsbn.org/15369.htm. [Accessed 16 June 2021].

Quality and Safety Education for Nurses (QSEN). (n.d.). Baccalaureate competencies. Retrieved from www.qsen.org/competencies/.

Clinical Judgment: Critical Thinking and Ethical Decision-Making

Chapter 4 examines the principles of ethical decision-making and the process for critical thinking. Both are essential foundational knowledge for you to make effective nursing clinical judgments to deliver safe, competent care. Clinical judgment ability is measured on the NCLEX State Board Examination allowing you to practice as a nurse. In addition to developing technical nursing skills, your ability to use critical thinking and ethical reasoning skills and to communicate these is a determining factor in your competency as a nurse. Ethical responsibility is a big aspect of nursing care. It is a much wider concept than legal responsibility, engaging not only your patients but also your entire community. Making ethical decisions requires that you understand the process. Ethical conflicts pervade our practice and have the potential to compromise quality of care if not resolved (Pavlish et al., 2011). In this book, we focus on bioethical principles as held in Western society. In addition to basic content presented in this chapter, an ethical dilemma is included in each subsequent chapter to help you begin applying your reasoning process.

Critical thinking is a learned skill that teaches you how to use a systematic process to make your clinical decisions. In the past, expert nurses accumulated this skill with on-the-job experience, through trial and error. But this essential nursing skill can be learned with continual practice and conscientious applications in educational programs. Studies show that practicing applications of evidence-based nursing increases your critical thinking abilities (Cui et al., 2018). The Applications section of this chapter specifically walks you through the reasoning process in applying the steps of critical thinking. Simulation exercises in each chapter help you practice applying these skills.

BASIC CONCEPTS

Types of Thinking

There are many ways of thinking (Fig. 4.1). Students often attempt to use total recall by simply memorizing a bunch of facts (e.g., memorizing the cranial nerves by using a mnemonic such as "On Old Olympus' Towering Tops …"). At other times, we rely on developing habits by repetition, such as practicing cardiopulmonary resuscitation (CPR) techniques. More structured methods of thinking, such as *inquiry*, have been developed in disciplines related to nursing. For example, you are probably familiar with the **scientific method**. As used in research, this is a logical, linear method of systematically gaining new information, often by setting up an experiment to test an idea. The nursing process uses a method of systematic steps: assessment before planning, planning before intervention, and evaluation.

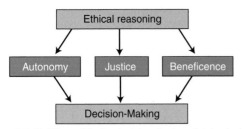

Figure 4.1 Guiding ethical principles that assist in decision-making.

CLINICAL JUDGMENT: DECISION-MAKING THEORETICAL MODELS

Clinical judgment is a combination of research, clinical expertise, and patient preferences. It requires both the ability to think critically and the knowledge as to how to apply ethical principles. Questions on the NCLEX Exam measuring clinical judgment abilities were developed based on a model they developed in 2019 (NCSBN, 2019). Components include the following:

- Recognizing cues
- Analyzing cues
- Developing and prioritizing hypotheses
- Generating solutions
- Making nursing interventions (acting)
- Evaluating patient outcomes

One characteristic of a critical thinker is self-reflection, a learned experience such as occurred in Ronnie Fox's case.

ETHICAL REASONING

In part, the quality nursing care depends on nursing values and ethics. In 2021, the International Council of Nurses (ICN) issued their newly revised Code of Ethics for Nurses. Nurses report patient well-being and dignity to be an important value related to giving care, yet often report feeling distress when forced to act contrary to what they believe is their patient's best interests. Most nurses report facing an **ethical dilemma** at least on a weekly basis. This became even more common during the recent COVID-19 pandemic when protective supplies were scarce and patient treatments were uncertain. As nurses, we frequently have to act in value-laden situations. For example, you may have patients who request abortions or who want "do not resuscitate" (DNR; "no code") orders. Willingness to comply with ethical and professional standards is a hallmark of a professional. Legal statutes that bind us are not to be confused with moral decisions, which theoretically are on a higher plain.

Organizational Barriers

Most healthcare agencies have ethics committees that often are the primary party involved in resolving difficult clinical case ethical dilemmas. Organizational rules and culture can constrain a nurse from following their professional principles, for example, a heavy workload or lack of policies about holding family conferences.

Personal Knowledge

Nursing is not the only healthcare profession struggling to apply ethical principles to clinical care situations. When tested, both physicians and nurses responded correctly to ethical dilemma questions less than half of the time. Is being ethically correct less than half the time acceptable? Practice in applying ethical principles is important. As a nurse, you will be called on to make ethical decisions. This requires clear understanding of the ethics of the nursing profession. Many nursing organizations have formally published ethical codes to promote ethical care and protect patient rights. In addition to ICN, examples include the Federation of European Countries or the American Nurses Association's Code of Ethics (ANA, 2015).

CASE STUDY: **Ronnie Fox, SN, Uses Journaling**

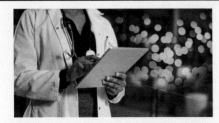

From iStock #1035963640, katleho Seisa. For an initial simulated lab experience, Ronnie was assigned to journal her own experiences, i.e., write an interpersonal process record of her talk with a standardized patient model from another culture. What felt comfortable? What was uncomfortable? Using self-reflection, she analyzed her conversation rating her conversation skills. Since her "patient" was an experienced elementary school teacher she was assigned to provide with predischarge teaching, Ronnie was asked to make suggestions for ways to change her own areas of discomfort.

During a pandemic, Ada Kelly, RN, is reassigned to work on an unfamiliar pulmonary intensive care unit. Patients there are highly infectious. Many have respiratory complications and are receiving mechanical ventilation. Ada worries that if she refuses this assignment, she could lose her job or even her license. But she also fears carrying this infection home to her two preschool children. This case highlights conflicting duties: employer/patient versus self/family. According to the ANA, nurses are obligated to care for all patients, unless a substitute nurse. There are limits to the personal risk of harm a nurse can be expected to accept, but care is a *moral duty* if patients are at significant risk for harm that her care can prevent. This situation becomes a *moral option* only if there are alternative sources of care (i.e., other nurses available).

Ethical Theories and Decision-Making Models

Ethical theories provide the bedrock from which we derive the principles that guide our decision-making. There is no one "right" answer to an ethical dilemma: The decision may vary depending on which theory the involved people subscribe to. The following section briefly describes the most common models currently used in Western bioethics. As we become a more culturally diverse society, other equally viable viewpoints may become acculturated. This discussion focuses on three decision-making models: utilitarian/goal-based, duty-based, and rights-based models.

The **utilitarian/goal-based model** says that the "rightness" or "wrongness" of an action is always a function of its consequences. Rightness is the extent to which performing or omitting an action will contribute to the overall good of the patient. Good is defined as maximum welfare or happiness. The rights of patients and the duties of a nurse are determined by what will achieve maximum welfare. When a conflict in outcome occurs, the correct action is the one that will result in the greatest good for the majority. An example of a decision made according to the goal-based model is forced mandatory institutionalization of someone with tuberculosis who refuses to take medicine to protect other members of the community. The patient's hospitalization produces the greatest balance of good over harm for the majority. Thus, "goodness" of an action is determined solely by its outcome.

The **deontological** or **duty-based model** is person centered. It incorporates Immanuel Kant's deontological philosophy, which holds that the "rightness" of an action is determined by other factors in addition to its outcome.

Respect for every person's inherent dignity is a consideration. For example, a straightforward implication would be that a physician (or nurse) may never lie to a patient. Do you agree? Decisions based on this duty-based model have a religious–social foundation. Rightness is determined by moral worth, regardless of the circumstances or the individual involved. In making decisions or implementing actions, the nurse cannot violate the basic duties and rights of individuals. Decisions about what is in the best interests of the patient require consensus among all parties involved. Examples are the medical code "do no harm" and the nursing duty to "help save lives."

The **human rights-based model** is based on the belief that each patient has basic rights. Our duties as healthcare providers arise from these basic rights. For example, a patient has the right to refuse care. Conflict occurs when the provider's duty is not in the best interests of the patient. The patient has the right to life, and the nurse has the duty to save lives, but what if the quality of life is intolerable and there is no hope for a positive outcome? Such a case might occur when a neonatal nurse cares for an infant with anencephaly (born without brain tissue in the cerebrum) in whom even the least invasive treatment would be extremely painful and would never provide any quality of life.

Ethical dilemmas arise when an actual or potential conflict occurs regarding principles, duties, or rights. Of course, many ethical or moral concepts held by Western society have been codified into law. Laws may vary by country and region, but a moral principle should be universally applied. Moral principles are shared by most members of a group, such as physicians or nurses, and represent the professional values of the group. Conflict arises when a nurse's professional values differ from the law. Conflict may also arise when you have not come to terms with situations in which your personal values differ from the profession's values. One example is doctor-assisted suicide (euthanasia). Consider the Ms French case.

Ms Francine French belongs to the "Socrates Society" whose members believe they have the right of self-termination. *Legally,* at the turn of the 21st century, such an act was legal in Oregon but illegal in Michigan. *Professionally,* the ANA Code of Ethics guides you to do no harm. You are a hospice nurse making a home visit. *Personally,* you believe euthanasia is morally wrong. Can you assist Francine at her request to hand her the suicide pill since she is now too weak to reach for her medicine?

1. Which ethical principle would you apply?
2. What could be the legal implications?

Bioethical Principles

To practice nursing in an ethical manner, you must be able to recognize the existence of a moral problem. Once you recognize a situation that puts your patient in jeopardy, you must be able to take action. Three essential, guiding, ethical principles have been developed from the theories cited earlier. The three principles that can assist us in decision-making are autonomy, beneficence (nonmaleficence), and justice.

Autonomy versus Medical Paternalism. Autonomy is the patient's right to self-determination. In the medical context, respect for autonomy is a fundamental ethical principle. It is the basis for the concept of informed consent, which means your patient makes a rational, informed decision without coercion. In the past, nurses and physicians often made decisions for patients based on what they thought was best for them. This *paternalism* sometimes discounted the wishes of patients and their families. The ethical concept of autonomy has emerged strongly as a right in Western countries. Aspects involving the individual's right to participate in medical decisions about his own care have become law in many places.

This moral principle of autonomy means that each patient has the right to decide about his or her healthcare. Patients who are empowered to make such decisions are more likely to comply with the treatment plan. Internal factors, such as pain, may interfere with a patient's ability to choose. External factors, such as coercion by a care provider, may also interfere. As a nurse, you and your employer must legally obtain the patient's permission for all treatment procedures. In the United States, under the Patient Self-Determination Act of 1991, all patients of agencies receiving Medicaid funds must receive written information about their rights to make decisions about their medical care. Nurses, as well as physicians, must provide them with all the relevant and accurate information they need to make an "informed" decision whether they agree to treatments. Nursing codes, such as the ANA Code, state that it is the nurse's responsibility to assist patients to make these decisions, as discussed in Chapter 3 in the section on informed consent.

Many of the nursing theories incorporate concepts about autonomy and empowering the patient to be responsible for self-care, so you may find this easy to accept as part of your nursing role. However, what happens if the patient's right to autonomy puts others at risk? Whose rights take precedence?

The concept of autonomy also has been applied to the way we practice nursing, but our professional autonomy has some limitations. For example, the American Medical Association's Principles of Medical Ethics says a physician can choose whom to serve, except in an emergency; however, the picture is a little different in nursing practice. According to the ANA Committee on Ethics, nurses are ethically obligated to treat patients seeking their care. A nurse has autonomy in caring for a patient, but this is somewhat limited because legally nurses must also follow physician orders and be subject to physician authority. Before the nurse or physician can override a patient's right to autonomy, they must be able to present a strong case for their point of view based on either or both of the following principles: beneficence and justice. Reflect on the case of Dorothy Newt.

Case Study: Dotty Newt and Autonomy

Ms Newt, 72 years of age, refuses physician-assisted suicide after being diagnosed with Alzheimer's disease. She also refuses entry into a long-term care facility, deciding instead to rely on her aged, disabled spouse to provide her total care as she deteriorates physically and mentally. As her home health nurse, you find Mr Newt is unable to provide the needed care.

1. What would you do?
2. Would it be ethical to ask her physician to transfer her to an extended care facility?

Beneficence and Nonmaleficence

Beneficence implies that a decision results in the greatest good or produces the least harm to the patient. This is based on the Hippocratic Oath and its concept of "do no harm." Avoiding actions that bring harm to another person is known as *nonmaleficence.* An example is the Christian belief of "do not kill," which has been codified into law but has many exceptions (e.g., soldiers sent to war are expected to kill the enemy).

In healthcare, beneficence is the underlying principle for Nursing Codes of Ethics, saying that the good of your patient is your primary responsibility. Nursing theorists have incorporated this into the nursing role, so you may find this easy to accept. Helping others may be why you chose to become a nurse. In nursing, you not only have the obligation to avoid harming your patients but also are expected to advocate for their best interests.

Beneficence is challenged in many clinical situations (e.g., requests for abortion or euthanasia). Currently, some of the most difficult ethical dilemmas involve situations where decisions may be made to withhold treatment. For example, decisions are made to justify such violations of beneficence in the guise of permitting merciful death. Is there a moral difference between actively causing death or in withholding treatment, when the outcome for the patient is the same death? There are clear legal differences.

In many places, a healthcare worker who intentionally acts to cause a patient's death is legally liable.

Other challenges to beneficence occur when the involved parties hold different viewpoints about what is best for the patient. Consider a case in which the family of an elderly, poststroke, comatose, ventilator-dependent patient wants all forms of treatment continued, but the healthcare team does not believe it will benefit the patient. The initial step toward resolution may be holding a family conference and really listening to the viewpoints of family members, asking them whether their relative ever expressed wishes verbally or in writing in the form of an advance directive or living will. Maintaining a trusting, open, mutually respectful communication may help avoid an adversarial situation. Consider Joe Harper's case.

Case Study: Joe Harper and Beneficence

Mr Harper, 62 years of age, is admitted with end-organ failure. You are expected to assess for any pain that he has and treat it. Do you seek a palliative order even though his liver cannot process drugs? It is estimated that more than 50% of conscious patients spend their last week of life in moderate to severe pain. Who is advocating for them?

1. Is it appropriate for you as a nurse to advocate for more pain medication for Mr Harper?

Justice

Justice is actually a legal term; however, in ethics, it refers to being fair or impartial. A related concept is equality (e.g., the just distribution of goods or resources, sometimes called *social justice* or *distributive justice*). Within the healthcare arena, this distributive justice concept might be applied to scarce treatment resources. As new and more expensive technologies that can prolong life become available, who has a right to them? Who should pay for them? If resources are scarce, how do we decide who gets them? Should a limited resource be spread out equally to everyone? Or should it be allocated based on who has the greatest need?

Unnecessary Treatment. Decisions made based on the principle of justice may also involve the concept of unnecessary treatment. Are all operations that are performed truly necessary? Why do some patients receive antibiotics for viral infections, when we know they do not kill viruses? Are unnecessary diagnostic tests ever ordered solely to document that a patient does not have condition X, just in case there is a malpractice lawsuit?

Social Worth. Another justice concept to consider in making decisions is that of social worth. Are all people equal? Are some more deserving than others? If Dan is 7

years old instead of 77 years old, and the expensive medicine would cure his condition, should these factors affect the decision to give him the medicine? If there is only one liver available for transplant today, and there are two equally viable potential recipients—Larry, age 54 years, whose alcoholism destroyed his own liver; or Kay, age 32 years, whose liver was destroyed by hepatitis she got while on a lifesaving mission abroad—who should get the liver?

Veracity. Truthfulness is the bedrock of trust. And trust is an essential component of the professional nurse–patient relationship. Not only is there a moral injunction against lying, but it is also destructive to any professional relationship. Generally, nurses would agree that a nurse should never lie to a patient. However, there is controversy about withholding information. We need clarity about truth telling. There will be times when we need to exercise some judgment about to whom to disclose information. We have an obligation to protect potentially vulnerable patients from information that would cause emotional distress. Although it is never acceptable to lie, nurses have evaded answering questions by saying, "You need to ask your physician about that." Can you suggest another response? Explain the Lee Smith case to other waiting patients.

Case Study: Lee Smith and Justice

Lee, age 18 years, is admitted to the emergency department (ED) bleeding from a chest wound. His blood pressure is falling, shock is imminent. Tomas, Sue, and Mary were registered ahead of Lee but do not have life-threatening complaints. ED's triage protocol says caring for the least stable patient is a priority. Is this a "just distribution" of ED resources?

Steps in Ethical Decision-Making

The process of moral reasoning and making ethical decisions has been broken down into steps. These steps are only a part of the larger model for critical thinking. If you are the moral agent making this decision, you must be skillful enough to implement the actions in a morally correct way.

In deciding how to spend your limited time with these patients, do you base your decision entirely on how much good you can do for each one? Under distributive justice, what should happen when the needs of these four conflict? You could base your decision on the principle of beneficence and do the greatest good for the most patients, but this is a very subjective judgment. In using ethical decision-making processes, nurses must be able to tolerate ambiguity and uncertainty. One of the most difficult aspects for the novice nurse to accept is that there often is no one "right" answer; rather, usually several options may be selected, depending on the person or situation, as in the Ruth Rae case.

Case Study: Mrs Ruth Rae and Ethical Decision-Making

You are assigned to four critical patients on your unit. Mrs Rae, 83 years of age, is unconscious and dying and needs suctioning every 10 min. Mr Jones, 47 years of age, has been admitted for observation for severe bloody stools. Mr Hernandez, 52 years of age, has newly diagnosed diabetes and is receiving intravenous (IV) drip insulin; he requires monitoring of vital signs every 15 min. Mr Martin, 35 years of age, is suicidal and has been told today he has inoperable cancer.

1. Would one of them benefit more from nursing care than the others?
2. Is there a better option (such as calling your supervisor for assistance)?

CRITICAL THINKING

Critical thinking is the basis of all our clinical reasoning, problem-solving, and decision-making. Critical thinking is a complex, analytical method of thinking, in which you purposefully use specific thinking skills to make clinical decisions. You are able to reflect on your own thinking process to make effective interventions that improve your patient's outcome. Although no consensus has been reached on a critical thinking definition in the nursing arena, we generally define critical thinking as the purposeful use of a specific cognitive framework to identify and analyze problems. Critical thinking enables us to recognize emergent situations, make clear, objective, clinical decisions, and intervene appropriately to give safe, effective care. It encompasses the steps of the nursing process, but possibly in a more circular loop than we usually envision the nursing process. By thinking critically, we can modify our care based on responses to these nursing interventions.

Characteristics of a Critical Thinker in Making Clinical Decisions

Process

Critical thinkers are skilled at using inquiry methods. They approach problem solutions in a systematic, organized, and goal-directed way when making clinical decisions. They continually use past knowledge, communication skills, new information, and observations to make these clinical judgments. Table 4.1 summarizes the characteristics of a critical thinker.

TABLE 4.1 Characteristics of a Critical Thinker	
Knowledge (thought processes)	• Be reflective and anticipate consequences • Combine existing knowledge and standards with new information (transformation) • Incorporate creative thinking • Recognize when information is missing and seek new input • Discard irrelevant information (discrimination) • Effectively interpret existing data • Consider alternative solutions
Skills	• Think in an orderly way, using logical reasoning in complex problem situations • Diligently persevere in seeking relevant information • Recognize deviations from expected patterns • Revise actions based on new input • Evaluate solutions and outcomes
Attitude	• Be inquisitive, desire to seek the truth • Seek to develop analytical thinking • Maintain open-mindedness and flexibility

Act

Expert nurses recognize that priorities change continually, requiring constant assessment and alternative interventions. When the authors analyzed the decision-making process of expert nurses, they all used the critical thinking steps described in this chapter when they made their clinical judgments, even though they were not always able to verbally state the components of their thinking processes. Expert nurses organized each input of patient information and quickly distinguished relevant from irrelevant information. They seemed to categorize each new fact into a problem format, obtaining supplementary data and arriving at a decision about diagnosis and intervention. Often, they commented about comparing this new information with prior knowledge, sometimes from academic sources and "best practice protocols" but most often from information gained from other nurses. They constantly scan for new information, and constantly reassess their patient's situation. This is not linear. New input is always being added. This contrasts with novice nurses who tend to think in a linear way, collect lots of facts but not logically organize them, and fail to make as many connections with past knowledge. Novice nurses' assessments are more generalized and less focused, and they tend to jump too quickly to a diagnosis without recognizing the need to obtain more facts.

Reflect

Critical thinking is more than just a *cognitive process* of the following steps. It also has an *affective component*—the willingness to engage in self-reflective inquiry. Most nurse educators say this sense of inquiry is crucial. As you learn to be a critical thinker, you improve and clarify your thinking process skills, reflect on this process, and learn from the situation so that you are more accurately able to solve problems based on available evidence. An attitude of openness to new learning is essential. Although cognitive thinking skills can be taught, you also need to be willing to consciously choose to apply this process.

Barriers to Thinking Critically and Reasoning Ethically

Attitudes and Habits

Barriers that decrease a nurse's ability to think critically, including attitudes such as "my way is better," interfere with our ability to empower patients to make their own decisions. Our thinking habits can also impede communication with patients or families making complex bioethical choices. Examples include becoming accustomed to acknowledging "only one right answer" or selecting only one option. Behaviors that act as barriers include automatically responding defensively when challenged, resisting changes, and desiring to conform to expectations. Cognitive barriers, such as thinking in stereotypes, also interfere with our ability to treat a patient as an individual.

Cognitive Dissonance

Cognitive dissonance refers to the mental discomfort you feel when there is a discrepancy between what you already believe and some new information that does not go along with your view. In this book, we use the term to refer to the holding of two or more conflicting values at the same time.

Personal Values versus Professional Values

We all have a personal value system developed over a lifetime that has been extensively shaped by our family, our religious beliefs, and our years of life experiences. Our values change as we mature in our ability to think critically, logically, and morally. Strongly held values become a part of self-concept. Our education as nurses helps us acquire a professional value system. In nursing school, as you advance through your clinical experiences, you begin to take on some of the

> **BOX 4.1   Five Core Values of Professional Nursing**
>
> Five *core values of professional nursing* have been identified by the American Association of Colleges of Nursing:
> - Human dignity
> - Integrity
> - Autonomy
> - Altruism
> - Social justice

values of the nursing profession as listed in Box 4.1. You are acquiring these values as you learn the nursing role. The process of this role socialization is discussed in Chapter 22. For example, maintaining patient confidentiality is a professional value, with both a legal and a moral requirement. We must take care that we do not allow our personal values to obstruct care for a patient who holds differing values.

Values Clarification and the Nursing Process

The nursing process offers many opportunities to incorporate *values clarification* into your care. During the assessment phase, you can obtain an assessment of the *patient's values* with regard to the health system. For example, you interview Mr Smith for the first time and learn that he has obstructive pulmonary disease and is having difficulty breathing, but he insists on smoking. Is it appropriate to intervene? In this example, you know that smoking is detrimental to a person's health and you, as a nurse, find the value of health in conflict with his value of smoking. It is important to understand your patient's values. When your values differ, you attempt to care for this patient within his or her reality. In this example, Mr Smith has the right to make decisions that are not always congruent with those of healthcare providers.

When identifying specific nursing diagnoses, it is important that your diagnoses are not biased. Examples of value conflicts might be spiritual distress related to a conflict between spiritual beliefs and prescribed health treatments, or ineffective family coping related to restricted visiting hours for a family in which full family participation is a cultural value. In the planning phase, it is important to identify and understand the patient's value system as the foundation for developing the most appropriate interventions. Plans of care that support rather than discount the patient's healthcare beliefs are more likely to be received favorably. Your interventions include values clarification as a guideline for care. You help patients examine alternatives. During the evaluation phase, examine how well the nursing and patient goals were met while keeping within the guidelines of the patient's value system.

In conclusion, when there is a conflict with own personal ethical convictions, nurses must put aside their own moral convictions to provide necessary assistance in a case of emergency when there is imminent risk to a patient's life. Ethical reasoning and critical thinking skills are essential competencies for making clinical judgments, in an increasingly complex healthcare system. To apply critical thinking to a clinical decision, we need to base our intervention on the best evidence available. Developing higher levels of critical thinking is a learned ability.

DEVELOPING AN EVIDENCE-BASED PRACTICE:

Intensive Care Units and Ethics

Patients are in critical condition when they are cared for in intensive care units (ICUs). Some patients will recover and go on to be discharged, but others are terminal. Crucial ethical conversations do not always occur. Pavlish and associates (2020) conducted a pre and post intervention evaluation to identify ethical concerns and implement staff support in six ICUs. The intervention consisted of an ethics video for staff, written support materials, and suggestions for improving 1649 staff nurse–patient interpersonal relationships. Researches taught staff nurses to integrate Early Action Ethics Protocol into their patient care.

Results

At a 3-month and a 6-month follow-up, there were significant increases in the likelihood of holding a family conference and obtaining a visit from a chaplain. The number of palliative care consultations also increased.
   Strength of this Research Evidence: High.

Application to Your Clinical Practice

1. Nurses are sometimes reluctant to initiate conversations about death issues. These findings support prior research, which shows that nurses do need to initiate such conversations rather than waiting for the patient to open discussions.
2. Establish routine protocols for frequent communication with critically ill patients and families.
3. Consider integrating the Early Action Ethics Protocol available in www.ajcconline.org/.
4. Introduce family conferences early, so referrals for supportive services can be made for family caretakers if necessary.

References

Pavlish, C.L., Henriksen, J., Brown-Saltzman, K., et al. (2020). A team-based early action protocol to address ethical concerns in the intensive care unit. *American Journal of Critical Care, 29*(1), 49–61.

APPLICATIONS

Problem-Solving

Clinical reasoning is a complex, cyclical process designed to solve problems. It embodies your ability to reason, to incorporate your existing knowledge, professional values, personal values, and your patient's values. You gather, update, and continually analyze patient information, weighing alternative actions to implement safe, competent care. Accepted methods for building your critical thinking abilities include case study analyses, questioning, reflective journaling, patient simulations, portfolios, concept mapping, and problem-based learning. Skills can be learned by participating in simulated patient case situations. According to Nelson (2017) and others, accepted teaching–learning methods for assessing critical thinking include use of case studies, questioning, reflective journalism, portfolios, concept maps, and problem-based learning.

SOLVING ETHICAL DILEMMAS AS PART OF CLINICAL DECISION-MAKING

Nurses indicate a need for more information about dealing with the ethical dilemmas they encounter, yet most say they receive little education in doing so. We need to remember that there is no one absolutely correct answer to an ethical dilemma. Simulation Exercises 4.1–4.3 give you opportunities to discuss ethical decision-making.

The ethical issues that nurses commonly face today can be placed in three general categories: moral uncertainty, moral or ethical dilemmas, and moral distress. *Moral uncertainty* occurs when a nurse is uncertain as to which moral rules (i.e., values, beliefs, or ethical principles) apply to a given situation. For example, should a terminally ill patient who is in and out of a coma and chooses not to eat or drink anything be required to have IV therapy for

---

SIMULATION EXERCISE 4.1   Autonomy

Purpose

To stimulate class discussion about the moral principle of autonomy.

Procedure

In small groups, read the three case examples in this chapter and discuss whether the patient has the autonomous right to refuse treatment if it affects the life of another person.

Reflective Discussion Analysis

Prepare your argument for an in-class discussion.

SIMULATION EXERCISE 4.2   Beneficence

Purpose

To stimulate discussion about the moral principle of beneficence.

Procedure

Read the following case example and prepare for discussion:

Dawn, a staff nurse, answers the telephone and receives a verbal order from Dr Smith. Ms Patton was admitted this morning with ventricular arrhythmia. Dr Smith orders Dawn to administer a potent diuretic, furosemide (Lasix) 80 mg, IV, STAT. This is such a large dose that she has to order it up from pharmacy.

As described in the text, you are legally obliged to carry out a doctor's orders unless they threaten the welfare of your patient. How often do nurses question orders? What would happen to a nurse who questioned orders too often? In a research study using this case simulation, nearly 95% of the time the nurses participating in the study attempted to implement this potentially lethal medication order before being stopped by the researcher!

Reflective Discussion Analysis

1. What principles are involved?
2. What would you do if you were this staff nurse?

SIMULATION EXERCISE 4.3   Justice

Purpose

To encourage discussion about the concept of justice.

Procedure

Consider that to contain costs, several years ago the state of Oregon attempted to legislate restrictions on what Medicaid would pay for. A young boy needed a standard treatment of bone marrow transplant for his childhood leukemia. He died when the state refused to pay for his treatment.

Read the following case example, and in a small group, answer the discussion questions:

Mr. Diaz, aged 74 years, has led an active life and continues to be the sole support for his wife and disabled daughter. He pays for healthcare with Medicare government insurance. The doctors think his cancer may respond to a very expensive new drug, which is not paid for under his coverage.

Reflective Discussion Analysis

1. Does everyone have a basic right to healthcare, as well as to life and liberty?
2. Does an insurance company have a right to restrict access to care?

hydration purposes? Does giving IV therapy constitute giving the patient extraordinary measures to prolong life? Is it more comfortable or less comfortable for the dying person to maintain a high hydration level? When there is no clear definition of the problem, moral uncertainty develops, because the nurse is unable to identify the situation as a moral problem or to define specific moral rules that apply. Strategies that might be useful in dealing with moral uncertainty include using the values clarification process, developing a specific philosophy of nursing, and acquiring knowledge about ethical principles.

Ethical or moral dilemmas arise when two or more moral issues are in conflict. An ethical dilemma is a problem in which there are two or more conflicting but equally right answers. Organ harvesting of a severely brain-damaged infant is an example of an ethical dilemma. Removal of organs from one infant may save the lives of several other infants. However, even though the brain-damaged child is definitely going to die, is it right to remove organs before the child's death? It is important for the nurse to understand that, in many ethical dilemmas, there is often no single "right" solution. Some decisions may be "more right" than others, but often what one nurse decides best differs significantly from what another nurse would decide.

The third common kind of ethical problem seen in nursing today is *moral distress*. Moral distress results when the nurse knows what is "right" but is bound to do otherwise because of legal or institutional constraints. When such situations arise (e.g., a terminally ill patient who does not have a "do not resuscitate" medical order and therefore resuscitation attempts must be made), nurses may experience inner turmoil. Nurses have reported that three of their most commonly encountered ethics problems have to do with resuscitation decisions for dying patients lacking clear code orders; patients and families who want more aggressive treatment; and colleagues who discuss patients inappropriately. Chapter 27 describes ways to moderate moral distress.

Because values underlie all ethical decision-making, nurses must understand their own values thoroughly before making an ethical decision. Instead of responding in an emotional manner on the spur of the moment (as people often do when faced with an ethical dilemma), the nurse who uses the values clarification process can respond rationally. It is not an easy task to have sufficient knowledge of oneself, of the situation, and of legal and moral constraints to be able to implement ethical decision-making quickly. Expert nurses still struggle and still have uncertainties. Taking time to examine situations can help you develop skills in dealing with ethical dilemmas in nursing, and the exercises in this book will give you a chance to practice. Each chapter in this book has included at least one ethical dilemma, so you can discuss what you would do.

As nurses, we advocate for our patient's best interests. To do so, we avoid a "paternalistic" imposing of what we think is in their best interests, instead listening and eliciting their preferences, to work collaboratively with the health-care team in developing an ethical patient-centered plan of care. Issues most frequently necessitating ethical decisions occur at the beginning of life and at the close of life.

Finally, reflect on your own ethical practice. How important is it for your patient to be able to always count on you? Consider the following journal entry (Milton, 2002):

I ask for information, share my needs, to no avail. You come and go ...

"Could you find out for me?" "Sure, I'll check on it." [But] check on it never comes ...

Who can I trust? I thought you'd be here for me ... You weren't. What can I do?

PROFESSIONAL VALUES ACQUISITION

Professional values or ethics consist of the values held in common by the members of a profession. Professional values are formally stated in professional codes. One example already mentioned is the ANA Code of Ethics for Nurses. Often, professional values are transmitted by tradition in nursing classes and clinical experiences. They are modeled by expert nurses and assimilated as part of the role socialization process during your years as a student and new graduate. Professional values acquisition should perhaps be the result of conscious choice by a nursing student.

APPLYING CRITICAL THINKING TO THE CLINICAL DECISION-MAKING PROCESS

This section discusses a procedure for developing critical thinking skills as applied to solving clinical problems. Different examples illustrate the reasoning process developed by several disciplines. Unfortunately, each discipline has its own vocabulary. Table 4.2 shows that we are talking about concepts with which you are already familiar. It also contrasts terms used in education, nursing, and philosophy to specify the steps to develop critical thinking skills. For example, the nurse performs a "patient assessment," which

TABLE 4.2 Critical Judgment Reasoning Process

Generic Reasoning Process	Diagnostic Reasoning in the Nursing Process	Ethical Reasoning	Critical Thinking Skill
Collect and interpret information	Gordon's functional patterns of health assessment	Obtain background information; identify ethical problem (parties, claim, basis)	1. Clarify concepts 2. Identify own, patient, and professional values and differentiate
Identify problem	Statement of nursing diagnosis	Consider ethical dilemma: • State the problem • Collect additional information • Develop alternatives for analysis	3. Integrate data and identify missing data 4. Collect new data 5. Identify problem 6. Examine skeptically 7. Apply criteria 8. Look at alternatives 9. Check for change in context
Plan for problem-solving	Prioritization of problems/interventions	Prioritized claims	10. Make decision, select best action plan, and act to implement
Implement plan	Nursing action	Apply moral principles and take action	
Evaluate	Outcome evaluation	Moral evaluation of outcome and reflect on the process used	11. Evaluate the outcome and reflect on the process

in education is referred to as "collecting information" or in philosophy may be called "identifying claims."

The process of critical thinking is systematic, organized, and goal directed. As critical thinkers, nurses are able to explore all aspects of a complex clinical situation. This is a learned process. Among many teaching–learning techniques helping you develop critical thinking skills, most are included in this book: reflective journaling, concept maps, role-playing, guided small group discussion, and case study discussion. An extensive case application follows. During your learning phase, the critical thinking skills are divided into 10 specific steps. Each step includes a discussion of application to the clinical case example provided.

To help you understand how to apply critical thinking steps, read the following case and then see how each of the steps can be used in making clinical decisions. Components of this case are applied to illustrate the steps and to stimulate discussion in the critical thinking process; many more points may be raised. From the outset, understand that, although these are listed as steps, they do not occur in a rigid, linear way in real life. The model is best thought of as a circular model. New data are constantly being sought and added to the process. Apply information in the ongoing case of Mrs Vilios:

Case Study: Unfolding Case With Mrs Vilios—Apply Clinical Judgment Concepts

Day 1—Mrs Vilios, a 72-year-old widowed teacher, has been admitted to your unit. Her daughter, Sara, lives 2 h away from her mother, but she arrives soon after admission. According to Sara, her mother lived an active life before admission, taking care of herself in an apartment in a senior citizens' housing development. Sara noticed that for about 3 weeks now, telephone conversations with her mother did not make sense or she seemed to have a hard time concentrating, although her pronunciation was clear. The admitting diagnosis is dehydration and dementia, rule out Alzheimer disease, organic brain syndrome, and depression. An IV drip of 1000 mL dextrose/0.45 normal saline is ordered at 50 drops/hour. Mrs Vilios's history is unremarkable except for a recent 10-pound weight loss. She has no allergies and is known to take acetaminophen regularly for minor pain.

Day 2—When Sara visits her mom's apartment to bring grooming items to the hospital, she finds the refrigerator and food pantry empty. A neighbor tells her that Mrs Vilios was seen roaming the halls aimlessly 2 days ago and could not remember whether she had eaten. As Mrs Vilios's nurse, you notice that she is oriented today (to time and person). A soft diet is ordered, and her urinary output is now normal.

Day 5—In the morning report, the night nurse states that Mrs Vilios was hallucinating and restraints were applied. A nasogastric tube was ordered to suction out stomach contents because of repeated vomiting. Dr Green tells Sara and her brother, Todos, that their mother's prognosis is guarded; she has acquired a serious systemic infection, is semicomatose, is not taking nourishment, and needs antibiotics and hyperalimentation. Sara reminds the doctor that her mother signed a living will in which she stated she refuses all treatment except IVs to keep her alive. Todos is upset, yelling at Sara that he wants the doctor to do everything possible to keep their mother alive.

Step 1: Clarify Concepts

The first step in making a clinical judgment is to identify whether a problem actually exists. Poor decision-makers often skip this step. To figure out whether there is a problem, you need to think about what to observe and what basic information to gather. If it is an ethical dilemma, you need to identify not only the existence of the moral problem but also all the interested parties who have a stake in the decision. Figuring out exactly what the problem or issue is may not be as easy as it sounds.

Look for Clues

Are there hidden meanings to the words being spoken? Are there nonverbal clues?

Identify Assumptions

What assumptions are being made?

Case Discussion

This case is designed to present both physiological and ethical dilemmas. In clarifying the problem, address both domains.

- Physiological concerns: Based on the diagnosis, the initial treatment goal was to restore homeostasis. By day 5, is it clear whether Mrs Vilios's condition is reversible?
- Ethical concerns: When is a decision made to initiate treatment or to abide by the advance directive and respect Mrs Vilios's wishes regarding no treatment?
- What are the wishes of the family? What happens when there is no consensus?
- Assumptions: Is the diagnosis correct? Does she have dementia? Or was her confusion a result of dehydration and a strange hospital environment?

Step 2: Identify Your Own Values

Values clarification helps you identify and prioritize your values. It also serves as a base for helping patients identify the values they hold as important. Unless you are able to identify your patient's values and can appreciate the validity of those values, you run the risk for imposing your own values. It is not necessary for your values and your patient's values to coincide; this is an unrealistic expectation. However, whenever possible, the patient's values should be taken into consideration during every aspect of nursing care. Discussion of the case of Mrs Vilios presented in this section may help you with the clarification process.

Having just completed the exercises given earlier should help your understanding of your own personal values and the professional values of nursing. Now apply this information to this case.

Case Discussion

Identify the values of each person involved:
- Family: Mrs Vilios signed an advance directive. Sara wants it adhered to; Todos wants it ignored. Why? (Missing information: Are there religious beliefs? Is there unclear communication? Is there guilt about previous troubles in the relationship?)
- Personal values: What are yours?
- Professional values: Nurses are advocates for their patients; beneficence implies nonmaleficence ("do no harm"), but does autonomy mean the right to refuse treatment? What is the agency's policy? What are the legal considerations? Practice refining your professional values acquisition by completing the values exercises in this chapter.

In summary, you need to identify which values are involved in a situation or which moral principles can be cited to support each of the positions advocated by the involved individuals.

Step 3: Integrate Data and Identify Missing Data

Think about knowledge gained in prior courses and during clinical experiences. Try to make connections between different subject areas and clinical nursing practice.
- Identify what data are needed. Obtain all possible information and gather facts or evidence (evaluate whether data are true, relevant, and sufficient). Situations are often complicated. It is important to figure out what information is significant to this situation. Synthesize prior information you already have with similarities in the current situation. Conflicting data may indicate a need to search for more information.
- Compare existing information with past knowledge. Has this patient complained of difficulty thinking before? Does she have a history of dementia?
- Look for gaps in the information. Actively work to recognize whether there is missing information. Was Mrs Vilios previously taking medications to prevent depression? For a nurse, this is an important part of critical thinking.

- Collect information systematically. Use an organized framework to obtain information. Nurses often obtain a history by asking questions about each body system. They could just as systematically ask about basic needs.
- Organize your information. Clustering information into relevant categories is helpful. For example, gathering all the facts about a patient's breathing may help focus your attention on whether they are having a respiratory problem. In your assessment, you note the rate and character of respirations, the color of nails and lips, the use of accessory muscles, and the grunting noises. At the same time, you exclude information about bowel sounds or deep tendon reflexes as not being immediately relevant to this patient's respiratory status. Categorizing information also helps you notice whether there are missing data. A second strategy that will help you organize information is to look for patterns. It has been indicated that experienced nurses intuitively note recurrent meaningful aspects of a clinical situation.

Case Discussion

Rely on prior didactic knowledge or clinical experience. Cluster the data. What was Mrs Vilios's status immediately before hospitalization? What was her status at the time of hospitalization? What information is missing? What additional data do you need?
- Physiology: Consider pathophysiological knowledge about the effects of hypovolemia and electrolyte imbalances on the systems such as the brain, kidneys, and vascular system. What is her temperature? What are her laboratory values? What is her 24-hour intake and output? Is she still dehydrated?
- Psychological/cognitive: How does hospitalization affect older adults? How do restraints affect them?
- Social/economic: Was weight loss a result of dehydration? Why was she without food? Could it be due to economic factors or mental problems?
- Legal: What constitutes a binding advance directive in the state in which Mrs Vilios lives? Is a living will valid in her state, or does the law require a health power of attorney? Are these documents on file at the hospital?

Step 4: Obtain New Data

Critical thinking is not a linear process. Expert nurses often modify interventions based on the response to the event, or change in the patient's physical condition. Constantly consider whether you need more information. Establish an attitude of inquiry and obtain more information as needed. Ask questions; search for evidence; and check reference books, journals, the ethics sources on the Internet, or written professional or agency protocols.

Evaluate conflicting information. There may be time constraints. If a patient has suspected "respiratory problems," you may need to set priorities. Obtain data that are most useful or are easily available. It would be useful to know oxygenation levels, but you may not have time to order laboratory tests. But perhaps there is a device on the unit or in the room that can measure oxygen saturation.

Sometimes you may need to change your approach to improve your chances of obtaining information. For example, when the charge nurse caring for Mrs Vilios used an authoritarian tone to try to get the sister and brother to provide more information about possible drug overdose, they did not respond. However, when the charge nurse changed his approach, exhibiting empathy, the daughter volunteered that on several occasions her mother had forgotten what pills she had taken.

Case Discussion

List sources from which you can obtain missing information. Physiological data such as temperature or laboratory test results can be obtained quickly; however, some of the ethical information may take longer to consider.

Step 5: Identify the Significant Problem
- Analyze existing information: Examine all the information you have. Identify all the possible positions.
- Make inferences: What might be going on? What are the possible diagnoses? Develop a working diagnosis.
- Prioritize: Which problem is most urgently in need of your intervention? What are the appropriate interventions?

Case Discussion

A significant physiological concern is sepsis, regardless of whether it is an iatrogenic (hospital-acquired) infection or one resulting from immobility and debilitation. A significant ethical concern is the conflict among family members and the patient (as expressed through her living will). At what point do spiritual concerns take priority over a worsening physical concern?

Step 6: Examine Skeptically

Thinking about a situation may involve weighing positive and negative factors, and differentiating facts that are credible from opinions that are biased or not grounded in true facts.
- Keep an open mind.
- Challenge your own assumptions.
- Consider whether any of your assumptions are unwarranted. Does the available evidence really support your assumption?

- Discriminate between facts and inferences. Your inferences need to be logical and plausible, based on the available facts.
- Are there any problems that you have not considered?

In trying to evaluate a situation, consciously raising questions becomes an important part of thinking critically. At times, there will be alternative explanations or different lines of reasoning that are equally valid. The challenge is to examine your own and others' perspectives for important ideas, complicating factors, other plausible interpretations, and new insights. Some nurses believe that examining information skeptically is part of each step in the critical thinking process rather than a step by itself.

Case Discussion

Challenge assumptions about the cause of Mrs Vilios's condition. For example, did you eliminate the possibility that she had a head injury caused by a fall? Could she have liver failure as a result of acetaminophen overdosing? Have all the possibilities been explored? Challenge your assumptions about outcome: Are they influenced by expected probable versus possible outcomes for this client? If she, indeed, has irreversible dementia, what will the quality of her life be if she recovers from her physical problems?

Step 7: Apply Criteria

In evaluating a situation, think about appropriate responses.
- Assess standards for "best practices" related to your patient's situation.
- Laws: There may be a law that can be applied to guide your actions and decisions. For example, by law, certain diseases must be reported to the state. If you suspect physical abuse, there is a state statute that requires professionals to report abuse to the Department of Social Services.
- Legal precedents: There may have been similar cases or situations that were dealt with in a court of law. Legal decisions do guide healthcare practices. In end-of-life decisions, when there is no legally binding healthcare power of attorney, the most frequent hierarchy is the spouse, then the adult children, then the parents.
- Protocols: There may be standard protocols for managing certain situations. Your agency may have standing orders for caring for Mrs Vilios if she develops respiratory distress, such as administering oxygen per face mask at 5 L/min.

Case Discussion

Many criteria could be used to examine this case, including the Nurse Practice Act in the area of jurisdiction; the professional organization code of ethics or general ethical principles of beneficence and autonomy; the hospital's written protocols and policies; state laws regarding living wills; and prior court decisions about living wills. Remember that advance directives are designed to take effect only when individuals become unable to make their own wishes known.

Step 8: Generate Options and Look at Alternatives

- Evaluate the major alternative points of view.
- Involve experienced peers as soon as you can to assist you in making your decision.
- Use clues from others to help you "put the picture together."
- Can you identify all the arguments—pros and cons—to explain this situation? Almost all situations will have strong counterarguments or competing hypotheses.

Case Discussion

The important concept is that neither the physician nor the nurse should handle this alone; rather, others should be involved (e.g., the hospital bioethics committee, the ombudsman patient representative, the family's spiritual counselor, and other medical experts such as a gerontologist, psychologist, and nursing clinical specialist).

Step 9: Consider Whether Factors Change If the Context Changes

Consider whether your decision would be different if there were a change in circumstances. For example, a change in their age, in the site of the situation, or in their culture may affect your decision. A competent nurse prioritizes the aspects of a situation that are most relevant and can modify her actions based on the patient's responses. A competent nurse anticipates consequences.

Case Discussion

If you knew the outcome from the beginning, would your decisions be same? What if you knew she had a terminal cancer? What if Mrs Vilios had remained in her senior housing project and you were the home health nurse? What if Mrs Vilios had remained alert during her hospitalization and refused IVs, hyperalimentation, nasogastric tubes, and so on? What if the family and Mrs Vilios were in agreement about no treatment? Would you make more assertive interventions to save her life if she were 7 years old, or a 35-year-old mother of five young children?

Step 10: Evaluate and Make the Intervention

After analyzing available information in this systematic way, you need to make a judgment or decision. An important part of your decision is your ability to communicate it coherently to others and to reflect on health status outcomes.

- Justify your conclusion.
- Evaluate outcomes.
- Test out your decision or conclusion by implementing appropriate actions.

As a critical thinker, you need to be able to accept that there may be multiple solutions that can be equally acceptable. In other situations, you may need to make a decision even when there is incomplete knowledge. Be able to cite your rationale or present your arguments to others for your decision choice and interventions. Revise interventions as necessary.

Clinical Decision-Making

While we have yet to arrive at a universal consensus for understanding **clinical decision-making**, many articles cite components of models developed by Levett-Jones et al. (2010), among others. Making clinical decisions is complex. As illustrated in Fig. 4.2, we could perhaps think of decision-making and intervention as striving to achieve P.A.R. We need to Process, Act, and Reflect to provide safe, competent, nursing care.

Process. As a nurse, you are faced with processing copious amounts of information quickly in using your critical thinking skills; we assess patient status and notice factors that characterize our patient's current situation. We incorporate our existing clinical knowledge to help us

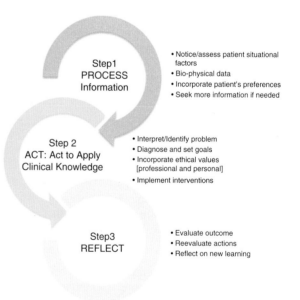

Figure 4.2 P.A.R.: The clinical decision-making process.

understand what is happening. This includes processing information from our assessment, biophysical data, our knowledge of patient preferences, and our understanding of current circumstances.

Act. Applying our clinical knowledge to identify problems, incorporate ethical values, and set goals, we make appropriate interventions. We recognize the need to continually gather and analyze new information.

Reflect. After you implement interventions, we examine outcomes. Was your assessment correct? Did you obtain enough information? Did the benefits to the patient and family outweigh the harm that may have occurred? In retrospect, do you know you made the correct decision? Did you anticipate possibilities and complications correctly? Did you communicate with the health team in a timely manner? This kind of self-examination can foster self-correction and learning. Reflecting on one's own thinking is the hallmark of a critical thinker. This self-reflection facilitates our learning.

This is a cyclical nursing care process in which constant reevaluation and reflection on one's actions and subsequent outcomes become new input. While the example of Mrs Vilios described a hospitalized situation, it is even more essential that nurses in the community be able to apply critical thinking to clinical decision-making so they may implement safer, evidence-based high-quality care in independent situations. Recognizing and treating deteriorations might prevent hospitalization.

Summarizing the Learning Process

Learning these steps in critical thinking results from repeated application. In addition to using peer discussions of the case studies, recording role-playing of simulated patient situations using standardized patient models or computer-generated problems gives opportunity for practice. A new graduate nurse must, at a minimum, be able to identify essential clinical data, know when to initiate interventions, know why a particular intervention is relevant, and differentiate between problems that need immediate intervention versus problems that can wait for action. Repeated practice in applying critical thinking can help a new graduate fit into the expectations of employers. In addition to lab situations, learning can occur through the analysis of interviews with experienced nurses about their decision-making.

▋ SUMMARY

Ethical reasoning and critical thinking are systematic, comprehensive processes to aide you in making clinical decisions. An important concept is to forget the idea that there is only one right answer in discussing ethical dilemmas. Accept that there may be several equally correct solutions depending on each individual's point of view.

Critical thinking is not a linear process. Analysis of the thinking processes of expert nurses reveals that they continually scan new data and simultaneously apply these steps in clinical decision-making. They monitor the effectiveness of their interventions in achieving desired outcomes for their patient. A nurse's moral reasoning and critical thinking abilities often have a profound effect on the quality of care given, which affects health outcomes. Functioning as a competent nurse requires that you have knowledge of medical and nursing content, "best practice" guidelines, an accumulation of clinical experiences, and an ability to think critically.

Almost daily, we confront ethical dilemmas and complicated clinical situations that require expertise as a decision-maker. We can follow the steps of the thinking process described in this chapter to help us respond to such situations. Developing clinical judgment is a learned process, one that requires repeated application.

NEXT-GENERATION NCLEX® EXAMINATION-STYLE CASE STUDY

Ethical Support of a Patient's Right of Autonomy
After learning of their cancer diagnosis, a patient has a long conversation about proposed treatment options with the oncologist. The next morning the patient shares with the nurse that he or she is very likely going to choose the option that includes a new chemotherapy treatment. The nurse responds with personal stories regarding the outcome of several patients with a similar diagnosis, adding that new therapies tend to be very expensive. The nurse stresses that while the decision is the patient's to make, it is worth considering that the traditional therapies have proven to be very effective.

In the aforementioned scenario, highlight the assessment findings that require immediate follow-up.

ETHICAL DILEMMA: What Would You Do?

The Moyers family has power of attorney over hospitalized, terminally ill Gail Midge, aged 42 years. They are consistently at her bedside and refuse to allow you and other nurses to administer pain medication ordered by Mrs M's physician, since they fear it will overdose her, causing her death. Gail often moans, cries with pain, and begs you for pain meds. The family threatens a lawsuit if she is given anything and then dies. What would you do?

DISCUSSION QUESTIONS

1. Consider the Quality and Safety Education for Nurses competency of patient-centered care and the concept of autonomy; apply this to a case QSEN (Level 2). When does a patient have the right to refuse treatment?

2. Use standards to analyze the characteristics of a **critical thinker** (Level 3). How did you develop these? Were they innate or when did you acquire them?

3. Construct an example showing when a nurse has an ethical obligation (Level 4). By choosing to become a nurse, do you assume an **ethical** obligation to treat any patient assigned to you? When are there exceptions?

REFERENCES

American Nurses Association (ANA). (2015). *Code of ethics for nurses with interpretive statements* (2nd ed.). Silver Spring, MD: ANA.

Cui, C., Li, Y., Geng, D., Zhang, H., & Jin, C. (2018). The effectiveness of evidence-based nursing on development of nursing students' critical thinking: A meta-analysis. *Nurse Education Today, 65*, 46–53.

Levett-Jones, T., Hoffman, K., Dempsey, J., et al. (2010). The "five rights" of clinical reasoning: An educational model to enhance nursing students' ability to identify and manage clinically "at risk" patients. *Nurse Education Today, 30*, 515–520.

Milton, C. L. (2002). Ethical implications for acting faithfully in nurse-person relationships. *Nursing Science Quarterly, 15*(1), 21–24.

National Council of State Boards of Nursing (NCSBN). (2019). *NCSBN clinical judgment measurement model*. Retrieved from www.ncsbn.org/14798.htm/. [Accessed 15 June 2021].

Nelson, A. E. (2017). Methods faculty use to facilitate nursing students' critical thinking. *Teaching and Learning in Nursing, 12*(1), 62–66.

Pavlish, C., Brown-Saltzman, K., Hersh, M., Shirk, M., & Rounkle, A. M. (2011). Nursing priorities, actions, and regrets for ethical situations in clinical practice. *Journal of Nursing Scholarship, 43*(4), 385–395.

SUGGESTED READING

International Council of Nurses (ICN). (2021). *The ICN code of ethics for nurses*. Geneva, Switzerland: ICN. Quality and Safety Education for Nurses (QSEN) Competencies. (n.d.). Retrieved from www.qsen.org/competencies.

5

Developing Patient-Centered Communication Skills

OBJECTIVES

At the end of the chapter, the reader will be able to:

1. Describe the elements of patient-centered communication.
2. Discuss active listening responses used in therapeutic communication.
3. Apply communication strategies and skills in patient-centered relationships to a simulation.
4. Analyze a recorded conversation to evaluate types and effectiveness of communication skills used.

Nurses communicate on many different levels—with patients, families, other professional disciplines, and a variety of external care providers involved with a patient's care. Although professional communication uses many of the same strategies as social communication, professional communication represents a specialized form of communication. It always has goals and a health-related purpose. High-quality care requires mastery of communication skills to have shared information.

Communicating as a professional nurse can be a challenge. Relational *and* informational aspects do not exist in the words themselves, but rather in their potential interpretations by the communicators engaged in the dialog. Consequently, professional communication is carefully thought out, and always considerate of how the recipient might respond to it. Effective communication represents a *combination* of relationship building, information sharing, and decision-making in communication, all of which are needed to achieve critically important clinical outcomes. Lack of effective communication is the most common patient complaint and actually interferes with care (Medendorp et al., 2021). Such skills are learned and take practice (Indeed.com, 2021). A good communicator

speaks in a way a patient can understand, with messages that are relevant and truthful (Kehoe, 2011). Professional conversations have health-related expectations and legal/ethical boundaries about what can and cannot be shared with others. Chapter 5 focuses on patient-centered communication skills, while Chapter 6 describes verbal and nonverbal styles.

BASIC CONCEPTS

Definitions

Communication refers to each transmission of information, whether intentional or not. Nonverbal behaviors, written communication, tone of voice, and words are forms of communication. The concept takes into consideration the values, words and ideas, emotions, and body language of sender, receiver, and context. Increasingly, people use media and other technology to communicate messages formally and informally. Try videoing a conversation with your smart phone.

Each message is intended to convey intended meaning, to exchange or strengthen ideas and feelings, and to share significant life experiences. Accompanying the message are nonverbal qualifiers in the form of gestures, body movements, eye contact, and personal or cultural symbols. Professional conversations differ from social conversations. Nurses need to competently communicate with physicians and other health professional colleagues, using professional technical or medical language. Nurses must learn to be equally skilled in turning technical and medical material into understandable information for patients and family members. Patients respond best when they believe their care providers understand their valuers and are paying attention to their concerns. Patient-centered communication involves informed consent, establishment of mutual goals, and shared decision-making regarding treatments. All conversations are confidential within the healthcare setting. Reflect on the Sue Fogty case.

CASE STUDY: Sue Fogty Has a Sexually Transmitted Disease

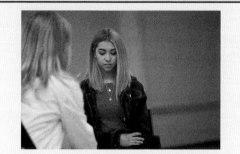

From iStock #1189837637, FatCamera.

Sue Fogty, 18 years old, comes to the student health center where Mary Braun, student nurse, is working. Ms Fogty complains of a white, thick, vaginal discharge that she also had last year when she was treated for chlamydia. She tells Mary that she is worried about talking with her since she is also a student. Mary reassures Ms Fogty that their conversation is confidential but that a report of her sexual partner contact will be sent to the health department by law for contact follow-up. Sue's name will remain confidential.

Functions of Professional Communication in Healthcare Systems

More than any other variable, effective interpersonal communication skills support safety and quality in healthcare delivery. Professional communication skills connect virtually all concepts and activities related to human health and well-being. Today's nurses should be equipped with a strong understanding of human biopsychosocial functioning, medical and nursing management of diverse health disorders, health-related ethical/legal issues, end-of-life care, and communication concepts and skills.

Collaborative Communication

Collegial conversations are collaborative. Such communication needs to be frequent, accurate, and directed toward achieving maximal health outcomes for patients. Frequent consultation with other team professionals involved in a patient's care helps ensure continuity of care.

Patient and Family Communication

As shown in Fig. 5.1, characteristics of ongoing collaborative conversations between patient/families and their healthcare providers have a direct impact on the quality and safety of clinical care, the achievement of meaningful clinical outcomes, and patient satisfaction. Optimizing health and patient/family satisfaction are considered critical outcomes intimately tied to communication. Specific ways that professional health communication impacts service quality are through the following:

- Understanding the patient's agenda and illness and needs from their perspective.
- Increased patient satisfaction and stronger, longer-lasting positive outcomes.
- More effective diagnosis, and earlier recognition of changes in health.
- More efficient utilization of health services.
- Development of collaborative professional relationships.

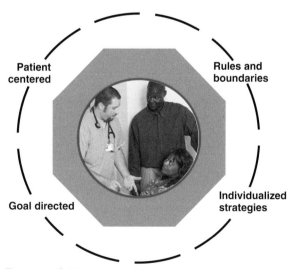

Figure 5.1 Collaborative nurse–patient–family communication.

CHARACTERISTICS OF PATIENT-CENTERED COMMUNICATION

Goals

Communication with patients should be health focused. Professional conversations are directed toward therapeutic outcomes and have rules and boundaries. Communication strategies are deliberately chosen to help patients reach goals. They terminate when the healthcare objective has been achieved or the patient has been discharged.

Content

At the core of patient-centered communication is exploring the patient's illness experience, its impact on the family, and relevance to beliefs and expectations. Honesty, clarity, and empathy are essential characteristics (Peplau, 1997). Building trust, alleviating anxiety, and enabling decision-making are content components. Box 5.1 identifies professional communication as a performance standard for nurses as defined by the American Nurses Association (ANA, 2007).

Empathy

This is an ability to understand and respond to another's attitude or experience. In clinical practice, use of **empathy** refers to being attuned to the patient's perspective of their health situation and to their psychological state (Lu & Zhang, 2021). Your patient's perspective might be very different from your own, but your aim is to find common ground upon which to base interventions. Examples of techniques include naming "It seems like you are saying … " or "some would feel [fill in appropriate word] in a similar situation." To foster empathy, you can acknowledge in words what the patient is feeling by saying "I can understand how this might upset you" or "This diagnosis is stressful to deal with."

Respect

Show your patients **respect** by calling them by surname and title, such as "Good morning, Mr Smith." Allow the patient to finish what they are saying. Avoid being distracted and multitasking. Respond fully and honestly. Speak in a calm, even tone of voice.

Boundaries

Professional conversations have defined interpersonal **boundaries** related to purpose and topic of conversation. Unlike social conversations when you speak spontaneously, professional conversations focus on the patient's thoughts or feelings related to health issues. Only the patient is expected to reveal personal information. Generally, nurses do not discuss their personal lives nor share opinions.

Factors That Influence Communication

Developing a common understanding of dialog is a crucial desired outcome of the professional conversation. Personal and environmental factors can affect dialog (Patel, 2019). For example, the patient might be in too much pain to concentrate on a conversation with you. Understanding your patient's point of view and responding with empathy, not sympathy, are key (Hashim, 2017). Being knowledgeable about your patient's educational level, cultural beliefs, or spiritual beliefs or personal values can affect the conversation. For example, consider a patient who speaks English as his or her second language. Can this affect meaning?

Barriers

Some patient circumstances that act as a barrier to communication include being in pain; values system at odds with your message; unfamiliar medical terms (jargon); strong feeling of defense or embarrassment; difficulty processing overwhelming amounts of information; or cognitive or physical limitations that impede message decoding. On the other hand, there are nurse characteristics that can act as a communication barrier, such as having an attitude that broadcasts disinterest; interrupting your patient

---

BOX 5.1   American Nurses Association Standards for Communication [Standard 11]

- Assesses communication format preferences of healthcare consumers, families, and colleagues.
- Assesses his or her own communication skills in encounters with healthcare consumers, families, and colleagues.
- Seeks continuous improvement of communication and conflict resolution skills.
- Conveys information to healthcare consumers, families, the interprofessional team, and others in communication formats that promote accuracy.
- Questions the rationale supporting care processes and decisions when they do not appear to be in the best interest of the patient.
- Discloses observations or concerns related to hazards and errors in care or the practice environment to the appropriate level.
- Maintains communication with other providers to minimize risks associated with transfers and transition in care delivery.
- Contributes to his or her own professional perspective in discussions.

TABLE 5.1 Communication Skills

	Communication Skill Strategy	Example
1	Active listening	Conveys attention using nonverbal behaviors such as leaning forward, nodding head.
2	Open-ended questions	"Can you tell me more about that?"
3	Focused questions	"How severe is your pain on a scale of 1:10 with 10 being worst ever?"
4	Closed-ended question	"Are you in any pain right now?"
5	Clarification	[Restate] "You seem to be saying you need to know more about this diagnosis" Or "I'm not sure I understand what you mean. Can you give me an example?"
6	Paraphrasing/restatement	[Restates] "You seem to be expressing frustration about your lack of progress."
7	Reflection	[Nurse mirrors back expressed emotion] "It sounds like you are frustrated by your lack of treatment options."
8	Summarizing	This is what we covered today. Tell me if I got it right.
9	Silence	[Nurse sits calmly while remaining therapeutically silent so patient can process data]
10	Providing or getting feedback	"Would you repeat back to me what you understand about your medicine?"
11	Validation	"How do you feel about what I just said?"
12	Using technology	[Texts a message to patient] remember to send me your blood glucose reading for today

repeatedly; thinking ahead to your next question instead of concentrating on the current one; biases or stereotypes leading to inaccurate assumptions about your patient; or feeling you are unable to help this patient. Some listening responses are listed in Table 5.1.

Communication Models

Models contain basic concepts of linear and transactional communication. The application section describes the use of active listening responses, verbal communication strategies, and other communication techniques that nurses and other health professionals consciously used to facilitate patient- and family-centered healthcare. Communication concepts and strategies presented in the chapter provide a practical methodology for connecting with patients and families to improve health outcomes.

Linear Model

The **linear model** is the simplest communication model, which consists of sender, message, receiver, channels of communication, and context. Linear models focus only on the sending and receipt of messages. They do not necessarily consider communication as enabling the development of cocreated meanings. Linear models are communication constructs, used in emergency health situations when time is of the essence to get immediate information.

Transactional Model

Transactional models are more complex. These models define communication as a reciprocal interaction process in which sender and receiver influence each other's messages and responses simultaneously as they converse. Each communicator constructs a mental picture of the other during the conversation, including perceptions about the other's attitude, and potential reactions to the message. Previous exposure to conversational concepts and ideas heightens the recognition and nature of the message interpretation. The outcome represents a new cocreated set of collaborative meanings.

Transactional models employ systems concepts in which a human system (patient/patient/family) receives information from the environment (**input**), internally processes it, and interprets its meaning (**throughput**). The result is new information or behavior referred to as ***output***. **Feedback** loops (from the receiver, or the environment) provide information about the output as it relates to the data received, and/or acted upon. This feedback either validates the received data or reflects a need to correct/modify original input information. Thus, transactional models draw attention to communication as being relational and having purpose and meaning-making attributes.

THERAPEUTIC COMMUNICATION FACTORS THAT AFFECT PROFESSIONAL COMMUNICATION SKILLS

Therapeutic communication, a term introduced by Jurgen Ruesch in 1961, refers to a dynamic interactive process entered into by healthcare providers, with their patients and significant others, for the purpose of achieving identified health-related goals (Ruesch, 1961). Therapeutic communication occurs in a variety of ways: through words, facial expressions, body language, e-mail, writing, and behaviors. Nurses and patients conduct treatment activities, collaborate with those involved in the patient's care, exchange information, and make shared decisions about all aspects of care with patients and families. What makes communication "therapeutic" is its purpose, its active engagement of the patient as a full partner in a health-related interactive process, and inclusion of relevant patient values and goals, emphasized throughout the dialog. Refer to Fig. 5.2 for a depiction of characteristics of therapeutic communication. A summary of communication skills and strategies is provided in Table 5.1.

NURSE SELF-AWARENESS

Nurses have ethical and professional responsibilities to develop awareness of their own characteristics that may impede communication. For example, we all grow up with stereotypes, often not even realizing it. We all have our own unique personality. For example, you might be shy and uncomfortable making conversation. Before approaching your patient to begin an interaction, think about the goals you want to achieve. Reflect on own personal beliefs that might affect the interaction. Developing self-awareness allows you to maintain authenticity, neutrality, and enough understanding to sustain this nurse–patient interaction.

ENVIRONMENTAL AWARENESS

Privacy

Privacy and space affect your conversations. Interviewing a patient when there is a lack of privacy may defeat your purpose. Environmental noise makes dialog difficult. Culturally, people need different amounts of space between speakers. Optimally, Western professional interviews need about 3 to 4 feet distance. If a patient is agitated, increasing this space may help. Of course, when nurses perform procedures, they intrude into personal space.

Time

Choosing a time when your patient is less stressed, not in pain or distracted, is important.

Cues

In face-to-face interactions, nurses have a rich range of visual and vocal cues, which provide additional data about the patient, if read correctly. Knowledge of patient habits, beliefs, preferences, cultural behaviors, and attitudes can support or contradict the spoken words. However, these cues may be easily misinterpreted, thus asking for

CHARACTERISTICS OF THE THERAPEUTIC PROCESS

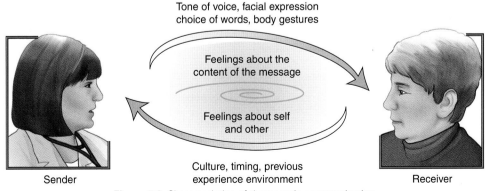

Figure 5.2 Characteristics of therapeutic communication.

clarifying feedback to ensure that all parties are looking at a situation from a similar perspective is essential. Try saying "I'd just like to check whether we both heard the same thing."

Nurses use words as a tool, a way to organize data around a health issue. The meaning of a message resides with the transaction, not just the words used. Terminology should be clear to both parties. Message should be complete, yet concise. Word choice, vocal tone, and nonverbal body language can all change the meaning of a message.

VERBAL RESPONSES IN SHORT ENCOUNTERS

As you ask clarifying questions, and share your own thinking responses about what you are seeing or hearing, you can develop a more in-depth understanding of the healthcare situation from the patient's perspective. Choice of words matters. Terminology should be clear, complete, concrete, and easily understandable to the listener. Words should neither overstate nor understate the situation. Since both words and nonverbal behaviors are subject to misinterpretation, nurses need to check in with their patients to ensure the accuracy of their perceptions. For example, "I'd just like to check in with you to make sure that I understand. Are you saying that … ?"

Factors That Influence Communication
Personal Factors
Developing a common understanding of the dialog, which occurs between nurses and patients, is a critical outcome of professional communication. Personal and environmental factors influence communication availability and readiness. For example, eye contact, full attention on the patient coupled with genuine respect, and clear, concise messages encourage patient participation. Words that respect a person's culture, spiritual beliefs, and educational level are more likely to capture the patient's attention.

Barriers
Obstacles to effective communication can occur within patients when they
- are preoccupied with pain, physical discomfort, worry, or contradictory personal beliefs;
- are unable to understand the nurse's use of language, terminology, or frame of reference;
- are struggling with a personal emotionally laden topic;
- are feeling defensive, insecure, or judged;
- are confused by the complexity of the message—too many issues, tangential comments;

- are deprived of privacy, especially if the topic is a sensitive one;
- have sensory or cognitive deficits that limit or compromise the receiving of accurate messages.

Barriers Within the Nurse
Obstacles within the nurse occur when the nurse is not fully engaged with the patient for one or more of the following reasons:
- Preoccupation with personal agendas
- Being in a hurry to complete physical care
- Making assumptions about patient motivations
- Cultural stereotypes
- Defensiveness, or personal insecurity about being able to help the patient
- Thinking ahead to the next question
- Intense patient emotion or aggressiveness
- Weak language that does not add value to the conversation
- Use of complex medical terminology, also known as "jargon"

Simulation Exercise 5.1 is designed to help students identify difficult communication issues in nursing practice.

SIMULATION EXERCISE 5.1 Complicated Communication Issues With Patients

Purpose: To help students identify common complicated communication issues with patients.

Procedure
In groups of three to four students:
1. In round-robin fashion, each student should share an "elevator version" of a nursing experience that illustrates a challenging communication encounter you have had or witnessed in a nurse–patient encounter.
2. Identify what components made the conversation difficult.
3. If you had the conversation, what might you do differently?

Reflective Discussion Analysis
1. Were there any common themes that your group found in the identified communication challenges?
2. Explore the insights you gained from doing this exercise.
3. How could you use what you learned from doing this exercise in your future nursing practice?

Self-Awareness

Nurses have an ethical and professional responsibility to resolve personal issues so that countertransference feelings do not affect communication. Patient-centered communication requires greater self-awareness. Before you begin, think about the goals you want to achieve with your patient. Remember to include areas of importance and concern to the patient. Self-awareness of personal vulnerabilities and prejudices allows nurses to maintain the authenticity, patience, neutrality, and understanding needed for therapeutic exploration of patient issues.

Environmental Factors

Privacy, space, and timing affect therapeutic conversations. Patients need privacy free from interruption and environmental noise for meaningful dialog to take place. "Noise" refers to any distraction, which interferes with being able to pay full attention to the discussion. It can be physical in the form of environmental distractions, even being tired. Semantic noise can occur in the form of cross-cultural language differences or psychological noise associated with mental illness. For example, TV or music can be distracting.

Proxemics

People require different amounts of personal space for conversational ease, defined as *proxemics*. Therapeutic conversations typically take place within a social distance (3–4 feet is optimal). Culture, personal preference, nature of the relationship, and the topic will influence personal space needs. DeVito (2016) identified four types of distance ranges typically associated with usual communication in the United States.

1. Close intimate relationships range from touch to 18 inches.
2. Personal distance ranges from 18 inches to 4 feet.
3. Social distance ranges from 4 to 12 feet.
4. Public distance ranges from 12 feet to more than 25 feet.

Patients experiencing anxiety usually need more physical space, whereas those experiencing a sudden physical injury, or undergoing a painful procedure, appreciate having the nurse in closer proximity. Sitting at eye level with bedridden patients is helpful.

Timing

Timing is important. Planning communication for periods when the patient is able to participate physically and emotionally is time-efficient and respectful of the patient's needs. Give your patients enough time to absorb material, to share their impressions, and to ask questions.

Patient behavior can cue the nurse about emotional readiness and available energy. The presence of pain or variations in energy levels, anger, or anxiety will require extra time to inquire about the change in the patient's behavior and its meaning, before proceeding with the healthcare dialog.

Communication as a Shared Partnership

Patient-centered care and collaborative partnerships in current healthcare deliverables require a broader span of collaborative communication skills to accomplish the active partnership needed for managing chronic disorders. Patients expect to be listened to and involved in their own care. But they also need support to do so. Functions of patient-centered communication include the following:

- Fostering healing relationships
- Exchanging information
- Responding to emotions
- Managing uncertainty
- Making decisions
- Enabling patient self-management

Patient-centered communication is an interactive reciprocal exchange of ideas in which nurses try to understand what it is like to be this person in this situation with this illness. Each patient and family has its unique set of values, patterns of behavior, and preferences that must be taken into account. How patients communicate with the nurse varies, based on culture and social background factors. Their readiness to learn, personal ways of relating to others, physical and emotional conditions, life experiences, and place in the life cycle are related factors in planning and implementing contemporary care through therapeutic conversations.

Patient-centered conversations include discussions needed for collaborative decision-making and for teaching patients self-management skills. Talking about complex personal health problems with a trained health professional allows patients and families to hear themselves, as they put health concerns into words. Feedback provided by the health professional ideally helps patients to realistically sort out their priorities and to determine the actions they want to take to effectively cope with their health circumstances.

APPLICATIONS

Effective communication is an art, as well as a professional competency. It is not only what you say, but also how you say it. Certain attitudes such as a nonjudgmental respectful attitude and maintaining a calm, thoughtful manner throughout the communication process are helpful.

DEVELOPING AN EVIDENCE-BASED PRACTICE

Active listening with empathetic caring is accepted as the foundation in building a therapeutic nurse–patient relationship in many health professions. A number of research studies have examined the impact of communication skill training, especially use of active listening, on skill use in relationships. McKenna (2020) measured empathy and listening styles in Australian student nurses to evaluate effective listening styles, while Brown (2020) conducted a similar study with occupationally therapy students. Gilligan (2021) more broadly examined 90 studies looking at effects of communication skill education on skill use by physicians.

Results
Study results showed increased use of communication skills including active listening following skill training. McKenna found nursing students preferred a listening style characterized by concern for patients and a focus on listening to what the patient was saying. Findings support earlier studies that show use of active listening correlates with a more positive provider–patient relationship (Pinto et al., 2012) and with greater patient-centered care (Haley et al., 2017).

Strength of research: Low. Studies tended to be surveys (cross-sectional samples) with no longitudinal measures.

Application to Your Clinical Practice
1. To develop communication skill use, students should have opportunities to practice skills such as active listening within their curricula.

2. Nurses need to actively transfer learning about communication skill development to the workplace.
3. Use of active listening and feedback about understanding what the patient feels should precede other interventions such as giving information.

References
Brown, T., Yu, M., & Etherington, J. (2020). Are listening and interpersonal communication skills predictive of professionalism in undergraduate occupational therapy students? *Health Professions Education, 6*(2), 187–200.
 Gilligan, C., Powell, M., Lynagh, M.C., et al. (2021). Interventions for improving medical students' interpersonal communication in medical consultations. *Cochrane Database of Systematic Reviews, 2*, CD012418.
 Haley, B., Heo, S., Wright, P., Barone, C., Rettigan, M. R., & Anders, M. (2017). Relationships among active listening, self-awareness, empathy and patient centered care in associate and baccalaureate degree nursing students. *NursingPlus Open, 3*, 11–16.
 McKenna, L., Brown, T., Williams, B., & Lau, R. (2020). Empathetic and listening styles of first year undergraduate nursing students: A cross-sectional study. *Journal of Professional Nursing, 36*(6), 611–615.
 Pinto, R. Z., Fereita, M., Oliveira, V., et al. (2012). Patient centered communication associated with therapeutic alliance: A systematic review. *Journal of Physiotherapy, 58*(2), 77–87.

Engaging the Patient

A patient-centered communication process starts with the first encounter. Your initial presentation of yourself will influence the communication that follows. Each patient should have your full attention. This means clearing your own mind of any preconceived notions, biases, and even your own thoughts. Entering the patient's space with an open, welcoming facial expression, respectful tone, and direct eye contact declares your interest and intent to know this person. Your posture immediately gives a message to the patient, either inviting trust or conveying disinterest. Whether you are sitting or standing, your posture should be relaxed, facing the patient and leaning slightly forward. Shaking the patient's hand with an open facial expression and a smile signals to the patient that he or she is the most important person in your orbit for the moment.

Introductions are important, especially if many health professionals are involved in the patient's care. Introduce yourself, and identify the patient by name before beginning the conversation. When more people than just the patient (family or other health team members) are involved in a discussion, expand the introductions. Center your attention on the patient, but do not ignore other participants. You can include family members with eye contact, physical cues, and so forth throughout the conversation.

Building Rapport

Begin with asking routine questions about the reason for admission, and other common information. Routine questions help to put the patient and family at ease. However, when you ask the patient to tell you about his or her health concerns and what prompted him or her to seek help at this time, keep this part of the conversation open. Allow the patient to tell you about his or her personal situation from a personal perspective, with few interruptions. Sequence questions going from easy general to more complex questions.

Keep in mind that patients will vary in their ability to effectively communicate their feelings, preferences, and concerns. Personal characteristics, culture, previous life and health experiences, and education level create differences. Considering these factors allows you to phrase questions and to interpret answers in more meaningful ways.

Being attentively present, providing relevant information, and actively listening to patient concerns help to build rapport. Patients who feel safe, accepted, and validated by their healthcare providers find it easier to collaborate with them. Although rapport building begins with the initial encounter, it continues as a thread throughout the nurse–patient relationship. Remember that patients are looking to you not only for competence but also for sincerity and genuine interest in them as individuals.

Developing a Shared Partnership

The idea of healthcare as a shared partnership in which the patient is an equal stakeholder and treatment partner in ensuring quality healthcare is relatively new. Building a shared, workable partnership alliance requires the following:

- Empathetic objectivity, which allows you to experience patients as they are, not the way you would like them to be.
- A "here and now" focus on the current issues and concerns important to the patient.
- Demonstration of respect, and asking questions about cultural and social differences that can influence treatment.
- Authentic interest in the patient and a confident manner that communicates competence.
- The capability to consider competing goals, and alternative ways to meet them.

Finding Common Ground

Patient-centered communication strategies allow patient and nurse to find common ground related to the patient's explanations of problems, their priorities, and their treatment goals. Before you can participate in the development of a shared approach to a problem, you have to give your full attention to what you are hearing from your patient.

The aspects of care that are most important to a patient and family, and what helps or hinders their capability to self-manage their health problems, are critical information. Look for themes revealing fears, feelings, and level of engagement. Patients also need to understand the full range of therapeutic choices available to them in treating and self-managing their illness. This is critical information, particularly for situations requiring informed consent.

COMMUNICATION SKILLS

Skilled strategies that nurses can use to guide therapeutic interventions include the following.

Active Listening

Active listening is defined as an *intentional* form of listening. It involves more than simply hearing words. The importance of listening in healthcare communication cannot be overestimated, a dynamically focused interpersonal process in which a nurse hears a patient's message, decodes its meaning, asks questions for clarification, and provides feedback to the patient. It is a transactional process that integrates the verbal and nonverbal components of a message.

Goal

The goal of active listening is to understand what the patient is trying to communicate through his or her story. Active listening requires full attention to understanding the patient's perspective without making any judgments. Using the listening responses presented later in the chapter increases understanding. If the interaction is very time limited, the nurse needs to verify information from the very first encounter. When the relationship develops, you can follow up and make time for patient questions: try saying "I'm wondering what questions you have?" or "One question I am frequently asked is …. " What do nurses listen for (Box 5.2)?

When a person is ill, listening requires extra effort. It also involves noting feelings and looking for underlying themes. The goal is mutual understanding of facts and emotions. Active listening contributes to fewer incidents of misunderstanding, more accurate comprehensive data, and stronger health relationships.

BOX 5.2 What the Nurse Listens For

- Content themes
- Communication patterns
- Discrepancies in message content, body language, and verbalization
- Feelings, revealed in a person's voice, body movements, and facial expressions
- What is not being said, as well as what is being said
- The patient's preferred representational system (auditory, visual, tactile)
- The nurse's own inner responses and personal ways of knowing
- The effect communication produces in others involved with the patient

SIMULATION EXERCISE 5.2 Practice With Active Listening

Purpose: To develop skill in the use of active listening and an awareness of elements involved.

Procedure
1. Break up into pairs. Each takes a turn describing an important experience, detailing their own emotions. The listening partner should use skills such as clarification, paraphrasing, reflection, alert body posture, eye contact, etc.
2. The listening partner indicates understanding by restating what was shared and summarizing observations about emotions expressed.

Reflective Discussion Analysis
In the large group, students should share their discoveries about active listening. What nurse behavior fosters active listening?

Listening responses in a patient-centered health environment ask about *all* relevant patient health concerns. They take into account the patient's values, preferences, and expectations related to treatment goals, priorities, and attitudes about treatment suggestions. Simulation Exercise 5.2 provides practice with active listening.

Listening responses can be integrated with asking for validation of patient preferences, for example, asking the patient, "How does the idea of _____ sound to you?" or "How easy will it be for you to learn to use your crutches?" Each of these questions and others along the same line can encourage a patient to explore potential concerns, expand on an idea, or voice confusion. This information is essential to achieve a shared understanding and realistic clinical expectations.

Open-Ended Questions

Open-ended questions are defined as questions that are open to interpretation and cannot be answered by "yes, or no," or a one-word response. They allow patients to express their problems or health needs in their own words. Open-ended questions usually begin with words such as "what," "how," or "can you describe for me …," etc. They provide a broader context for each patient's unique health concerns and are likely to yield more complete information. Open-ended questions invite patients to think and reflect on their situation. They help connect relevant elements of the patient's experience (e.g., relationships, impact of the illness on self or others, environmental barriers, and potential resources or concerns). Open-ended questions, such as the ones identified below, are core clinical questions:

- "What is important to you now?"
- "What do you see as the next step?"
- "What are you hoping will happen with this treatment?"

Open-ended questions are used to elicit the patient's thoughts and perspectives without influencing the direction of an acceptable response. For example:

Can you tell me what brought you to the clinic (hospital) today?

What has it been like for you since the accident?

Where would you like to begin today?

How can I help you?

Ending the dialog with a general open-ended question, such as "Is there anything else concerning you right now?" or "Is there anything we have overlooked today?" can provide relevant information that might otherwise be overlooked. Simulation Exercise 5.3 gives practice with asking open-ended questions.

Focused Questions

Focused questions require more than a yes or no answer, but they place limitations on the topic to be addressed. They are useful in emergencies and in other situations when immediate concise information is required. Focused questions can clarify the timing and sequence of symptoms, and concentrate on details about a patient's health

SIMULATION EXERCISE 5.3 Asking Open-Ended Questions

Purpose: To develop skill in the use of open-ended questions to facilitate information sharing.

Procedure
1. Break into pairs. Role-play a situation in which one student takes the role of facilitator and the other the sharer. (If you work in the clinical area, you may want to choose a clinical situation.)
2. As a pair, select a topic. The facilitator begins asking open-ended questions.
3. Dialog for 5 min on the topic.
4. In pairs, discuss perceptions of the dialog and determine which questions were comfortable and open-ended.

Reflective Discussion Analysis
As a class, give examples of open-ended questions used. Summarize. Discuss how open-ended questions can be used sensitively with uncomfortable topics.

concerns. For example, they can include when symptoms began, what other symptoms the patient is having, and what a patient has done to date to resolve the problem.

Patients with limited verbal skills sometimes respond better to focused questions because they require less interpretation. Examples of focused questions include the following:

Can you tell me more about the pain in your arm?

Can you give me a specific example of what you mean by … ?

When did your stomach pain begin?

These help patients to organize data and to prioritize immediate concerns; for example, you might ask a question at the end of the conversation such as "Of the concerns we talked about today, which has been the most difficult for you?"

Circular questions are a form of focused questions that look at how other people within the patient's support circle respond to a patient's health issues. These questions are designed to identify differences in the impact of an illness on individual family members, and to explore changes in relationships brought about by the health circumstances. For example, "When your dad says he doesn't want hospice care because he is a fighter, what is that like for you?"

Closed-Ended Questions

Closed-ended questions are defined as narrowly focused questions, for which a single answer, for example, "yes," "no," or a simple phrase answer serves as a valid response. They are useful in emergency situations when the goal is to obtain information quickly, and the context or patient's emotional reactions are of secondary importance because of the seriousness of the immediate situation. Examples of closed-ended questions include the following:

Does the pain radiate down your left shoulder and arm?

When was your last meal?

Clarification

Clarification is defined as a brief question or a request for validation. It is used to better understand a patient's message; for example, "You stated earlier that you were concerned about your blood pressure. Tell me more about what concerns you." The tone of voice used with a clarification response should be neutral, not accusatory or demanding. Failure to ask for clarification when part of the communication is poorly understood means that you might act on incomplete or inaccurate information. You can practice clarification in Simulation Exercise 5.4.

SIMULATION EXERCISE 5.4   Using Clarification

Purpose: To develop skill in the use of clarification.

Procedure
1. Write a paragraph related to a clinical experience you have had.
2. Place all the student paragraphs together and then pick one (not your own).
3. Develop clarification questions you might ask about the selected clinical experience.

Reflective Discussion Analysis
Share with the class your chosen paragraph and the clarification questions you developed. Discuss how effective the questions are in clarifying information. Other students can suggest additional clarification.

Paraphrasing/Restatement

Paraphrasing is a response used to check whether the nurse's translation of the patient's words represents an accurate interpretation of the message. The strategy involves the nurse *taking* the patient's original message and transforming it into his or her own words, without losing the meaning. A paraphrase should be shorter and more specific than the patient's initial statement so that the focus is on the core elements of the original statement. Your objective in using paraphrasing is to find a common understanding of issues important to your patients. Paraphrasing allows you to summarize or streamline a message, and/or highlight key points of the longer message. Try Simulation Exercise 5.5 to practice paraphrasing.

Restatement is a strategy used to broaden a patient's perspective or when the nurse needs to provide a sharper focus on a specific part of the message. For example, you might say, "Let me see if I have this right …" (followed by a restatement of the patient's words). Restatement is effective when a patient overgeneralizes, or seems stuck in a repetitive line of thinking. When sparingly implemented in a questioning manner, a restatement strategy focuses the patient's attention on the possibility of an inaccurate or global assertion.

Reflection

Reflection is a response that focuses on the emotional part of a message. It offers nurses a way to empathetically mirror their sense of how a patient may be emotionally

SIMULATION EXERCISE 5.5   Role-Play Practice With Paraphrasing and Reflection

Purpose: To practice the use of paraphrasing and reflection as listening responses.

Procedure

1. The class forms into groups of three students each. One student takes the role of patient, one the role of nurse, and one the role of observer.
2. The patient shares with the nurse a recent health problem he or she encountered and describes the details of the situation and the emotions experienced. The nurse responds, using paraphrasing and reflection in a dialog that lasts at least 5 min. The observer records the statements made by the helper. At the end of the dialog, the patient writes his or her perception of how the helper's statements affected the conversation, including what comments were most helpful. The helper writes a short summary of the listening responses he or she used, with comments on how successful they were.

Reflective Discussion Analysis

1. Share your summary and discuss the differences in using the techniques from the helper, patient, and observer perspectives.
2. Discuss how these differences related to influencing the flow of dialog, helping the patient feel heard, and the impact on the helper's understanding of the patient from both the patient and the helper positions.
3. Identify places in the dialog where one form of questioning might be preferable to another.
4. How could you use this exercise to understand your patient's concerns?
5. Were you surprised by any of the summaries?

experiencing their health situation. There are several ways to use reflection, for example:

- Reflection on vocal tone: "You seem to have some anger and frustration in your voice as you describe your accident" or "You sound happy when you talk about your grandson."
- Reflection example, linking feelings with content: "It sounds like you feel _____ because _____."
- Linking current feelings with past experiences: "It seems as if this experience reminds you of feelings you had

with other healthcare providers, when you didn't feel understood."

A reflective listening response should be a simple observational comment, expressed tentatively, not an exhaustive comment about the patient's emotional reaction. It offers an opportunity for the patient to validate or to change the narrative. When reflecting on an emotional observation, students sometimes feel they are putting words into the patient's mouth when they "choose" an emotion from their perception of a patient's message. This would be true if you were choosing an emotion out of thin air, but not when you empathetically mirror what you are hearing from the patient. You can simply present potential underlying feelings present in the patient's narrative, without interpreting its meaning.

Summarization

Summarization is a skill used to review content and process. Summarization pulls several ideas and feelings together, either from one interaction or from a series of interactions, into a few brief sentences. This would be followed by a comment seeking validation, such as "Tell me if my understanding of this agrees with yours." A summary statement can also be useful as a bridge to change the topic or focus of the conversation. The summarization should be completed before the end of the conversation, but with enough time before you leave the room, for validation or questions.

Silence

Silence, delivered as a brief pause, is a powerful listening response. Intentional pauses can allow the patient to think. A short pause lets the nurse step back momentarily and process what has been heard, before responding. Silence can be used to emphasize important points that you want the patient to reflect on. By pausing briefly after presenting a key idea and before proceeding to the next topic, it encourages a patient to reflect on what has just been discussed.

When a patient falls silent, it can mean many things: something has touched the patient, the patient is angry or does not know how to respond, or the patient is thinking about *how* to respond. A verbal comment to check on the meaning of the message is helpful.

Not all responses are helpful. Nurses need to recognize when their responses are interfering with objectivity or are inviting premature closure. Table 5.2 provides definitions of negative listening responses that block communication.

TABLE 5.2 Negative Listening Responses

Category of Response	Explanation of Category	Examples
False reassurance	Using pseudo-comforting phrases in an attempt to offer reassurance	"It will be okay." "Everything will work out."
Giving advice	Making a decision for a patient; offering personal opinions; telling a patient what to do (using phrases such as "ought to," "should")	"If I were you, I would ..." "I feel you should ..."
False inferences	Making an unsubstantiated assumption about what a patient means; interpreting the patient's behavior without asking for validation; jumping to conclusions	"What you really mean is you don't like your physician." "Subconsciously, you are blaming your husband for the accident."
Moralizing	Expressing your own values about what is right and wrong, especially on a topic that concerns the patient	"Abortion is wrong." "It is wrong to refuse to have the operation."
Value judgments	Conveying your approval or disapproval about the patient's behavior or about what the patient has said using words such as "good," "bad," or "nice"	"I'm glad you decided to ..." "That really wasn't a nice way to behave." "She's a good patient."

Evaluation of the patient's present overall pattern of interaction with others includes strengths and limitations, family communication dynamics, and developmental and educational levels. Culture, role, ways of handling conflict, and ways of dealing with emotions also reflect and influence communication patterns. For example, AJ is a patient with chronic mental illness. She frequently interrupts and presents with a loud, ebullient opinion on most things. This is AJ's communication pattern. To engage successfully with her, you would need to listen, while accepting her way of communicating as a part of who she is, without being judgmental, joining in with arguing the validity of her position, or getting lost in detail. Remember that patients who are anxious often use a controlling form of communication and are preoccupied with their own version of events. They may have difficulty listening to or assimilating information. Taking a little extra time to establish rapport and gently set limits on what is open for discussion can help patients like AJ remain focused in conversations.

Giving Feedback

Feedback is a message a nurse gives to the patient in response to a question, verbal message, or observed behavior. Feedback can focus on the content, the relationship between people and events, the feelings generated by the message, or parts of the communication that are not clear. Feedback should be specific and directed to the behavior.

It should not be an analysis of the patient's motivations. Verbal feedback provides the receiver's understanding of the sender's message and personal reaction to it. Effective feedback offers a neutral mirror, which allows a patient to view a problem or behavior from a different perspective. Feedback is most relevant when it only addresses the topics under discussion and does not go beyond the data presented by the patient. Effective feedback is clear, honest, and reflective. Feedback supported with realistic examples is believable, whereas feedback without documentation to support it can lack credibility.

Effective feedback is specific rather than general. Telling a patient he or she is shy or easily intimidated is less helpful than providing a behavioral example, "I noticed when the anesthesiologist was in here that you didn't ask her any of the questions you had about your anesthesia tomorrow. Do you want to look at what you might want to know so you can get the information you need?" With this response, the nurse provides precise information about an observed behavior and offers a potential solution. The patient is more likely to respond with validation, or correction, and the nurse can provide specific guidance.

Feedback can be about the nurse's observations of nonverbal behaviors; for example, "You seem (angry, upset, confused, pleased, sad, etc.) when ..." Request for feedback can be framed as a question, requiring the patient to elaborate; for example, "I want to be sure that we have the same understanding of what we have talked about. Can you tell me in your own words what we discussed?"

Not all feedback is equally relevant, nor is it always accepted. A benchmark for deciding whether feedback is appropriate is to ask yourself, "Does this feedback advance the goals of the relationship?" and "Does it consider the individualized needs of the patient?" If the answer to either question is "no," then while the feedback may be accurate, it may be inappropriate in the current context. Most people find "why" questions difficult to answer. In general, avoid asking "why" questions to patients as an initial questioning strategy. Motivation is typically multidetermined, so often it is more difficult to answer. Asking "how" or "what" questions is usually focused, and these questions are more easily answered.

Timing

Feedback given as soon as possible after a behavior in need of change is observed is most effective. Other factors (e.g., a patient's readiness to hear feedback, privacy, and the availability of support from others) contribute to effectiveness. Providing feedback about behaviors over which the patient has little control only increases the personalized feelings of low self-esteem and leads to frustration. Feedback should be to the point and empathetic. Most patients are not looking for brilliant answers from the nurse. Rather, they seek feedback and want caring support that suggests a compassionate understanding of their particular dilemma. No matter what level of communication exists in the relationship, the same needs—"hear me," "touch me," "respond to me," "feel my pain and experience my joys with me"—are fundamental themes. These are the themes addressed by patient-centered communication.

Validation

This special form of feedback is used to ensure that both participants have the same basic understanding of messages. Word meanings lie within people, not in the words themselves. The meaning of the same word has cultural and contextual implications that can be different for each communicator. Simply asking patients whether they understand what was said is not an adequate method of validating message content. Instead, you might ask, "How do you feel about what I just said?" or "I'm curious what your thoughts are about what I just told you." If the patient does not have any response, you can suggest that the patient can respond later, "Many people do find they have reactions or questions about [the issue] after they have had a chance to think about it. I would be glad to discuss this further." Validation can provide new information that helps the nurse frame comments

that are more responsive to the patient's need. Notice the differences in the nature of the following responses in the Jim Cay case.

Case Study: Jim Cay Talks With His Nurse Ann Cain, RN

Jim: "I feel so discouraged. No matter how hard I try, I still can't walk without pain on the two parallel bars."

Ann: "Are you saying you want to give up because you don't think you will be able to walk again?" At this point, it is unclear that the patient wants to give up, so Ann's comment expands on the patient's meaning without having sufficient data to support it. Although it is possible that this is what Jim means, it is not the only possibility. The more important dilemma for Jim may be whether his efforts have any purpose. The next response focuses only on the negative aspects of the communication and ignores the patient's comment about his efforts.

Ann: "So you think you won't be able to walk independently again."

In the following final response example, Ann addresses both parts of Jim's message and makes the appropriate connection. Ann's statement invites Jim to validate her perception.

Ann: "It sounds to me as if you don't feel your efforts are helping you regain control over your walking."

OTHER COMMUNICATION SUGGESTIONS

Avoid Overload

People can absorb only so much information at one time, particularly if they are tired, fearful, or discouraged. Introducing new ideas *one at a time* allows the patient to more easily process data. Repeating key ideas and reinforcing information with concrete examples facilitate understanding and provide an additional opportunity for the patient to ask questions. Paying attention to nonverbal response cues from the patient that support understanding or that reflect a need for further attention is an important dimension of successful communication.

Focus

In today's healthcare delivery system, nurses must make every second count. It is important for nurses and patients to select the most pressing or relevant healthcare topics for discussion.

Sensitivity to patient needs and preferences should be factors to take into consideration. You should not force a patient to focus on an issue that he or she is not yet willing to discuss unless it is an emergency situation. You can always go back to a topic when the patient is more receptive. For example, you might say, "I can understand that this is a difficult topic for you, but I am here for you if you would like to discuss [identified topic] later."

Present Reality

Presenting reality to a patient who is misinterpreting, it can be helpful as long as the patient does not perceive that the nurse is criticizing the patient's perception of reality. A simple statement, such as "I know that you feel strongly about _____, but I don't see it that way," is an effective way for the nurse to express a different interpretation of the situation. Another strategy is to put into words the underlying feeling that is being implied but is not stated.

Use Metaphors

Familiar images promote understanding. Metaphors represent an unrelated figure of speech that can help patients and families process difficult, new, or abstract information by comparing it with more familiar images from ordinary life experience. Sometimes a metaphor example can be more persuasive than a medical explanation. For example, chronic lung disease as "emphysema is like having lungs similar to 'swiss cheese'" and the airways in asthma are like "different sized drainpipes that can get clogged up and need to be unclogged." A familiar concrete image can help a patient connect with an abstract medical diagnosis that is harder to comprehend. Data supported by a metaphoric explanation can be more persuasive than a literal explanation. The choice of metaphor is important.

Use Humor

Humor is a powerful patient-centered communication technique when used for a specific therapeutic purpose. Humor recognizes the incongruities in a situation, or an absurdity present in human nature or conduct. Humor lightens the mood and puts a tense situation in perspective. A good laugh can bond communicators together in a shared conversation in ways that might not happen otherwise. Humor works best when rapport is well established, and a level of trust exists between the nurse and patient. A humorous comment should fit the situation, not dominate it. When using humor, it is best to focus on an idea, event, or situation, or something other than the patient's personal characteristics. Humor and laughter have healing purposes. Laughter generates energy and activates β-endorphins, a neurotransmitter that creates natural highs and reduces stress hormones. The surprise element in humor can cut through an overly intense situation and put it into perspective.

The following factors contribute to the successful use of humor:
- Knowledge of the patient's response pattern
- An overly intense situation
- Timing
- Situation lending itself to an imaginative or paradoxical solution
- Gearing the humor dynamics to the patient's developmental level and interests
- Focus on the humor in a situation or change in circumstance rather than a patient's personal characteristics

USING TECHNOLOGY IN PATIENT-CENTERED RELATIONSHIPS

The many uses of technology in communication are detailed in Chapters 25 and 26. Increasingly, nurses are incorporating technology to communicate in digital encounters with patients and families. Although technology can never replace face-to-face time with patients, voice mail, e-mail, and telehealth virtual home visits help connect patients with care providers and provide critical information. As health-related technology becomes ever more sophisticated, nurses will be expected to acquire new communication skills.

SUMMARY

This chapter discusses basic therapeutic communication skills that nurses can use with patients across clinical settings. Nurses use active listening, open-ended questions, clarification, paraphrasing, reflection, summarization, silence, and feedback to elicit complete information. Other strategies include the use of metaphors, reframing, humor, confirming responses, feedback, and validation. Feedback provides a patient with needed information.

ETHICAL DILEMMA: What Would You Do?

You have a wonderful relationship with a patient and family. They have revealed issues they had never talked about before and raised questions that extend beyond the scope of the current health problem. You are about to rotate off the unit. What professional and ethical issues do you consider to provide ongoing care for this family?

DISCUSSION QUESTIONS

1. Of the therapeutic communication skills described, which ones are most effective, in your opinion?

2. Give examples of factors that impede communication and suggest remedies.

REFERENCES

American Nurses Association (ANA). (2007). *Scope and standards of practice* (3rd ed.). Silver Spring, MD: American Nurses Association.

DeVito, J. (2016). *The interpersonal communication book* (14th ed.). Edinburgh Gate Essex: Pearson Education Limited.

Hashim, M. J. (2017). Patient-centered communication: Basic skills. *American Family Physician*, 95(1), 29–34.

Indeed.com, Resumes & Cover Letters, & Communication skills for Career Success. (2021). *Indeed career guide*. Retrieved from www.indeed.com/career-advice/resumes-cover-letters/communication-skills/. [Accessed 7 May 2021].

Kehoe, D. (2011). *Effective communication skills*. Chantilly, VA: The Great Courses.

Lu, X., & Zhang, R. (2021). Impact of patient information behaviours in online health communities on patient compliance and the mediating role of patients' perceived empathy. *Patient Education and Counseling, 104*(1), 186–193.

Medendorp, N. M., van den Heuvel, L., Han, P., Hillen, M. A., & Smets, E. M. A. (2021). Communication skills training for healthcare professionals providing genetic counseling: A scoping literature review. *Patient Education and Counseling, 104*(1), 20–32.

Patel, D. (2019). *Communication strategies. 14 proven ways to improve your communication skills*. Retrieved from https://www.entrepreneur.com/article/300466. [Accessed 7 May 2021].

Peplau, H. E. (1997). Peplau's theory of interpersonal relations. *Nursing Science Quarterly, 10*(4), 162–167.

Ruesch, J. (1961). *Therapeutic communication*. New York: Norton.

6

Variation in Communication Styles

OBJECTIVES

At the end of this chapter, the reader will be able to:

1. Describe the component systems of communication, describing congruence between verbal and nonverbal messages.
2. Discuss how metacommunication messages may affect patient responses.

3. Apply examples of body cues that convey nonverbal messages.
4. Analyze research studies for evidence-based clinical practices that improve communication.

Communication is a multidimensional, dynamic, complex process (Keutchafo, 2020). Every one of us has different preferred methods for giving and receiving communication. These vary depending on the particular individual and specific situation. This chapter explores styles of communication that serve as a basis for building a relationship to provide safe, effective patient-centered care. Patient-centered communication is an underlying component of all six of the prelicensure competencies identified in the Quality and Safety Education for Nurses (QSEN) project. Your communication style is a combination of specific speech-related characteristics cueing others about how to interpret a message. For patients, effective communication has been shown to produce better health outcomes, greater satisfaction, increased understanding, shorter hospital stays, and decreased costs. What is your style? Some of us tend to be more assertive, imposing our desires on others, whereas others of us seek more of an equal partnership, negotiating in a give-and-take fashion. At the other end of the personal style spectrum, some individuals tend to withdraw or even put all of the other person's desires ahead of their own needs. In developing a style suitable to professional nurse–patient or nurse–team–patient relationships, we modify our personal style to fit our professional role. As learners, students are monitored in the clinical setting as we demonstrate expected communication styles that convey warmth, trustworthiness, and respectful assertiveness and use our newly acquired therapeutic communication skills.

BASIC CONCEPTS

Metacommunication

Communication is a combination of verbal and nonverbal behaviors integrated for the purpose of sharing information. Within the nurse–patient relationship, any exchange of information between two individuals also carries messages about how to interpret the communication. It is important not only to understand the message but also to recognize the underlying feelings.

Metacommunication is a broad term used to describe all of the factors that influence how the message is perceived. It is a message about how to interpret what is going on. Metacommunicated messages may be hidden within verbalizations or be conveyed as *nonverbal* gestures and expressions. Some studies report greater compliance to requests when they are accompanied by a metacommunication message asking for a response to the appropriateness of the request. Sydney's case should clarify this concept.

Style Factors

Factors in our verbal style include pitch, tone, and frequency. Nonverbal style includes facial expression, gestures, body posture and movement, eye contact, distance from the other person, and so on. These nonverbal behaviors are clues patients give us to help us understand their words as depicted in Fig. 6.1. Sharpening our observational skills helps us gather data needed for nursing assessments and interventions. Both of us, patient and nurse,

CASE STUDY: Sydney Leiu, Student Nurse, and Metacommunication

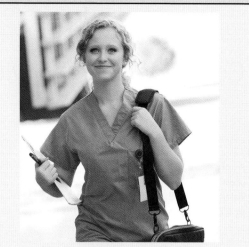

From iStock #520686505; SDI Productions.

Sydney: (smiling, making eye contact, and using warm tone): Hi, I am Sydney. We nursing students are trying to encourage community awareness in promoting environmental health and are looking for people to hand out fliers. Would you be willing?

(Metacommunication): I realize that this is a strange request, seeing that you do not know who I am, but I would really appreciate your help. I am a nice person.

In this metacommunicated message about how to interpret meaning, the student nurse used both verbal and nonverbal cues. She conveyed a verbal message of caring; making appropriate, encouraging responses; and sending a nonverbal message by maintaining direct eye contact, presenting a smooth face without frowning, and using a relaxed and fluid body posture without fidgeting.

A student studying American Sign Language for the deaf was surprised that it was not sufficient merely to make the sign for "smile" but that she had to actually show a smile at the same time. This congruence helped to convey her message. You can communicate your acceptance, interest, and respect nonverbally. What style can we use to most positively affect our patients' health practices? A comprehensive review shows that we have inadequate information about this.

VERBAL COMMUNICATION

Words are symbols used by people to think about ideas and to communicate with others. Choice of words is influenced by many factors (e.g., your age, race, socioeconomic group, educational background, and gender) and by the situation in which the communication is taking place.

The interpretation of the meaning of words may vary according to the individual's background and experiences. It is dangerous to assume that words have the same meaning for all persons who hear them. Language is useful only to the extent that it accurately reflects the experience it is designed to portray. Consider, for example, the difficulty an American would have in communicating with a person who speaks only Vietnamese, or the dilemma of the young child with a limited vocabulary who is trying to tell you where it hurts. One's voice can be a therapeutic part of treatment, as in Mrs. Garcia's case.

Case Study: Mrs Garcia Is Unconscious

For weeks, while giving care to Mrs Garcia, a 42-year-old unconscious woman, her nurse, Sue Shabana, used soothing touch and conversation. She also encouraged Mr Garcia to do the same. When the woman later regained consciousness, she told Sue that she recognized her voice!

enter this new relationship with our own specific styles of communication.

Some individuals depend on a mostly verbal style to convey their meaning, whereas others rely on nonverbal strategies to send the message. It is estimated that 70%–90% of messages are conveyed nonverbally (Keutchafo, 2020). Some communicators emphasize giving information; others have as a priority the conveying of interpersonal caring. Longer nurse–patient relationships allow each person to better understand the other's communication style.

In a professional relationship, verbal and nonverbal components of communication are intimately related.

Meaning

There are two levels of meaning in language: denotation and connotation. Both are affected by one's culture. **Denotation** refers to the generalized meaning assigned to a word; **connotation** points to a more personalized meaning of the word or phrase. For example, most people would agree that a dog is a four-legged creature, domesticated, with a characteristic vocalization referred to as a bark. This would be the denotative, or explicit, meaning of the word. When the word is used in a more personalized way, it reveals the connotative level of meaning. "What a dog" and "His bark is worse

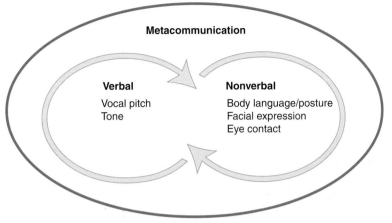

Figure 6.1 Factors in communication styles.

than his bite" are phrases some people use to describe personal characteristics of human beings rather than animals. We need to be aware that many messages convey only a part of the intended meaning. Do not assume that the meaning of a message is the same for the sender and the receiver until mutual understanding is verified. To be sure you are getting your message across, ask for feedback.

VERBAL-STYLE FACTORS THAT INFLUENCE NURSE-TO-PATIENT PROFESSIONAL COMMUNICATION

The following six *verbal* styles of communication are summarized in Table 6.1:

1. *Moderate pitch and tone in vocalization.* The oral delivery of a verbal message, expressed through tone of voice, inflection, sighing, and so on, is referred to as **paralanguage.** It is important to understand this component of communication because it affects how the verbal message is likely to be interpreted. For example, you might say, "I would like to hear more about what you are feeling" in a voice that sounds rushed, high-pitched, or harsh. Or you might make this same statement in a soft, unhurried voice that expresses genuine interest. In the first instance, the message is likely to be misinterpreted by the patient, despite your good intentions. Your caring intent is more apparent to the patient in the second instance. Voice inflection (pitch and tone), loudness, and rate of speaking either support or contradict the content

TABLE 6.1 Styles That Influence Professional Communications in Nurse–Patient Relationships	
Verbal	**Nonverbal**
Moderates pitch and tone	Allows therapeutic silences; listens
Varies vocalizations	Uses congruent nonverbal behaviors
Encourages involvement	Uses facilitative body language
Validates worth	Uses touch appropriately
Advocates for patient as necessary	Proxemics—respects patient's space
Appropriately provides needed information: briefly and clearly, avoiding slang	Attends to nonverbal cues

of the verbal message. Varying your pitch helps others perceive you more positively. Ideas may be conveyed merely by emphasizing different portions of your statement. When the tone of voice does not fit the words, the message is less easily understood and is less likely to be believed. Some, especially when upset, communicate in an emotional rather than intellectual manner. A message conveyed in a firm, steady tone is more reassuring than one conveyed in a loud, emotional, abrasive, or uncertain manner. In contrast, if you speak in a flat, monotone voice when you are upset, as though the matter were of no consequence, you confuse your patient, making an appropriate response difficult.

2. *Vary vocalizations.* In some cultures, sounds are punctuated, whereas in others, sounds have a lyrical or singsong quality. We need to orient ourselves to the characteristic voice tones associated with other cultures.

3. *Encourage involvement.* Professional styles of communication have changed over time. We now partner with our patients in promoting their optimal health. We expect and encourage them to assume responsibility for their own health. Consequently, provider–patient communication has changed. Paternalistic, "I'll tell you what to do" styles are no longer acceptable.

4. *Validate patient's worth.* Styles that convey caring send a message of individual worth that sustains the relationship. For example, some prefer providers who use a "warm" communication style to show caring, give information, and talk about their own feelings. Confirming responses validate the intrinsic worth of the person. These are responses that affirm the right of the individual to be treated with respect. They also affirm autonomy (i.e., the patient's right, ultimately, to make his or her own decisions). Disconfirming responses, in contrast, disregard the validity of patients' feelings by either ignoring them or by imposing a value judgment. Such responses take the form of changing the topic, offering reassurance without supporting evidence, or presuming to know what patients mean without verifying the message with them. More experienced nurses use more confirming communication. These communication skills are learned.

5. *Advocate for the patient when necessary.* Our personalities affect our style of social communication; some of us are naturally shy. But in our professional relationships, we must often assume an assertive style of communicating with other health providers or agencies to obtain the best care or services for our patient.

6. *Provide needed information appropriately.* Providing accurate information in a timely manner in understandable amounts is discussed throughout this book. In our social conversations, there is often a rhythm: "You talk, I listen," then "I get to talk, you listen." However, in professional communications, the content is more goal-focused. Self-disclosure from the nurse must be limited. It is not appropriate to tell a patient your problems or your own weight struggles, as in Ms. Kahama's case.

Case Study: Kay Kelly and Ms Kahama's Weight Loss

Nurse practitioner Kay Kelly, FNP, sitting in the exam room with Ms Kahama, is typing into the Electronic Health Record on her tablet. She says "You are still 40 pounds overweight, but are making progress losing!" She shares the screen to show a basal metabolic weight graph contrasting Ms Kahama's body mass with the norm. Is this paternalistic? Or is this potentially a way of engaging her patient in a weight loss discussion? Initial studies show that when providers gazed at computer screens instead of maintaining eye contact with their patients, the patients became detached. The *Journal of the American Medical Association* and other publications have suggested sharing pertinent screen images with patients as a strategy for getting them to be more involved.

NONVERBAL COMMUNICATION

As we noted, most of our person-to-person communication is **nonverbal communication**. All our words are accompanied by nonverbal cues that offer meaning about how to interpret the message. Think of the most interesting lecturer you ever had. Did this person lecture by making eye contact? By using hand gestures? By moving among the students? By conveying enthusiasm?

The function of nonverbal communication is to give us cues about what is being communicated. We give meaning about the purpose or context of our message nonverbally; this can increase the accuracy and efficiency of its impact on the listener. Some of these nonverbal cues are conveyed by tone of voice, facial expression, and body gestures or movement. Skilled use of nonverbal communication through therapeutic silences, use of congruent nonverbal behaviors, body language, touch, proxemics, and attention to nonverbal cues such as facial expression can build rapport. Emotional meanings are communicated through body language.

Aspects of Nonverbal Style That Influence Nurse–Patient Professional Communication

We must be aware of the ways in which our nonverbal messages are conveyed. The position of your hands, the look on your face, and the movement of your body all give cues regarding your meaning. It is important to use attending behaviors, such as leaning forward slightly, to convey to the patient that his or her conversation is worth listening to. Think of the last time an interviewer kept fidgeting in his seat, glanced frequently at his wall clock, or shuffled his papers while you were speaking. How did this make you feel? What nonverbal message was being conveyed? Read about nonverbal behaviors of a competent nurse:

1. *Allow silences.* In our social communications, the norm is a question–response sequence. The goal is to have no overlap and no gap between turns. We often become uncomfortable if conversation lags. There is a tendency to rush in to fill the void. But in our professional nurse–patient communication, we use silence therapeutically, allowing needed time to think about things.

2. *Use congruent nonverbal behaviors.* Nonverbal behavior should be congruent with the message and should reinforce it. If you knock on your instructor's office door to seek help, do you believe her when she says she would love to talk if you see her grimace and roll her eyes at her secretary? In another example, if you smile while telling your nurse-manager that your assignment is too much to handle, the seriousness of your message will be negated. Try to give nonverbal cues that are congruent with the message you are verbally communicating. When nonverbal cues are incongruent with the verbal information, messages are likely to be misinterpreted. When your verbal message is inconsistent with the nonverbal expression of the message, the nonverbal expressions assume prominence and are generally perceived as more trustworthy than the verbal content. You need to comment on any incongruence to help your patient. For example, when you enter a room to ask Mr Sala if he is having any postoperative pain, he may say "No," but he grimaces and clutches his incision. After you comment on the incongruent message, he may admit that he is having some discomfort. Can you think of a clinical situation in which you changed the meaning of a verbal message by giving nonverbal "don't believe what I say" cues?

3. *Use facilitative body language. Kinesics* is an important component of nonverbal communication. Commonly referred to as ***body language***, it is defined as involving the conscious or unconscious body positioning or actions of the communicator. Words direct the content of a message, whereas emotions accentuate and clarify the meaning of the words. Some nonverbal behaviors, such as tilting your head or facing your patient at an angle, promote communication. Pay attention to our body position, commenting that turning away conveys nervousness. Try viewing Amy Cuddy's, 2012 TED talk.

   • **Posture.** Leaning forward slightly communicates interest and encourages your patient to keep the conversation going. Keep your arms uncrossed with palms open, knees uncrossed, and body loose, not tight and tense. Your relaxed posture conveys openness. Turning away indicates lack of interest, whereas directly and closely facing the patient, crossing your arms and staring unblinkingly, or jabbing your finger in the air suggests aggression.

   • **Facial expression.** Six common facial expressions (surprise, sadness, anger, happiness/joy, disgust/contempt, and fear) represent global, generalized interpretations of emotions common to all cultures. Facial expression either reinforces or modifies the message the listener hears. The power of the facial expression far outweighs the power of the actual words. It is considered to be a reliable indicator of a person's true emotion (Kee, 2018). So try to maintain an open, friendly expression without being boisterously cheerful. Avoid furrowing your forehead or assuming a distracted or bored expression.

   • **Eye contact.** Making direct eye contact, but not staring, generally conveys a positive message. Most patients interpret direct eye contact as an indication of your interest in what they have to say, although there are cultural differences. *Keep* wide open eyes and maintaining direct eye contact with your patient promotes closeness. Has anyone every rolled their eyes while talking with you? What message does this convey?

   • **Gestures.** Some gestures, such as affirmative head nodding, help to facilitate conversation by showing interest and attention. The use of open-handed gestures can also facilitate communication. Avoid folding your arms across your chest or fidgeting. Movements of extremities may give cues to feelings. Making a fist can convey how angry someone is, just as the use of stabbing, abrupt hand gestures may suggest distress, whereas hugging one's arms closely (self-embracing gestures) may suggest fear. *Observe hand movements.* If someone is speaking with you but twiddling their thumbs, what does that convey? Throwing up your hands could be interpreted as a "what's the use" message. Be careful of cultural meaning of gestures. What seems friendly to you might be considered obscene in another culture.

4. *Touch.* Touching is one of the most powerful ways you have of communicating nonverbally. Within a professional relationship, affective touch can convey caring, empathy, comfort, and reassurance. Brief touching can be comforting as in Fig. 6.2. When a nurse touches patients, this contact can be perceived by the patient as either an expression of caring or negatively as a threat. Care must be taken to abide by the patient's cultural proscriptions about the use of touch. The literature

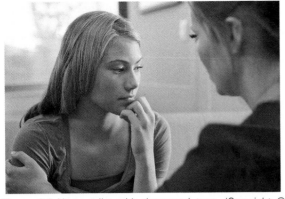

Figure 6.2 Nurse talks with depressed teen. (Copyright © monkeybusinessimages/iStock/Thinkstock.)

cites variations across cultures, such as the proscription some Muslim and Orthodox Jewish men follow against touching women other than family members. They might be uncomfortable shaking the hand of a female healthcare provider. In another example, some Native Americans use touch in healing, so that casual touching may be taboo. The vast majority of patients report feeling comforted when a professional health provider touches them.

The "best" type of touch cited by patients is holding one of their hands. All nurses giving direct care use touch to assess and to assist. We touch to help our patient walk, roll over in bed, and so on. However, just as you would be careful about invading someone's personal space, you must be careful about when and where on the body you touch your patients. Your use of touch can elicit misunderstanding if it is perceived as invasive or inappropriate. Gender and culture determine perceptions about being touched.

5. *Proxemics.* We can use physical space to improve our interactions. **Proxemics** refers to the perception of what is a proper distance to be maintained between oneself and others as prescribed by one's culture.

Each culture prescribes expectations for appropriate distance depending on the context of the communication. As discussed in Chapter 5, the "proper" social distance for an interpersonal relationship as 1.5–4 feet in Western cultures. Americans, Canadians, and other Westerners tend to become uncomfortable if someone stands closer than 3 feet. In almost all cultures, zero distance is shunned except for loving or caring interactions. In giving physical care, nurses enter this "intimate" space. Caution is needed when you are at this closer distance, lest your actions be misinterpreted, since violating personal space can be threatening.

6. *Attend to nonverbal body cues.*
   • **Posture.** Often, the emotional component of a message can be indirectly interpreted by observing body language. Rhythm of movement and body stance may convey a message about the speaker. For example, when patients speak while directly facing you, this conveys more confidence than if they turn their bodies away from you at an angle. A slumped, head-down posture and slow movements might give you an impression of lassitude or low self-esteem, whereas an erect posture and decisive movement suggest confidence. Rapid, diffuse, agitated body movements may indicate anxiety. Forceful body movements may symbolize anger. When someone bows her head or slumps her body after receiving bad news, it conveys sadness. Can you think of other cues that body posture might give you? An attentive posture, sitting face-to-face and leaning slightly forward or tilting your head slightly conveys attentiveness to what the patient is saying. But tapping your fingers or feet and crossing your arms over your chest or slouching convey negative messages to the patient. Head down position can be interpreted as disinterest or rejection, while turning your head away says, "I'm done listening."
   • **Facial expression.** Facial characteristics such as frowning or smiling add to the verbal message conveyed. Almost instinctively, we use facial expression as a barometer of another person's feelings, motivations, approachability, and mood. From infancy, we respond to the expressive qualities of another's face, often without even being aware of it. Therefore, assessing facial expression together with other nonverbal cues may reveal vital information that will affect the nurse–patient relationship. For example, a worried facial expression and lip biting may suggest anxiety. In Kee's study (2018), a negative facial expression by doctors was interpreted by patients as disinterest and led some to doubt their doctor's competency. A bored or frowning face conveys disinterest or disapproval. Tightly clenched lips suggest anger. Absence of a smile in greeting or grimacing may convey a message about how ill your patient feels.
   • **Eye contact.** Research suggests that individuals who make direct eye contact while talking or listening create a sense of confidence and credibility, whereas downward glances or averted eyes signal submission, weakness, or shame. In addition to conveying confidence, maintaining direct eye contact communicates honesty. Failure to maintain eye contact, known as *gaze aversion*, is perceived as a nonverbal cue meaning

that the person is lying to you. If your patient's eyes wander around during a conversation, you may wonder if he is being honest. Even young children are more likely to attribute lying to those who avert their gaze.

Interpretation of Nonverbal Behaviors

Assessing the extent to which nonverbal cues communicate emotions can help you to communicate better. Studies repeatedly show that the failure to acknowledge nonverbal cues is often associated with inefficient communication by the health provider.

It is best if we verify our assessment of the meaning of observed nonverbal behaviors. Body cues, although suggestive, are imprecise. When communication is limited by the state of a person's health, pay even closer attention to nonverbal cues. Your patient's pain, for example, can be assessed through facial expression even when he or she is only partially conscious. What would you say in the Mr Geeze case?

Case Study: Mr Geeze and Metacommunication

Mr Geeze smiles but narrows his eyes and glares at the nurse. An appropriate comment for the nurse to make might be, "I notice you are smiling, but you say that you would like to kill me for mentioning your fever to the doctor. It seems that you might be angry with me."

Use of an incompatible communication style or failing to validate what patients are communicating nonverbally can adversely affect the level of support you can offer, leaving your patient feeling anxious or even hopeless. In this situation the patient may reject your well-meaning advice.

COMMUNICATION ACCOMMODATION THEORY

Giles and Ogay (2007) theorized that people adapt or adjust their speech, vocal patterns (diction, tone, rate of speaking), dialect, word choice, and gestures to accommodate others. This theory suggests that it is desirable to adjust one's speech to our conversational partners to help facilitate our interaction, increase our acceptance, and improve trust and rapport. This is known as *convergence*. Convergence is thought to increase the effectiveness of your communication.

Accommodation can occur unconsciously or can be a conscious choice. For example, when you are speaking to a child, you might deliberately assume a more assertive, commanding style to get the child to obey. Choice of a distinctly different style is known as *divergence*. Conversely, you might choose convergence when you want to teach something about a disease condition. You might attempt to match your patient's speed and speech cadence. You definitely adapt or accommodate by choosing to match your vocabulary in an effort to be better understood. In general, if the person choosing to use convergence has more power in the relationship, he or she may be perceived as patronizing. This theory assumes that people are communicating in a rational manner. During a conflict, people can become unreasonable or irrational; this would not a time to choose the use of an accommodation style.

EFFECTS OF SOCIOCULTURAL FACTORS ON COMMUNICATION

Communication is also affected by such style factors as cultural background, age cohort, gender, ethnicity, social class, and location. Of course, not everyone communicates in the manner described. These are broad generalizations as described in the literature.

Age Cohort and Generational Diversity

The members of today's nursing workforce now span four generations. As might be expected, members of different generations hold differing views regarding work motivation, personal values, and attitudes toward their work; they also have differing communication styles and preferences. Differences exist in people's communication styles when they are interacting with authority figures. Differences also occur in learning styles and commitment to the organization (QSEN, n.d.). If ignored, generational differences can become a source of conflict in the workplace.

Each age cohort, born approximately every 20 years, has some communication style characteristics in common, which differentiate each group from prior generations. Communication Accommodation Theory, as described earlier, has been used to explore intergenerational communication problems. In considering the generation gap, beliefs about communication and goals for interactions differ among cohorts. For example, accommodation theory has been used to explore ageism, the negative evaluation of the elderly by those who are younger. In society, youth may deliberately choose divergence, purposely amplifying differences as by talking more rapidly, using slang, or emphasizing difference in values. In healthcare settings, studies of the generation gap and ageism stereotypes have found miscommunication outcomes in intergenerational interactions between providers and patients. How well would you respond to a patronizing style?

Some nurses might prefer digital communication via secure texting on cell phones, whereas others might prefer face-to-face communication.

Younger nurses and physicians, raised in the digital age, may rely on the Internet and social medial for information, social interaction, and communication. The nursing literature suggests that agencies and supervisors need to determine a person's preferred method of communication. People learn and communicate best if they are engaged in their preferred style.

Gender

Communication patterns are integrated into gender roles, which are defined by an individual's culture. In communication studies, gender differences have been shown to be greatest in terms of the use and interpretation of nonverbal cues. This may reflect gender differences in intellectual style as well as culturally reinforced standards of acceptable role-related behaviors. Of course, there are wide variations within the same gender.

We are now questioning whether traditional ideas about male and female differences in communication are as prevalent as previously thought. Is there really a major difference in communication according to gender?

What is factual and what is a stereotype? More healthcare communication studies need to be done before we will really know. Because traditional thinking about gender-related differences in communication content and process in both nonverbal and verbal communication are being revised, consider what you read critically.

Traditionally, women in most cultures were said to tend to avoid conflict and to want to smooth over differences. They were said to demonstrate more effective use of nonverbal communication and to be better decoders of nonverbal meaning. Feminine communication was thought to be more person-centered, warmer, and more sincere. Studies show that women tend to use more facial expressiveness, to smile more often, to maintain eye contact, to touch more often, and to nod more often. Women have a greater range of vocal pitch and also tend to use different informal patterns of vocalization than men. They use more tones signifying surprise, cheerfulness, and unexpectedness. Women tend to view conversation as a connection to others.

Traditionally, men in Western cultures were thought to communicate in a more task-oriented, direct fashion, to demonstrate greater aggressiveness, and to boast about their accomplishments. They have also been viewed as more likely to express disagreement. Studies show that men prefer a greater interpersonal distance between themselves and others and that they use gestures more often. Men are more likely to maintain eye contact in a negative encounter, although overall they maintain less direct eye contact; they also use less verbal communication than women in interpersonal relationships. Men are more likely to initiate an interaction, talk more, interrupt more freely, talk louder, disagree more, use hostile verbs, and talk more about issues.

Gender Differences in Communication in Healthcare Settings

The effects of gender on communication have long been discussed in the literature. But do these differences actually affect performance? It has been suggested that more effective communication occurs when provider and patient are of the same gender, although this was not found to be true in some studies. In professional healthcare settings, women have been noted to use more active listening, using

---

DEVELOPING AN EVIDENCE-BASED PRACTICE

Keutchafo et al. (2020) reviewed 22 South African studies of nurse communication with older adults to identify nonverbal behaviors and perceptions of nonverbal messaging.

Results

A content analysis showed the nurses choose these nonverbal behaviors to enhance listening and display interest: tactile contact (shaking hands, touching, stroking); kinesthetics (smiling, friendly facial expression, eye movement, head nodding, leaning forward slightly); demonstrating presence (sitting face-to-face); and demonstrating active listening (showing respect and positive regard). Reports from the senior adult's perspective showed perceptions of negative communication as lack of eye contact, speaking too loud or from too far away.

Strength of research evidence: Low to moderate, since methodology data was not supplied. The authors stated that the quality of these studies was high.

Application to Your Clinical Practice

1. Identify your own style of nonverbal communication.
2. Senior adults are attentive to nonverbal communication.
3. Validate whether the patient has interpreted your nonverbal messaging correctly, perhaps by requesting feedback.

References

Keutchafo, E. L. W., Kerr, J., & Jarvis, M.A. (2020). Evidence of nonverbal communication between nurses and older adults: A scoping review. *BMC Nursing, 19*, 53.

encouraging responses such as "Uh-huh," "Yeah," and "I see," and to use more supportive words.

Location

Rural citizens tend to be underserved by healthcare facilities and providers. Patients in urban areas have reported poorer communication by their healthcare providers. One factor that might affect these results is that rural patients tend to be cared for by the same providers. In a clinic or other busy location, lack of privacy certainly affects the style as well as the content of communications.

Perceptions

Patients might not always have the same perceptions as you do regarding the message you sent. Were your verbal and nonverbal messages congruent? Did your communication covey your trustworthiness? Did the patient perceive you as empathetic?

APPLICATIONS

Knowing Your Own Communication Style

The style of communication you use can influence your patients' behaviors and their ability to reach their health goals. An aggressive communication style from a healthcare provider tends to create hostility or antipathy, whereas the use of an assertive, empathic style while seeking to make a point may lead to best outcomes. Users of a passive communication style are basically not active in helping patients to achieve their goals, whereas users of a more persuasive style wait to listen to before trying to make their points.

Patients report being dissatisfied with poor communication more than with other aspects of their care. Simulation exercises in prior chapters should give you the basic skills you need in your nurse–patient relationships, but remember that you bring your own communication style with you, as does your patient. Because we differ widely in our personal communication styles, it is important for you to identify your style and to know how to modify it for certain patients. Try Simulation Exercise 6.1 for a quick profile of your personal communication style. How does your affective style come across? Do patients view you as empathic, caring, and reassuring? Experienced nurses adapt their innate social style so that their professional communications fit the patient and the situation. You too must modify your style to be sure that it is compatible with your patients' needs. Think about the potential for incompatibility in the following Michaels case.

Case Study: Mr Michaels–Nurse Green Interaction

Ms Green (in a firm tone): Mr Michaels, it's time to take your medicine.

   Mr Michaels (in a complaining tone): You are so bossy!

Empathy. Empathic communication is crucial to your nursing care and may improve a patient's health outcome. Recognize how others perceive you. Consider all the nonverbal factors that affect their perceptions of you, such as gender, manner of dress, appearance, skin tone, hairstyle, age, role as a student, gestures, and mannerisms. Simulation Exercise 6.2 may increase your awareness of gender bias.

Own communication style assessment. The initial step in identifying your own style may be to compare your style with those of others. Ask yourself, "What makes someone perceive a nurse either as authoritarian or as accepting and caring?" Video recording yourself in an interaction might be revealing. The Simulation Exercise 6.3 video may help you to compare your style with those of others.

Assess need to change own style. Develop an awareness of alternative styles that you can comfortably assume if the occasion warrants. For example, Watts et al. (2017) suggests assessing whether changing your style to speak more slowly, using more nonverbal communication, and involving family members will help get the message across to people of other ethnic groups. It is important to figure out whether some other factors may be influencing your style toward a particular patient and if that is appropriate. How might the other person's age, race, socioeconomic status, or gender affect his or her responses to you? We must continually work to update our communication competencies. Internal organizational communication is rapidly becoming electronic. Some hospital agencies are increasingly relying on digital communication, eliminating many of the nuances communicated nonverbally.

INTERPERSONAL COMPETENCE

Nurse–patient communication processes are based on the nurse's interpersonal competence and the situations that nurses find themselves in. Higher levels of anxiety affect your communication. **Interpersonal competence** develops as you come to understand the complex cognitive, behavioral, and cultural factors that influence communication. This understanding, together with the use of a broad range of communication skills, can help you to interact positively with your patients as they attempt to cope with multiple demands. Developing good communication skills will

SIMULATION EXERCISE 6.1 My Communication Style: Quick Profile

Purpose
To develop self-reflection.

Procedure
Answer the following:
1. I prefer to
   - Get my way.
   - Follow the rules.
   - Avoid confrontation.
2. My verbal tone is most often
   - Warm.
   - Enthusiastic.
   - Determined.
3. If we have a difference of opinion, I usually want to
   - Dominate.
   - Compromise.
   - Give in.
4. In a social group situation, I sometimes
   - Fail to give my opinion.
   - Am very, very polite.
   - Digress from the topic.
   - Become irritated with those who disagree with me.
5. My friends have told me that
   - I talk using my hands.
   - I smile a lot.
   - I can't sit still.

Reflective Discussion Analysis
Compare your answers with book content on style. Analyze how these factors might affect your nurse–patient relationships.

SIMULATION EXERCISE 6.2 Gender Bias

Purpose
To create discussion about gender bias.

Procedure
In small groups, read and discuss the following comments that are made about care delivery on a geriatric psychiatric unit by staff and students: "Male staff tend to be slightly more confident and to make quicker decisions. Women staff are better at the feeling things, like conveying warmth."

Reflective Discussion Analysis
1. Reflect as to the effect of gender on perceptions of comments. Determine whether these comments are made by male or female staff.
2. Analyze their accuracy. Be sure to support with evidence from the text.
3. Can you truly generalize attributes to any male and female individuals?

SIMULATION EXERCISE 6.3 Self-Analysis of Video Recording

Purpose
To increase awareness of students' own style.

Procedure
With a partner, role-play an interaction between nurse and patient. Use the video capacity of your cell phone to record a 1–2-min interview with the camera focused on you. The topic of the interview could be "identifying health promotion behaviors" or something similar.

Reflective Discussion Analysis
Analyze playbacks in a group. What postures were used? What nonverbal messages were communicated? How? Were verbal and nonverbal messages congruent?

increase your competent communication. Such skills are identified as among the attributes of expert nurses with the most clinical credibility. In dealing with a patient in the sociocultural context of the healthcare system, two kinds of abilities are required: social cognitive competency and message competency.

Social cognitive competency is the ability to interpret message content within interactions from the point of view of each of the participants. By embracing your patients' perspectives, you begin to understand how they organize information and formulate goals. This is especially important when your patients' ability to communicate is impaired by a mechanical barrier such as a ventilator. Patients who have recovered from critical illnesses requiring ventilator support report that they felt fear and distress during this experience.

Message competency refers to the ability to use language and nonverbal behaviors strategically in the intervention phase of the nursing process to achieve the goals of the interaction. Communication skills are used as a tool to influence patients to maximize their adaptation. Think how it feels when your patient sees you smile and hears you say, "That's impressive; you have successfully self-injected your insulin!"

NONVERBAL-STYLE FACTORS THAT INFLUENCE COMMUNICATION AND RELATIONSHIPS

Nonverbal communication is widely perceived as the way to convey emotion. Nonverbal characteristics we need to interpret include the following:

- Proxemics: As we have discussed, this refers to the use of space and distance.
- Haptics: Haptics refers to the therapeutic use of touch to communicate nonverbally providing comfort, reassurance. Comment on the quality of the nurse's touch in Fig. 6.3.
- Kinesics: Sometimes encompassed in the broader term of "body language," these are body movements we described that convey meaning.
- Posture: What cues did we discuss?
- Facial expression: A pleasant, smiling, alert facial expression conveys interest.

VERBAL-STYLE FACTORS THAT INFLUENCE RELATIONSHIPS

Vocalics

Vocalics refers to aspects of the voice. The tone, volume, pitch, and rhythm can alter message meaning. Speaking rapidly may make it difficult for your patient to understand. But speaking overly slowly can be interpreted as patronizing. Box 6.1 contains suggestions to improve your own professional style of communicating.

Slang and Jargon

Different age groups even in the same culture may attribute different meanings to the same word. For example, an adult who says "That's cool" might be referring to the temperature, whereas another might be conveying satisfaction. In healthcare, the "food pyramid" is understood by nurses to represent the basic nutritional food groups needed for health; however, the term may have limited meaning for others.

Beginning nursing students often report confusion while learning all the medical terminology required for their new role. Remembering our own experiences, we can empathize with patients who are attempting to understand the **medical jargon** involved in healthcare. Careful explanations help overcome this communication barrier. For successful communication, the words we use should have a similar meaning to both individuals in an interaction. An important part of the communication process is the search for a common vocabulary so that the message sent is the same as the one received. Consider the oncology nurse who develops a computer databank of cancer treatment terms.

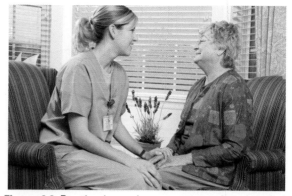

Figure 6.3 Emotional meanings are communicated through body language, particularly facial expression.

BOX 6.1   Suggestions to Improve Your Communication Style

- Adapting yourself to your patient's cultural values
- Using nonverbal communication strategies, such as follows:
  - Maintaining eye contact
  - Displaying pleasant, animated facial expressions
  - Smiling often
  - Nodding your head to encourage talking
  - Maintaining an attentive, upright posture and sitting at the patient's level, leaning forward slightly
  - Attending to proper proximity and increasing space if the patient shows signs of discomfort, such as averting his or her gaze, or swinging his or her legs.
- Using touch if appropriate to the situation
- Using active listening and responding to patient's cues
- Using verbal strategies to engage your patient
  - Using humor, but avoiding gender jokes
  - Attending to proper tone and pitch, avoiding an overly loud voice
  - Avoiding jargon
  - Using nonjudgmental language and open-ended questions
  - Listening and avoiding jumping in too soon with problem-solving
  - Verbalizing respect
  - Asking permission before addressing a client by his or her first name
  - Conveying caring comments
  - Using confirming, positive comments

While she is admitting Mr Michaels as a new patient, the nurse uses an existing template model on her computer to create an individualized terminology sheet with just the words that would be encountered by him during his course of chemotherapy.

Responsiveness of Participants

How responsive the participants are affects the depth and breadth of communication. Reciprocity affects not only the relationship process but also patient health outcomes. Some people are naturally more verbal than others. It is easier to have a therapeutic conversation with extroverted patients who want to communicate. You will want to increase the responsiveness of those who are less verbal and enhance their responsiveness. Verbal and nonverbal approval encourages patients to express themselves. Elsewhere, we discuss skills that promote responsiveness, such as active listening, demonstrations of empathy, and acknowledgment of the content and feelings of messages.

Respect

Sometimes acknowledging the difficulty your patients are having in expressing their feelings, praising your patients' efforts, and encouraging them to use more than one route of communication will help. Such strategies demonstrate interpersonal sensitivity. Listening to the care experience of a patient, responding to verbal or nonverbal cues, and avoiding "talking down" encourage communication and may improve compliance with the treatment regimen. Providers who fail to introduce themselves may be perceived as rude. Simulation Exercise 6.4 will help you practice the use of confirming responses.

SIMULATION EXERCISE 6.4   Observing Nonverbal Cues

Purpose
To increase skill in interpreting nonverbal communication.

Procedure
Observe a brief dramatic scene from a movie or TV show with the sound off. Make note of the nonverbal body language seen and what interpretations you made.

Reflective Discussion Analysis
Share observations with a group. Focus discussion on the variations in the way nonverbal was interpreted. Discuss ways in which nurses can use their observations of patient nonverbal behaviors to gain a better understanding of the message.

Roles of Participants

Paying attention to the *roles relationship* among the communicators may be just as important as deciphering the content and meaning of the message. The relationships between the roles of the sender and those of the receiver influence how the communication is likely to be received and interpreted. The same constructive criticism made by a good friend and by one's immediate supervisor is likely to be interpreted differently, even though the content and style are similar. Communication between subordinates and supervisors is far more likely to be influenced by power and style than by gender. When roles are unequal in terms of power, the more powerful individual tends to speak in a more dominant style. This is discussed in Chapters 22 and 23.

Context of the Message

Communication is always influenced by the environment in which it takes place. It does not occur in a vacuum but is shaped by the situation in which the interaction occurs. Taking time to evaluate the physical setting and the time and space in which the contact takes place—as well as the psychological, social, and cultural characteristics of each individual involved—gives you flexibility in choosing the most appropriate context.

Involvement in the Relationship

Relationships generally need to develop over time because communication changes during different phases of the relationship. Studies show that physicians, nurses, and other healthcare workers respond to patients' concerns less than half the time. Responses tend to focus on physical care and often do not address social-emotional care. These days, nurses working with hospitalized patients have less time to develop relationships, whereas community-based nurses may have greater opportunities. To begin to explore ethical problems in your nursing relationships, consider the ethical dilemma provided.

Use of Humor

As discussed elsewhere, research has associated the use of humor with stress relief, diffusion of conflict, enhancement of learning, and improved communication in nurse–patient relationships. Can you incorporate humor into your relationships without using disparagement?

ADVOCATE FOR CONTINUITY OF CARE

We have learned that in patients, evaluation of positive healthcare communication is higher when they consistently relate to the same individuals providing their care. These providers are more likely to listen to them, to explain things clearly, to spend enough time with them, and to show them respect. Because physicians, nurses, and other team members communicate differently with patients, it is crucial for them to pool information.

SUMMARY

Communication style involves more than an exchange of verbal and nonverbal information. As our population becomes more diverse, we are challenged to provide patient-centered care that is sensitive to culture, race, ethnicity, gender, and sexual orientation. The recurring theme in this chapter is that you can adapt your communication style to better suit individual patients. Modifying your style to provide more effective communication promotes safer care and better health outcomes. This chapter offers suggestions for styles of verbal and nonverbal communication as well as a beginning discussion of cultural and gender differences. Style factors that affect the communication process include the responsiveness and role relationships of the participants, the types of responses and context of the relationships, and the level of involvement in the relationship. Both verbal and nonverbal skills are suggested.

ETHICAL DILEMMA: What Would You Do?

Katy Collins, RN, is a new grad who learns that a serious error that harmed a patient has occurred on her unit. She realizes that if staff continues to follow the existing protocol, this error could occur again. In a team meeting led by an administrator, Katy raises this issue in a tentative manner. The leader speaks in a loud, decisive voice and states that he wants input from the staff nurses. However, he glances at the clock, gazes over Katy's head, and maintains a bored expression. Katy gets the message that the administration wants to smooth over the error, bury it, and go on as usual rather than using resources and time to correct the underlying problem.

1. What ethical principle is being violated in this situation?
2. What message does the administrator's behavior convey?
3. Explain the congruence. Draw conclusions about how you would change the nonverbal message to make it congruent.

DISCUSSION QUESTIONS

1. Use Simulation Exercise 6.2 to apply your knowledge about the influence of gender on communication.
2. In a loud, commanding voice, a nurse tells an immediate postoperative patient to take deep breaths every 20 min despite the pain it causes. Describe three possible reactions that might occur. Formulate ways to make this intervention more effective.

REFERENCES

Cuddy, A. (2012). *Your body language may shape what you are*. TED Talks. [website]. Retrieved from www.ted.com/search?q=amy+cuddy. [Accessed 24 May 2021].

Giles, H., & Ogay, T. (2007). Communication accommodation theory. In B. B. Whaley, & W. Samter (Eds.), *Explaining communication: Contemporary theories and exemplars* (pp. 293–310). Mahwah, NJ: Lawrence Erlbaum.

Kee, J. W. Y., Khoo, H. S., Lim, I., & Koh, M. Y. H. (2018). Communication skills in patient-doctor interactions: Learning from patient complaints. *Health Professions Education*, 4(2), 97–106.

Keutchafo, E. L. W., Kerr, J., & Jarvis, M. A. (2020). Evidence of nonverbal communication between nurses and older adults: A scoping review. *BMC Nursing*, 19, 53.

Quality and Safety Education for Nurses (QSEN). (n.d.). *Teamwork & collaboration (QSEN competencies: Online teaching modules)*. Retrieved from www.QSEN.org/.

Watts, K. J., Meiser, B., Zilliacus, E., et al. (2017). Communication with patients from minority backgrounds: Individual challenges experienced by oncology health professionals. *European Journal of Oncology Nursing*, 26, 83–90.

7

Intercultural Communication and Patient Diversity

OBJECTIVES

At the end of the chapter, the reader will be able to:
1. Describe the concept of cultural competence.
2. Discuss key dimensions of intercultural communication with diverse patients.
3. Apply the concept of culturally competent communication to a case study.
4. Cultural competence is an essential skill for nurses and part of our code of ethics (ANA, 2015; Smith, 2018).

Healthcare professionals and their patients each bring a personalized cultural background and diverse perspectives, with associated values and beliefs, to each healthcare encounter. A person's culture will influence the way relevant information is interpreted and acted upon by patients and their families. Each patient's social class, religious beliefs and spirituality, education, and family norms also influence patient preferences and values. National Standards for Culturally and Linguistically Appropriate Services (CLAS) in Health and Health Care, discussed in this chapter, mandate close attention to honoring diversity in all aspects of health communication. The recent pandemic exposed urgent need to rectify the healthcare disparities that have long existed for people of color in our country (National Academies, 2021). Nurses need to view care through a health equity lens, consistently incorporating an attitude of providing care within the patient's cultural context.

Understanding cultural variations in communication is basic to our nursing care. This chapter discusses culturally competent communication concepts that may help you deal effectively with culturally diverse patients encountered in healthcare settings. We recognize that within a given culture, there is wide variation partly affected by the individual's degree of acculturation.

BASIC CONCEPTS

Nursing of the future will be shaped not only by social changes, such as employment moving into the community setting and by technical advances, but also by cultural challenges. Care of culturally diverse patients requires modifications to nursing assessments, diagnoses, treatment planning and interventions, and patient teaching. Increasing your cultural knowledge and skills and cultivating an accepting attitude will help you become more comfortable and capable.

Definitions

Current literature and government reports use a mixture of terms when discussing ethnicity: Black or African Americans; Hispanic or Latino or LatinX Americans; Asian Americans or name of country of origin, such as Chinese American; Indigenous or Native Americans are some terms used. Until standardization occurs, this book also uses a mix of terms.

- *Culture:* This is a complex social concept consisting of family customs, health beliefs, values, and ethnic identities held by individuals and groups. Communication is more than language and nonverbal behaviors. It is about the way we view other people, family expectations, and cultural norms. Each culture has its own beliefs about health and illness and treatment. These differences will impact on effectiveness of your healthcare delivery. Culture is also a term applied to designate professional and organizational system values.
- *Diversity:* Variations occur among and across groups in race, ethnicity, gender, cultural background, sexual orientation, physical and mental abilities, socioeconomic status, experiences, and beliefs.
- *Cultural competency:* In nursing, we define cultural competence as having a knowledgeable and accepting open attitude that enables us to work effectively with diverse

CASE STUDY: The Kimi Poua Case About Communication

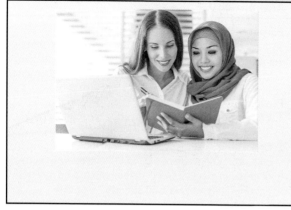

Kimi is a 19-year-old nursing student raised in a Southern Asian culture. English is her second language. She struggles with her instructor's expectations that she will use communication skills with her patients. She cannot grasp the casual talk her patients offer about families and activities. Kimi says her brain is totally focused with the physical care skills required, leaving her little mental energy to translate the colloquialisms her patients use in conversations. Patients interpret her silence as coldness of lack of interest.

1. What other dynamics affect Kimi's behavior? Consider that her culture of origin does not value "small talk."
2. What advice would you give to Kimi?

patients. Cultural competence is a legal and ethical standard, an essential skill of nursing care (IOM, 2003).

Incidence

The racial and ethnic distribution of the US population today reports a 62.6% non-Latino Caucasian majority population; 17% Hispanic or Latino ethnicity (rising to 29% by 2050); 13% African American (rising to 14% by 2050); and 5% Asian (rising to 14% by 2050); and slightly less than 2% Native American (declining to 1% by 2050). Overall, by 2050, today's minority groups are projected to make up approximately 54%–58% of the population in the United States.

Cultural Variation

Each cultural group develops shared stories, values, beliefs, and practices, which are shaped by both their history and geography. This chapter discusses cultural values about access to care, health treatment options, or ethnic and religious beliefs about key issues such as dietary habits influence health behaviors and clinical outcomes. Significant health disparities exist among the culturally and linguistically diverse population groups. Reflect on the Kimi Poua case.

How Culture Is Learned

We are born into a culture; however, culture is not an inborn characteristic. Initially, culture is learned through family and then through other social institutions, such as school, church affiliations, and community contacts. As children learn language from their primary caregivers, and later refine their language skills in school, they simultaneously integrate the cultural attitudes, meanings, values, and thought patterns that inform their words. Immigrants acquire a cultural identity through a two-step interpersonal process in which the person transitions from adhering to traditional cultural beliefs and values in a country of origin toward full adoption of the values and beliefs of culture.

- *Cultural pattern:* The social customs, expected behaviors, cultural beliefs, values, and language passed down from generation to generation by a group of people are their **cultural patterns.** These patterns are informally transmitted through the family, and formally through other affiliations such as school, work, and church. Cultural patterns and beliefs dictate personal preferences and influence how people process and interpret incoming communication. Social factors, such as class and literacy level, further distinguish individual response patterns within a culture. Cultural patterns become an essential part of personal identity. This is because we learn them from the people who are important to us and/or through events that touch us deeply. Patients from other cultures may disagree with the Western view of correct medical treatment. Their own views need to be taken into account when providing advice and care.

- *Acculturation:* This describes how immigrants from a different culture learn and choose to adapt to the behavior and norms of a different, new culture, which holds different expectations. This can be a complicated process because it includes embracing new social, hierarchal, and kinship relationships, consistent with an unfamiliar cultural context. Becoming acculturated creates stress due to the competing pressures of reconciling a familiar cultural identity with the need to adopt new customs essential to functioning effectively in the adopted culture. Exploring your patient's level of acculturation as it relates to culturally based explanatory models of illness, traditional health behaviors, and their potential impact on healthcare matters.

- *Assimilation:* **Assimilation** occurs when an individual from a different culture fully adopts the behaviors, customs, and values of the mainstream culture as part of his or her social identity. To become fully assimilated, immigrants must conform and adapt to the norms of the new culture. This is a gradual process. By the third generation, many immigrants may have little knowledge of their traditional culture and language or allegiance to their original heritage. Box 7.1 summarizes points of cultural diversity in healthcare.

Simulation Exercise 7.1, examining authenticity in personal cultural patterns, offers you an opportunity to reflect on your own cultural heritage and examine what is fundamental about its influence on you. Box 7.2 lists tips for your intercultural communication consideration when caring for someone from another culture.

Theoretical Frameworks

Frameworks provide a structure to organize and explain behaviors. Among the many, we highlight:

Szalay's Process Model of Intercultural Communication

Lorand Szalay (1981) views intercultural communication as an interactive process between representational systems of communication, i.e., the sender and the receiver. The meaning attached to words is influenced by each person's cultural knowledgebase. Their interpretation of messages is shaded by their own history and cultural frame of reference. In this manner, differences in cultural experiences affect coding and decoding of messages, producing different interpretations. To bridge intercultural communication differences, Szalay advocates adapting communication content to the cultural meanings and frame of reference held by the other person. Carefully select words to bridge gaps between two different frames of reference. Miscommunication results when interpretations differ.

SIMULATION EXERCISE 7.1   Cultural Authenticity

Purpose

To help students appreciate the importance of understanding your own culture as a basis for understanding culture relationships in healthcare.

Procedure

1. Write a one-page story about your own culture and/or ethnic background as you understand it.
2. Describe in what ways family and social customs or culture-bound traditions have influenced your sense of personal development, career and leisure choices, opportunities, values, and so forth.
3. Discuss how personal understanding of your cultural background has changed over time.
4. Identify how knowing about one's own culture informs cultural sensitivity to others in healthcare situations.
5. Briefly answer the question, "Does my story represent my cultural authenticity?"

Reflective Discussion Analysis

1. Share your culture story in small groups of three to four students.
2. As a class, discuss how personal culture can influence health behaviors.
3. Identify common themes.
4. Discuss how culturally authentic knowledge prevents unconscious projection of a personal cultural context on a patient from a different culture.

Purnell's Model of Cultural Competence

Larry Purnell (2013) considers cultural competence from a macrolevel (global society, community, family, down to the microlevel of the person). Using Purnell's domains as a framework for understanding individual differences allows for a comprehensive cultural assessment, leading to a culturally congruent, individualized, patient-centered approach to patient care. Understanding the patient's cultural explanation for the health problem is essential, as different cultures frame illness and its causes in various ways. For example, in Asian cultures, depression is characterized as "sadness," rather than a mental disorder. Table 7.1 provides Purnell's domains of assessment when your patient is from a different culture.

Madeleine Leininger's Theory of Cultural Nursing Care

Leininger was a nurse anthropologist who founded the field of study known as transcultural nursing. Her "Theory of Culture Care" asks us to examine culture from our patient's

BOX 7.2 Tips for Your Intercultural Communication Consideration

- Be aware of own cultural biases.
- Be respectful, establish trust by frequently sharing information.
- Recognize patient values may differ from your own.
- Learn about others' cultural health-related norms.
- Be open-minded.
- Adapt your behaviors to avoid offensive or negative interpretations.
- Listen carefully and check patient understanding by having them "talk back."
- Be aware of prohibitions, such as dietary limitations.
- Identify who the decision-maker is in this family and include them in discharge teaching.
- Abide by cultural restrictions, for example, prohibitions about touch or sustained eye contact.
- Understand that there is wide variation within each cultural group.
- Use your understanding of culture to elicit your patient's perspective and beliefs.

point of view, attending to their valuers and beliefs about health and illness. Leininger viewed the concept of "care" as the essence of nursing, a view shared by most of the major nursing theorists (Leininger, 1988). A second major construct is that "caring" is basic to well-being, health, and facing death. A third construct of this theory is "culture care." This is defined as willingness to be open to alternative thinking that is of benefit and is useful to the patient. There are many other components to this theory, but one worth mentioning for purposes of this book is "Culture Care Restructuring" by which a culturally sensitive nurse helps patients adapt to develop a shared goal of health outcome and modify health behaviors to achieve optimal health (Leininger & McFarland, 2006).

Nursing. Using Leininger's framework, we give patient-centered care. Acknowledging our patient's cultural beliefs, we use interventions congruent with that culture's norms. Nurses who fail to adapt to their patient's culture greatly reduce the quality of care (Alligood, 2022). Nurses who provide culturally congruent care contribute to their patient's well-being. Are you open to listening to new ideas, different ways of viewing illness? Are you willing to be changed at least a little bit by your patient's point of view?

Cultural Diversity

Definition

Cultural diversity is a term used to describe social variations between cultural groups. Unrecognized and/or unaccepted differences among different cultural groups can present significant difficulties in communication. Lack of exposure to and/or understanding of the normal patterns of people from other cultures decreases acceptance, reinforces stereotypes, and creates prejudice. People tend to notice differences related to language, manners, mannerisms, and behaviors in people of different cultures in ways that do not happen with people from their own culture.

Diversity can exist *within* a culture. In fact, more differences occur among individuals within a culture than between cultural groups, related to differences in educational and socioeconomic status (SES), age, gender, and life experiences. Within the same culture, individuals with radically different philosophies, social patterns, and sanctioned behaviors coexist, sometimes peacefully, and other times in conflict with each other. Consider, for example, the divisive political differences between liberal and conservative voters, the disagreements between faith beliefs, and different social expectations of the very poor versus the very rich.

Despite historic legislation designed to make quality healthcare opportunities available to everyone, progress has been slow, and prejudicial attitudes continue to play a role in not ending unequal treatment for minority populations. The National Academies (2021) says nurses need to improve their knowledge and skills, addressing the social determinants of health.

Professional Health Education Lacks Cultural Diversity

Culture diversity is an issue within the healthcare profession. Minority nurses account for only 16.8% of the professional nursing workforce. Minorities comprise only about 3% of medical school faculty and about 16% of nursing faculty (Beard, 2021). Increasing the number of culturally diverse health professionals in the workforce must be an area of emphasis to help ensure equity and understanding in healthcare. Simulation Exercise 7.2 provides an opportunity for reflection on components of cultural diversity within the profession while interviewing a nurse from another culture.

Lack of Diversity in Healthcare Providers

Lack of cultural diversity continues to be an issue within our nursing profession. Minority nurses comprise just 16.8% of the professional nursing workforce. Do you think increasing the number of diverse workers needs to become a priority in healthcare?

CULTURE IN HEALTHCARE

Beliefs

In healthcare, culture provides a relevant context for understanding how patients and families experience

TABLE 7.1 Purnell's Domains of Cultural Assessment

Domains of Cultural Assessment	Sample Areas for Inquiry
Personal heritage	Country of origin, reasons for migration, politics, class distinctions, education, social and economic status
Communication	Dominant language and dialects, personal space, body language and touch, time relationships, greetings, eye contact
Family roles and organization	Gender roles; roles of extended family, elders, head of household; family goals, priorities, and expectations; lifestyle differences
Workforce issues	Acculturation and assimilation, gender roles, temporality, current and previous jobs, variance in salary and status associated with job changes
Bioecology	Genetics, hereditary factors, ethnic physical characteristics, drug metabolism
High-risk health behaviors	Drugs, nicotine and alcohol use, sexual behaviors
Nutrition	Meaning of food, availability and food preferences, taboos associated with food, use of food in illness
Pregnancy and childbearing	Rituals and constraints during pregnancy, labor and delivery practices, newborn and postpartum care
Death rituals	How death is viewed, death rituals, preparation of the body, care after death, use of advance directives, bereavement practices
Spirituality	Religious practices, spiritual meanings, use of prayer
Healthcare practices	Traditional practices, religious healthcare beliefs, individual versus collective responsibility for health, how pain is expressed, transplantation, mental health barriers
Healthcare practitioners	Use of traditional and/or folk practitioners, gender role preferences in healthcare

Adapted from Purnell, J. D., & Paulanka, B. J. (2013). *Transcultural health care: A culturally competent approach* (4th ed.). Philadelphia: F.A. Davis.

health and illness. Cultural beliefs and values help explain how people approach shared decision-making and participate in patient-centered self-management care. In high-context cultures, such as Asian and Latino cultures, family involvement in decision-making is desirable, and family-centered decision-making tends to prevail over self-determination.

Genetic versus Cultural Determinants of Health Status

Physiological risk factors and vulnerabilities are often attributed to ethnic groups. For example, do you think Native Americans have a higher incidence of alcoholism? Or do you associate sickle cell disease with African Americans? Poor socioeconomic status is a social determinant of health. Do you think the higher occurrence of heart disease, diabetes, cancer among indigenous populations is due to their genetic heritage or a reflection of socioeconomic variables? Understanding embedded cultural considerations in healthcare delivery enhances compliance with treatment. Culture acts as a crucial filter through which we view others.

Economics

The nation's health agenda, *Healthy People 2030*, says **health disparity** is closely linked with a person's socioeconomic status. The inequity present in health disparities influences a person's capacity to achieve positive health outcomes, experience satisfaction with treatment, and achieve healthy well-being through normal channels.

Access

Laurencin and McClinton (2020) say minorities continue to have limited access to healthcare clinics or providers.

Outcomes

Culturally competent care is said to result in higher levels of patient satisfaction and perception of equality, better adherence to the treatment plan, and improved health outcomes.

Health Disparities

The Institute of Medicine (2002b) reported that people of color and ethnic minorities receive a lower quality of care even when insurance and income were considered.

SIMULATION EXERCISE 7.2 An Interview to Reflect on Diversity in the Nursing Profession

Purpose

To help students learn about the experience of nurses from a different ethnic group.

Procedure

1. Each student will interview a registered nurse from an ethnic minority group different from his or her own ethnic origin.
2. The following questions serve as an interview guide:
   a. In what ways was your educational experience more difficult or easier as a minority student?
   b. What do you see as the barriers for minority nurses in our profession?
   c. What do you see as the opportunities for minority nurses in our profession?
   d. What do you view as the value of increasing diversity in the nursing profession for healthcare?
   e. What do you think we can do as a profession and personally to increase diversity in nursing?
3. Write a one- to two-page narrative report about your findings to be presented in a follow-up class.

Reflective Discussion Analysis

1. What were the common themes that seemed to be present across narratives?
2. In what ways, if any, did doing this exercise influence your thinking about diversity?
3. Did you find any of the answers to the interview questions disturbing or surprising?
4. How could you use this exercise to become culturally competent?

The *National Healthcare Quality and Disparities Report* (AHRQ, 2020) confirms that racial minorities that comprise 30% of our population continue to have higher mortality and morbidity rates. The US Preventive Services Task Force (Doubeni et al., 2021) acknowledges that preventive healthcare services are not equitably available to minorities. Despite legislation designed to create equitable care available to all, progress has been slow. Inequities were further exposed during the recent pandemic. Health disparities create an increased health burden on certain segments of the population, particularly those with the least ability to correct their health situation. The IOM (2002a) identified economic status and social class as components of diversity related to health risk.

Etiology

Healthcare inequities are not as much related to cultural identity as to lower income, making it more difficult is a fee-for-use medical system.

Social Determinants of Health

People use many different terms to describe healthcare access and use, including social issues (WHO, n.d.). Common factors, including those identified in *Healthy People 2030* (USDHHS, n.d.) include the following:

- *Insurance status:* Lack of insurance coverage impedes use of healthcare.
- *Economic status:* Poorer people are less able to afford care, especially preventive care, adequate housing, prescribed medications, and so on. Lack of stable housing is cited in the *Future of Nursing 2020–30* report as impeding care delivery.
- *Housing instability:* Delivering healthcare in the community becomes a challenge when people of limited financial means lack stable housing (Fauteux, 2021).
- *Educational status:* People with low health literacy are less able to navigate the system or to incorporate health teaching.
- *Attitudes:* Much has been written about lack of trust in the healthcare system, about the implicit biases of providers, and about discriminatory practices against minorities.

Incidence

According to the National Health Care Quality and Disparities Report of 2019, we have made some gains in access to care by minorities. But on 30%–40% of the quality measures, Blacks, American Indians, Alaskan Natives, Hispanics, and Asians received worse care than whites. Freedland sees this higher risk pattern as systemic, result of many decades of lower quality care (Freedland et al., 2020). The US Congress receives an annual report on the nation's health, yet many were struck by the overt inadequacies in care exposed by the COVID-19 pandemic.

Cultural Determinants of Healthcare

Health disparities adversely affect certain populations and groups of people who have systematically experienced greater obstacles to healthcare. Disparities can reflect an ethnic group; a religion; SES; education, gender, and age; mental health; and cognitive, sensory, or physical disability. Sexual orientation or gender identity, geographic locale, and physical or mental disability create informal disparities, historically linked to discrimination, but not always recognized as a challenge to equity in healthcare.

- *Poverty:* Poverty is a primary determinant of childhood intellectual, emotional, and social developmental factors and is an excellent predictor of nearly every adult disease (Raphael, 2009). People living in poverty think carefully about seeking medical attention. Often the emergency department is their only source for care. The idea that the poor can exercise choice or implement health promotion activities is not necessarily part of their worldview. Care strategies need to overcome a sense of hopelessness through proactive and patient-oriented approaches. It means treating each patient as a culturally unique person who has formed opinions about their disease process and its treatment.

- *Racism:* Racism is defined as acceptance of biases and stereotypes attributed to a group. The incidence is widespread. In fact, the National Academies Future of Nursing Report (2021) states that nurses must be prepared to deal with structural racism. Roberts writes about the pain African American nurses experience when they are subjected to demeaning comments from patients, peers, or supervisors (Roberts, 2020). If you observed an incident, how would you deal with it?
- *Mistrust:* America has a long history of misuse of minorities by government entities, in terms of healthcare, unethical medical experiments, and lack of funding for needed health services (Warren et al., 2017).

Ethnicity and Related Concepts

Ethnicity

This is a description of a person's awareness of a shared cultural heritage with others based on common racial, geographic, ancestral, religious, or historical bonds. People develop a sense of identity associated with a particular heritage that passes from generation to generation. **Ethnicity** creates a sense of belonging and inspires a strong commitment to associated values and practices. Ethnicity is a social construct, not a descriptor of race or physical features. People with similar skin color and features can have a vastly different ethnic heritage.

Ethnocentrism

Ethnocentrism is defined as a belief that one's own culture is superior to others. The concept of ethnocentrism can foster the belief that one's culture has the right to impose its standards of "correct" behavior and values on another culture.

Cultural Relativism

Cultural relativism holds that each culture is unique, and its merits should be judged only on the basis of its own values and standards. Behaviors viewed as unusual from outside a culture can make perfect sense when they are evaluated within a cultural context.

World View

Following Leininger's definition, we mean the outlook a person develops through when they consider others in groups, nations, and globally.

Intercultural Communication in Healthcare

Intercultural communication refers to conversations taking place between people from different cultures. The concept embraces differences in perceptions, language, and nonverbal behaviors and results in a recognition of different interpretive contexts. It is a primary means of sharing meaning and developing relationships between people of different cultures. Effective intercultural interactions take place within transcultural caring relationships. This means that the patient's *perception* of his or her relationship with the nurse can be just as important as the words used in the communication. Reflect on the Mrs Sou case.

Case Study: Mrs Sou is Admitted to the Obstetrics Unit

A Chinese first-time mother, tense and afraid as she entered the transition phase of labor, speaks no English. Her husband speaks very little and considers birthing as women's work. Callister's (2001) example describes the palpable tension that fills the room. The nurse, Beth, could not speak Chinese, but she tries to convey a sense of caring, touching the woman, speaking softly, modeling supportive behavior for her husband, and helping her to relax as much as possible. The atmosphere in the room changes considerably with the calm competence and quiet demeanor projected by Beth. Following the birth, the father conveyed to her how grateful he was that she spoke Chinese. She tactfully said, "Thank you, but I don't speak Chinese." He looked at her in amazement and said with conviction, "You spoke Chinese."
1. Why did Mr Sou think this?
2. How did Beth communicate?

Language

Developing a common understanding of the issues that speaking different languages creates involves more than understanding vocabulary and grammar is not enough. Cultural language competence requires knowing what to say, and how, when, where, and why to say it.

Within the same language, words can have more than one meaning. For example, the words *hot, warm,* and *cold* can refer to temperature, to impressions of strong personal characteristics, or to responses to new ideas. Idioms are particularly problematic because they represent a nonliteral expression of an idea. Neuliep (2015) describes how, in the United States, the word *bomb* is used not to only to refer to an explosive device but slangily to express doing poorly on an examination. Nonverbal behaviors, particularly gestures and eye contact, can have very different meanings in various cultures. What is appropriate in one culture can be thought of as discourteous or insulting in another culture.

Even when a patient speaks good English, it is best to use clear, simple language rather than complex words and to speak slowly. Despite having relatively strong verbal skills in an adopted language, many people with English as a second language lack the complex vocabulary in

---

DEVELOPING AN EVIDENCE-BASED PRACTICE

Even though recent nursing literature has many articles on healthcare inequity, relatively few research studies are available. The researchers at the Agency for Health Care Research and Quality (AHRQ, 2019) systematically reviewed 120 published research studies to examine, in part, barriers to preventive healthcare for populations adversely affected by disparities: Asians, African Americans, Hispanics, rural, and other low-income patients. They examined barriers to screenings for colorectal cancer, breast cancer, and cervical cancer, also looking at smoking cessation programs. Various outreach interventions to reduce disparities were examined.

Findings

Supplementary reminders to patients navigating screening appointments such as mail or phone reminders, educational materials, and educational videos with physician reminders improved the rates of screenings (colorectal = high; breast = moderate; cervical cancer = moderate).

Strength of the evidence: AHRQ states the strength of evidence is low, mostly due to lack of quality research.

Implications for Your Clinical Practice

1. Recognize that many do not have regular primary care providers, so reminders for screening preventive care needs require extra outreach. One study found reminders to adult parents during pediatric well child visits were effective! So include reminders in all your patient education efforts.
2. Facilitate community engagement, enlist professional and social organizations such as churches.
3. Lack of insurance can discourage people from getting needed screenings, so free clinics, safety net clinics, or screening programs at health departments can be publicized.

Reference

Agency for Healthcare Research and Quality (AHRQ). (2019). Achieving health equity in preventive services: Evidence summary. *Comparative effectiveness review number 222*. Retrieved from https://effectivehealthcare.ahrq.gov /sites/default/files/cer-222-evidence-summary-health-equity.pdf. (Accessed 23 June 2021).

English needed to quickly grasp what is being said. Think about your own experiences learning a foreign language in school. You probably were more comfortable expressing yourself in simple terms, basically because you did not have the more complex vocabulary needed to understand language nuances and multiple meanings. You could attend to the conversation better when the words were spoken slowly with spacing between words. Frequent checks for understanding facilitate communication with culturally diverse patients.

APPLICATIONS

Importance of Culture in Healthcare Communication

We live in a global society, created by dramatic changes in immigration patterns and instant technological connectivity creating an environment where cross-cultural awareness and intercultural communication competence are a necessity. In the United States, the healthcare system is extremely complex and fragmented (Braithwaite et al., 2020). Cultural differences and speaking English as a second language make it even more difficult to navigate the system.

The Institute of Medicine (2002b, 2003) identifies ineffective communication as a significant source of health disparities, that is, unequal care and health outcomes among minority populations in the United States. This makes the nurse's ability to communicate and function effectively with culturally diverse patients even more important, as nurses frequently have the most consistent and continuous contact with people seeking medical treatment and health information. Can you accommodate health beliefs that differ from your more mainstream, scientifically based ones? Reflect on the Gupta case as you read the next few pages.

Case Study: Mrs Barrete Gupta's Cultural Heritage

Mrs Gupta is a 47-year-old woman, a practicing Hindu, who emigrated 30 years ago from India. She is seen in your clinic for uncontrolled hypertension. Sarah Rey, RN, is a home health nurse working out of this clinic. Her mission is to make scheduled follow-up home visits to reinforce antihypertension treatment options. She works with Mrs Gupta to establish trust, answering all her questions and seeking information about the homeopathic treatments she is self-administering. While encouraging her to take the doctor-prescribed antihypertensive medication, she is open to those patients' homeopathic

TABLE 7.2 Assessing Patient Preferences When the Patient Is from a Different Culture

Areas to Assess	Sample Assessment Questions
Explanatory models of illness	"What do you think caused your health problem? Can you tell me a little about how your illness developed?"
Traditional healing processes	"Can you tell me something about how this problem is handled in your country? Are there any special cultural beliefs about your illness that might help me give you better care? Are you currently using any medications or herbs to treat your illness?"
Lifestyle	"What are some of the foods you like? How are they prepared? What do people do in your culture to stay healthy?"
Type of family support	"Can you tell me who in your family should be involved with your care? Who is the decision-maker for healthcare decisions?"
Spiritual healing practices and rituals	"I am not really familiar with your spiritual practices, but I wonder if you could tell me what would be important to you so we can try to incorporate it into your care plan."
Cultural norms about personal care	"A number of our patients have special needs around personal care, of which we are not always aware. I am wondering if this is true for you and if you could help me understand what you need to be comfortable."
Truth-telling and level of disclosure	Ask the family about cultural ways of talking about serious illness. In some cultures, the family knows the diagnosis/prognosis, which is not told to the ill person (e.g., Hispanic, Asian).
Ritual and religious ceremonies at time of death	Ask the family about special rituals and religious ceremonies at time of death.

treatments that are not incompatible. Sarah helps Mrs Gupta select low-sodium foods that still meet her culturally preferred vegetarian diet.

1. What other information does Sarah need to learn about this culture and her patient's beliefs?

Care of the Culturally Diverse Patient

Communication must be considered within the context of overall care. Intercultural care requires effective communication. Nurses need cultural *knowledge*; ability to select appropriate communication *skills*; and ability to have an *attitude* of acceptance of differences.

Nursing

Knowledge. A component of effective intercultural communication relates to developing knowledge of common behavioral response patterns associated with different cultures and worldviews.

Culturally Competent Communication. Intercultural communication requires effort and places increased demands on a nurse's time (Hemberg & Vilander, 2017). Knowledge of cultural norms is essential for nurses. Awareness of cultural differences is basic as is sensitivity to differences in beliefs about one's body, health, or

treatment. Finding ways to bridge these differences and form a partnership with your patient is crucial.

Language. Recent immigrants or those who may not speak English appreciate a nurse who takes the time to find translation or refers them to case managers or social workers who can arrange this. Ask simple questions during assessment as listed in Table 7.2. Nurses demonstrate cultural sensitivity by using neutral words and behaviors, which are respectful of the patient's culture, and avoiding could be interpreted as offensive (AACN, 2008). A valuable way to learn about another person's culture is to spend time with them and to ask frequent questions about what is important to them about their culture. Even if the patient speaks English, always allow additional time for communication processing. People with English as a second language tend to think and process information in their native language, translating back and forth from English.

Nonverbal Cultural Differences. Be aware that gestures can have less acceptable connotations in other cultures. An example is pointing, which is considered rude by some. Eye contact and touch can also be misinterpreted. An example might be a recent emigrant from the Middle East who interprets such behavior from a female nurse as disrespectful.

Nursing Skills

Assessment. When meeting a patent for the first time, your goal is to build rapport. You should introduce self and identify your role; call the patient by name to show respect (ask how to pronounce it if unsure); speak clearly, allowing time for translation or processing and spending more time; avoid assumptions until validated; allow more time to assess language use and understanding; inquire about patient's health beliefs about current illness in your position as an open-minded learner; and ask permission for use of tools for assessment and treatment, explaining their use if necessary.

Interventions. The ability to understand the patient's traditional healthcare interventions can help you make decisions about which can be incorporated into your care plan and which may be harmful and need to be discouraged. For example, placing a medicine bundle at the bedside of a traditional Native American patient does not interfere with the treatment plan. On the other hand, how would you handle it if a patient from Haiti refuses medication for his HIV-positive treatment in favor of traditional herbs?

Evaluation of Care and Teaching. Does your patient's culture have strong beliefs about family involvement in decision-making? When your patient expresses preference for their healthcare decisions and disclosure of diagnostic information, their preferences should be honored. For example, some Asian, Hispanic, and Black-American families prefer decisions be made by the family. Thus, inclusion of family in health teaching is essential.

Framing Patient Teaching With Culturally Diverse Patients

The LEARN model is used to frame clinical teaching and coaching encounters with culturally diverse patients.

- **L**isten carefully to patient perceptions and the words the patient uses. Ask the patient to describe the illness or injury, how it occurred, and what the patient believes caused it.
- **E**xplain what the patient needs to understand about his or her condition or treatment, incorporating patient's words and explanatory models.
- **A**cknowledge cultural differences between nurse and patient viewpoints, without devaluing the patient's viewpoint. Respect cultural sources of healthcare, and incorporate culturally acceptable treatments and interventions when possible. Ask about cultural and family treatment considerations. Use frequent validation to ensure the cultural appropriateness of provider assumptions.
- **R**ecommend what the patient should do. Frame treatment suggestions using a culturally acceptable care process. Invite patient participation in developing a plan that is culturally authentic and therapeutic.
- **N**egotiate with the patient to culturally adapt constructive self-management strategies based on patient input. Negotiation of cultural acceptability is fundamental to

patient compliance. Familiarity with formal and informal sources of healthcare, such as churches, shamans, medicine men and women, curanderos, and other faith healers, provides additional patient support.

Improving Culturally Competent Care

Cultural competence is defined as a set of cultural behaviors and attitudes integrated into the practice methods of a system, agency, or its professionals that enables them to work effectively in cross-cultural situations. The concept represents a process, not an event. Fig. 7.1 provides a graphic depiction of this process for improving cultural care competence. The IOM (2003) and the American Association of Colleges of Nursing (AACN, 2008) identify cultural competence as an essential skill set required for professional nurses and other healthcare providers.

Minority populations, especially new immigrants, have special problems with access and continuity of healthcare. They are often marginalized economically, occupationally, and socially in ways that adversely affect their access to mainstream healthcare. Accessing healthcare can be so frustrating that they give up when they meet even small obstacles. A secondary issue is a lack of knowledge and experience with how to obtain services. Undocumented immigrants have an added burden of fearing deportation if their legal status is revealed. Nurses can help patients successfully navigate the healthcare system. Patients also appreciate providers who orient them to the clinical setting and set the stage for a comfortable encounter.

The Institute of Medicine (IOM, 2002a) report on *Speaking of Health* established guidelines to promote more effective communication practices in diverse communities. Nurses need to view cultural diversity as a solid dimension of effective healthcare. It is important to avoid making assumptions about the degree to which patients embrace particular cultural beliefs because of issues such as acculturation and significant life experiences. Understanding cultural patterns helps normalize behaviors, attitudes, and values as being different, rather than as being wrong or inferior.

National Culturally and Linguistically Appropriate Services Standards

In April 2017, the Office of Minority Health of the DHHS published a revised culturally and linguistically appropriate services (CLAS) policies and practices document. Known as the National Standards for Culturally and Linguistically Appropriate Services in Health and Health Care, the CLAS document provides a national blueprint for advancing health equity by reducing health disparities (USDHHS, 2017).

The overarching CLAS standard is to provide effective, equitable, understandable, and respectful quality care and services that are responsive to diverse cultural health beliefs

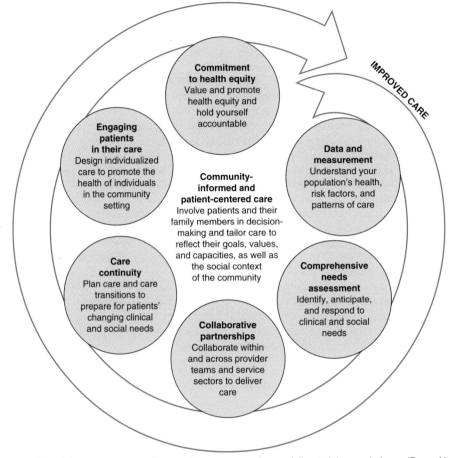

Figure 7.1 Promising systems practices to improve care for socially at-risk populations. (From National Academies of Sciences, Engineering, and Medicine. (2016). *Systems practices for the care of socially at-risk populations*. Washington, DC: The National Academies Press.)

and practices, preferred languages, health literacy, and other communication needs. Five population groups were identified, including people with disabilities, low health literacy, limited English proficiency, racial/ethnic minorities, and sexual and gender minorities.

Specific objectives are designed to improve the accessibility and quality of service for diverse populations. A related goal is to provide services in a manner that respects the personalized cultural perspectives of diverse populations. Simulation Exercise 7.3 examines values and perceptions associated with different cultures.

Characteristics of a Culturally Competent Nurse

Knowledge

Cultural competence is a learned process. Learning about every different culture would be impossible, but developing knowledge about one or two that many of your patients come from is doable. Focus on common behavioral responses. For example, our midwestern emergency department had many pediatric patients recently relocated from Appalachia. The father in these families was often nonverbal during the visit but actually was the decision-maker, so he needed to be addressed regarding diagnosis and treatment.

Skills

We deliberately select communication that is sensitive to a patient's cultural preference, using neutral words. We abide by nonverbal prohibitions, such as a desire to not be touched. We explain clearly the Western medical treatment regimen, but evaluate efficacy of use of alternative, culturally derived regimens.

Validation is an important communication strategy with culturally diverse patients, as word meanings are not

SIMULATION EXERCISE 7.3 Conducting a Culturally Sensitive Assessment

Purpose
To practice assessment related to cultural issues and to improve your cultural competence.

Procedure
Watch any social justice media presentation. Suggested possibilities are short vignettes on YouTube.

Reflective Discussion Analysis
1. In a small group, discuss the main idea presented.
2. What were your thoughts and feelings following viewing a video?

---

the same even within a culture. In many cultures, there is a tendency to view health professionals as authority figures, treating them with deference and respect. This value can be so strong that a patient will not question the nurse or in any way indicate mistrust of professional recommendations. They just do not follow the professional advice. Using teach-back and having patients repeat process instructions improve compliance. Families from other cultures might rely on folk medicines or other alternative healthcare remedies. We need to understand the patient's healthcare traditions, which are fundamental in an individual's culture.

Attitude
Culturally competent nurses are aware of their own cultural biases and recognize the need to adapt their communication to fit into their patient's expectations. We all harbor bias, even if unintentionally. Often we feel our culture or our knowledge of medicine gives us the "right" answer. Can you cite an example? McGee-Avila (2018) suggests that while healthcare team members have medical expertise, we need to recognize that each patient has unique life experience expertise.

Nurses need to practice self-reflection and be open to learning. Nurses dealing with patients from a different culture value a willingness to acknowledge their own missteps (Warren, 2017).

Cultural sensitivity is an integral part of competence. The Office of Minority Health (USDHHS, 2018) defines *cultural sensitivity* as the ability to be appropriately responsive to the attitudes, feelings, or circumstances of groups of people that share a common and distinctive racial, national, religious, linguistic, or cultural heritage. Cultural sensitivity emphasizes an openness to different cultural beliefs and values, with a corresponding willingness to incorporate the patient's cultural values in care whenever possible. Cultural sensitivity

facilitates care and self-management of health conditions. It is hard for patients to overlook a significant tradition. When health recommendations conflict with their worldview, patients are less likely to follow them.

Can you accept the legitimacy of patient concerns, even if they are outside your cultural experience? Perkins (2021) says it is necessary to acknowledge any minority patients expression of fears, distrust, and concerns, even if our forebears did not have the same discriminatory historical experiences.

Cultural Humility
Recent literature suggests that cultural humility is a better term than cultural competency. **Cultural humility** is defined as a process of openness, self-awareness, being egoless, and incorporating self-reflection and critique after willingly interacting with diverse individuals. The results of achieving cultural humility are mutual empowerment, respect, partnerships, optimal care, and lifelong learning (Foronda et al., 2018). This terminology pinpoints an attitude that is characterized by openness and a willingness to learn from patients about their beliefs. While we and healthcare team members have the medical expertise, we recognize that patients are the expert in their own health.

Use of Interpreters
Federal law (Title VI of the Civil Rights Act) mandates the use of a trained interpreter for any patient experiencing communication difficulties in healthcare settings due to language. Interpreters should have a thorough knowledge of the culture and the language. Interpreters are available virtually, or by telephone, or employed by agencies. Try to avoid using family or friends, as there are quality assurance and ethical issues.

Time Orientation
Culturally, clock time versus activity time can reflect cultural standards. This can be a major issue when appointments or medications are involved. Precise time frames are important in low-context cultures (North America and Western Europe). People in these cultures are accustomed to setting and meeting exact time commitments for appointments and taking medications. In high-context cultures, individuals do not consider commitment to a future appointment as important as attending to what is happening in the moment. Time is a more flexible concept in such cultures.

SUMMARY

This chapter explores the intercultural communication situations that occur when the nurse and patient are from different cultures. Culture is defined as a common collectivity of beliefs, values, shared understandings, and patterns of behavior of a designated group of people. Culture needs to be viewed as a human structure with many variations in meaning.

Intercultural communication is defined as a communication in which the sender of a message is a member of one culture and the receiver of the message is from a different culture. Different cultures create and express different personal realities.

A *culturally sensitive assessment* is defined as a systematic appraisal of beliefs, values, and practices conducted to determine the context of patient needs and to tailor nursing interventions. It is composed of three progressive, interconnecting elements: a general assessment, a problem-specific assessment, and the cultural details needed for successful implementation.

Knowledge and acceptance of the patient's right to seek and support alternative healthcare practices dictated by culture are important. They can make a major difference in compliance and successful outcome. Healthcare professionals sometimes mistakenly assume that illness is a single concept, but illness is a personal experience strongly colored by cultural norms, values, social roles, and religious beliefs. Characteristics of a culturally sensitive

nurse were discussed, specific to knowledge, skills, and attitudes. Interventions that take into consideration the specialized needs of the patient from a culturally diverse background follow the mnemonic LEARN: Listen, Explain, Acknowledge, Recommend, and Negotiate.

> **ETHICAL DILEMMA: What Would You Do?**
> Antonia Martinez is admitted to the hospital and needs immediate surgery. She speaks limited English, and her family is not with her. She is frightened by the prospect of surgery and wants to wait until her family can be with her to help her make the decision about surgery. As a nurse, you feel there is no decision to be made: She must have the surgery, and you need to get her consent form signed now. What would you do?

DISCUSSION QUESTIONS

1. In what ways does your cultural identity influence the way you think, feel, and act toward someone of another culture?
2. Think of a person or a patient from another culture, and describe how you think that this person perceives or responds to you as someone from a different culture.
3. In what ways is your patient's culture similar or different from yours?

NEXT-GENERATION NCLEX® EXAMINATION–STYLE CASE STUDY

Addressing Communication Barriers

A 19-year-old Latino migrant worker presents at the local hospital's emergency department (ED) after sustaining a three-inch laceration to the right forearm. The patient neither speaks nor understands English sufficiently to give a medical history or details concerning the accident leading to the wound. The patient appears nervous and teary eyed. After the wound is cleansed and bleeding is controlled, it is determined that stitches and an antibiotic will be required. Postdischarge care will include wound care and follow-up appointment for stitch removal in 2 weeks.

Complete the following sentences by choosing from the list of options.

At this time, to best address the patient's needs, the nurse would first _____(1)_____ to _____(2)_____.

Options for 1	Options for 2
Arrange for a medical translator to be present	Provide emotional support as well as supplement missing medical history information
Request that a friend or family member be called to the ED to translate	Ensure the patient is able to effectively participate in care planning
Contact the hospital's social services department	Assist with post-discharge recovery care needs

REFERENCES

Agency for Healthcare Research and Quality (AHRQ). (2020). *2019 national healthcare quality and disparities report.* AHRQ Publication 20(21)-0045-EF Rockville, MD: AHRQ. Retrieved from: https://www.ahrq.gov/sites/default/files/wysiwyg/research/findings/nhqrdr/2019qdr.pdf. [Accessed 23 June 2021].

Alligood, M. R. (2022). *Nursing theorists and their work* (10th ed.). St. Louis: Elsevier.

American Association of Colleges of Nursing (AACN). (2008). *The essentials of baccalaureate education for professional nursing practice.* Washington, DC: AACN. Retrieved from: https://www.aacnnursing.org/portals/42/publications/baccessentials08.pdf. [Accessed 23 June 2021].

American Nurses Association. (2015). *Code of ethics for nurses with interpretative statements.* Silver Spring, MD: ANA.

Beard, K. V. (2021). Moderator: American Nurses Association Webinar Report (2021). Get our house in order. *American Journal of Nursing*, 121(1), 18–20.

Braithwaite, J., Vincent, C., Garcia-Elorrio, E., et al. (2020). Transformational improvement in quality care and health systems: The next decade. *BCM Medicine*, 18(1), 340.

Callister, L. C. (2001). Culturally competent care of women and newborns: Knowledge, attitude, and skills. *Journal of Obstetric, Gynecologic, and Neonatal Nursing*, 30(2), 209–215.

Doubeni, C. A., Simon, M., & Krist, A. H. (2021). Addressing systemic racism through clinical preventive services:

Recommendations from the U.S. Preventive Services Task Force. *Journal of the American Medical Association, 325*(7), 627–628.

Fauteux, N. (2021). Beyond screening: Health systems invest in social determinants of health. *American Journal of Nursing, 121*(2), 53–55.

Foronda, C. L., Baptiste, D. L., Pfaff, T., et al. (2018). Cultural competency and cultural humility in simulation-based education: An integrative review. *Clinical Simulation in Nursing, 15*, 42–60.

Freedland, K. E., Dew, M. A., Sarwer, D. B., et al. (2020). Health psychology in the time of COVID-19. *Health Psychology, 39*(12), 1021–1025.

Hemberg, J. A. V., & Vilander, S. (2017). Culture and communicative competencies in the caring relationship with patients from another culture. *Scandinavian Journal of Caring Sciences, 31*(4), 822–929.

Institute of Medicine (IOM). (2002a). *Speaking of health: Assessing health communication strategies for diverse populations*. Washington, DC: National Academy Press.

Institute of Medicine (IOM). (2002b). *Unequal treatment. What healthcare providers need to know about racial and ethnic disparities in healthcare*. Washington, DC: National Academy Press.

Institute of Medicine (IOM). (2003). *Unequal treatment: Confronting racial and ethnic disparities in health care*. Washington, DC: National Academy Press.

Laurencin, C. T., & McClinton, A. (2020). The COVID-19 pandemic: A call to action to identify and address racial and ethnic disparities. *Journal of Racial and Ethnic Health Disparities, 7*(3), 398–402.

Leininger, M. M. (1988). Leininger's theory of nursing: Cultural care diversity and universality. *Nursing Science Quarterly, 1*(4), 152–160.

Leininger, M., & McFarland, R. (Eds.). (2006). *Culture care diversity and universality: A worldwide nursing theory*. Sudbury, MA: Jones & Bartlett.

McGee-Avila, J. (2018). *Practicing cultural humility to transform health care*. [Blog post] Robert Wood Johnson Foundation [website]. Retrieved at: https://www.rwjf.org/en/blog/2018/06/practicing-cultural-humility-to-transform-healthcare.html. [Accessed 23 June 2021].

National Academies of Science, Engineering, and Medicine. (2021). *The Future of Nursing 2020–2030: Charting a path to achieve health equity*. Washington, DC: The National Academies Press.

Neuliep, J. (2015). *Intercultural communication: A contextual approach*. Thousand Oaks, CA: Sage Publications.

Perkins, D. E. (2021). A COVID-19 vaccination challenge. *American Journal of Nursing, 121*(3), 11.

Purnell, L. D. (2013). *Transcultural healthcare: A culturally competent approach* (4th ed.). Philadelphia: F.A. Davis.

Raphael, D. (2009). Poverty, human development, and health in Canada: Research, practice, and advocacy dilemmas. *Canadian Journal of Nursing Research, 41*(2), 7–18.

Roberts, D. C. (2020). The elephant in the room. *Nursing, 50*(12), 42–46.

Smith, L. S. (2018). A nurse educator's guide to cultural competence. *Nursing Management, 49*(2), 11–14.

Szalay, L. B. (1981). Intercultural communication—a process model. *International Journal of Intercultural Relations, 5*(2), 133–146.

U.S. Department of Health and Human Services (USDHHS). (n.d.). *Healthy people 2030 [website]*. Social determinants of health. Retrieved from: https://health.gov/healthypeople/objectives-and-data/social-determinants-health. [Accessed 23 June 2021].

U.S. Department of Health and Human Services, Office of Minority Health (USDHHS). (2017). *National standards for culturally and linguistically appropriate services in health care*. Washington, DC: Author.

U.S. Department of Health and Human Services, Office of Minority Health (USDHHS). (2018). *Culturally competent nursing care: A cornerstone of caring*. Retrieved from: https://ccnm.thinkculturalhealth.hhs.gov/. [Accessed 23 June 2021].

Warren, N., Baptiste, D. L., Foronda, C., & Mark, H. D. (2017). Evaluation of an intervention to improve clinical nurse educators' knowledge, perceived skills, and confidence related to diversity. *Nurse Educator, 42*(6), 320–323.

World Health Organization (WHO). (n.d.). *Social determinants of health*. Retrieved from: https://www.who.int/health-topics/social-determinants-of-health#tab=tab_1. [Accessed 23 June 2021].

8

Communicating in Groups

OBJECTIVES

At the end of the chapter, the reader will be able to:

1. Identify the characteristics of small group communication in contemporary healthcare.
2. Discuss the stages of small group development.
3. Compare and contrast different types of therapeutic groups.
4. Apply group concepts in therapeutic groups.
5. Apply evidence-based intervention to group simulation.

Group membership is routine in all aspects of human life. We work together in school, at our jobs in clinical practice, in community activities, and in many other areas. As part of social identification, we behave in accordance with the norms of our identified groups (van den Broek et al., 2021). In healthcare, group communication format is a major means for communicating with both patients in treatment groups and coworkers in work groups.

Communication formats are used extensively as a major means of communication for clinical knowledge sharing and decision-making. The group format provides us with opportunities to provide information, express ideas, take positions, share our perspectives, and learn from others' perspectives. Meeussen et al. (2018) do note that diversities among group members may affect group dynamics, potentially leading to innovation and creativity. This chapter focuses on group communication in healthcare.

BASIC CONCEPTS

Definition

Human communication within a group is defined as an interdependent system of three or more individuals, interacting for the achievement of some common goal. They influence one another through multiple inputs and responses, with each group member's contribution having an influence on the behavior and responses of other group members. Over time, a group culture emerges. Every group has its own identity and structure, but we will discuss some commonalities. Reflect on the Mary Tyler case.

CASE STUDY: Mary Tyler and Her Student Support Group

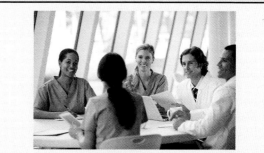

Copyright © monkeybusinessimages/iStock/Thinkstock.

Mary Tyler is 18 years old and in her second year as a student nurse. She is assigned to a clinical rotation with six other students under the guidance of an instructor who is not her clinical supervisor. The group meets weekly this first semester as a support group to facilitate adjustment to working in the hospital and to reflect on communication skill learning. It is not a clinical postconference group to discuss patients. Observe this picture of a student group; if you were the leader, how would you engage these students?

Structure

Primary Groups

Primary groups are characterized by an informal structure and close personal relationships. Group membership in primary groups is automatic such as being born into a family. Or it can be voluntarily chosen because of a strong common interest such as long-term school friendships. There are no previously determined end dates and primary groups are a source of socialization.

Secondary Groups

Secondary groups are time-limited. Group size is determined by goals and functions. They have a prescribed formal structure, a designated leader, and specific goals and functions. When the group completes its task, or achieves its goals, the group ends.

Group Communication in Healthcare

Counseling and therapy groups, psychoeducation, work groups, and interprofessional clinical teams functioning within a larger healthcare system setting rely on aspects of group communication to achieve designated goals in healthcare settings. Multiple informational inputs available in small groups are an invaluable input resource in professional clinical education.

Nurses are involved in task forces and committees to help strengthen health systems and improve clinical outcomes within the profession, on interprofessional healthcare teams, and in groups within the larger community. Group communication provides a central means of communicating with others within and between clinical settings. As you work with others in small group formats to complete educational projects or engage in related reflective analysis discussions of simulated and experiential clinical scenarios, you are using group communication skills. Interprofessional education and practice collaboration uses small group communication as a fundamental form of interaction. Types of groups are listed in Table 8.1.

CHARACTERISTICS OF SMALL GROUP COMMUNICATION THERAPY

Group Purpose

The group purpose provides the rationale for a group's existence and direction for group decisions. In patient healthcare, types of groups include therapy groups, support groups, activity groups, and health education groups. We also have many staff work groups. Purpose influences the type of communication and activities required to meet group goals. For example, the purpose of group therapy would be to improve the interpersonal functioning of individual members, while a support group seeks and provides emotional assistance. An example would be Alcoholics Anonymous meetings. Health education groups meet to share information and often include family members.

TABLE 8.1 Group Type and Purpose

Group	Purpose
Therapy	Reality testing, encouraging personal growth, inspiring hope, strengthening personal resources, developing interpersonal skills
Support	Giving and receiving practical information and advice, supporting coping skills, promoting self-esteem, enhancing problem-solving skills, encouraging patient autonomy, strengthening hope and resiliency
Activity	Getting people in touch with their bodies, releasing energy, enhancing self-esteem, encouraging cooperation, stimulating spontaneous interaction, supporting creativity
Health education	Learning new knowledge, promoting skill development, providing support and feedback, supporting development of competency, promoting discussion of important health-related issues

In a work group, the purpose would support a better solution to implementation of a specific work-related issue, such as wait times, transfer processes, or introduction of a new program or protocol. Health teams are groups of professionals from several disciplines who meet to coordinate and share communication to enhance delivery of quality healthcare to assigned patients.

Group Goals

Group goals define expected therapeutic outcomes in a process group or describe a defined work outcome in a task group, indicating goal achievement. Goals serve as benchmarks for successful achievement. Matching group goals with member needs and characteristics is essential in counseling and therapeutic groups. In work groups, the match should be between group members' expertise/skills, interests, and goal requirements.

General group goals should be of interest to the group members. Group members need to understand and commit to achieving group goals. Goals need to be achievable, measurable, and within the capabilities of group membership. A good match energizes a group; members develop commitment and interest because they perceive the group as having value.

BOX 8.1 Communication Principles to Facilitate Cohesiveness

- Group tasks should be within the membership's range of ability and expertise.
- Comments and responses should be nonevaluative, focused on behaviors rather than on personal characteristics.
- The leader should point out group accomplishments and acknowledge member contributions.
- The leader should be empathetic and teach members how to give effective feedback.
- The leader should help group members view and work through creative tension as being a valuable part of goal achievement.

Cohesion

Group unity or **cohesion** results when members desire to work together to accomplish their goals. Cohesiveness is described in Box 8.1. Sources of cohesiveness include shared goals, working through and solving problems, and the nature of group interaction. A sense of interconnection is the basis for group identity and is an essential characteristic of optimum group productivity.

Group Size and Composition

Group purpose dictates group size. Patient-centered therapeutic groups consist of six to eight members. With fewer than five members, deep sharing tends to be limited. Education-focused groups, such as medication, psycho-education, diagnosis, skill training, and treatment groups, can have 10 or more members. Membership on interdisciplinary teams varies, depending in part on patient needs. They typically reflect the essential number of healthcare professionals needed to coordinate and share care responsibility for a common patient population.

Careful selection of group members should be based on functional similarity, commitment to identified group goals, and basic knowledge of how group communication processes enable goal achievement. A person's capacity to derive benefit from the group and to contribute to group goals is a critical requirement for patient therapy groups.

Functional similarity is defined as choosing the group members who are similar enough—intellectually, emotionally, and experientially—to interact with one another in a meaningful way.

Participation can be compromised by a "one-of-a-kind" significant emotional difference, for example, acute psychosis that would interfere with meaningful communication. Group therapy is contraindicated for an acutely psychotic, actively suicidal, paranoid, excessively hostile, or

SIMULATION EXERCISE 8.1   Exploring Functional Similarity

Purpose
To provide an experiential understanding of functional similarity.

Procedure
1. Break class into groups of four to six people.
2. One person should act as a scribe.
3. Identify two characteristics or experiences that all members of your group have in common other than that you are in the same class.
4. Identify two things that are unique to each person in your group (e.g., only child, never moved from the area, born in another country, unique skill or life experience).
5. Each person should elaborate on both the common and different experiences.

Reflective Discussion Analysis
1. What was the effect of finding common ground with other group members?
2. In what ways did finding out about the uniqueness of each person's experience add to the discussion?
3. Did anything in either the discussion of commonalities or differences in experience stimulate further group discussion?
4. How could you use what you have learned in this exercise in your clinical practice?

impulsive patient until symptoms are brought under control. Simulation Exercise 8.1 teaches you about functional similarities.

In work (task) groups, functional similarity consists of choosing members with complementary experiential knowledge or skill sets, plus the interest, commitment, and essential skills to contribute to group goals. This type of functional match produces a higher level of group performance and member satisfaction.

Interpersonal compatibility among group members can enhance task interdependence and the desire to work together as a group. On the other hand, differences in outlook and opinion can enrich group conversation, if not extreme. Working through differences to achieve consensus makes the group process a richer experience, and the outcome will reflect a broader consensus.

Norms

Group norms refer to the unwritten behavioral rules of conduct expected of group members. Norms provide needed predictability for effective group functioning and make the group safe for its members. There are two types of norms: universal and group specific.

Universal. **Universal norms** are explicit behavioral standards, which must be present in all groups to achieve effective outcomes. Examples include confidentiality, regular attendance, and using the group as the forum for discussion rather than individual discussion with members outside of the group. Unless group members in process groups believe that personal information will not be shared outside the group setting (confidentiality), trust will not develop. Regular attendance at group meetings is critical to group stability and goal achievement. Even if the member is a perfect fit with group goals, he or she must fully commit to regular attendance and full participation. Personal relationships between group members outside of the group also threaten the integrity of the group.

Group-specific. **Group-specific norms** are constructed by group members. They represent the shared beliefs, values, and unspoken operational rules governing group functions. Norms help define member interactions. They are often implicit. Examples include the group's tolerance for lateness, use of humor, or confrontation, and talking directly to other group members rather than about them. Simulation Exercise 8.2 can help you develop a deeper understanding of group norms.

Group Role Positions

A person's role position in the group corresponds with the status, power, and internal image that other members in the group hold of the member. Group members assume, or are ascribed, roles that influence their communication and the responses of others in the group. They usually have trouble breaking away from roles they have been cast in despite their best efforts. For example, people will look to the "helper" group member for advice, even when that person lacks expertise or personally needs the group's help. That identified "helper" member may suffer because he or she does not always receive the help he or she needs. Other times, group members project a role position onto a particular group member that represents a hidden agenda or an unresolved issue for the group as a whole. Projection is largely unconscious, but it can be destructive to group functioning. For example, if the group as a whole seems to scapegoat, ignore, defer to, or consistently idealize one of its members, this group projection can compromise the group's effectiveness because of an unrealistic focus on one group member. Simulation Exercise 8.3 considers group role-position expectations with a fun "Headbands" simulation exercise.

Group Dynamics

Group dynamics is a term used to describe the communication processes and behaviors that occur during the life of the group. These underlying forces represent a complex blend of individual and group characteristics that interact with each other to achieve the group purpose. The primary forces operating in groups are individual dynamics (member variables), interpersonal dynamics (group communication variables), and group as a whole dynamics related to purpose and norms. The group leader is charged with integrating these multiple variables into a workable group process. Group work can enhance member confidence, interpersonal skills, and cultural awareness.

Theoretical Concepts: Group Process

Group process refers to the structural development of small group relationships.

Tuckman (1965, 1977) with Jensen developed a *five-stage model of small group development* (forming, storming, norming, performing, and adjourning) that remains the most commonly used framework for the structural development and relationship process of small groups. Stages of group development are applicable to work groups and therapeutic groups. Each sequential phase of group development has its own set of tasks, which build and expand on the work of previous phases. Yalom and

---

SIMULATION EXERCISE 8.2   **Identifying Norms**

Purpose
To help identify norms operating in groups.

Procedure
1. Divide a piece of paper into three columns.
2. In the first column, write the norms you think exist in your class or work group. In the second column, write the norms you think exist in your family. Examples of norms might be as follows: no one gets angry, decisions are made by consensus, assertive behaviors are valued, missed sessions and lateness are not tolerated.
3. Share your norms with the group, first related to the school or work group and then to the family. Place this information in the third column.

Reflective Discussion Analysis
1. What were some of the differences in existing norms for school and work and family?
2. Were there any universal norms on either of your lists?
3. Was there more or less consistency in overall student responses about class and work group norms and family norms? If so, what would account for it?

SIMULATION EXERCISE 8.3 Headbands: Group Role Expectations

Purpose

To experience the pressures of role expectations on group performance.

Procedure

1. Break the group up into a smaller unit of six to eight members. In a large group, a small group performs while the remaining members observe.
2. Make up mailing labels or headbands that can be attached to or tied around the heads of the participants. Each headband is lettered with directions on how the other members should respond to the role. Examples:
   - Comedian: laugh at me
   - Expert: ask my advice
   - Important person: defer to me
   - Stupid: sneer at me
   - Insignificant: ignore me
   - Loser: pity me
   - Boss: obey me
   - Helpless: support me
3. Place a headband on each member in such a way that the member cannot read his or her own label, but the other members can see it easily.
4. Provide a topic for discussion (e.g., why the members chose nursing, the women's movement), and instruct each member to interact with the others in a way that is natural for him or her. Do not role-play; be yourself. React to each member who speaks by following the instructions on the speaker's headband. You are not to tell one another what the headbands say, but simply to react to them.
5. After about 20 min, the facilitator halts the activity and directs each member to guess what his or her headband says and then to take it off and read it.

Reflective Discussion Analysis

Initiate a discussion, including any members who observed the activity. Possible questions include the following:

1. What were some of the problems of trying to be yourself under conditions of group role pressure?
2. How did it feel to be consistently misinterpreted by the group—to have them laugh when you were trying to be serious or ignore you when you were trying to make a point?
3. Did you find yourself changing your behavior in reaction to the group treatment of you—withdrawing when they ignored you, acting confident when they treated you with respect, giving orders when they deferred to you?

Modified from Pfeiffer, J., & Jones, J. (1977). *A handbook of structured experiences for human relations training* (Vol. VI). La Jolla, CA: University Associate Publishers.

Leszcz (2005) developed a similar model to explain group dynamics. Yalom's process explanations are similar to Tuckman's, but the phases of group development use different names. Group structure includes interpersonal interactions, while content often falls into the realm of task activity.

Forming (Orientation Phase)

The forming phase begins when members come together as a group. Members enter group relationships as strangers to one another. The leader orients the group to the group's purpose and asks members to introduce themselves. The information each person shares about himself or herself should be brief and relate to personal data relevant to achieving the group's purpose.

During the forming phase, the leader introduces universal norms (group ground rules) for attendance, participation, and confidentiality. Getting to know one another, finding common threads in personal or professional experience, and acceptance of group goals and tasks are initial group tasks. Members have a basic need for acceptance, so communication is more tentative than it will be later when members know and trust one another.

Storming (Conflict or Catharsis Phase)

The storming phase focuses on power and control issues. Members use testing behaviors around boundaries, communication styles, and personal reactions with other members and the leader. Remember there will be some resistance to change. Characteristic behaviors may include disagreement with the group format, topics for discussion, the best ways to achieve group goals, and comparisons of member contributions. Setting group goals evolves from a brainstorming discussion of alternative concerns generated by its members that the group might pursue. The next step is to choose the most promising issues to focus on as top priority concerns the group feels it can address. According to Freeman et al. (2019), group leaders successfully deal with resistance through relationship building. Although the storming phase is uncomfortable, successful resolution leads to the development of group-specific norms.

Norming (Cohesion or Focus Phase)

In the norming phase, individual goals become aligned with group goals. Group-specific norms help create a supportive group climate characterized by dependable fellowship and purpose. These norms make the group "safe," and members begin to experience the cohesiveness of the group as "their group." The group holds its members accountable and challenges individual members who fail to adhere to expected norms.

Brainstorming. This consists of the group members thinking of as many ideas as possible related to resolving an identified issue. Criticism of any ideas and/or statements of judgment are not permitted in the early stages of brainstorming. Later, the group members will begin to prioritize which potential solutions are the most workable.

Performing (Working Phase)

Most of a group's work gets accomplished in the performing phase. This phase of group development is characterized by interdependence, acceptance of each member as a person of value, and the development of group cohesion. Members feel loyal to the group and engaged in its work. They are comfortable taking risks and are invested enough in one another and the group process to offer constructive comments without fearing censure from other members.

Adjourning (Termination Phase)

Tuckman introduced the adjourning phase as a final phase of group development at a later date (Tuckman & Jensen, 1977). This phase is characterized by reviewing what has been accomplished, reflecting on the meaning of the group's work together, creating deliverables, and making plans to move on in different directions.

Group Role Functions

Functional roles differ from the positional roles that group members assume. Group roles relate to the type of member contributions needed to achieve group goals. Roles are the behaviors members choose to use to move toward goal achievement (task functions) and behaviors designed to ensure personal satisfaction (maintenance functions).

Balance between task and maintenance functions increases group productivity. When task functions predominate, member satisfaction decreases, and a collaborative atmosphere is diminished. When maintenance functions override task functions, members have trouble reaching goals. Members do not confront controversial issues, so the creative tension needed for successful group accomplishment is compromised. Task and maintenance role functions found in successful small groups are listed in Box 8.2.

BOX 8.2   Task and Maintenance Functions in Group Dynamics

Task Functions: Behaviors Relevant to the Attainment of Group Goals

- **Initiating**: Identifies tasks or goals; defines group problem; suggests relevant strategies for solving problem.
- **Seeking information or opinion**: Requests facts from other members; asks other members for opinions; seeks suggestions or ideas for task accomplishment.
- **Giving information or opinion**: Offers facts to other members; provides useful information about group concerns.
- **Clarifying, elaborating**: Interprets ideas or suggestions placed before group; paraphrases key ideas; defines terms; adds information.
- **Summarizing**: Pulls related ideas together; restates key ideas; offers a group solution or suggestion for other members to accept or reject.
- **Consensus taking**: Checks to see whether group has reached a conclusion; asks group to test a possible decision.

Maintenance Functions: Behaviors That Help the Group Maintain Harmonious Working Relationships

- **Harmonizing:** Attempts to reconcile disagreements; helps members reduce conflict and explore differences in a constructive manner.
- **Gatekeeping:** Helps keep communication channels open; points out commonalties in remarks; suggests approaches that permit greater sharing.
- **Encouraging:** Indicates by words and body language unconditional acceptance of others; agrees with contributions of other group members; is warm, friendly, and responsive to other group members.
- **Compromising:** Admits mistakes; offers a concession when appropriate; modifies position in the interest of group cohesion.
- **Setting standards:** Calls for the group to reassess or confirm implicit and explicit group norms when appropriate.

Note: Every group needs both types of functions and needs to work out a satisfactory balance of task and maintenance activity.

Dysfunction

Sometimes a group member acts in ways that do not advance the purpose of the group. An example of a dysfunctional role is known as *"self-role."* The person unconsciously acts to meet self-needs at the expense of other

TABLE 8.2   Nonfunctional Self-Roles

Role	Characteristics
Aggressor	Criticizes or blames others, personally attacks other members, uses sarcasm and hostility in interactions
Blocker	Instantly rejects ideas or argues an idea to death, cites tangential ideas and opinions, obstructs decision-making
Joker	Disrupts work of the group by constantly joking and refusing to take group task seriously
Avoider	Whispers to others, daydreams, doodles, acts indifferent and passive
Self-confessor	Uses the group to express personal views and feelings unrelated to group task
Recognition seeker	Seeks attention by excessive talking, trying to gain leader's favor, expressing extreme ideas or demonstrating peculiar behavior

members' needs, group values, and goal achievement. As identified in Table 8.2, nonfunctional self-roles detract from the group's work and compromise goal achievement by taking time away from group issues and creating discomfort among group members.

APPLICATIONS TO HEALTH-RELATED GROUPS

In clinical settings, a health-related group purpose and goals dictate group structure, membership, and format. For example, a medication group would have an educational purpose. A group for parents with critically ill children would have a family support design, while a therapy group would have restorative healing functions. Activity groups are used therapeutically with children and with chronically mentally ill patients who have difficulty fully expressing themselves verbally. Exploration of personal feelings would be limited and related to the topic under discussion in an education group. In a therapy group, such probing would be encouraged.

Group Membership

Therapeutic and support groups are categorized as closed or open groups, and as having homogeneous or heterogeneous membership. *Closed therapeutic* groups have a selected membership with an expectation of regular attendance for an extended time period. Group members

may be added, but their inclusion depends on a match with group-defined criteria. Most psychotherapy groups fall into this category. *Open groups* do not have a defined membership. Most community support groups are open groups. Individuals come and go depending on their needs. One week the group might consist of two or three members and the next week 15 members. Some groups, such as Alcoholics Anonymous, have open meetings that anyone can attend and "closed" meetings that only alcoholic members can attend.

Having a homogeneous or heterogeneous membership identifies member characteristics. *Homogeneous* groups share common characteristics, for example, diagnosis (e.g., breast cancer support group) or a personal attribute (e.g., gender, or age). Twelve-step programs for alcohol or drug addiction, eating disorders, and gender-specific consciousness-raising groups are familiar examples of homogeneous groups. Psychoeducation (e.g., medication groups) groups often have a homogeneous membership related to particular medications or a diagnosis.

Heterogeneous groups represent a wider diversity of member characteristics and personal issues. Members vary in age, gender, and psychodynamics. Most psychotherapy and insight-oriented personal growth groups have a heterogeneous membership.

Creating the Group Environment

Privacy and freedom from interruptions are key considerations in selecting an appropriate location. A sign on the door indicating that the group is in session is essential for privacy. Seating should be comfortable and arranged in a circle so that each member has face-to-face contact with all other members. Being able to see facial expressions and to respond to several individuals at one time is essential to effective group communication. Often, group members choose the same seats in therapy groups. When a member is absent, that seat is left vacant.

Therapy groups usually meet weekly at a set time. Support groups meet at regular intervals, more often monthly. Educational groups meet for a predetermined number of sessions and then disband. Unlike individual sessions, which can be convened spontaneously in emergency situations, therapeutic groups meet only at designated times. Most therapeutic and support groups meet for 60–90 min on a regular basis with established, agreed-on meeting times. Groups that begin and end on time foster trust and predictability.

GROUP LEADERSHIP

Group leadership is based on two assumptions: (1) group leaders have a significant influence on group process; and

(2) most problems in groups can be avoided or reworked productively if the leader is aware of and responsive to the needs of individual group members, including the needs of the leader.

Effective leadership requires adequate knowledge of the topic, preparation, professional attitudes and behavior, responsible selection of members, and an evidence-based approach. Personal characteristics demonstrated by effective group leaders include commitment to the group purpose; self-awareness of personal biases and interpersonal limitations, careful preparation of the group, and an accepting attitude toward group members. Knowledge of group dynamics, training, and supervision are additional requirements for leaders of psychotherapy groups. Health education group leaders need to have expertise about the topic to be discussed. A major difference between group and individual communication is that the leader relates to the group as a whole, instead of with only one person. The leader joins member responses and themes together and/or points to conversational differences as providing broader information.

Leadership Styles

Throughout the group's life, the group leader models an attitude of caring, objectivity, and integrity. There are three general styles: authoritarian, democratic, and laissez-faire.

The **authoritarian group leader** takes full responsibility for group direction and controls interactions. This style works best when there is limited time to make decisions.

The **democratic group leader** invites member participation encouraging active discussions and shared decision-making. Democratic leaders are good listeners; they can adapt their leadership style to fit the changing needs of the group. They respectfully support the reliability of group members as equal partners in meeting group goals. Democratic leaders are goal-directed but flexible.

Laissez-faire group leaders are somewhat disengaged and do not control decision-making.

Successful leaders trust the group process enough to know that group members can work through conflict and difficult situations. They might vary their leadership style based on the task. Leaders know that even mistakes can be temporary setbacks and can be used for discussion to promote group member growth. Ideally, group leadership is a shared function of all group members, with many opportunities for different informal leaders to divide up responsibility for achieving group goals. The bonds that build between group members are real. It is important that all group members feel some ownership of group solutions.

Informal Group Leaders

Informal power is given to members who best clarify the needs of the other group members or who move the group toward goal achievement. Informal leaders develop within the group because they have a good grasp of the situational demands of the task at hand. They are not always the group members making the most statements. Some individuals, due to the force of their personalities, knowledge, or experience, will emerge as informal leaders within the group.

Emergent informal leaders become the voice of the group. Their comments are equated with those of the designated leader. Emergent leaders are more willing to take an active role in making a recommendation and generally move the group task forward. Reflect on the case of Al Smith.

Case Study: Al Smith and Cancer Support Group

Mr Smith is a powerful informal leader in a cancer survivors' support group. Although he makes few comments, he has an excellent understanding of and sensitivity to the needs of individual members. When these are violated, Al speaks up, and the group listens.

Coleadership

Coleadership represents a form of shared leadership found primarily in therapy and support groups. It is desirable for several reasons. The coleader adds another perspective related to processing group dynamics. Coleaders can provide a wider variety of responses and viewpoints that can be helpful to group members. When one leader is under fire, it can increase the other leader's confidence, knowing that an opportunity to process the session afterward is available.

Respecting and valuing each other, with sensitivity to a coleader's style of communication, is characteristic of effective coleadership. Problems can arise when coleaders have different theoretical orientations or are competitive with each other. Needing to pursue solo interpretations rather than explore or support the meaning of a coleader's interventions is distracting to the group.

APPLICATIONS

There are many types of groups that nurses can lead. Some are within healthcare agencies but more are out in the community, or even online. Suggestions for communication vary with the type of group.

Therapeutic Groups

The term "therapeutic" connotes more than treatment of mental or behavioral disorders. Within group, contributions of others are able to resonate with a member's

---

DEVELOPING AN EVIDENCE-BASED PRACTICE

A number of studies have examined work groups and leadership styles. To succeed in reaching goals, members need to develop cohesion. The literature divides leadership styles into task accomplishment issues and relationship issues. Leadership is one factor contributing to cohesion. Cummings (2018) did a metaanalysis of 129 studies of nursing leadership styles and effects on the staff nurse work force.

Results

Outcomes were congruent with other studies showing that relational leadership styles promote more positive outcomes, as opposed to focusing only on task accomplishment. Effective leaders were found to have encouraged and supported group members to agree to work toward the common goal, refocusing members when necessary thus fostering more group cohesion (Burlingame, 2018; Cruz, 2020).

Strength of research: Moderate. More nursing studies are needed of nurse managers.

Application to Your Clinical Practice

1. Nurses functioning as group leaders need to incorporate relationship skills and provide support to members as well as encouraging them to move toward meeting group goals.
2. Nurses can foster a sense of group cohesion by encouraging members to talk with each other in front of the whole group circle, while other members actively listen.
3. Leaders model normative behavior such as civility and active interest in each other.

References

Burlingame, G. M., McClendon, D. T., & Yang, C. (2018). Cohesion in group therapy: A meta-analysis. *Psychotherapy (Chic), 55*(4), 384–398.

Cruz, M., Osilla, K. C., & Paddock, S. M. (2020). Group cohesion and climate in cognitive behavioral therapy for individuals with a first-time DUI. *Alcoholism Treatment Quarterly, 38*(1), 68–86.

Cummings, G. G., Tate, K., Lee, S., et al. (2018). Leadership styles and outcome patterns for the nursing workforce and work environment: A systematic review. *International Journal of Nursing Studies, 85*, 19–60.

---

experience, change behaviors, and strengthen emotions. Making important connections among multiple realities offers different possibilities to individual patients to learn about and test out new interpersonal communication skills. Generally, in therapy groups, members share their own experiences in an effort to seek help and help others. Through their feedback, they are able to help other members adopt new behaviors.

Responsibilities of nurse leaders of these types of groups include organizational arrangements such as room reservations, meeting times, and agenda setting. Leaders set operating behavior ground rules. At the end of each session, the leader should summarize achievements. Leaders of therapy groups encourage participation of each member, bring new information, moderate disputes, and most importantly connect responses together to highlight different options for meeting goals. Nurses usually have advanced preparation for conducting therapy groups and need a clinical consultant for oversight. Table 8.3 displays factors found in therapeutic group formats.

- *Reminiscence groups.* These groups are designed to aide persons, usually elderly, who would benefit from a life review process. They do not attempt to bring new insights but are focused on helping members retrieve past, pleasant memories. These groups are meant to provide a supportive, ego-enhancing experience. Each

member in turn talks about today's theme such as recalling school days, or family celebrations, or favorite pets.
- *Reality orientation groups.* Often comprised of confused, institutionalized patients, reality orientation groups are directed at helping members remain in contact with their environment. Hopefully, participation will reduce confusion about time, place, and person. Props can be introduced such as calendars or pictures of the seasons to stimulate interest. Such groups can meet briefly each day. The theme can be reinforced throughout the day. For example, the leader could post a picture of "younger self" on a patient's door.
- *Remotivation groups.* These groups stimulate thinking about skills needed for activities of daily living. The purpose of these groups is to attempt to reach a part of a cognitively disturbed mind that is still functioning. Each meeting focuses on a theme such as art appreciation, music, or plants. Visual props may stimulate greater participation.

Support Groups

Support groups can provide a place for a member to share concerns with others who are having a similar experience or a similar diagnosis. Group conversation is more complicated than individual conversation, because each member

TABLE 8.3 Therapeutic Factors in Groups

Installation of hope	Occurs when members see others who have overcome problems and are successfully managing their lives.
Universality	Sharing common situations validates member experience, decreases sense of isolation: "Maybe I am not the only one with this issue."
Imparting information	New shared information is a resource for individual members and stimulates further discussion and the learning of new skills.
Imitative behavior	Members learn new behaviors through observation and the modeling of desired actions and gain confidence in trying them, e.g., managing conflict, receiving constructive criticism.
Socialization	Group provides a safe learning environment in which to take interpersonal risks and try new behaviors.
Interpersonal learning	Group acts as a social microcosm; focus is on members learning about how they interact and getting constructive feedback and support from others.
Cohesiveness	Sense of we-ness. Emphasizes personal bonds and commitment to the group. Members feel acceptance and trust from others. Cohesiveness serves as the foundation for all curative factors.
Catharsis	Expression of emotion that leads to receiving support and acceptance from other group members.
Corrective recapitulation of primary family	Allows for recognition and handling of transference issues in therapy groups. This helps group members to avoid repeating destructive interaction patterns in the "here and now."
Altruism	Providing help and support to other group members enhances personal self-esteem.
Existential factors	Highlights primary responsibility for taking charge of one's life and the consequences of their actions, creating a meaningful existence.

Adapted from Yalom, I. & Leszcz, M. (2005). *The theory and practice of group psychotherapy* (5th ed.). New York: Basic Books.

brings his or her own unique experiences. The nurse leader provides organizational protocols, provides information about the purpose and the need to give feedback, and works to ensure this is a safe environment for members to function in.

- *Discussion groups.* The usual format is a didactic presentation about a topic followed by group discussion. The expectation is that each member contributes. Elements of a successful discussion group are listed in Table 8.4.

Activity Groups

There are many types of activity groups, such as follows:

- *Occupational therapy.* Members work on a project or work with others to learn a new skill. Examples might include cooking classes, ceramics classes, or art classes. Each activity is chosen for its therapeutic value such as strengthening balance or improving muscle strength.
- *Exercise therapy.* The nurse leader models an exercise, and members copy it.
- *Artistic groups.* Such groups encourage patients to get in touch with inner feelings.

Health Education Groups

Agencies may organize a time-limited group to provide a group of similar patients with needed information. Examples could include lifestyle changes, childbirth preparation classes, parenting education, etc.

Professional Work Groups

Work groups are task oriented, created to address an employing organization's needs. Generally, their charge is to identify problems and plan changes to rectify problems. There is no focus on changing behavior of group members. Group communication and dynamics may be somewhat similar to other groups we have discussed. Characteristics of effective work groups are listed in Table 8.5.

- *Leadership of work groups.* Work group leaders do the organizational tasks of time, place, and agenda. They keep members on the task and summarize progress at the conclusion of each meeting. Allowing members to submit agenda items helps members buy into ownership of our task, usually producing a better outcome.

TABLE 8.4   Elements of Successful Discussion Groups

Element	Rationale for Problem-Solving
Careful preparation	Thoughtful agenda and assignments establish a direction for the discussion and the expected contribution of each member.
Informed participants	Each member should come prepared so that all members are communicating with relatively the same level of information, and each is able to contribute equally.
Shared leadership	Each member is responsible for contributing to the discussion; evidence of social loafing is effectively addressed.
Good listening skills	Concentrates on the material, listens to content. Challenges, anticipates, and weighs the evidence; listens between the lines to emotions about the topic.
Relevant questions	Focused questions keep the discussion moving toward the meeting objectives.
Useful feedback	Thoughtful feedback maintains the momentum of the discussion by reflecting different perspectives of topics raised and confirming or questioning others' views.

TABLE 8.5   Characteristics of Effective and Ineffective Work Groups

Effective Groups	Ineffective Groups
Goals are clearly identified and collaboratively developed.	Goals are vague or imposed on the group without discussion.
Open, goal-directed communication of feelings and ideas is encouraged.	Communication is guarded; feelings are not always given attention.
Power is equally shared and rotates among members, depending on ability and group needs.	Power resides in the leader or is delegated with little regard to member needs. It is not shared.
Decision-making is flexible and adapted to group needs.	Decision-making occurs with little or no consultation. Consensus is expected rather than negotiated based on data.
Controversy is viewed as healthy because it builds member involvement and creates stronger solutions.	Controversy and open conflict are not tolerated.
There is a healthy balance between task and maintenance role functioning.	There is a one-sided focus on task or maintenance role functions to the exclusion of the complementary function.
Individual contributions are acknowledged and respected. Diversity is encouraged.	Individual resources are not used. Conformity and being a "company person" is rewarded. Diversity is not respected.
Interpersonal effectiveness, innovation, and problem-solving adequacy are evident.	Problem-solving abilities, morale, and interpersonal effectiveness are low and undervalued.

- *Member responsibilities.* Members need to commit to achieving goals, prepare information ahead of each meeting, demonstrate respect for each other's ideas, and positively affirm the contributions of other members. This helps create cohesiveness.

Structural Group Development Communication Strategies

Forming Phase

How well leaders initially prepare themselves and group members has a direct impact on building the trust needed within the group. The forming phase in therapeutic groups focuses on helping patients establish trust in the group and with one another. Communication is tentative. Even when members know each other, it is helpful to have each do a brief introduction, which includes past experiences that might contribute to meeting group goals or shares a little of their reason for coming to the group. An introductory prompt such as "What would you most like to get out of this group?" helps the patients link personal goals to group goals.

In the first session, the leader introduces group goals. Clear group goals are particularly important to provide a frame for the group in its initial session. Unclear goals breed boredom or frustration. The leader clarifies how the group will be conducted and what the ground rules are, such as confidentiality, regular attendance, and mutual respect.

Storming Phase

This stage might be characterized by some disagreements among group members. This is normal behavior as group members feel more comfortable with expressing authentic opinions. The leader plays an important facilitative role in the storming phase by accepting differences in member perceptions as being expected and growth producing. By affirming genuine but different strengths in individual members, leaders model handling conflict with productive outcomes. Linking constructive themes while identifying the nature of the disagreement is an effective modeling strategy. Disagreements usually die down when members accept the common goal.

Norming Phase

To be successful, group norms should support accomplishment of group goals. Tasks in the norming phase center on the development of the implicit group-developed rules governing their group behaviors. Group-specific norms develop spontaneously through group–member interactions. They represent the group's shared expectations of its members. For example, lateness may not be tolerated. The group leader encourages member contributions and emphasizes cooperation in recognizing each person's talents and contributions related to group goals. If administrators are group members, they should attend all sessions. Few circumstances are more disrupting than having an administrator enter or exit the group at will.

Performing Phase

Most of the group's work gets accomplished during this phase. Members focus on problem-solving and developing new behaviors.

Leader Communication. The group leader is responsible for keeping the group on task to accomplish group goals. Leader interventions should be consistent and supportive. If group members seem to be moving off track, asking open-ended questions or verbally observing group processes can restore forward movement. Modeling respect, empathy, appropriate self-disclosure, and ethical standards helps ensure a supportive group climate. Effective group leaders trust group members to develop their own solutions, but they call attention to important group dynamics when needed. This can be introduced with a simple statement, such as "I wonder what is going on here right now."

Members. Group members are responsible for helping to maintain a supportive group-work environment.

Working together and participating in another person's personal growth allows members to experience one another's personal strengths and the collective caring of the group. Of all the possibilities that can happen in a group, individual members report feeling affirmed and respected by other group members as being most valuable. Because members function interdependently, they are able to work through disagreements and difficult issues in ways that are acceptable to each individual and the group. Feedback should be descriptive and specific to the immediate discussion. As with other types of constructive feedback, the feedback should focus only on modifiable behaviors.

Group Think as a Barrier. This phenomenon occurs when a member values approval from other members above reasonable decision-making. Is this "going along to get along"? To reduce occurrence of group think, allow members to hold different opinions and acknowledge contrary opinions.

Monopolizing as a Barrier. Monopolizing the conversation is a negative form of power communication used to advance a personal agenda without considering the needs of others. It may not be intentional, but rather a member's way of handling anxiety. When one member monopolizes the conversation, there are several ways the leader can respond. Acknowledging this person's contribution and broadening the input with a short open-ended question such as "Has anyone else had a similar experience?" can redirect the attention to the larger group.

Adjourning Phase

The final phase of group development, termination or adjournment, ideally occurs when the group members have achieved desired outcomes. The termination phase is about task completion and disengagement. The leader summarizes the goals accomplished or clarifies previous comments to connect cognitive and feeling elements that need to be addressed.

Groups versus Teams

Teams and groups have certain characteristics in common, but there are also some clear differences. Team communication occurs as a continuous process. Collaborative, multiskilled interdisciplinary healthcare teams are needed when caring for complex care patients. Team members are expected to provide ideas and care skills to reach patient goals as discussed in Chapter 23. Team members need to achieve consensus and constructively manage conflict, focus on collaborative problem-solving, coordinate their actions, and offer interpersonal support to one another. Implementation takes place through actions related to specified health goals. Communication takes place through electronic channels and face-to-face communication. The involved patient and family are considered part of the health team.

SUMMARY

This chapter describes ways in which a group experience enhances patients' abilities to meet therapeutic self-care demands. The rationale for providing a group experience for patients is described. Group dynamics include individual member commitment, functional similarity, and leadership style. Group concepts related to group dynamics consist of purpose, norms, cohesiveness, roles, and role functions. Communication suggestions and role responsibilities were discussed. Tuckman's phases of group development—forming, storming, performing, and adjourning—provide guidelines for group leaders.

ETHICAL DILEMMA: What Would You Do?

Mrs Murphy is 39 years old and has had multiple admissions to the psychiatric unit for bipolar disorder. She wants to participate in group therapy but is disruptive when she is in the group. The group gets angry with her monopolization of their time. She says she has just as much right as a group member to talk if she chooses. Mrs Murphy's symptoms could be controlled with medication, but she refuses to take it when she is "high" because it makes her feel less energized. How do you balance Mrs Murphy's rights with those of the group? Should she be required to take her medication? Or should she be excluded from the group if her behavior is not under her control? How would you handle this situation from an ethical perspective?

DISCUSSION QUESTIONS

1. How would you describe the differences between a work task group and a collaborative healthcare team?
2. How do active listening strategies differ in group communication versus individual communication?
3. What do you see as potential ethical issues in group communication formats?

REFERENCES

Freeman, B. J., Bess, G., Fleming, C. M., & Novins, D. K. (2019). Transforming through leadership: A qualitative study of successful American Indian Alaska native behavioral health leaders. *BMC Public Health, 19*(1), 1276.

Meeussen, L., Agneessens, F., Delvaux, E., & Phalet, K. (2018). Ethnic diversity and value sharing: A longitudinal social networking perspective on interactive group process. *British Journal of Social Psychology, 57*(2), 428–447.

Tuckman, B. W. (1965). Developmental sequence in small groups. *Psychological Bulletin, 63*, 384–399.

Tuckman, B. W., & Jensen, M. A. C. (1977). Stages of small-group development revisited. *Group & Organization Management, 2*(4), 419–427.

van den Broek, S., Tielemans, C., ten Cate, O., & Kruitwagen, C. (2021). Professional and interpersonal group identities of final year medical and nursing students. *Journal of Interprofessional Education & Practice, 22*(9756), 100392.

Yalom, I., & Leszcz, M. (2005). *The theory and practice of group psychotherapy.* New York: Basic Books.

9

Self-Concept in Professional Interpersonal Relationships

OBJECTIVES

At the end of this chapter, the reader will be able to:

1. Define the concept of self-concept and describe its characteristics.
2. Apply the nursing process in caring for patients with disturbances in the pattern of self-concept as related to body image, personal identity, and social role.
3. Evaluate therapeutic communication interventions related to self-esteem issues.
4. Apply therapeutic communications that meet patient spiritual needs to a case in healthcare.

This chapter focuses on self-concept as a key dynamic in communication, therapeutic relationships, and self-management strategies. This chapter identifies basic concepts and frameworks related to the development of self-concept and describes its impact on individual development. The Application section discusses communication strategies nurses can use with patients to empirically enhance self-concept in healthcare situations.

BASIC CONCEPTS

Definition
Self-Concept
Self-concept is defined as the totality of each person's beliefs about their inner self. It represents an integration of one's cultural heritage, environment, gender roles, ethnic and spiritual beliefs, education, basic personality traits, and cumulative life experiences.

This multidimensional construct mirrors an integration of individual's personal beliefs, values, attitudes, and behaviors. The self-concept has physical, emotional, social, and spiritual dimensions linked to functional well-being and health behaviors. It also incorporates feedback from others.

Physical Appearance. Physicality, especially in adolescents, plays a large part in America society as to how people perceive us and give us feedback, which reinforces our self-perceptions.

Constructing the self-concept requires a cultural foundation. Therefore, self-identity usually incorporates ethnic identity.

Body Image. Part of one's concept of self is our image of body size and function. The study of Shpigelman & HaGani (2019) pointed out that an individual with observable disability may develop either a positive body image or a negative one, whereas individuals with hidden disabilities such as mental illness have been found to develop a more negative self-image. Body image can be a major component of one's concept of self (Ramadhanty & Hamid, 2021).

Self-Esteem. Closely intertwined with self-concept is **self-esteem,** defined as a person's personal sense of worth and well-being. The terms *self-image, self-concept,* and *self-perception* are often used interchangeably to refer to the way individuals view and assess themselves. Abundant essays have been written about self-esteem, especially regarding the importance of a high self-esteem among American teens, particularly young women. Reflect on the Kali Rotoga case.

115

CASE STUDY: **Kali Rotoga and Low Self-Esteem**

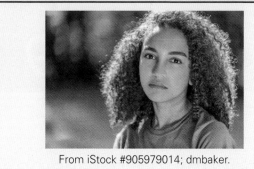

From iStock #905979014; dmbaker.

Kali Rotoga, 17 years old, comes to your outpatient clinic. She is a tall, slender, and beautiful young woman who is complaining of stomach pain. She has a flat affect and blank facial expression. Things are slow so you have plenty of time for conversation after obtaining her history. She tells you she feels lost, has dropped out of school, and has no plans for the future. All her school life her classmates made fun of her skin tone, saying she is not "black" enough. As the conversation continues, it is apparent that she has very poor self-esteem.

1. What other questions might you ask?
2. What should your main concern be?

Self-Clarity. An important feature of self-concept involves **self-clarity,** which is defined as the extent to which sense of self is stable and well defined. Self-concept clarity is clearly intertwined with healthy identity development. This relates to the individual's beliefs about their ability to accomplish a task and to deal with the challenges of life. This feature of the self-concept helps people to confront control issues and cope with the many facets of life. Self-efficacy plays a major part in determining our chances for success; in fact, some psychologists rate self-efficacy above talent in the recipe for success (Bandura, 1997).

A healthy self-concept including the aforementioned features, regardless of culture, reflects attitudes, emotions, and values that are realistic, congruent with one another, and consistent with a meaningful purpose in life. Fig. 9.1 identifies characteristics of a healthy self-concept. Each of these features is discussed further in the applications.

Self-Concept in Healthcare. A strong sense of self has been described as a protective factor in coping with chronic illness. When people experience a major health disruption, it alters the way they think, feel, value their sense of self, and the way they communicate with others.

Features and Functions of Self-Concept. A person's self-concept is fluid. It consists of various coexisting self-images. Different aspects of the self-concept become visible, depending on the situation. For example, a student might be a marginal student in English literature but a star in a mathematics course on differential equations. Which is the true self, or are both valid?

Self-concept helps people to make sense of their past and present; it helps them to communicate across varied situations and to imagine what they are capable of becoming physically, emotionally, intellectually, socially, and spiritually in relation to others in the future.

Over the course of a lifetime, self-concept changes and develops in complexity. As one ages, the "self" develops

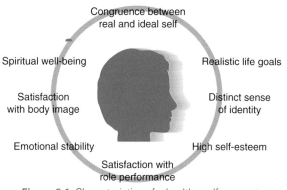

Figure 9.1 Characteristics of a healthy self-concept.

and becomes shaped by personal experiences and personally developed values and beliefs. Simulation Exercise 9.1 provides an opportunity for you to practice self-awareness by examining your self-concept.

Self-Fulfilling Prophecies. **Possible selves** is a term used to explain the future-oriented component of self-concept. Personal wishes and desires are valuable influences in goal setting and motivation, when they lead to realistic actions. For example, a nursing student might think, "I can see myself becoming Dean of nursing." Such thoughts help the novice nurse work harder to achieve professional goals. Negative possible selves can also become a self-fulfilling prophecy. For example, Martha receives a performance evaluation indicating a need for improved self-confidence. Seeing this criticism as a negative commentary on her "self," she fulfills the attribution by performing awkwardly when she is being assessed in the clinical area.

Development of Self-Concept and Self-Esteem. Self-concept represents an interaction between the life experiences and challenges that occur and the individual's response to them. Life experiences, social status,

SIMULATION EXERCISE 9.1   Who Am I?

Purpose
To help students understand some of the self-concepts they hold about themselves.

Procedure
1. Spend 10–15 min reflecting about how you would have defined yourself during middle school or high school and how you would define yourself today.
2. What has changed in your sense of self, and if there were changes, why did they occur?
3. Using only **three one-word** descriptors, describe yourself today. There are no right or wrong answers.
4. Pick the one descriptor that you believe defines yourself best.
5. In small groups of four to six students, share your results.

Reflective Discussion Analysis
1. Were you surprised with the changes from your earlier descriptors as a teen or preteen?
2. Were you surprised with any of your choices as current descriptors?
3. How hard was it to pick the one best descriptor out of the five?
4. How did you describe yourself? Could your self-descriptors be categorized or prioritized in describing your overall self-concept?
5. What did you learn about the process of examining your self-concept from doing this exercise? What situational factors seemed to impact your descriptor choice?
6. How could you use this information in professional interpersonal relationships with patients?

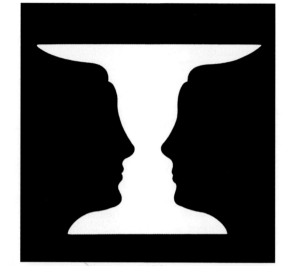

Figure 9.2 The figure-ground phenomenon. Where you focus your attention makes a difference in your perception of the figures. (From the Westinghouse Learning Corporation: Self-instructional unit 12: perception, 1970. Reprinted with permission.)

significant relationships, and opportunities influence how people define themselves throughout life. Interactions in the family environment were previously considered the primary source in the development of self-esteem. Some studies have suggested that genetic factors play a significant role in the etiology of self-esteem. The external social context into which a child is born, as well as their physical development, and relationships contributes to shaping their self-concept.

Social environment plays an important role in shaping and supporting one's personal self-concept. Current research supports the idea that a nurturing home environment, sports participation, academic success, religious affiliation, professional opportunities, praise for successful accomplishments, and supportive mentors tend to encourage the development of a positive self-concept (Arnett, 2018). Factors such as poverty, a chaotic upbringing, loss of a parent, poor educational opportunities, and adverse life events contribute to the development of a negative self-concept. However, there are individuals who experience unfortunate social circumstances yet develop a dynamic self-concept as a reaction to their circumstances, creating a resiliency to the impact of negativity. They are interested in improving their environment and serve as role models to others about what is possible against all odds. Others with more fortunate life circumstances may develop negative self-concepts or overinflated positive self-concepts with little grounding in reality. At times, these individuals may be at risk for having difficulty accepting negative events in life. This further illustrates how understanding an individual's self-concept assists nurses to individually determine which therapeutic intervention will help during health events. When life presents individuals with unpredictable trauma or devastation, nurses can play a critical role in helping patients to reframe a potentially incapacitating sense of self into one including more hope and broader options. In an effort to enhance resilience, nurses can help patients revisit personal strengths, consider new possibilities, incorporate new information, and seek out appropriate resources as a basis for making sound clinical decisions for themselves and taking constructive actions. Sometimes just a nurse being present can help a patient.

Self-Concept in Interpersonal Relationships. Self-concept is formed in relation to others. When two people communicate, each person's perceptions are influenced by their self-concept and level of self-esteem. Fig. 9.2 illustrates how perceptions can differ from person to person.

Negative Attributions. Language is influential in forming perceptions of the self and others and reflects society's values. Self-concept can easily be shaken by **negative attributions** of communication; therefore, it is vital for nurses to be sensitive to the impact of language in interactions with patients. **Microaggressions** involve communicating subtle and often unintentional discrimination pertaining to self-concepts of race, ethnicity, gender, or any other demographic. This type of communication can be viewed as affecting self-concept by implying a negative attribution.

Sue's work (2007) in professional communications also describes **microassaults** as explicit negative verbal or nonverbal communication that offends an individual through criticism, slighting, or purposeful prejudicial actions, for example, identifying someone as a "Medicaid patient" when the cost of a generic drug is being discussed. This might influence a patient's self-concept and might shut down further communication related to education about drug dosage.

Microinsults are subtle unintended rebuffs, but the insinuation would clearly offend the recipient. For example, during the nutritional assessment of a female patient with diabetes, a nurse comments that "all diabetics cheat on their diet." This not only demeans patients' efforts to control glucose levels but also reduces identity to a diagnosis.

Microinvalidations are communications that discount or invalidate a person's values, feelings, or lifestyle. For example, stating to a single mother, "It must be difficult managing child rearing by yourself as a single mom." This message conveys that this patient represents a deficit model of child rearing. Rather than empowering the mother, the statement implies a lesser standard of parenting, which does not enhance the mother's self-esteem.

Although these nurse–patient communications seem harmless, they clearly communicate an expectation or attribution that can lead to increased levels of anger, mistrust, and loss of self-esteem. They impede further communication.

Cultural Identity. A clear **cultural identity** is positively related to a clear self-concept and self-esteem. An understanding of the fundamental differences in cultural worldviews within the context of globalization can help nurses to frame supportive interventions in ways that support ethnocultural variations and patients' self-concepts (see Chapter 7). Individual differences also exist within cultures, and each individual is unique.

Gender. **Gender roles** refer to socially constructed roles and behaviors that occur in a historical and cultural context and that vary across societies and over time. Self-perceptions regarding gender evolve from socially learned behaviors that are constructed by the prevailing culture.

There may also be genetic components. Despite progressive feminist changes, subtle gender differences are still evidenced in the form of social expectations, career options, pay differentials, and so forth. LGTB individuals have long fought for equal recognition. Many individuals do not fit into traditional gender categories and genuinely do not feel related to the socially constructed roles of society. Transgendered and intersexed people struggle with a society that may hold rigid boundaries around the constructs of sex and gender. Nurses working with patients need to approach gender identity as distinct from biology and consider the individual's subscribed gender identity.

Case Study: Leslie Morgan and Gender Issues

Struggling to complete the health intake questionnaire demographic information, Leslie Morgan, age 16 years, tells nurse Mary Kane, "If I go to the doctor, I'm labeled a 'female,' but in everyday life at school, most people think I'm a 'male.' I have always felt different, not wanting dresses or dolls."

Discussion: Nurses need to be supportive in this genuine aspect of identity and understand a patient's reluctance to refuse identification as male or female.

Theoretical Frameworks
Frameworks Within Personality Theory

The self is a central construct in theories of personality. These theories argue that our self-concept develops from and is influenced by social interactions with others. Sullivan (1953) refers to *self-concept* as a self-system that people develop to (1) present a consistent image of self, (2) protect themselves against feelings of anxiety, and (3) maintain their interpersonal security.

Humanism (Rogers, 1959) defines the *self* as an organized, fluid, but consistent conceptual pattern of perceptions of characteristics and relationships or the "I" and the "me" together with values attached to these concepts. When the "actual self" (who we believe we are) and the "ideal self" (how a person would ideally like to be) are similar, the person is likely to have a positive self-concept and self-esteem. Rogers equated having a coherent well-integrated self-concept with being mentally healthy and well adjusted.

Cognitive Approaches. Is a child born without a concept of self? The child learns to differentiate self from others in the intimate sphere of family, in friendships, and in cultural practices. This requires relating to others and having vast interaction in the environment.

Behaviorists believe that early childhood interactions foster self-concepts of a *good me* (resulting from reward and approval experiences), a *bad me* (resulting from punishment and disapproval experiences), and a *not me* (resulting from anxiety-producing experiences that are dissociated by the person as not being a part of his or her self-concept). These influences continue through adulthood and color a person's responses to life. Having a therapeutic relationship can help patients develop a different, more positive sense of self.

George Mead applies a sociological approach to the study of self-concept. The self-concept affects and is influenced by how people experience themselves in relation to others. Mead's model emphasizes the influence of culture, moral norms, and language in framing self-concepts through interpersonal interactions (symbolic interactionism).

Erikson's Theory of Psychosocial Development

Erik Erikson's (1968, 1982) theory of psychosocial self-development is a well-known model. His theory emanated from his work as a therapist, and his theory has stimulated a wealth of research and application. Central to his framework is the concept of identity formation. He believed that identity formation is lifelong development (Erikson, 1959). Personality develops

as a person responds to evolving developmental challenges (psychosocial crises) during the life cycle. As individuals pass through ascending stages of ego development, with mastery of each developmental task, a personal sense of identity evolves. This is most obvious during adolescence, when teens experiment with different roles as they seek to establish a strong, comfortable personal identity. This development is not linear, nor does it occur across physical, emotional, and social development in the same sequential order. This is seen in the physically mature adolescent who may behave in a less mature fashion socially and emotionally.

The first four stages of Erikson's model serve as building blocks for his central developmental task of establishing a healthy ego identity (identity vs. identity diffusion). Erikson's stages of ego development are outlined in Table 9.1. Erikson believed that stage development is never final. Reworking of developmental stages can occur any time during the life span. Erikson's model can help nurses to analyze the age appropriateness of behavior from an ego development perspective. For example, a teenager giving birth is still coping with issues of self-identity rather than generativity.

TABLE 9.1   Erikson's Stages of Psychosocial Development, Clinical Behavior Guidelines, and Stressors

Stage of Personality Guidelines	Ego Strength or Virtue	Clinical Behavior Guidelines	Stressors
Trust versus mistrust	Hope	Appropriate attachment behaviors Ability to ask for assistance with an expectation of receiving it Ability to give and receive information related to self and health Ability to share opinions and experiences easily Ability to differentiate between how much one can trust and how much one must distrust	Unfamiliar environment or routines Inconsistency in care Pain Lack of information Unmet needs (e.g., having to wait 20 min for a bedpan or pain injection) Losses at critical times or accumulated loss Significant or sudden loss of physical function (e.g., a patient with a broken hip being afraid to walk)
Autonomy versus shame and doubt	Willpower	Ability to express opinions freely and to disagree tactfully Ability to delay gratification Ability to accept reasonable treatment plans and hospital regulations Ability to regulate one's behaviors (overcompliance, noncompliance, suggest disruptions) Ability to make age-appropriate decisions	Overemphasis on unfair or rigid regulation (e.g., putting patients in nursing homes to bed at 7 p.m.) Cultural emphasis on guilt and shaming as a way of controlling behavior Limited opportunity to make choices in a hospital setting Limited allowance made for individuality

Continued

TABLE 9.1   Erikson's Stages of Psychosocial Development, Clinical Behavior Guidelines, and Stressors—cont'd

Stage of Personality Guidelines	Ego Strength or Virtue	Clinical Behavior Guidelines	Stressors
Initiative versus guilt	Purpose	Ability to develop realistic goals and to initiate actions to meet them Ability to make mistakes without undue embarrassment Ability to have curiosity about healthcare Ability to work for goals Ability to develop constructive fantasies and plans	Significant or sudden change in life pattern that interferes with role Loss of a mentor, particularly in adolescence or with a new job Lack of opportunity to participate in planning of care Overinvolved parenting that does not allow for experimentation Hypercritical authority figures No opportunity for play
Industry versus inferiority	Competence	Work is perceived as meaningful and satisfying Appropriate satisfaction with balance in lifestyle pattern, including leisure activities Ability to work with others, including staff Ability to complete tasks and self-care activities in line with capabilities Ability to express personal strengths and limitations realistically	Limited opportunity to learn and master tasks Illness, circumstance, or condition that compromises or obliterates one's usual activities Lack of cultural support or opportunity for training
Identity versus identity diffusion	Fidelity	Ability to establish friendships with peers Realistic assertion of independence and dependence needs Demonstration of overall satisfaction with self-image, including physical characteristics, personality, and role in life	Lack of opportunity Overprotective, neglectful, or inconsistent parenting Sudden or significant change in appearance, health, or status Lack of same-sex role models
Identity versus isolation	Fidelity	Ability to express and act on personal values Congruence of self-perception with nurse's observation and perception of significant others	Lack of opportunity to interact with others Lack of guidance about socially proactive behaviors Loss of significant others Loss of memory Impaired hearing
Intimacy versus isolation	Love	Ability to enter into strong reciprocal interpersonal relationships Ability to identify a readily available support system Ability to feel the caring of others Ability to act harmoniously with family and friends	Competition Communication that includes a hidden agenda Projection of images and expectations onto another person Lack of privacy Loss of significant others at critical points of development

TABLE 9.1 Erikson's Stages of Psychosocial Development, Clinical Behavior Guidelines, and Stressors—cont'd

Stage of Personality Guidelines	Ego Strength or Virtue	Clinical Behavior Guidelines	Stressors
Generativity versus stagnation and self-absorption	Caring	Demonstration of age-appropriate activities Development of a realistic assessment of personal contributions to society Development of ways to maximize productivity Appropriate care of whatever one has created Demonstration of a concern for others and a willingness to share ideas and knowledge Evidence of a healthy balance among work, family, and self-demands	Aging parents, separately or concurrently with adolescent children Obsolescence or layoff in career "Me generation" attitude Inability or lack of opportunity to function in a previous manner Children leaving home Forced retirement
Integrity versus despair	Wisdom	Expression of satisfaction with personal lifestyle Acceptance of growing limitations while maintaining maximum productivity Expression of acceptance of certitude of death, as well as satisfaction with one's contributions to life Lack of opportunity	Rigid lifestyle Loss of significant other Loss of physical, intellectual, and emotional faculties Loss of previously satisfying work and family roles

Cognitive Behavioral Model

Pioneered in the 1960s by Beck and Beck (2011), this model is a blend of cognitive and behavioral theories that provides a psychosocial structure for therapy. This model states that thoughts, feelings, and behaviors are all connected. The premise is that individuals develop a mental organizational schema through their experiences over time. New experiences and information are then fitted into this existing schema. In some individuals, cognitive distortions occur secondary to biased, negative interpretations, which lead to problematic behaviors, for example, depression or anxiety (Wilde & Dozois, 2019). These individuals are not as able as others to recognize their own emotional state, thus leading them toward maladaptive behaviors (Stuart, 2020). One example might be compulsive overeating. Therapy focuses on cognitive restructuring: recognizing inaccurate thinking and negative concepts of self; challenging these thoughts and beliefs; and modeling development of better coping skills. Hopefully, the individual develops new information processing skills to deal with the immediate problem; observes and imitates new behavior; and is shaped, that is, rewarded for desired behavior.

APPLICATIONS

Role of Self-Concept in Patient-Centered Relationships

This section identifies strategies to strengthen self-concept, self-efficacy, and self-esteem in healthcare relationships and communication. It is important to initiate caring relationships with the premise that each patient is a unique person with strengths, values, cultural beliefs, and experiential life concerns. What health providers say, how they say it, and what they do matter in establishing relationships supportive of patients' identities and patient-centered care.

DEVELOPING AN EVIDENCE-BASED PRACTICE

Much has been written about nurses' well-being, burnout, and mediating factors. The National Academy of Medicine created the Action Collaborative on Clinician Well-being and Resilience to explore evidence-based solutions. Among studies, Gabriel's 2020 research looked at whether nurse sense of control of events during their shift affected emotional exhaustion. Cochrane scholars did a metaanalysis on 44 studies to find variables that increased nurse resilience and decreased depression.

Results

Gabriel reported a negative relationship between harmful effects of less control and emotional exhaustion. Importantly, they found emotional exhaustion is buffered by higher self-esteem. The Cochrane analysis found use of short-term cognitive behavioral therapy to be an effective intervention. They concluded that offering resilience training programs and coaching from a team of expert nurses would be somewhat effective in mediating emotional exhaustion, a finding that includes DeGrazia's 2021 research.

Strength of research: Unknown, interventions need to be more rigorously tested.

Application to Your Clinical Practice

Most findings point to a need for agency changes, such as offering support programs for nurses and physicians.

1. Nursing administrators should advocate for support programs, for allowing nurses more control over their workflow, for offering programs using cognitive behavioral intervention.
2. Report all cases of burnout (per the National Academy of Medicine).
3. Nurses actively seek social support from family, friends, or colleagues in person or online.

References

DeGrazia, M., Porter, C., Sheehan, A., et al. (2021). Building moral resiliency through the nurse education and support team initiative. *American Journal of Critical Care, 30*(2), 95–102.

Gabriel, A. S., Erickson, R. J., Diefendorff, J. M., & Krantz, D. (2020). When does feeling in control benefit well-being? The boundary conditions of the identity commitment and self-esteem. *Journal of Vocational Rehabilitation, 119*, 103415.

Kunzler, A. M., Helmreich, I., Chmitorz, A., et al. (2020). Psychological interventions to foster resilience in healthcare professionals. *Cochrane Database of Systematic Reviews, 7*(7), CD012527.

National Academy of Medicine. Action collaborative on clinician well-being and resilience. Retrieved from https://nam.edu/initiatives/clinician-resilience-and-well-being/. (Accessed 22 June 2021).

Self-concept is an essential starting point for understanding patients' behaviors related to coping, engagement in meaningful activities, and improved mood. Self-concept variables can act as facilitators or barriers to a patient's efforts to engage in healthier lifestyle behaviors and the self-management of chronic disorders.

Patterns and Nursing Diagnosis Related to Self-Concept

Gordon (2007) identifies related functional health patterns as self-perception, self-concept, and value belief patterns. Injury, illness, and treatment can challenge these functional health patterns regardless of specific medical diagnosis. As a person's perception of self-concept is disturbed, perception of the future becomes uncertain and unpredictable.

Body Image Issues

Body image involves people's perceptions, thoughts, and behaviors associated with their appearance. Perception of one's body image changes throughout life, influenced by aging, the appraisals of others, cultural and social factors, and physical changes resulting from illness, injury, and even treatment effects. For example, the potential for impotence and incontinence with prostate surgery can, secondary to treatment, create a body image issue for men. This body image issue may have further implications for nurses' assessment of self-esteem issues.

Self-esteem is a critical dimension of body image, the value people place on their appearance, or biological or functional intactness. For example, individuals with an eating disorder may see themselves as "fat" despite being dangerously underweight. Ideal body image reflects sociocultural norms and popular media portrayals. Research consistently finds that physical appearance is strongly related to overall high self-esteem; therefore, nurses need to be cognizant of patients' perceptions of physical changes.

Cultures differ in their value of specific physical characteristics. Sociocultural theories of body image suggest that body dissatisfaction results from a person's inability to meet unrealistic societal ideals. Any changes in physical appearance or function can challenge self-concept (Arnett, 2018).

Permanent and even temporary changes in appearance influence attributions that others may make, and how individuals perceive these responses. Discrimination can be subtle or overt, and the experience of a distorted body image can be long-lasting. In a study of overweight adolescents, a primary theme that emerged was forever describing self as overweight, even if the excess weight is lost in adult years. Less overt body images disturbance, for example, infertility or epilepsy, not obvious to others can still affect self-concept.

Nursing Strategies and Body Image

The *meaning* of body image is highly individual. Some, such as Helen Keller or Stephen Hawking, frame a potentially negative body image as a positive feature of their identities. Others let a physical deviation become their defining feature. Patients with the same medical condition can have different body image issues. Assessment should take the following into account:

- Negative communications about the body
- Preoccupation with or no mention of changes in body structure and function following medical interventions
- Reluctance to look at or touch a changed body structure
- Social isolation and loss of interest in friends and work after a change in body structure, appearance, or function
- Expressed concerns or fears about changes.

Assessment. Patient-centered assessment includes the patient's strengths, expressed needs and goals, the nature and accessibility of the patient's support system, and the perception of the impact the changes have on lifestyle. Frequently deficits are magnified, and compensatory personal resources are overlooked. Nurses can use a strength-based approach. Simply listening to the patient's response to changes in health can provide insight into its effect on self-concept, as is the situation in the Ms Tulley case.

Case Study: Ms Tina Tulley

Ms Tulley, age 28 years, is 1-day postmastectomy. Even though she has been shown arm exercises to reduce swelling, she refuses. She appears sad and seems to be grieving.

Nurses can model acceptance for patients experiencing an altered body image. Acceptance is a process, and patients need time to reconcile body image issues. Open-ended questions about what the patient expects and helping patients identify social supports can facilitate acceptance. Talking with others who have similar changes can provide credible, practical advice. For example, a "Reach to Recovery" volunteer visit with a mastectomy patient and referrals to support groups can assist a patient to accept help and advice.

Personal Identity

Identity is described as an intrapersonal psychological process consisting of a person's beliefs and values, characteristics and abilities, relationships with others, how they fit into the world, and personal growth potential. Spirituality is a significant resource and an essential component of personal identity. The identity develops and changes over time in relation to stage of life, situations, and experiences. There are multiple dimensions to personal identity, just as there are in self-concept: gender and sexual identities, social role identity (parent, student, widow, etc.), cultural and ethnic identity, economic contextual identity, and so forth. Each facet affects a person's world view, sense of self, and communication patterns with others.

Individuals pass through each life stage as outlined by Erikson; our perceptions of personal identity change to reflect who we are in the present moment physically, psychologically, contextually, and spiritually.

When a major and/or sudden change in health status forces a reappraisal of personal identity, its impact on a patient can be swift, life-altering, and compelling.

Nursing Strategies to Provide Support and Strengthen Identity

Changes in self-perception occur with change in health status. In addition to accepting an illness and learning new self-management skills, many people have to adapt to an altered social identity and renegotiate relationships. This activity involves a degree of emotional discomfort because things are not the same for the patient or for those with whom the patient interacts. Renegotiating relationships can be awkward and anxiety-producing, and patients often need the nurse's support in determining how to respond.

Developing self-perceptions of achieving personal health and well-being may be as important as objective data for predicting health outcomes over time. Nurses can help patients reestablish a more positive self-identity by encouraging the patient and family to engage in open-ended questions in a spirit of mutual discovery related to the following:

- What is this patient coping with in relation to their current circumstances?
- What is needed to support this patient in reconnecting with the person that they are capable of being?

Including a significant family member in this discussion is essential. Family may not anticipate or have an awareness of a change in personal identity, as often the focus of return to health is more physically defined. Benner (2003) advocates exploring what matters to the patient and *emphasizing a person's strengths* as a basis for developing and enhancing creative meaning. This strength-based approach creates a climate where patients *can* improve their situation and creates new possibilities for enhancing personal identity during illness. Even the smallest positive movement toward change can make a difference in a patient's self-image.

Box 9.1 describes patient-centered interventions to enhance personal identity. Think about applying these strategies to your colleagues as well as to your patients. Read the Lee case.

Case Study: Linda Lee, RN, and Job Defining Sense of Self

Linda Lee has worked in a busy surgical unit for 4 years. Returning to work after a hospitalization for major depression, she finds she has been relieved of her position as charge nurse. Other staff are highly protective of her. She is carefully watched to ensure that she is not going to relapse, and she is given simpler tasks to avoid stressing her out. Linda cannot understand why her coworkers do not see her as the same person she was before. Although her depression is in remission, Linda has been "reclassified" as a mentally ill person in the eyes of her coworkers. Her colleagues' efforts are well intentioned, but they have a negative effect on Linda's sense of personal identity.

Perception

Perception is a process through which we interpret sensory information and whereby a person transforms sensory data into connected personalized understanding. According to self-perception theory, we interpret our own actions in the same way as we interpret others' actions, and our actions are often socially influenced and not produced of our own free will, as we might expect.

Helping patients to refocus their attention in contemplating difficult circumstances, or using a new perspective, can alter meaning and suggest different options. Perceptions differ because people develop mindsets that alter data in personal ways. Patients with delirium or psychoactive drug reactions experience global perceptual distortions, whereas those with mental illness can experience personalized perceptual distortions. Distorted perceptions influence interpretation of communication, whether sending, receiving, or interpreting verbal messages and nonverbal behaviors. Simple perceptual distortions can be challenged with compassionate questioning and sometimes targeted humor. Validation of perceptual data is needed because the nurse and the patient may not be processing the same reality. What do you think about the Mrs Hummer case?

BOX 9.1 Patient-Centered Interventions to Enhance Personal Identity: Perceptions and Cognition

- Explain to newly admitted patients their clinical environment, patient rights, and expected care routine.
- Actively listen and facilitate the patient's "story" of the present healthcare experience, including concerns about coping, impact on self and others, and hopes for the future.
- Remember that each patient is unique. Respect and tailor responses to support individual differences in personality, identity, responses, intellect, values, culture, and understanding of medical processes.
- Encourage as much patient input as is realistically possible into diagnostic and therapeutic regimens.
- Provide information as it emerges about changes in treatment, personnel, discharge, and after care. Include family members whenever possible and desired, particularly when giving difficult news.
- Explain treatment procedures including rationale and allow ample time for questions and discussion.
- Encourage family members to bring in familiar objects, pictures, or a calendar particularly if the patient is in the hospital or care facility for an extended period.
- Encourage as much independence and self-direction as possible.
- Avoid sensory overload and repeat instructions if the patient appears anxious.
- Use perceptual checks to ensure you and the patient have the same understanding of important material.
- Encourage older patients and seniors to maintain an active, engaged lifestyle in line with their interests, capabilities, and values.

Case Study: Mrs Hummer Expresses Sadness to Bobby Way, RN

Grace Ann Hummer is a 65-year-old widow with arthritis, a weight problem, and failing eyesight. Admitted for a minor surgical procedure, Mrs Hummer says she does not know why she is putting herself through all of this. Nothing can be done for her because she is too old and decrepit.

Bobby: As I understand it, you came in today for removal of your bunions. Can you tell me more about your problem as you see it? *(Asking for this information separates the current situation from an overall assessment of ill health.)*

Mrs Hummer: Well, I've been having trouble walking, and I can't do some of the things I like to do that require extensive walking. I also have to buy "clunky" shoes that make me look like an old woman.

Bobby: So you are not willing to be an old woman yet? (Taking the patient's statement and challenging the cognitive distortion presented in her initial comments with humor allows the patient to view her statement differently.)

Mrs. Hummer (laughing): Right, there are a lot of things I want to do before I'm ready for a nursing home.

Discussion: Questioning perceptions and active listening help patients make sense of perceptual data in a more conscious way, and the patient feels heard. A cognitive appraisal of personal identity in the face of illness can contribute to treatment adherence and an enhanced sense of well-being. Keeping communication simple, delivering straightforward messages with compassion, and making interactions participatory with a back-and-forth dialog reduce the potential for acting on perceptual distortions.

Cognition

Cognition represents the thinking processes people use in making sense of the world. What people *think* about their perceptions is the throughput that connects perceptions with associated feelings and directly influences clinical outcomes. Faulty perceptions of a situation can stimulate automatic negative thoughts, which may not be realistic. Referred to as cognitive distortions, automatic thoughts about self-constructed realities create negative feelings, which can have a powerful impact on communication and behavior. Conscious reality-based thought processes are essential to acquiring and sustaining an accurate interpretation of self. Nurses can use supportive strategies to assist patients to examine cognitive distortions so that they are better able to develop realistic solutions to difficult health problems.

Supportive Nursing Strategies Using the Cognitive Behavioral Model

Cognitive behavioral approaches focus on encouraging patients to reflect on difficult situations from a broader perspective. Cognitive distortions are viewed by us as "thinking errors." Reflection on a variety of explanations provides patients with more options to realistically interpret the meaning of their perceptions. Cognitive approaches help patients identify, reflect on, and challenge negative automatic thinking processes instead of accepting them as reality. Common cognitive distortions are identified in Box 9.2.

Modeling cues to behavior and coaching patients to challenge cognitive distortions with positive self-talk and mindfulness are also helpful.

> **BOX 9.2   Examples of Cognitive Distortions**
>
> 1. "All or nothing" thinking—the situation is all good or all bad; a person is trustworthy or untrustworthy.
> 2. Overgeneralizing—one incident is treated as if it happens all the time; picking out a single detail and dwelling on it.
> 3. Mind reading and fortune telling—deciding a person does not like you without checking it out; assuming a bad outcome with no evidence to support it.
> 4. Personalizing—seeing yourself as flawed instead of separating the situation as something you played a role in but did not cause.
> 5. Acting on "should" and "ought to"—deciding in your mind what is someone else's responsibility without perceptual checks; trying to meet another's expectations without regard for whether it makes sense to do so.
> 6. "Awfulizing"—assuming the worst, that every situation has a catastrophic interpretation and anticipated outcome.

Self-Esteem

Self-esteem is defined as the *emotional* value a person places on his or her self-concept. People who view themselves as worthwhile and of value have high self-esteem. They challenge negative beliefs that are unproductive or interfere with successful functioning. With a positive attitude about self, an individual is more likely to view life as a glass half full rather than half empty. People with low self-esteem do not value themselves and do not feel valued by others. Self-esteem can be related to either a specific dimension of self, "I am a good writer," or it may have a more global meaning, "I am a good person who is worth knowing." Try Simulation Exercise 9.2 to define what matters to you.

Self-esteem is related to happiness. Low self-esteem is more likely to lead to depression under some circumstances. Some studies support the buffer hypothesis, which is that high self-esteem mitigates the effects of stress, but other studies come to the opposite conclusion, indicating that the negative effects of low self-esteem are mainly felt in good times. Still others find that high self-esteem leads to happier outcomes regardless of stress or other circumstances. A person with high self-esteem views life's inevitable problems as challenges from which one can learn and grow. Table 9.2 identifies behaviors associated with high versus low self-esteem.

Self-esteem is closely linked to our emotions, particularly those of pride or shame, and our sense of control (self-efficacy) over life events. Verbal and nonverbal behaviors presenting as powerlessness, frustration, inadequacy, anxiety, anger, or apathy suggest low self-esteem. This pattern tends to be defensive in relationships and seeks

SIMULATION EXERCISE 9.2 **What Matters to Me?**

Purpose
To help students understand the relationship between self-concepts and what is valued.

Procedure
This exercise may be done as a homework exercise and shared with your small group.
- Spend 10 min reflecting about the three activities, roles, or responsibilities you value most in your life. (There are no right or wrong answers.)
- Now prioritize them and identify the one that you value the most. (This is never easy.)
- In one to two paragraphs, explain why the top contender is most important to you.
- In small groups of four to six students, share your results.

Reflective Discussion Analysis
1. Were you surprised by any of your choices or what you perceived as being most important to you?
2. In what ways do your choices affirm self-concept and self-esteem?
3. What are the implications of doing this exercise for your helping patients understand what they value and how this reflects self-esteem?

constant reassurance from others because of self-doubt. Instead of taking constructive actions that could raise self-esteem, people worry about issues they cannot control and see life's challenges as problems rather than opportunities. People with low self-esteem are less likely to correctly identify the informational value of their feelings. This is important, as they are easily influenced by what is referred to as "an affective margin of distortion" that can color communication.

Self-esteem increases gradually throughout adulthood, peaking around the late 60s. Over the course of adulthood, individuals increasingly occupy positions of power and status, which might promote feelings of self-worth. Many life span theorists have suggested that in midlife, people are concerned with trying to figure out how they want to spend their later years and what is important to them personally. Self-esteem declines in old age. The few studies of self-esteem in old age suggest that self-esteem begins to decline around age 70. This decline may be due to the dramatic confluence of changes that occur in old age, including changes in work (e.g., retirement), relationships (e.g., the loss of a spouse), and physical functioning (e.g., health problems) as well as a decline in socioeconomic status. The old-age decline may also reflect a shift toward a more modest, humble, balanced view of the self in old age (Erikson, 1985).

The experience of success or failure can also cause fluctuations in self-esteem. Sources of situational challenges include loss of a job; loss of an important relationship; and negative changes in one's appearance, role, or status. Longstanding issues of verbal or physical abuse, neglect, chronic illness, codependency, and criticism by significant others

TABLE 9.2 **Behaviors Associated With High Versus Low Self-Esteem**

People With High Self-Esteem	People With Low Self-Esteem
Expect people to value them	Expect people to be critical of them
Are active self-agents	Are passive or obstructive self-agents
Have positive perceptions of their skills, appearance	Have negative perceptions of their skills, appearance, sexuality, and behaviors
Perform equally well when being observed as when not being observed	Perform less well when being observed
Are nondefensive and assertive in response to criticism	Are defensive and passive in response to criticism
Can accept compliments easily	Have difficulty accepting compliments
Evaluate their performance realistically	Have unrealistic expectations about their performance
Are relatively comfortable relating to authority figures	Are uncomfortable relating to authority figures
Express general satisfaction with life	Are dissatisfied with their lot in life
Have a strong social support system	Have a weak social support system
Have a primary internal locus of control	Rely on an external locus of control

can result in lowered self-esteem. Illness, injury, and other health issues also challenge a person's self-esteem. Findings from a sizable number of research studies demonstrate an association with changes in health status, functional abilities, emotional dysfunction, and lowering of self-esteem.

Self-esteem can also be enhanced through social support. Rebuilding relationships with family, friends, and teachers as well as participation in social activities and clubs can promote the process of achieving self-esteem. Nurses can help patients sort out and clarify the beliefs and emotions that get in the way of an awareness of their intrinsic value. Note how the patient describes achievements. Does the patient devalue accomplishments, project blame for problems onto others, minimize personal failures, or make self-deprecating remarks? Does the patient express shame or guilt? Does the patient seem hesitant to try new things or situations or express anxiety about coping with events? Observe defensive behaviors. Lack of culturally appropriate eye contact, poor hygiene, self-destructive behaviors, hypersensitivity to criticism, a need for constant reassurance, and the inability to accept compliments are behaviors associated with low self-esteem. Table 9.2 identifies characteristic behaviors related to self-esteem.

Therapeutic Strategies and Self-Esteem Issues

When people have low self-esteem and low self-worth, notions that no one really cares predominate. By understanding these underlying feelings as a threat to self-esteem (e.g., intense fear, anguish about an anticipated loss, and lack of power in an unfamiliar situation), nurses can facilitate opportunities for sharing the patient's story. The nurse might identify a legitimate feeling by saying, "It must be frustrating to feel that your questions go unanswered," and then asking, "How can I help you?"

Nurses also help patients increase self-esteem by being psychologically present as sounding boards. The process of engaging with another human being who offers a different perspective and demonstrates control in responding to events can enhance self-esteem. The implicit message the nurse conveys with personal presence and interest, information, and a guided exploration of the problem is twofold. The first is confirmation of the patient: "You are unique, you are important, and I will stay with you through this uncomfortable period."

The second is the introduction of the possibility of hope: "There may be some alternatives you haven't thought of that can help you cope with this problem. Would you ever consider … ?" Once a person starts to take control over his or her responses to events, a higher level of well-being can result. Vital to implementation of this intervention is to not minimize the energy required to change. As clear as the pathway to hope may be, the nurse needs to understand that it is not a simple road for the patient.

Using a strength-based approach offers the patient some control. It is helpful to say, for example, "The thing that impresses me about you is …" or "What I notice is that although your body is weaker, it seems as if your spirit is stronger. Would you say this is true?" Such questions help the patient focus on positive strengths. Behaviors suggestive of enhanced self-esteem include the following:
- Taking an active role in planning and implementing self-care
- Verbalizing personal psychosocial strengths
- Expressing feelings of satisfaction with self and ways of handling life events

Self-Efficacy

Self-efficacy is the belief in one's capabilities to organize and execute the courses of action required to manage prospective situations (Bandura, 2007). In other words, self-efficacy is a person's belief in his or her ability to succeed in a particular situation. People who believe that they can make changes and take control over their situation value their competence and ability to succeed. They are less likely to harbor self-doubts or dwell on personal deficiencies when difficulties arise. Successful self-management depends on developing self-efficacy.

Support of self-efficacy is critical to helping people with mental illness live successfully in the community. Self-efficacy improves motivation and helps patients sustain their efforts in the face of temporary setbacks.

Self-management support should include specific problem-solving skills and processes patients need to cope. Breaking difficult tasks down into achievable steps and completing them reinforce self-efficacy. Explain why each step is important to the next, and remind patients of progress toward a successful outcome.

Identify Patient Strengths

Skills training in areas where patients have deficits while also sincerely noting patients' efforts and persistence will encourage patients to take their next steps. Work with patients to use solutions and resources within their means. For example, exercise may become an acceptable option if patients know of free or low-cost exercise programs for seniors living in the community. Encourage significant others in the patient's life to give support and approval. Families appreciate receiving specific suggestions and opportunities to give appropriate support.

Self-help and support groups can be useful adjuncts to treatment. Discovering that others with similar issues have found ways to cope encourages patients and reinforces self-efficacy that they too can achieve similar success. The understanding, social support, and reciprocal learning found in these groups can provide opportunities for valuable information sharing and role modeling.

Role Performance

Role performance requires self-efficacy with links to self-concept. Professional identity can be conceptualized as a logical consequence of self-identity. Quality of life, a priority goal in *Healthy People 2030*, and role performance are also interrelated. How effectively people are able to function within expected roles influences their value within society and affects personal self-esteem.

Role performance and associated role relationships matter to people, as evidenced in symptoms of depression, feelings of emptiness, and even suicide when a significant personal or professional role ceases to exist.

Nurses need to be sensitive to the changes in role relationships that illness and injury produce for self, family, and relationships. An individual's social role can rapidly transform from independent self-sufficiency to vulnerability and dependence on others. New role behaviors may be uncomfortable and anxiety-producing. Asking open-ended and focused questions about the patient's relationships, across family, work, and social groups is a useful strategy for assessing role change. Box 9.3 presents suggestions that can be integrated into patient assessments.

Preconceived notions of role disruption for an ill or disabled person arise more commonly when the illness is protracted, recurrent, or seriously role-disruptive. When patients have to leave paid employment because of a chronic illness, it affects self-concept, because many people's social and personal identities are tied to their work roles. Nurses can coach patients about how to present themselves when they return to work. They can help patients learn how to respond to subtle and not-so-subtle discriminatory actions associated with others' lack of understanding of the patient's health situation.

Spiritual Aspects of Personal Identity

Spirituality is a unified concept, closely linked to a person's world view, providing a foundation for a personal belief system about the nature of a higher power, moral–ethical conduct, and reality. One's spiritual self-concept is concerned with one's relationship to a higher power and the vital life forces that support wholeness. When health fails or circumstances seem beyond control, it is often the spiritual that sustains peoples' sense of self, facilitates the will to live, and helps maintain a positive outlook and a sense of peace.

The term *spirituality* is often used synonymously with *religion*, but it is a much broader concept. A key difference is that religion involves beliefs and values within an

---

> **BOX 9.3   Sample Assessment Questions Related to Role Relationships**
>
> **Family**
> 1. "Who do you see in your family as being supportive of you?" or "Who can you rely on to help you through any changes?"
> 2. "Who do you see in your family as being most affected by your illness (condition)?" or "Who do you think will need to adjust more than any other family member?"
> 3. "What changes do you anticipate as a result of your illness (condition) in the way you function in your family?" or "Will your health change how things get done in the family?"
>
> **Work**
> 1. "What are some of the concerns you have about your job at this time?"
> 2. "Who do you see in your work situation as being supportive of you?"
>
> **Social**
> 1. "How has your illness affected the way people who are important to you treat you?"
> 2. "Is there anyone outside of family you turn to for support?"
> 3. "If (name)_____ is not available to you, who else might you be able to call on for support?"

---

organized faith community, whereas spirituality describes self-chosen beliefs and values changing over time that give personal meaning to one's life. Try Simulation Exercise 9.3 to practice responses to patients in spiritual distress.

Spiritual aspects of self-concept can be expressed through the following:
1. Membership in a specific religious faith community
2. Mindfulness, meditation, or other personalized lifeways and practices
3. Cultural and family beliefs about forgiveness, justice, human rights, social justice
4. Crises or existential situations that stimulate a search for purpose, meaning, and values beyond the self

The Joint Commission mandates that healthcare agencies, including long-term hospice and home care services, assess patients' spiritual needs, provide for the spiritual care of them and their families, and supply appropriate documentation of that care. Health crises can be a time of spiritual renewal, when one discovers new inner resources, strengths, and capacities never before tested. Alternatively, it can signal a period of spiritual desolation, leaving the

SIMULATION EXERCISE 9.3   Responding to Issues of Spiritual Distress

Purpose
To help students understand responses in times of spiritual distress.

Procedure
Review the following case situations and develop an appropriate response to each.
1. Mary is 16 years old and has just found out she has a sexually transmitted disease. Her family belongs to a Christian church in which sex before marriage is not permitted. Mary feels guilty about her current status and sees it as "God punishing me for fooling around."
2. Kema is married to an abusive, alcoholic husband. She reads the Quran daily during Ramadan and prays for her husband's healing. She feels that God will turn the marriage around if she continues to pray for changes in her husband's attitude. "Praised be God … guide us to the right path" she implores.
3. Ari tells the nurse, "I feel that God has let me down. I was taught that those who follow the law or do good are rewarded while those who don't are punished. I have been a good rabbi, husband, father, and son. Now the doctors tell me I'm going to die and I am 50 years old. That doesn't seem fair to me."

Reflective Discussion Analysis
1. Share your answers with others in your group. Did you have to explore spiritual beliefs beyond your own?
2. Give and get feedback on the usefulness of your responses.
3. In what ways can you use this new knowledge in your nursing care?

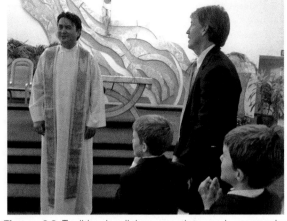

Figure 9.3 Traditional religious practices and ceremonies strengthen value systems that are integral to personal self-concepts.

- Sources of hope and support
- Desire for visitation from clergy or pastoral chaplain

Spirituality can be a powerful resource in families, and it is important to incorporate questions about the family's spirituality if they are involved in supporting the patient.

Nursing Strategies That Foster Spirituality

Providing privacy and quiet times for spiritual activities is important. An important component of nursing care is helping patients address their spiritual identity by providing time for spiritual practices and referral to chaplains or spiritual directors. This also includes advocating for the patient's spiritual practice related to dietary restrictions, mindfulness settings, holy day activities, meditating or praying, and end-of-life cultural practices. For example, in some forms of the Jewish religion, turning lights on or off or adjusting the position of an electric bed is not permitted. Traditional rituals can bring comfort (Fig. 9.3).

Praying with a patient, even when the patient is of a different faith, can be a soothing intervention.

individual feeling abandoned, angry, and powerless to control or change important life circumstances.

Assessment should take account of the patient's
- Willingness to talk about personal spirituality or beliefs
- Belief in a personal god or higher power
- Relevance of specific cultural or religious practices to the individual
- Changes in religious practices or beliefs
- Areas of specific spiritual concern activated by the illness, for example, is there an afterlife?
- Extent to which illness, injury, or disability has had an effect on the patient's spiritual beliefs

▮ SUMMARY

This chapter focuses on the self-concept as a key variable in the nurse–patient relationship. *Self-concept* refers to an acquired constellation of thoughts, feelings, attitudes, and beliefs that individuals have about the nature and organization of their personality. Self-concept develops through the interaction between experiences with the environment and personal characteristics.

Aspects of self-concept discussed in the chapter include body image, personal identity, role performance, self-esteem, self-efficacy, self-clarity, and spirituality. The self-concept is a dynamic construct, composed of many features, capable of developing new paths to help answer such question as, "Who am I?" "What is important to me in this situation or phase of life?" As a professional nurse, you will have many opportunities to help patients answer these questions.

Disturbances in body image refer to issues related to changes in appearance and physical functions, both overt and hidden. Personal identity is constructed through cognitive processes of perception and cognition. Serious illnesses such as dementia and psychotic disorders threaten or crush a person's sense of personal identity. Self-esteem is associated with the emotional aspect of self-concept and reflects the value a person places on his or her personal self-concept and its place in the world. Self-efficacy pertains to the control individuals feel they have to make changes in the face of challenges to self-clarity, which relates to the stability of the defined self. Self-esteem hopefulness and spirituality have been shown to be positively related to health-related quality of life. Understanding elements of self-concept and their critical role in managing behavior is key to working effectively with patients of all ages. It is a core variable to consider in therapeutic communication, nurse–patient relationships, and interventions.

ETHICAL DILEMMA: What Would You Do?

Jimmy is a 68-year-old man with diabetes; he was brought to the emergency room in kidney failure. The doctor has indicated that he needs Jimmy to agree to dialysis, but Jimmy refuses, saying "this only prolongs the final result." He refuses to listen to any long-term plan of care, and his wife is confused about options beyond dialysis. The doctor wants you to get Jimmy's consent for immediate dialysis. As the nurse caring for this patient, what would you do?

DISCUSSION QUESTIONS

1. What role do the various modalities of social media play in the development and/or validation of a person's self-concept?
2. In what ways are spirituality and world view connected in defining self-concept?
3. Drawing on your experience, what are some specific ways in which you can help another person develop a stronger sense of self?

ACKNOWLEDGMENT

Thanks to Eileen O'Brien, who wrote the previous edition of this chapter.

REFERENCES

Arnett, J. J. (2018). *Adolescence and emerging adulthood: A cultural approach* (6th ed.). Hoboken, NJ: Pearson.

Bandura, A. (1997). *Self-efficacy. The exercise of control.* New York: W.H. Freeman and Company.

Bandura, A. (2007). Self-efficacy in health functioning. In S. Ayers (Ed.), *Cambridge handbook of psychology, health and medicine* (2nd ed.) (pp. 191–193). New York: Cambridge University Press.

Beck, J., & Beck, A. (2011). *Cognitive conceptualization: Cognitive behavior therapy.* New York: Guilford Press.

Benner, P. (2003). Reflecting on what we care about. *American Journal of Critical Care, 12*(2), 165–166.

Erikson, E. (1959). *Identity and the life cycle: Selected papers.* Oxford, UK: International Universities Press.

Erikson, E. (1968). *Identity: Youth and crisis.* New York: Norton.

Erikson, E. (1982). *The life cycle completed: A review.* New York: Norton.

Erikson, E. H. (1985). *The life cycle completed.* New York: Norton.

Gordon, M. (2007). Self-perception-self-concept pattern. In *Manual of nursing diagnoses* (11th ed.). Chestnut Hill, MA: Jones & Bartlett.

Ramadhanty, R. P., & Hamid, A. Y. S. (2021). Body image perception is related to self-esteem of the adolescents with acne vulgaris. *Enfermeria Clinica, 31*(Suppl. 2), S326–S329.

Rogers, C. (1959). A theory of therapy, personality and interpersonal relationships as developed in the client-centered framework. In S. Koch (Ed.), *Psychology: A study of a science. Vol. 3: Formulations of the person and the social context.* New York: McGraw Hill.

Shpigelman, C. N., & HaGani, N. (2019). The impact of disability type and visibility on self-concept and body image: Implications for mental health nursing. *Journal of Psychiatric and Mental Health Nursing, 26*(3–4), 77–86.

Stuart, G. (2020). *Principles and practice of psychiatric nursing.* St. Louis: Elsevier.

Sue, D. W., Capodilupa, C., Torino, G., et al. (2007). Racial microaggressions in everyday life. Implications for clinical practice. *The American Psychologist, 62*(4), 271–286.

Sullivan, H. S. (1953). *The interpersonal theory of psychiatry.* New York: Norton.

Wilde, J. L., & Dozois, D. J. A. (2019). A dyadic partner-schema model of relationship distress and depression: Conceptual integration of interpersonal theory and cognitive-behavioral models. *Clinical Psychology Review, 70*, 13–25.

10

Developing Patient-Centered Therapeutic Relationships

Patient- and family-centered care models of healthcare delivery support the inclusion of the patient and the patient's family as essential members of the interprofessional care team. The Academy of Sciences considers PCC a pillar of care. One of the six QSEN competencies identified as essential for a beginning nurse is ability to give PCC (Disch & Barnsteiner, 2021). Patients are expected to take an active role in self-managing the care of their chronic diseases. While they cannot always defeat a disorder, they can, with our help, learn to live successfully with a chronic illness. Nurses strive to communicate support and information in a culturally sensitive manner. Consideration of a patient's preferences should be a hallmark of healthcare. Chapter 10 explores core concepts and essential features of patient-centered therapeutic relationships.

BASIC CONCEPTS

The importance of patient-centered relationships as a major component of safe, quality healthcare delivery cannot be overemphasized. Research indicates that effective relationships are a significant predictor of positive health outcomes (Hibbard et al., 2017).

Definition

A patient-centered relationship between provider and patient is categorized as a purposeful therapeutic alliance, linked to helping patients achieve identifiable health goals. The National Council of State Boards of Nursing defines a **therapeutic relationship** as one that allows nurses to apply their professional knowledge, skills, abilities, and experiences toward meeting the health needs of the patient. Therapeutic relationships in healthcare can take place in a variety of venues, ranging from preventive care through intensive care management of an acute medical or psychological condition, and follow-up care of patients, posthospitalization.

Goals

Nurses engage their patient in a therapeutic relationship to help them achieve self-management, develop a healthier lifestyle, and provide care that helps restore them to maximum possible health. The importance of putting PCC concepts into practice cannot be overemphasized. Reflect on the Ruiz case.

Patient-Centered Therapeutic Relationships

PCC relationships represent a subset of professional therapeutic relationships, in which nurses and other health professionals engage with their patients to
- understand the patient's experience of an illness;
- help them learn to self-manage chronic health problems;
- develop healthy lifestyle behaviors to prevent or minimize the development of chronic disorders; and
- increase their satisfaction with clinical outcomes and well-being.

CASE STUDY: Mary Ruiz and Colitis

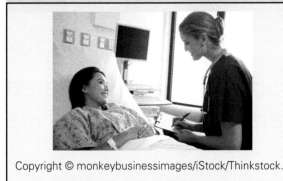

Copyright © monkeybusinessimages/iStock/Thinkstock.

Mary Ruiz, age 18 years, is admitted for treatment of a flare-up of her colitis. She is especially upset about the ongoing diarrhea. Carol Gard, RN, works with Mary on admission day to develop a mutual, realistic plan of care, which includes Ms Ruiz's preferences. Carol's vocal tone and facial expression convey genuine empathy and interest in her patient. Ms Ruiz comes to feel valued, as this professional relationship continues. Notice the eye contact, sitting posture, and pleasant expression on Carol's face.

PCC relationships begin with the expectation that patients will take an active participatory role in self-managing their chronic health condition(s). They are characterized as a clinical partnership that recognizes the patient as a source of control and a full partner. Nurses provide compassionate and coordinated care based on respect for patients' preferences, values, and needs. Considering care from a patient's perspective helps develop trust, respect, and consistent care. The patient is the best informant about the meaning of their illness to their life.

The correlation between therapeutic relationship and patient centeredness is portrayed in Fig. 10.1. The continuum of patient-centered relationships ranges from those found in critical care, to relationships supporting primary care self-management of chronic conditions, to settings for preventive and urgent care. Home-based and long-term care settings involve documentation of PCC at a higher level of intervention than ever before.

Structure

The underlying premise is that each patient is unique and different. Communication is basic to establishing a patient-centered relationship (ANA, 2010). Communication needs to be individualized, wholistic, and empowering. Relationships are time limited, subject to treatment and other regulatory concerns. A relationship can span an 8-hour shift. It can occur episodically, or at regularly scheduled times; as a single encounter, or as an emergency care contact. Longer-term relationships can last over a period of days, weeks, or months as in a home healthcare patient or one with a patient in a mental health inpatient setting or rehabilitation center. Regardless of the amount of time spent, each relationship can, and should, be meaningful. The relationship typically terminates when identified clinical objectives are achieved, or the patient is transferred to a different care setting.

Barriers

New graduate nurses have had limited opportunities to develop professional communication skills. Much initial energy is focused on mastering the technical skills needed in their care. Practice with Simulation Exercises helps begin this process. It can be uncomfortable at first to discuss with a patient their poor prognosis or end-of-life condition. Kantor and Stadelman (2020) comment that student preference for electronic communication can also be a barrier to therapeutic interaction. Nurses develop comfort with their use of communication skills over time.

Self-Disclosure

This is a limited sharing of personal data on the nurse's part, just enough to facilitate the relationship. Limit your self-revelation to brief general comments such as how many years experience you have in nursing or where you went to school, but do not share intimate details of your life (NCSBN, 2018; Valente, 2017). Avoid implying your experience is exactly the same as the patient's experience. Table 10.1 outlines the differences between helping therapeutic relationships and social relationships.

Characteristics of Patient-Centered Care Relationships

Patient

These relationships are based on the premise that each person's experience of an illness, injury, or disease is a unique holistic human experience, and much more than simply a biomedical process. Patient- and family-centered care applies to patients of all ages and can be practiced in any healthcare setting. Such relationships are subject to legal and ethical standards.

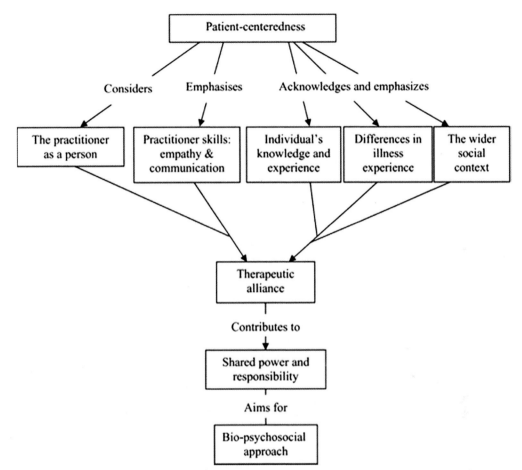

Figure 10.1 Model of patient centeredness in nurse–patient relationships. (From Lhussier, M., Eaton, S., Forster, N., Thomas, M., Roberts, S., & Carr, S. M. (2015). Care planning for long-term conditions—a concept mapping. *Health Expectations, 18*(5), 605–624.)

Nursing Support

Relational connections in patient-centered relationships offer supportive intervention that is respectful, individualized, and empowering. Each relationship is based on the importance of understanding the patient as a unique individual with a health need or functional capacity that interferes with one or more aspects of their life in a meaningful way. In addition to a patient's physical and clinical needs, nurses need to consider each patient's cognitive, sociocultural, and emotional context, as these data frame the patient's personalized experience of health issues. Addressing situational, cultural, religious, and family circumstances allows for a more inclusive *holistic* targeted understanding of the patient's preferences and life goals.

These data allow nurses to individualize, support, and understand the fuller dimensions of a patient's health issues. Listening to what a patient identifies as primary concerns provides stronger information about the patient's values and preferences.

Respect

Respectful care starts with careful listening and emphasizes the patient's strengths, abilities, wishes, and goals. Respect assumes, until proven otherwise, that patients are interested in bettering their health, and are willing to make positive efforts, even when those efforts are not clearly visible. Nurses demonstrate respectful care when they support patient autonomy and realistic care goals.

TABLE 10.1   Differences Between Helping Relationships and Social Relationships

Helping Relationships	Social Relationships
Healthcare provider takes responsibility for the conduct of the relationship and for maintaining appropriate boundaries	Both parties have equal responsibility for the conduct of the relationship
Relationship has a specific health-related purpose and goals	Relationship may or may not have a specific purpose or goals
Meeting the professional health-related needs and goals of the patient determines the duration of the relationship	Relationship can last a lifetime or terminate spontaneously at any time
Focus of the relationship is on the needs of the patient	The needs of both partners can receive equal attention
Relationship is entered into because of a patient's healthcare need	Relationship is entered into spontaneously for a wide variety of purposes
Choice of who to be in relationship is not available to either the helper or the patient	Behavior for both participants is spontaneous; people choose companions
Self-disclosure by the nurse is limited to data that facilitate the health-related relationship. Self-disclosure by the patient is expected and encouraged.	Self-disclosure for both parties in the relationship is expected and encouraged

Individualized Care

Listening to what the patient identifies as his or her main concern provides contextual data about patient values and preferences within the family and community. Once you have a composite picture of each patient, and of what matters to the patient and family, it becomes easier to develop a care plan based on individual patient goals and values. Motivation and interest are significant contributors to relevant goal development and continued efforts to achieve personally relevant life and health goals.

The experience of "becoming a patient" varies from person to person. In a professional health relationship, neither clinician nor patient exists independently of the other. A patient-centered relationship seeks to understand the patient as a person with emotional, physical, and spiritual needs coping with health-related life issues. What happens within this relationship becomes the shared product of their interaction. Patient-centered interactions take place within the context of the nurse/patient culture, personal worldviews, previous life experiences, the nature of the illness and its impact on other relationships, and personal values—all of which are important to the patient.

Elements of the Patient-Centered Relationship Model

PCC is basically examining healthcare from the patient perspective of their care and their relationships with the health professionals caring for them. A patient-centered relationship considers each individual patient as a *person* first and foremost, with distinctive personally held values, beliefs, and life goals. Second, this person

is a "patient with a medical or psychiatric diagnosis," requiring treatment and tangible professional support to resolve a chronic illness, or to improve preventive care. In crisis situations, immediate life-sustaining issues take precedence. Personal factors, especially those related to patient dignity and individuality, should still be incorporated.

A major value of this model is that it can be integrated across multiple care settings. The inclusion of transitional care initiatives helps offset potential gaps in service. In addition to patient education and traditional care provision, nurses work with patients and families to help them develop the self-management skills and strategies they need to cope with chronic disorders such as diabetes, arthritis, and cardiac issues.

The Patient-Centered Care Process

Orientation/Assessment Phase. In this phase, the nurse obtains information and tries to engage the patient in management of their illness (Fite et al., 2019). The orientation phase of the relationship defines the purpose, roles, and rules of the process and provides a framework for assessing patient needs. The nurse builds a sense of trust through consistency of actions. A patient-centered assessment seeks an integrated understanding of each patient's contextual world—including emotional needs and life issues. These data form a relational informational platform that "fits" the patient and provides a common ground for developing mutually agreed upon self-management and health-related clinical strategies. Refer to the assessment guidelines in Box 10.1.

BOX 10.1 Guidelines for Effective Initial Assessment Interviews

- Tune in to the physical and psychological behaviors that express the patient's point of view.
- Do self-checks for stereotypes or premature understanding of the patient's issues, and set aside personal biases.
- Be tentative in your listening responses, and ask for validation frequently.
- Mentally picture the patient's situation, and ask appropriate questions to secure information about any areas or issues you are not clear about.
- Give yourself time to think about what your patient has said before responding or asking the next question.
- Mirror the patient's level of energy and language.
- Be authentic in your responses.
- Assume responsibility for personal actions, if choosing to refuse treatment.
- Follow hospital regulations regarding safety and conduct.

Working Phase. Developing a mutual patient-centered plan encourages patient autonomy. The nurse encourages the patient to develop self-efficacy in all aspects of care. Self-efficacy plays an important role in personal motivation (Bandura, 2012). Self-efficacy is defined as the confidence that a person holds about personal ability to achieve goals or to complete a task. Self-efficacy beliefs affect the quality of human functioning through cognitive, motivational, affective, and decisional processes. Specifically, people's beliefs in their efficacy will influence whether they have confidence in their abilities to achieve the goals they set for themselves. Once a patient and clinician(s) agree on a workable action plan, nurses provide therapeutic interventions and treatments as ordered.

Nurses also initiate applicable patient education; nurses provide therapeutic interventions and treatment. Compassionate coaching and informed support of targeted self-management strategies become an important focus of the care partnership. These communication strategies are specifically designed to incorporate patient values and preferences as an essential component of care, to whatever extent is possible.

Communication. Professional relationships and informational transfer are major communication tools used to meet one or more of the following care goals:

- Understanding the patient's experience of an illness

- Helping patients to effectively self-manage chronic health problems
- Encouraging patients to develop healthy lifestyle behaviors to prevent or minimize the development of chronic disorders

Termination Phase. All the team members help plan for discharge to home or community care. Sometimes there is a case manager who writes the discharge plan and makes referrals to community facilities of home health agencies. The case manager or primary nurse assumes responsibility for follow-up verification to avoid gaps in service. The discharge plan needs to be expedited to notify the patient's primary physician about on-going treatment plans, medications needed, etc.

Collaborative Patient-Centered Relationships

Collaborative interprofessional care approaches embedded in designated healthcare teams, rather than single practitioners assuming responsibility for the patient-centered healthcare of patients, have become the new norm in healthcare delivery. This paradigm shift is based on the premise that no single healthcare discipline can provide complete care for a patient with today's multiple chronic healthcare needs. Interprofessional collaborative relationships bring together the sophisticated medical, nursing, pharmacy, rehabilitative, psychological, and social work skills needed to support desired patient-centered outcomes. The relationship aspect develops from mutual respect and power sharing among all team members, including the patient, to achieve clinical outcomes.

Care coordination among multiple care providers is an essential component of interprofessional patient-centered relationships (WHO, 2010). Contemporary practice requires that nurses lead, coordinate, and integrate their professional nursing skills with those of other health team members (depending on the circumstances) for maximum effectiveness.

Duration

Time spent with patients varies. A patient-centered relationship can span an 8-hour full shift in a hospital. They occur at regularly scheduled times, as a single encounter, or as an emergency care contact. Longer-term relationships can last over a period of days, weeks, or months in a mental health inpatient setting, or in a rehabilitation center. Patient-centered relationships increasingly take place in community-based medical homes, in the patient's home, or as a one-time encounter in an urgent care center.

Depending on the geographic area, some relationships can take place digitally. Patients have the capability to communicate with providers through secure patient portals, as described on Chapters 25 and 26.

BOX 10.2 Peplau's Six Nursing Relationship Roles

- *Stranger* role: Receives the patient the same way one meets a stranger in other life situations; provides an accepting climate that builds trust.
- *Resource* role: Answers questions, interprets clinical treatment data, and gives information.
- *Teaching* role: Gives instructions and provides training; involves analysis and synthesis of the learner experience.
- *Counseling* role: Helps the patient understand and integrate the meaning of current life circumstances; provides guidance and encouragement to make essential changes.
- *Surrogate* role: Helps the patient clarify domains of dependence, interdependence, and independence; acts on the patient's behalf as an advocate.
- *Leadership* role: Helps the patient assume maximum responsibility for meeting treatment goals in a mutually satisfying way.

Theoretical Frameworks

Theoretical frameworks that support the study of patient-centered relationships in nursing practice include caring as a core theme in nursing theories: Peplau's interpersonal nursing theory, Carl Rogers' person-centered theory, and Maslow's needs theory.

Caring. Caring represents a core foundational value in professional nursing relationships. It is this component of professional relationships that is best remembered by patients, families, and nurses. The caring involved in patient-centered relationships is not so much about the words themselves, or about specific tasks. Rather, it is about a sustained connection, and the meaning that caring connection holds for the recipient. Caring as a key characteristic of professional nursing should be embodied as a visible component of each nurse's relationship, with patients and families, and with each other. The concept of *"caring"* is valued by NSBON and is integrated into NCLEX testing for licensure (Ignatavicius, 2021). You demonstrate caring by showing respect, being attentive, and showing interest in the patient's point of view. You work to build a mutually trusting relationship with physical, psychological, educational, and spiritual interventions.

Hildegard Peplau's Interpersonal Nursing Theory. Hildegard Peplau's (1992; 1997) interpersonal nursing theory is a well-known theory of interpersonal relationships in nursing. She identifies four sequential phases of a nurse–patient relationship: *preinteraction, orientation,*

working phase (problem identification and exploitation), and *termination.* These phases are an overlapping part of a holistic relationship. Each phase serves to broaden as well as deepen the emotional connection between nurse and patient. Peplau identified six professional roles the nurse can assume during the course of the nurse–patient relationship as listed in Box 10.2.

Carl Rogers's Client-Centered Model. Carl Rogers's model states that each person has within himself or herself the capacity to heal if given support and treated with respect and unconditional positive regard in a caring, authentic, and therapeutic relationship (Rogers, 1958). Rogers presents a person-centered approach to the study of therapeutic relationships and the relevant concepts supporting it. He identifies three major provider attributes of person-centered relationships in therapeutic setting, as follows:
- authenticity (being "real" in a relationship without artificial facades)
- prizing (trust and respect)
- empathetic understanding

Abraham Maslow's Needs Theory. According to the International Council of Nurses (ICN), human needs guide the work of nursing (ICN, 2011). Abraham Maslow's (1970) needs theory offers a motivational framework that nurses use to prioritize patient needs in planning their care. Fig. 10.2 shows Maslow's model as a pyramid, with need requirements occurring in an ascending fashion from basic survival needs through to self-actualization.

Maslow defines first-level needs as *deficiency* needs, meaning that these are fundamental needs required for human survival. First-level *basic physiological needs* include hunger, thirst, sexual appetites, and sensory stimulation. Maslow's second-level *safety and security needs* describe basic physical safety and emotional security, for example, financial safety, freedom from injury, safe neighborhood, and freedom from abuse. Until basic deficiency needs are met, people cannot attend to personal growth needs.

Satisfaction of basic deficiency needs allows for attention to the fulfilment of growth needs. *Love and belonging needs* relate to emotionally connecting with, and experiencing, oneself as being a part of a family and/or community. The next level *self-esteem needs* refers to a person's need for recognition and appreciation. A sense of dignity, respect, and approval by others for oneself is a hallmark of successfully meeting self-esteem needs. Maslow's highest level of need satisfaction, *self-actualization*, refers to a person's need to achieve his or her (self-defined) human potential. Self-actualized individuals are not superhuman; they are subject to the same feelings of insecurity that all individuals experience. The difference is that they accept

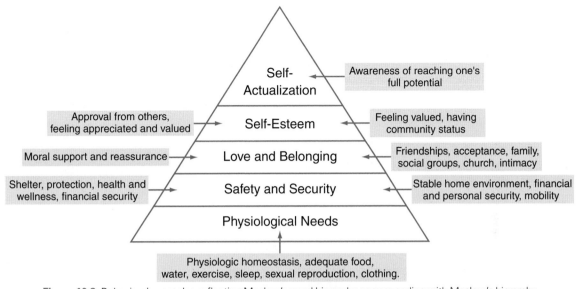

Figure 10.2 Behavioral examples reflecting Maslow's need hierarchy corresponding with Maslow's hierarchy of needs.

this vulnerability as part of their human condition. Not everyone reaches this developmental stage.

Nurses use Maslow's theory with patients and families to prioritize nursing interventions that best match with patient needs and priorities.

Elements to Consider in Caring Relationships

Self-Awareness. As you focus on caring, maintain a realistic outlook that outcomes for some patients are beyond your control. Focus on what you think the patient can change, but recognize change is a hard task for many patients. Always maintain awareness of boundaries and of your limitations. Circumstances such as death of your patient can take an emotional toll. On some units, nurse managers hold debriefing meetings to offer support to staff. Take your "emotional temperature" to recognize your own stress as discussed in Chapter 27.

Therapeutic Use of Self. The therapeutic relationship is not simply about what the nurse does, but who the nurse *is* in relation to patients and their families. Use of self is an important tool. Nurses cultivate an attitude of interest in the whole person. Developing optimal connection implies authenticity. This genuineness is recognized as a precondition for the therapeutic use of self in the nurse–patient relationship. Being genuine or authentic is closely aligned with honesty. The concept builds on a person's values and is influenced by a person's culture.

APPLICATIONS

The term "patient-centered care" was initially developed by the Picker Institute (n.d.), shifting focus from a disease model to one emphasizing inclusion of the patient and family as full partners in planning and implementing meaningful healthcare. Providers hold a genuine desire to support the patient to achieve maximum health and well-being through an action plan tailored to patient needs, values, and preferences.

Level of Involvement

Overinvolvement

Sometimes a nurse losses essential objectivity needed to support the patient. Warning signs that the nurse is becoming overinvolved can include giving extra time and attention to certain patients; visiting patients during off-duty hours; doing things for patients that they could do for themselves; discounting the actions of other professionals or believing that they are the only one who understands the patient's needs.

Disengagement

The opposite of overinvolvement is *disengagement,* which occurs when a nurse emotionally or physically withdraws from having more than a superficial contact with a patient. Disengagement can be related to either the patient's behavior or intensity of suffering. It can be a symptom

---

DEVELOPING AN EVIDENCE-BASED PRACTICE

Nurse–Patient Caring Relationships

Effective therapeutic interpersonal relationships with patients is a core concept in nursing clinical practice aimed toward helping patients achieve maximum outcomes. Caring and trust are commonly identified as major components, with many tools available that attempt to measure relationships. However, Hartley and colleagues' review (2020) shows this concept is poorly understood. Carley et al. (2021) also found that lack of knowledge interfered with relationships, specifically interfered with establishment of trust. This finding is substantiated by many others who describe a lack of research into nurse–patient relationship components. Hartley analyzed eight published research studies of interventions to promote stronger nurse–patient relationships, including professional development workshops and continuing education sessions; group-based programs to encourage reflection; self-education or assigned readings; application of interaction protocols in nurse–patient dyads. Helt et al. (2020) examined effects of clinical simulations to increase nurse knowledge.

Results

No one method was found to significantly improve nurse–patient relationships over time except the clinical simulation strategy. Didactic presentations and clinical simulations were found to significantly increase nurse knowledge and self-efficacy. One study of beginning nursing students showed they questioned how to demonstrate caring within the nurse–patient relationship.

Strength of research: Low. Most studies were descriptive rather than experimental. Reviewers advocated the need for research and wondered how concepts so fundamental to the practice of nursing can be so untested.

Application to Your Clinical Practice

1. Use many modalities to learn about effective nurse–patient therapeutic relationships. Encourage use of clinical simulation methods.
2. Nurses need to consciously be aware of communication skills that build meaningful relationships and become aware of challenges to developing these relationships.
3. Caring as a basic relationship component should be actively demonstrated from initial contact and consistently throughout the relationship with patients (Albinsson et al., 2021).

References

Albinsson, G., Carlsson-Blomster, M., & Lindqvist, G. (2021). In search of a caring relationship: Nursing students' notions of interactions in the nurse-patient relationship. *Nurse Education in Practice, 50*, 102954.

Carley, A., Melrose, S., Rempel, G., Diehl-Jones, W., & Schwarz, B. A. (2021). Professional development needs of non-radiology nurses: An exploration of nurses' experiences caring for interventional radiology patients. *Journal of Radiology, 40*(2), 146–151.

Hartley, S., Raphael, J., Lovell, K., & Berry, K. (2020). Effective nurse-patient relationships in mental health care: A systematic review of interventions to improve the therapeutic alliance. *International Journal of Nursing Studies, 102*, 103490.

Helt, J., Gilmer, M.J., & Connors, L. (2020). Clinical simulation training in nurses caring for pediatric oncology patients. *Clinical Simulation in Nursing, 47*, 73–81.

---

of burnout or heightened stress on the nurse's part. For example, an increased number of deaths or high stress levels on a unit can create compassion fatigue, which can lead to disengagement as a self-protective mechanism. Signs of disengagement include withdrawal, limited perfunctory contacts, minimizing the patient's suffering, and engaging in defensive or judgmental communication.

Helpful Levels of Involvement

Maintaining a helpful level of involvement is always the responsibility of the professional nurse. To sustain a helpful level of professional connection and/or to regain perspective in a relationship:

- Focus on the process of care while acknowledging that the outcome may or may not be within your control.
- Focus on the things that you can change while acknowledging that there are things over which you have no control.
- Be aware and accepting of your professional limits and boundaries.
- Monitor your reactions and seek assistance when you feel uncomfortable about any aspect of the relationship.
- Balance giving care to a patient with taking care of yourself, without feeling guilty.

Developing a Collaborative Relationship

Engaging the Patient

Both the patient and the nurse have rights and responsibilities. Trust is essential to patient engagement and to effective decision-making in PCC. The American Hospital

BOX 10.3 Patient Rights and Responsibilities

All patients have the following rights:

- Impartial access to the most appropriate treatment regardless of race, age, sexual preference, national origin, religion, handicap, or source of payment for care
- To be treated with respect, dignity, and personal privacy in a safe, secure environment
- Confidential treatment of all communication and other records related to care or payment, except as required by law or signed insurance contractual arrangements (all patients should receive Notice of Privacy Practices)
- Active participation in all aspects of decision-making regarding personal healthcare
- To know the identity and professional status of each healthcare provider
- To have treatments and procedures explained to them in ways they can understand
- To receive competent interpreter services, if required, to understand care or treatment
- To refuse treatment, including lifesaving treatment, after being told of the potential risks associated with such refusal
- To receive appropriate pain management
- To express grievances regarding any violation of patient rights internally and/or to the appropriate agency

All patients have the following responsibilities:

- To treat their care providers with respect and courtesy, including timely notification for appointment cancellations
- To provide accurate, complete information about all personal health matters
- To follow recommended treatment plans

Association (AHA, 2003) has developed a brochure outlining the rights and responsibilities of patient care partnerships. The document is accessible in multiple languages on the AHA website. Hospitals today have copies of comprehensive patient rights posted on their websites. Written copies are given to patients on admission. A sample listing of common patient rights and responsibilities is provided in Box 10.3.

Setting Realistic Goals for Self-Management

Self-management strategies work best when they are linked to a patient's values, interests, capabilities, and resources.

The patient has to believe that a goal is both meaningful and achievable. Nurses need to get an idea about patient and family motivation to make changes.

Patients are expected to be active agents in supporting their own healthcare processes.

Self-Awareness

Self-awareness is an intrapersonal process, which allows nurses to self-reflect on aspects of their personal feelings and beliefs. A common definition of self-awareness includes the nurse's conscious recognition of personal thoughts, motivations, strengths, and emotions, and how each can influence their behavior in the professional relationship. This gives the nurse more options to be therapeutic. For example, in a situation when a nurse realized that the respiratory therapist would be better equipped to explain the process of weaning the patient from a ventilator, she arranged for the therapist to provide the explanation, while providing her presence and support by staying with the patient during the explanation and the weaning process.

To remain authentic, nurses need to be clear about their personal values, beliefs, stereotypes, and personal perspectives, because of their potential influence on patient decisions. Self-awareness of bias or value conflicts is important to acknowledge because these factors can sabotage relationship goals. The reality is that there are some patients who are difficult to work with productively. Much of the time, patients who are difficult are also in psychological pain, which colors how they feel about themselves and about life. Being calm, interested, but not pushy helps to make for a better interpersonal encounter. A useful strategy in such situations is to seek further understanding of the patient as a person.

Case Study: Brian Haggarty, a Homeless Man

Brian Haggarty tells the nurse, "I know you want to help me, but you can't understand my situation. You don't know what it is like out on the streets." Instead of responding defensively, the nurse responds, "You are right; I don't know what it is like to be homeless, but I would like to know more about your experiences. Can you tell me what it has been like for you?" With this listening response, the nurse invites the patient to share his experience. The data might allow the nurse to appreciate and address the loneliness, fear, and helplessness the patient is experiencing, which are universal feelings.

SIMULATION EXERCISE 10.1   Introductions in the Nurse-Patient Relationship

Purpose

To provide simulated experience with initial introductions.

Procedure

The introductory statement forms the basis for the rest of the relationship. Effective contact with a patient helps build an atmosphere of trust and connectedness with the nurse. The following statement is a good example of how one might engage the patient in the first encounter:

"Hello, Mr Smith. I am Sally Parks, a nursing student. I will be taking care of you on this shift. During the day, I may be asking you some questions about yourself that will help me to understand how I can best help you."

Role-play the introduction to a new patient with one person taking the role of the patient; another, the nurse; and a third person, an involved family member, with one or more of the following patients:

1. Mrs Dobish is a 70-year-old patient admitted to the hospital with a diagnosis of diabetes and a question about cognitive impairment.

2. Thomas Charles is a 19-year-old patient admitted to the hospital following an auto accident in which he broke both legs and fractured his sternum.

3. Barry Fisher is a 53-year-old man who has been admitted to the hospital for tests. The physician believes he may have a renal tumor.

4. Marion Beatty is a 9-year-old girl admitted to the hospital for an appendectomy.

5. Barbara Tangiers is a 78-year-old woman living by herself. She has multiple health problems including chronic obstructive pulmonary disease and arthritis. This is your first visit.

Reflective Discussion Analysis

1. In what ways did you have to modify your introductions to meet the needs of the patient and/or circumstances?

2. What were the easiest and hardest parts of doing this exercise?

3. How could you use this experience as a guide in your clinical practice?

Presence

Presence involves the nurse's capacity to know when to provide help, when to stand back, when to speak frankly, and when to withhold comments because the patient is not ready to hear them. The nurse's ability to be "present" in the relationship (rather than adopting a work persona), to expose themselves fully to understanding the patient's and their own experiences, to be open and truthful in their dealings, and to be generous in committing to the patient's best interests, aides in the development of a therapeutic relationship.

Peplau's developmental phases parallel the nursing process. The orientation phase correlates with the assessment phase of this process. The identification component of the working phase corresponds to the planning phase, whereas the working phase parallels the exploitation component of the implementation phase. The final resolution phase of the relationship corresponds to the evaluation phase of the nursing process.

Key Concepts

Nurses enter interpersonal relationships with patients in the "*stranger*" *role*. The patient does not know you, and you do not know the patient as a person. Nurses have an advantage, as the care environment is familiar to them. This is not necessarily true for patients. Many patients not only need an introduction to the nurse but also need an orientation to the setting and what to expect in the assessment phase.

You can begin the process of developing trust by providing the patient with basic information about yourself such as name and professional status (Peplau, 1997). This can be a simple introduction: "Good morning, Mrs. Kenney, I am Susan Smith, a registered nurse, and I am going to be your nurse on this shift." Nonverbal supporting behaviors of a handshake, eye contact, and a smile can reinforce your words.

Introductions are important even with patients who are confused, aphasic, comatose, or unable to make a cogent response because of mental illness or dementia. Starting with the first encounter, patients begin to assess the trustworthiness of each nurse who cares for them. Sustained attention is probably the single most important indicator of relationship interest.

After introducing yourself, the next query should be: "How would you prefer to be addressed?" Simulation Exercise 10.1 is designed to give you practice in making introductory statements.

Clarifying the Purpose of the Relationship

Clarity of purpose related to identifiable health needs is an essential dimension of the nurse–patient relationship. It is difficult to fully participate in *any* working partnership without understanding its purpose and expectations.

Patients need basic information about the purpose and nature of the assessment interview, including what information is needed, how the information will be used, how the patient can participate in the treatment process, and what the patient can expect from the relationship. To understand the importance of orientation information, consider the value of your having a clear syllabus and expectations for your nursing courses. It can make all the difference in actively engaging your interest.

The length and nature of the relationship dictate the depth of the orientation. An orientation given to a patient by a nurse assigned for a shift would be different from that given to a patient when the nurse assumes the role of primary care nurse over an extended period. When the relationship is of longer duration, the nurse should discuss its parameters (e.g., length of sessions, frequency of meetings, and role expectations of the nurse and patient). It is important to give the patient sufficient orientation information to feel comfortable, but not so much that it overloads the initial getting-to-know-you process.

Assessment interview meetings should have two outcomes. First, the patient should feel that the nurse is interested in him or her as a person, apart from their diagnosis. Second, the patient and nurse should emerge from the encounter with a better understanding of the most relevant health issues, and know what will happen next. At the end of the contact, the nurse should thank the patient for his or her participation and provide the patient with easy ways to access professional help, if needed.

Establishing Trust

Trust is defined as a relational process, one that is dynamic and fragile, yet involving the deepest needs and vulnerabilities of individuals. Patients intuitively assess the nurse's trustworthiness through their "presence," focused attention, and actions. Data regarding the level of the nurse's interest, knowledge base, and competence are factored into the patient's decision to trust and to engage actively in the relationship. Kindness, competence, and a willingness to be actively involved get communicated through the nurse's words, tone of voice, and actions. Does the nurse seem to know what he or she is doing? Is the nurse tactful and respectful of cultural differences? Confidentiality, sensitivity to patient needs, and honesty help to confirm your trustworthiness and to strengthen the relationship.

Assessing Patients' Emotional Needs in Communication

A patient's level of trust can fluctuate with illness, age, and the influence of past successful or unsuccessful encounters with others. Modifications in your approach make a difference. For example, you would hold a different conversation

with an adolescent than you would with an elderly patient. The acutely ill patient will need short contacts that are to the point, empathic, and related to providing comfort and care. Patients with mental illness typically require more time and patience to engage in a trusting relationship. The idea of having a professional person care about them—in fact, any person—in any "real way" can be incomprehensible. Having this awareness helps the nurse look beyond the bizarre behaviors that some patients present in response to their fears about helping relationships.

Case Study: Mrs O'Connell, a Psychiatric Patient

Nurse (with eye contact and enough interpersonal space for comfort): "Good morning, Mrs. O'Connell. My name is Karen Martin. I will be your nurse today." (Patient looks briefly at the nurse, and looks away, then gets up and moves away.)

Nurse: "This may not be a good time to talk with you. Would you mind if I checked back later with you?" (The introduction coupled with an invitation for later communication respects the patient's need for interpersonal space and allows the patient to set the pace of the relationship.)

Later, the nurse notices that Mrs O'Connell circles around the area the nurse is occupying, but she does not directly approach the nurse. The nurse smiles encouragingly and repeats nondemanding invitations to the patient, which give the patient the time and space to become more comfortable.

Schizophrenic patients often enter and leave the space occupied by the nurse, almost circling around a space that is within visual distance of the nurse. With patience and tact, the nurse engages the patient slowly with a welcoming look and brief verbal contact. Over time, brief meetings that involve an invitation and a statement as to when the nurse will return help reduce the patient's anxiety, as indicated in the dialogue in the following case example. Many mentally ill patients respond better to shorter, frequent contacts until trust is established.

Participant Observation

Peplau describes the role of the nurse in all phases of the relationship as being that of a "participant observer." This means that the nurse simultaneously actively participates in and observes the progress of the relationship as it unfolds. Observations about changes in the patient's behavior, and feedback, help direct subsequent dialogue and actions in the relationship. According to Peplau, observation includes self-awareness on the part of the nurse. This self-reflection is as critical to the success of the relationship as is the assessment of the patient's emerging responses in the relationship. Self-awareness is a critical component of participant observation. According to Peplau (1997), nurses must observe their own behavior, as well as the patient's, with unflinching self-scrutiny and total honesty in assessment of their behavior in interactions with patients. In some ways, nurses act as a mirror for the patient, reflecting back to the patient a fuller picture of the human experience of illness and its contextual dimensions.

Self-awareness in therapeutic relationships is a reflective intrapersonal process. This introspective process helps nurses get in touch with their personal values, feelings, attitudes, motivations, strengths, and limitations—and how these reflections might color or affect the relationship with individual patients. Critically examining their own behaviors and the impact on the relationship helps nurses create a safe, trustworthy, and caring relational structure.

Understanding the Patient's Perspective

PCC requires understanding each patient's illness experience with the broader framework of

- life history, including unique personal and developmental issues;
- family history and level of social support;
- employment, school, and community background;
- cultural background and spiritual connections; and
- quality of life, financial resources, and knowledge of support services.

All involved care providers have a legal and ethical responsibility to participate in helping patients understand the nature of an illness as a basis for developing meaningful options in resolving it. Once the nurse and patient develop a working definition of the problem, the next step is to brainstorm the best ways to meet treatment goals. The brainstorming process occurs more easily when you as a nurse are relaxed and are willing to understand views different from your own. Brainstorming involves generating multiple ideas, while suspending judgment until all possibilities are presented. However, having evidence-based knowledge of potential treatment goals, risk/benefit ratios, and other options is an essential component of effective relationships.

The next step is to look realistically at ideas that could work, given the resources that the patient has available right now, and patient preferences. Resistance can be worked through with the empathetic reality testing of various options. Peplau suggests that a general rule of thumb in working with patients is to struggle with the problem, not with the patient.

Assess what help is needed. The last component of the assessment process relates to determining the kind of help needed, and who can best provide it. Careful consideration of the most appropriate sources of help is an important, but often overlooked, part of the assessment process needed in the planning phase.

Communication Strategies During Phases of the Patient-Centered Relationship

Relationship-centered care recognizes that the provider–patient relationship is the unique product of its participants and its context. Technology can be off-putting if it becomes the primary focus of the interaction. It is important to demonstrate during patient interviews that you value the person as a human being over technology. This is an area commented on by patients.

Preinteraction Phase Communication

This is the only phase that does not involve direct communication with the patient. You gather data from records and colleagues. Having background information can make a difference in your approach. For example, two women are admitted to labor and delivery. One is happily married and looking forward to using what she has learned in Lamaze classes, while the other is unwed and planning to give her baby up for adoption. Would this make a difference in your initial conversations?

Orientation/Assessment Phase Communication

You use communication strategies that convey your interest. Greet your patient with respect and positive interest. The patient should be comfortable, alert, and not in pain. Ensure the initial interaction takes place in a private area. Sit at eye level and maintain eye contact. The patient's current health situation is a good starting place for choice of topic. Some fundamental differences such as age and first experience with a medical diagnosis are self-evident from observation and chart review, but should be verified for accuracy. Other less obvious differences may emerge as the patient tells their story.

Sharing Information. Open, honest communication and two-way sharing of information are essential for effective planning. The trust that develops within the relationship is incremental, based on mutual respect for what each person brings to the therapeutic alliance. Remember, therapeutic relationships should directly revolve around the patient's needs and preferences. Simulation Exercise 10.2 helps you practice identifying patient strengths.

You can begin to elicit data about the patient by simply asking why they are seeking treatment at this time. Using questions that follow a logical sequence, when there is something you do not understand, and asking only one

SIMULATION EXERCISE 10.2   **Shared Decision-Making**

Purpose

To develop awareness of shared decision-making in treatment planning.

Procedure

1. Read the following clinical situation.
2. Mr Singer, aged 48 years, is a white, middle-class professional recovering from his second myocardial infarction. After his initial attack, Mr Singer resumed his 10-hour workday, high-stress lifestyle, and usual high-calorie, high-cholesterol diet of favorite fast foods, alcohol, and coffee. He smokes two packs of cigarettes a day and exercises once a week by playing golf. Mr Singer is to be discharged in 2 days. He expresses impatience to return to work but also indicates that he would like to "get his blood pressure down and maybe drop 10 pounds."
3. Role-play this situation in dyads, with one student taking the role of the nurse, and another student taking the role of the patient.
4. Develop treatment goals that seem realistic and achievable, considering Mr Singer's preferences, values, and health condition.
5. After the role-playing is completed, discuss some of the issues that would be relevant to Mr Singer's situation and how they might be handled.
6. What are some concrete ways in which you could engage Mr Singer's interest in changing his behavior to facilitate a healthier lifestyle?

question at a time help a patient feel more comfortable. This strategy is likely to elicit more complete data. You can periodically check in with the patient with a simple statement such as "I wonder if you have any questions so far …" or "is there anything you would like to add?"

Working (Exploitation/Active Intervention) Phase Communication

With relevant patient-centered goals to guide nursing interventions and patient actions, the conversation turns to active problem-solving related to assessed healthcare needs. Patients are better able to discuss deeper, more difficult issues, and to experiment with new roles and actions in the working phase, and the relationship with provider nurses is judged to be trustworthy as a guide to action. Corresponding to the *implementation phase* of the nursing process, the working phase focuses on self-directed actions related to personal health goals, the self-monitoring of changes, and the self-management of

personal healthcare, to whatever extent is possible in promoting the patient's health and well-being.

Supporting patient self-management strategies. **Self-management** is defined as a patient's ability to manage the symptoms and consequences of living with a chronic condition, including treatment, physical, social, and lifestyle changes. Helping patients develop realistic self-management strategies is a key concept in caring for patients experiencing chronic disorders. Patients are expected to actively participate in health-related decision-making and behaviors. Asking, "what is the most important outcome you hope to accomplish in managing your health issues?" is a good lead into this discussion. Avoid taking more responsibility for actions than the patient or situation requires. For example, it may seem more efficient time-wise to give a bath to a stroke victim, but what happens when this patient goes home and lacks either the confidence or the skills to complete this task safely?

Throughout the working phase, nurses need to be sensitive about whether the patient is still responding at a useful level. Looking at difficult problems and developing strategies to resolve those problems is not an easy process, especially when resolution requires significant behavioral changes. If the nurse is perceived as inquisitive, rather than facilitative, communication breaks down. Warning signs that the pace may need adjustment include changes in facial expression, loss of eye contact, fidgeting, abrupt changes in subject, or asking to be left alone.

Health disruptions create distress and usually require adaptive changes in more than one life domain. In addition to providing direct care, nurses need to help patients and families cope with unique emotional and reality challenges associated with the patient's health disruption. Most problems, should they arise, should be treated as temporary setbacks that provide new information about what needs to happen next. Helping patients develop alternative strategies to successfully cope with unexpected responses can strengthen a patient's problem-solving abilities. Alternative options (i.e., a plan B) when an original plan does not bring about the desired results can be empowering.

Shared Decision-Making. The pinnacle of PCC, effective decision-making represents both a cognitive and an interpersonal process. This concept requires transparent communication because of the active involvement of patients and families that is needed to consider the pros and cons of treatment options. Decisions should reflect patient priorities, preferences, and values, as well as the reality of the clinical situation. In addition to providing patients with information about their disease process or injury, patients need to have a clear understanding of treatment options related to the side effects and the potential consequences of each option, including what happens if no treatment is given.

Elwyn et al. (2012) outlines three key steps in an effective shared decision process. They label these as follows:

- *Choice talk* consists of finding out what information the patient has, how much information the patient wants, and who should be involved in the decision-making process. Inquiry into patient goals and concerns can help frame the option talk in the next step. Choice talk also requires assessing whether or not the information a patient already has is the correct information.
- *Option talk* consists of providing sufficient and relevant information about potential treatment options, the risks involved, the pros and cons of one option versus another. This discussion should consider what the health provider knows about the patient's values, preferences, priorities, and concerns. The extent of risk and the potential for outcome uncertainty should be included in the discussion. It is important to check in with patients about their potential fears, expectations, and other ideas that they may have about different options.
- *Decision talk* involves participatory active engagement, because this is when the patient needs to make a decision. Whenever possible, patients should not be forced to make a choice without being ready to make one. It is helpful to ask, "Are you ready to make a decision, or do you need more time to think about it?" Some patients need not only time, but also more information. They may want to consult with others who would be affected. This is particularly true for patients from a high context culture. It is critical that the decision be based on each patient's informed choice. Having additional opportunities to revisit what led to the decision helps to confirm that the patient is comfortable with the decision. Simulation Exercise 10.3 gives insight into identifying patient strengths.

Giving Constructive Feedback. Constructive feedback involves drawing the patient's attention to the existence of unacceptable behaviors or contradictory messages while respecting the fragility of the therapeutic alliance, and the patient's need to protect the integrity of his or her self-concept. To be effective, constructive confrontations are best attempted when the following criteria have been met:

- The nurse has established a firm, trusting bond with the patient.
- The timing and environmental circumstances are appropriate.
- The confrontation is delivered in a private setting, in a nonjudgmental, calm, and empathetic manner.
- Only those behaviors capable of being changed by the patient are up for discussion.
- The nurse supports the patient's autonomy and right to self-determination as long as it does not interfere with the rights of others.

SIMULATION EXERCISE 10.3   Identifying Patient Strengths

Purpose

To identify personal strengths in patients with serious illness.

Procedure

1. Think about a patient you have had with a serious or prolonged chronic illness.
2. What personal strengths does this person possess that could have a healing impact? For example, strengths can be courage, patience, fighting spirit, family, and so on.
3. Write a one-page description of the patient and the personal strengths observed, despite the patient's medical or psychological condition.

Reflective Discussion Analysis

1. If you did not have to write the description, would you have been as aware of the patient's strengths?
2. How could you help the patient maximize his or her strengths to achieve quality of life?
3. What did you learn from this exercise that you can use in your future clinical practice?

Family. Engaging the patient's family early in the treatment process is also essential. Nurses must be familiar enough with the patient's symptoms and behaviors so they can accurately communicate the meaning of symptoms and suffering to family members, or other healthcare colleagues and team members. This is also important from the perspective of discharge as most patients have to manage their recovery in home environments with less supervision and coaching.

Termination Phase Communication

Unlike social relationships, therapeutic relationships have a predetermined ending. They typically end when treatment outcomes have been achieved, the patient has been discharged, or the number of visits authorized by insurance has been achieved. In the termination phase, the nurse and patient jointly evaluate the patient's responses to treatment and explore the meaning of the relationship and what goals have been achieved. Discussing patient achievements and patient-centered plans for the future is the activity with relevance for the termination phase.

Termination is a significant issue in long-term settings such as skilled nursing facilities, bone marrow transplant units, rehabilitation hospitals, and state psychiatric facilities. Meaningful long-term relationships can and do develop in these settings. If the relationship has been effective, real work has been accomplished. Nurses need to be sufficiently aware of their own feelings so that they may use them constructively without imposing them on the patient. It is appropriate for nurses to share some of the meaning the relationship held for them, as long as such sharing fits the needs of the interpersonal situation and is not excessive or too emotionally intense. Reflect on the Allyshia Green case.

Case Study: Allyshia Green Is Discharged

Allyshia Green is 16 and has spent many months on a bone marrow transplant unit. She developed a real attachment to her primary nurse, who had stood by her during the frightening physical assaults to her body and appearance occasioned by the treatment. She was unable to verbally acknowledge the meaning of the relationship with the nurse directly, despite having been given many opportunities to do so by the nurse. She was heard to say that she could not wait to leave this awful hospital and that she was glad she did not have to see the nurses anymore. Yet, later she was found sobbing in her room the day she left. The relationship obviously had meaning for the patient, but she was unable to express it verbally.

Adaptation for Brief Relationships

Four essential qualities are needed to establish relatedness in short-term relationships: a sense of belonging, reciprocity, mutuality, and synchrony.

Orientation Phase

By necessity a short interaction requires us to focus on the "here and now" essentials such as problem identification and an emphasis on quickly understanding the context in which the problem is embedded. Start with the patient's chief concern, followed by the patient's symptoms and the personal and emotional context in which they occur. A simple statement posed at the beginning of each shift, such as "What is your most important need today?," or "What is the most important thing I can do for you today?" helps focus the relationship on immediate concerns.

Working Phase

Brief relationships should be solution-focused right from the start. Giving patients your undivided attention and using concise active listening responses are essential to understanding the complexity of issues facing patients. Action plans should be as simple and specific as possible. Changes in the patient's condition or other circumstances may require treatment modifications that should be expected in short-term relationships. Keeping patients and families informed,

and working with them on alternative solutions, is essential to maintaining trust in short-term relationships.

Termination Phase

This last phase includes discharge planning, agency referrals, and arranging follow-up appointments in the community for the patient and family. Anticipatory guidance in the form of simple instructions, written guidelines, and a review of important skills is appropriate.

Difficult Discussions

Developing skills to manage difficult discussions requires practice. In clinical settings, you will deal with patients who have received a poor prognosis or who are facing end-of-life issues. Sometimes it is up to the nurse to initiate these conversations without waiting for the patient. Also refer to the chapter on palliative care. Other times, in established relationships, your patient wants to share thoughts, as in the case of Kelly Whit.

Case Study: Kelly Whit and End-of-Life Issues

Mrs Whit, age 40 years, has been diagnosed with terminal ovarian cancer. Her nurse, Barb Suarez, RN, is administering morphine but notices a frowning face, commenting "You seem sad today." Mrs Whit responds "It's not that I mind dying so much as it is not knowing what to expect, what's going to happen to me during the process." Barb paraphrases "It sounds like you can accept the dying but fear what the experience will be. Tell me more about what worries you."

1. How does this nurse link the emotional context to the content of the message? Ms Suarez demonstrates her desire to understand. By acknowledging cues, she normalizes the feelings and can use this opening to provide needed support and some information.

Communication skills for difficult discussions may include the following:
- Managing some quiet time for uninterrupted discussion.
- Conveying empathy and caring, showing warmth and interest, using congruent nonverbal communication skills such as positioning at same height and maintaining eye contact.
- Eliciting your patient's level of understanding. Traditionally, it is the physician who gives the prognosis, but patients often ask their nurse to explain. Generally, if your patient asks, they are ready to hear.
- Loss is a universal feeling you have in common, so you can relay your feelings without specifying why.
- Clarifying misinformation.

- Asking patient about their main concern. How will their condition affect their family roles?
- Assessing current coping and strengths. What support systems are available?
- Offering reasonable reassurance but not giving false hope.
- Being sensitive to your patient's reaction, noting verbal and nonverbal cues. Give information in small doses, allowing them time to process. At the conclusion of a difficult conversation, summarize main points. Usually, these difficult conversations are not a one-time occurrence but require communication over time to process.
- Evaluation of communication.

Nurses need time for reflection to examine outcomes of their patient relationships. Were your interventions effective? Did your patient progress toward maximum possible health or toward acceptance of their condition or impending death? Remember the analogy of the glass half full. You need to replenish your spirit of resiliency. Try exercises in Chapter 27 for help.

SUMMARY

The nurse–patient relationship represents a purposeful use of self in conversations with patients and their families. Therapeutic relationships demonstrate caring and interest in helping patient achieve maximum possible benefit. These relationships have boundaries and must conform to legal and ethical standards. Purpose guides the relationship communication, always directed toward meeting patient needs and advancing their well-being. This chapter describes four stages: preintervention, organization/assessment, working phase, and termination. Communication intervention strategies were discussed. Suggestions were also provided for handling difficult conversations.

ETHICAL DILEMMA: What Would You Do?

A patient with lymphoma refused a blood transfusion after her first round of chemotherapy. Her physician was upset that she would not accept this logical treatment. The nurse in this case example said, "I explained to him what her beliefs were and why she refused blood." He continued to look confused, and I said, "We may not understand it fully, but we have to respect her decision and not let our personal opinions impede our care." He looked at me and said I was absolutely right.

DISCUSSION QUESTIONS

1. In what ways do organizational structure and expectations in your clinical setting enhance or impede development of therapeutic relationships in nursing care?

REFERENCES

American Hospital Association (AHA). (2003). *The patient care partnership: Understanding expectations, rights and responsibilities.* Retrieved from http://www.aha.org/content/00-10/pcp_english_030730.pdf. [Accessed 22 June 2021].

American Nurses Association (ANA). (2010). *Nursing scope and standards of practice* (2nd ed.). Silver Spring, MD: ANA.

Bandura, A. (2012). On the functional properties of perceived self-efficacy revisited. *Journal of Management, 38*(1), 9–44.

Disch, J., & Barnsteiner, J. (2021). QSEN in an Amazon world. *American Journal of Nursing, 121*(3), 40–46.

Elwyn, G., Frosch, D., Thompson, R., et al. (2012). Shared decision making: A model for clinical practice. *Journal of General Internal Medicine, 27*(10), 1361–1367.

Fite, R. O., Assefa, M., Demissie, A., & Belachew, T. (2019). Predictors of therapeutic communication between nurses and hospitalized patients. *Heliyon, 5*(10), e02665.

Hibbard, J. H., Mahoney, E., & Sonet, E. (2017). Does patient activation level affect the cancer journey? *Patient Education and Counseling, 100*(7), 1276–1279.

Ignatavicius, D. D. (2021). Preparing for the new nursing licensure exam: The next-generation NCLEX. *Nursing, 51*(5), 34–41.

International Council of Nurses (ICN). (2011). *Position statement: Nurses and human rights.* Geneva, Switzerland: ICN. Retrieved from https://www.icn.ch/sites/default/files/inline-files/E10_Nurses_Human_Rights%281%29.pdf. [Accessed 22 June 2021].

Kantor, D. P., & Stadelman, A. (2020). Preparing nursing graduates to engage in difficult conversations with patients. *American Journal of Nursing, 120*(8), 11–15.

Maslow, A. (1970). *Motivation and personality* (2nd ed.). New York: Harper & Row.

National Council of State Boards of Nursing (NCSBN). (2018). *A nurse's guide to professional boundaries.* Chicago: NCSBN. Retrieved from: https://www.ncsbn.org/ProfessionalBoundaries_Complete.pdf. [Accessed 22 June 2021].

Peplau, H. E. (1992). Interpersonal relations: A theoretical framework for application in nursing practice. *Nursing Science Quarterly, 5*(1), 13–18.

Peplau, H. E. (1997). Peplau's theory of interpersonal relations. *Nursing Science Quarterly, 10*(4), 162–167.

Picker Institute. (n.d.). Principles of person-centred care [website]. Retrieved from https://www.picker.org/about-us/picker-principles-of-person-centred-care/. [Accessed 22 June 2021].

Rogers, C. R. (1958). The characteristics of a helping relationship. *The Personnel & Guidance Journal, 37*(1), 6–16.

Valente, S. M. (2017). Managing professional and nurse-patient relationship boundaries in mental health. *Journal of Psychosocial Nursing and Mental Health Services, 55*(1), 45–51.

World Health Organization (WHO). (2010). *World Health Organization: Framework for action on interprofessional education and collaborative practice.* Geneva, Switzerland: WHO Press.

11

Bridges and Barriers in Therapeutic Relationships

OBJECTIVES

At the end of the chapter, the reader will be able to:

1. Describe which nursing actions can promote patient-centered communication: respect, caring, empowerment, trust, empathy, mutuality, veracity, and confidentiality.
2. Describe personal and organizational barriers to the development of effective communication.
3. Apply nursing actions that best reduce barriers to communication to simulated cases.
4. Analyze findings from research studies for use in clinical practice to foster communication in clinical practice.

Health communication is a multidimensional process. It includes aspects from the sender and the receiver of a message. To be effective communication, it has to be a two-way dialog (Wune, 2020). This chapter focuses on the communication components of the nurse–patient relationship acting as bridges to promote patient health and safety outcomes. Effective communication improves patient satisfaction, facilitates patient decision-making, and promotes adherence to treatment protocols. Nurses apply the concepts of respect, caring, empowerment, trust, empathy, and mutuality, as well as confidentiality and veracity. We actively engage patient participation in health decisions and abide by their rights in providing informed consent as recognized by the World Health Organization WHO (n.d.).

Implementing actions that convey feelings of respect, caring, warmth, acceptance, and understanding to the patient is an interpersonal skill that requires practice. Novice students may encounter interpersonal situations that leave them feeling helpless and inadequate. Such feelings are common. Through practice, discussion of these feelings in peer groups, and simulation learning activities, you gain skills to deal with these feelings.

BASIC CONCEPTS

Bridges to the Relationship

Accurate nursing communication about the patient's condition is crucial to the efficient provision of high-quality, safe care. It improves patient outcomes. Safety issues are reliant on uses of communication tools that nurses use as bridges to better communication. Communication also affects us as providers in terms of our job satisfaction and stress levels. The following concepts describe methods to help you improve your communication and barriers to avoid.

Respect

Conveying genuine respect for your patients assists in building professional relationships. Because your mutual goal is to maximize your patient's health status, you need to convey respect for their values and opinions. Asking them what they prefer to be called and always addressing them as such is a correct initial step. Of course, you avoid the sort of casual addresses portrayed in bad television shows, such as "How are you feeling, honey?" "Mom, hold your baby," or "How are we feeling today?" We try to remember that hospitalized patients feel a loss of control in relation to interpersonal relationships with staff.

Lack of Respect

Patients report feeling devalued when they perceived that staff were avoiding talking with them or were unfriendly; they felt comforted when a little "chit-chat" was exchanged.

Collaborative Communication

In a true collaborative model, each team member conveys respect and assumes responsibility for initiating clear

CASE STUDY: Mr Syds in ICU

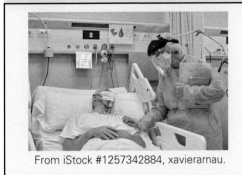

From iStock #1257342884, xavierarnau.

Mr Syds is recovering from pulmonary distress in an intensive care unit. This morning as the team gathers at his bed for rounds, he confides in his nurse about feeling a "sense of doom." Noting his anxious expression, falling oxygenation levels, and slight temperature, the nurse uses the CUS TeamSTEPPS communication tool, saying "I am concerned about these changes." Mr Syds's feedback taken together with physiological data prompts pattern recognition among team members. They explore the possibility that his pressure ulcer (local infection) may be evolving into sepsis (a systemic infection).

communication. Lack of respect among team members is associated with poor communication, leading to adverse patient outcomes. In establishing patient-centered care, we should treat every patient as a respected member of the team (a QSEN competency), as suggested in Mr Syds's case.

Caring

Caring is an intentional human action characterized by commitment and a sufficient level of knowledge and skill to allow you to support basic integrity. You offer caring to your patient by means of the therapeutic relationship. Nursing theorists, especially Watson, describe the need to develop and sustain a helping, trusting, caring relationship. Your ability to care develops from a natural response to help those in need, from the knowledge that caring is a part of nursing ethics, and from respect for self and others. As a caring nurse, you give patient-centered care, recognizing and assisting the patients in their struggle for health and well-being rather than simply doing things for them. They detect care and empathy from your behaviors.

Provision of a caring relationship that facilitates health and healing is identified as an essential feature of contemporary nursing practice in the Social Policy Statement of the American Nurses Association (ANA, 2010). In the professional literature, the focus of the caring relationship is clearly placed on meeting patient needs. Patient-centered care is a QSEN competency. The behavior of "caring" is not an emotional feeling. Rather, it is a chosen response to need. You willingly give of yourself as an ethical responsibility, as pictured in Fig. 11.1.

Patients want us to understand why they are suffering. Healthcare workers tend to speak in a medical language that values facts and events. In contrast, patients tend to value associations and causes. To bridge this potential gap, you need to convey a sense that you truly care about their perspective. Families also need to experience a sense of caring

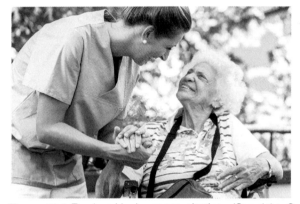

Figure 11.1 Touch adds in communication. (Copyright © kzenon/iStock/Thinkstock.)

from the nurse. Many families do not believe healthcare workers have a clear understanding of the problems they are encountering while caring for their ill family member. "Caring" interventions in the form of conferences where family members could express emotions and talk with experts, in conjunction with being given written materials, may help decrease anxiety. Refer to Table 16.2 in Chapter 16 for interventions to reduce family anxiety.

Lack of Caring

Although nursing has had a long-standing commitment to patient-focused care, sometimes you may observe a situation in which you feel a nurse is apathetic, trying to meet his or her own needs rather than the patient's needs. Some nurses develop a detachment that interferes with expressions of caring behaviors. At other times, nurses can be so rushed to meet multiple demands that they seem unable to focus on the patient. Simulation Exercise 11.1 will help you focus on the concept of caring.

SIMULATION EXERCISE 11.1 Application of Caring

Purpose
To help you apply caring concepts to nursing.

Procedure
Identify some aspects of caring that might be applied to nursing practice. Work in a group to compile a list.

Reflective Discussion Analysis
Discuss examples of how this form of caring could be implemented in a nurse–patient situation.

Empowerment

Empowerment is defined as assisting patients to take charge of their lives. Our nursing goal is to use communication skills to build bridges to form partnerships, a QSEN competency. We use the interpersonal process to provide information, tools, and resources that help patients build skills to reach their health goals. Empowerment is an important aim in every nurse–patient relationship and is addressed by nursing theories such as Orem's view of the patient as an agent of self-care. Empowered patients feel valued and are more likely to adopt successful coping methods. Studies demonstrate that the more involved people are in their own care, the better the health outcome.

Lack of Empowerment

Unempowered patients do not take responsibility for their own health. In the past, many providers exhibited a paternalistic attitude toward their patients characterized by the attitude of "I know what is best for you or I can do it better." Empowerment should extend to families. Lack of information about giving care, managing medicines, or recognizing approaching crises can be a major impediment to those who care for sick relatives. Failure to assist patients and their families to assume personal responsibility, or failure to provide appropriate resources and support, undermines empowerment.

Trust

Establishing **trust** is the foundation in all relationships. The development of a sense of interpersonal trust, a sense of feeling safe, is the keystone in the nurse–patient relationship. Trust provides a nonthreatening interpersonal climate in which people feel comfortable revealing their needs. The nurse is perceived as dependable. Establishment of this trust is crucial toward enabling you to make an accurate assessment of needs.

Trust is also the key to establishing effective work team relationships. Lack of trust in the workplace has detrimental effects for the organization and coworkers, undermining performance and commitment. According to Erikson (1963), trust is developed by experiencing consistency, sameness, and continuity during care by a familiar caregiver. Trust develops based on past experiences. In the nurse–patient relationship, maintaining an open exchange

BOX 11.1 Techniques Designed to Promote Trust

- Convey respect.
- Consider the patient's uniqueness.
- Show warmth and caring.
- Use the patient's proper name.
- Use active listening.
- Give sufficient time to answer questions.
- Maintain confidentiality.
- Show congruence between verbal and nonverbal behaviors.
- Use a warm, friendly voice.
- Use appropriate eye contact.
- Smile.
- Be flexible.
- Provide for allowed preferences.
- Be honest and open.
- Give complete information.
- Provide consistency.
- Plan schedules.
- Follow through on commitments.
- Set limits.
- Control distractions.
- Use an attending posture: arms, legs, and body relaxed; leaning slightly forward.

of information contributes to trust. For the patient, trust implies a willingness to place oneself in a position of vulnerability, relying on health providers to perform as expected. Honesty is a basic building block in establishing trust. Studies show that patients or their surrogates want "complete honesty," and most prefer complete disclosure. Box 11.1 lists interpersonal strategies that help promote a trusting relationship.

Mistrust

Mistrust has an effect not only on communication but also on healing process outcomes. Trust can be replaced with mistrust, as might occur if the nurse violates patient confidentiality. Just as some agency managers treat employees as though they are not trustworthy, some

---

SIMULATION EXERCISE 11.2 **Techniques That Promote Trust**

Purpose
To provide practice in using trust promoting skills.

Procedure
1. Read the list of interpersonal techniques designed to promote trust (see Box 11.1).
2. Individual: Describe the relationship with your most recent patient. Was there a trusting relationship? How do you know? Which techniques did you use? Which ones could you have used?
3. Small group: Break class up into groups of three. Have students interview another group member to obtain a

brief health history. The third member observes and records trusting behaviors. Interviews should last 5 min; then share findings.

Reflective Discussion Analysis
Share findings in class with a focus on techniques and outcomes observed. Consider relative effectiveness. Alternative exercise: Have dyads do the BACKWARD FALL in which one student falls backward and the student behind catches him or her.

---

nurses treat some patients as though they are misbehaving children. An example might be a community health nurse who is inconsistent about keeping patient appointments or a pediatric nurse who indicates falsely that an injection will not hurt. Such behaviors create mistrust. It is hard to maintain trust in any situation when one person cannot depend on another. Having confidence in the nurse's skills, commitment, and caring allows the patient to place full attention on the health situation requiring resolution. Of course, patients can also jeopardize the trust a nurse has in them. Sometimes patients "test" a nurse's trustworthiness by sending the nurse on unnecessary errands or talking endlessly on superficial topics. As long as nurses recognize testing behaviors and set clear limits, it is possible to develop trust. Simulation Exercise 11.2 is designed to help students become more familiar with the concept of trust.

Empathy

Empathy is the ability to be sensitive to and communicate understanding of the patient's feelings. Empathy is the ability to put yourself into another's position. Empathy and empathetic communication are crucial to the practice of nursing, characteristic of a helping relationship. Empathy is an important element of a therapeutic relationship. The ability to effectively communicate empathy is associated with improved satisfaction and patient adherence to treatments. A policy statement from the American Academy of Pediatrics extends this communication component to your patient's family (Levetown, 2008).

An empathetic nurse perceives and *understands* the patient's emotions *accurately*. Some nurses might term this as *compassion,* which has been identified by staff nurses as being crucial to the nurse–patient relationship. Communication skills are used to convey respect and empathy. Although expert nurses recognize the emotions

a patient feels, they hold on to their objectivity, maintaining their own separate identities. As a nurse, you try not to overidentify with or internalize the feelings of your patient. If internalization occurs, objectivity is lost, together with the ability to help the patient move through their feelings. It is important to recognize that these feelings belong to them, not to you.

Communicate your understanding of the meaning of a patient's feelings by using both verbal and nonverbal communication behaviors. Maintain direct eye contact, use attending open body language, and keep a calm tone of voice. Acknowledging your patients' message about their feelings, difficulties, or pain helps create a positive connection. Remember to validate accuracy by restating what you understand the patient to be conveying, and have them confirm verbally that this is accurate. If you need more information about their feelings, ask them to expand on their message, perhaps asking, "Are there other things about this that are bothering you?" Now that you have full information, you can directly make interventions to address their needs.

Lack of Empathy

A failure to understand patient needs may lead you to fail to provide essential education or to provide needed emotional support. Major *organizational* barriers to empathy exist in the clinical environment, including a lack of time *associated with heavy workloads.* Several studies suggest that a lack of empathy will affect the quality of care, result in less favorable health outcomes, and lower patient satisfaction. As providers, we can consciously choose to express empathy.

Mutuality

Mutuality is the recognition of reciprocity in which we value and support the well-being of patients. It means

SIMULATION EXERCISE 11.3   Evaluating Mutuality

Purpose
To identify behaviors and feelings on the part of the nurse and the patient that indicate mutuality.

Procedure
Complete the following questions by answering yes or no after terminating with a patient; then bring it to class. Discuss the answers. How were you able to attain mutuality, or why were you unable to attain it?
1. Was I satisfied with the relationship?
2. Did the patient express satisfaction with the relationship?

3. Did the patient share feelings with me?
4. Did I make decisions for the patient?
5. Did the patient feel allowed to make his or her own decisions?
6. Did the patient accomplish his or her goals?
7. Did I accomplish my goals?

Reflective Discussion Analysis
In groups, analyze vignettes for mutuality.

---

that the nurse and patient agree on the patient's health problems and the means for resolving them. Both parties are committed to enhancing the patient's well-being. This is characterized by mutual respect for the autonomy and value system of the other. In developing mutuality, you maximize your patient's involvement in all phases of the nursing process. Mutuality is collaboration in problem-solving and drives the communication at the initial encounter. Evidence of mutuality is seen in the development of individualized patient goals and nursing actions that meet identified, unique health needs. Simulation Exercise 11.3 provides practice in evaluating mutuality.

As nurses, we respect interpersonal differences. We involve our patients in the decision-making process. We accept their decisions even if we do not agree with them. Effective use of values clarification assists patients in decision-making. Those who clearly identify their own personal values are better able to solve problems effectively. Decisions then have meaning to the patient. There is a greater probability that they will work to achieve success. When a mutual relationship is terminated, both parties experience a sense of shared accomplishment and satisfaction.

Veracity

Veracity or truthfulness in communication is the most important aspect in upholding a high standard of ethical nursing (ANA, 2015). Legal and ethical standards mandate specific nursing behaviors, such as confidentiality, beneficence, and respect for patient autonomy. These behaviors are based on professional nursing values that stem from ethical principles. By adhering to these "rules," nurses build their therapeutic relationships. When patients know they can expect the truth, the development of trust is promoted and helps build your relationship.

Barriers to Veracity

Sometimes it is not as easy to maintain truthfulness as we would hope. For example, the physician or the family may not have told the patient all that you know. Any deception (lies or omissions) erodes trust in care providers, but there may be a need to balance truth-telling with the need to preserve some hope. Avoid demeaning comments about other health providers, so you do not damage trust. When questioned by a patient, you can support their desire to seek a second medical opinion.

PATIENT-CENTERED COMMUNICATION

Within conversations between patient and nurse, the patient should remain the focus. We should focus our energy on what our patient is trying to tell us. We strive to use the "unconditional regard" advocated by Carl Rogers, accepting our patient's comments as we do a valued person.

In social conversations, it is common to take turns. When the other person speaks, we may mentally rehearse our response. However, in professional patient–nurse communication, this means that we are not listening with 100% attention directed toward what the patient is trying to tell us.

Acceptance

Everyone has **biases**. We need to make it a goal to reduce bias by recognizing a patient as a unique individual, both different from and similar to self. Acceptance of the other person needs to be total. The authors believe unconditional acceptance, as described by Rogers (1961), is essential in the helping relationship. It does not imply agreement or approval; acceptance occurs without judgment. Fred Rogers, the children's television show host, ended his programs by telling his audience, "I like you just the way you

SIMULATION EXERCISE 11.4   Reducing Clinical Bias by Identifying Stereotypes

Purpose

To identify and reduce nursing biases. Practice identifying professional stereotypes and how to reduce them is one component of maintaining high-quality nursing care.

Procedure

Each of the following describes a stereotype. Identify the stereotype and how it might affect nursing care. As a nurse, what would you do to reduce the bias in the situation? Are there any individuals or groups of people for whom you would not want to provide care (e.g., homeless women with foul body odor and dirty nails)?

Situation A

Mrs Daniels, an obstetric nurse who believes in birth control, comments about her client, "Mrs Gonzales is pregnant again. You know the one with six kids already! It makes me sick to see these people on welfare taking away from our tax dollars. I don't know how she can continue to do this."

Situation B

Mrs Brown, a registered nurse on a medical unit, is upset with her 52-year-old female patient. "If she rings that buzzer one more time, I'm going to disconnect it. Can't she understand that I have other patients who need my attention more than she does? She just lies in bed all day long. And she's so fat; she's never going to lose any weight that way."

Situation C

Mrs Waters, a staff nurse in a nursing home, listens to the daughter of a 93-year-old resident, who says, "My mother, who is confused most of the time, receives very little attention from you nurses, while other patients who are lucid and clear-minded have more interaction with you. It's not fair! No wonder my mother is so far out in space. Nobody talks to her. Nobody ever comes in to say hello."

are." How wonderful if we, as nurses, could convey this type of acceptance through our words and actions. Simulation Exercise 11.4 examines ways of reducing clinical bias.

Stereotyping acts as a communication barrier. This is the process of attributing characteristics to a group of people as though all persons in the identified group possessed them. People may be stereotyped according to ethnic origin, culture, religion, social class, occupation, age, and other factors. Even health issues can be the stimulus for stereotyping individuals. For example, alcoholism, mental illness, and sexually transmitted diseases are fertile grounds for the development of stereotypes. Stereotypes have been shown to be consistent across cultures and somewhat across generations, although the value placed on a stereotype changes. Stereotypes are learned during childhood and reinforced by life experiences.

Stereotypes are never completely accurate. No attribute applies to every member of a group. All of us like to think that our way is the correct way, and that everyone else thinks about life experiences just as we do. The reality is that there are many roads in life, and one road is not necessarily any better than another. Emotions play a role in the value we place on negative stereotypes. Stereotypes based on strong emotions are called prejudices. Highly emotionally charged stereotypes are less amenable to change. In the extreme, this can result in discrimination.

Confidence

TeamSTEPPS talks about the need for each team member to practice competently. Nursing competence comes from education and experience. So practice those skills, but also be aware of communicating confidence in your competence to patients. In the second most watched TED talk, Amy Cuddy says, "fake it until you make it." She is discussing nonverbal behaviors that convey confidence. Seek out opportunities to hone your competence. A mild level of **anxiety** heightens one's awareness of the surrounding environment and fosters learning and decision-making. Therefore, it may be desirable to allow a mild degree of anxiety. It is not prudent, however, to prolong even a mild state of anxiety. Asking for help is not a sign of weakness, but rather is a sign of strength.

Anxiety

Such feelings can become a personal barrier to communication in a patient-centered relationship. **Anxiety** is a vague, persistent feeling of impending doom. It is a universal feeling; no one fully escapes it. The impact on the self is always uncomfortable. It occurs when a threat (real or imagined) to one's self-concept is perceived. Lower satisfaction with communication is associated with increased patient anxiety. Anxiety is usually observed through the physical and behavioral manifestations of the attempt to relieve the anxious feelings. Although individuals experiencing anxiety may not know they are anxious, specific behaviors provide clues that anxiety is present. Simulation Exercise 11.5 identifies behaviors associated with anxiety. Table 11.1 shows how an individual's

SIMULATION EXERCISE 11.5   Identifying Verbal and Nonverbal Behaviors Associated With Anxiety

Purpose

To broaden the learner's awareness of behavioral responses indicating anxiety.

Procedure

List as many anxious behaviors as you can think of. Each column has a few examples to start. Discuss the lists in a group, and then add new behaviors to your list.

Verbal	Nonverbal
Quavering voice	Nail biting
Rapid speech	Foot tapping
Mumbling	Sweating
Defensive words	Pacing

Reflective Discussion Analysis

Construct other examples.

TABLE 11.1   Levels of Anxiety With Degree of Sensory Perceptions, Cognitive and Coping Abilities, and Manifest Behaviors

Level of Anxiety	Sensory Perceptions	Cognitive and Coping Ability	Behavior
Mild	Provides heightened state of alertness; increased acuity of hearing, vision, smell, touch	Enhanced learning, problem-solving; increased ability to respond and adapt to changing stimuli; enhanced functioning[a]	Walking, singing, eating, drinking, mild restlessness, active listening, attending, questioning
Moderate	Decreased sensory perceptions; can adapt with guidance to enable expansion of sensory fields for limited periods	Loss of concentration; decreased cognitive ability; cannot identify factors contributing to the anxiety-producing situation; with directions can cope, reduce anxiety, and solve problems; inhibited functioning	Increased muscle tone, pulse, respirations; changes in voice tone and pitch, rapid speech, incomplete verbal responses; engrossed with detail
Severe	Greatly diminished perceptions; decreased sensitivity to pain	Limited thought processes; unable to solve problems even with guidance; cannot cope with stress without help; confused mental state; limited functioning	Purposeless, aimless behaviors; rapid pulse, respirations; high blood pressure; hyperventilation; inappropriate or incongruent verbal responses
Panic	No response to sensory perceptions; rapid respirations and possible chest pain	No cognitive or coping abilities; without intervention, death is imminent	Immobilization

[a]Functioning refers to the ability to perform activities of daily living for survival purposes.

---

sensory perceptions, cognitive abilities, coping skills, and behaviors relate to the intensity and level of anxiety experienced. Suggestions for reducing your anxiety or for destressing are listed in Box 11.2. Some of these can be taught to patients.

Proxemics

As we noted, **proxemics** is the study of an individual's use of space. Intrusion potentially *impacts negatively on patient-centered communication.* Personal space is an invisible boundary around an individual. The emotional personal space boundary provides a sense of comfort and protection. It is defined by past experiences, current circumstances, and culture.

In most cultures, men need more space than women do. People generally need less space in the morning. The elderly need more control over their space, whereas small children generally like to touch and be touched by others. Although the elderly appreciate human touch, they generally do not like it to be applied indiscriminately. Reflect on the photo in Fig. 11.1. Does this elder look open to being touched?

BOX 11.2   Nursing Strategies to Reduce Anxiety

For Patient:
- Use active listening to show acceptance.
- Be honest; answer all questions at the patient's level of understanding.
- Explain procedures, surgery, and policies, and give appropriate reassurance based on data.
- Act in a calm, unhurried manner.
- Speak clearly, firmly (but not loudly).
- Give information regarding laboratory tests, medications, treatments, and rationale for restrictions on activity.
- Set reasonable limits and provide structure.
- Encourage self-affirmation through positive statements such as "I will" and "I can."
- Use drawings or play therapy with dolls, puppets, and games with youth.
- Use a therapeutic touch.
- Initiate recreational activities, such as physical exercise, music, card games, board games, crafts, and reading.
- Teach deep breathing and relaxation exercises.
- Use guided imagery.

For Nurses:
- Treat sleep as a precious medicine.
- Eat healthy, fuel up.
- Exercise daily.
- Meditate daily (even if only for 5 min).
- Use guided imagery, positive attitude, and positive affirmations.
- Listen to music.
- Do chair yoga.
- Download the Breathe app, and have it remind you to do deep breathing periodically.
- Take your assigned breaks to do some of the above!

Data from Gerrard, B., Boniface, W., & Love, B. (1980). *Interpersonal skills for health professionals.* Reston, VA: Reston Publishing; TeamSTEPPS National Conference, June 2017; and others.

Situational anxiety causes a need for more space. Persons with low self-esteem prefer more space, as well as some control over who enters their space and in what manner. Usually, people will tolerate a person standing close to them at their side more readily than directly in front of them. Direct eye contact causes a need for more space. Placing oneself at the same level (e.g., sitting while patients are sitting, or standing at eye level when they are standing)

allows more access to the patient's personal space because such a stance is perceived as less threatening.

Violations of Personal Space as a Communication Barrier

Hospitals are not home. Many nursing care procedures are a direct intrusion into your patient's personal space. Commonly, procedures that require tubes (e.g., nasal gastric intubation, administration of oxygen, catheterization, and intravenous initiation) restrict mobility, resulting in loss of control over personal territory. When more than one health professional is involved, the impact of the intrusion on the patient may be even stronger. In many instances, personal space requirements are an integral part of a person's self-image. When patients lose control over personal space, they may experience a loss of identity and self-esteem. It is recommended that you maintain a social physical body distance of 4 feet when not actually giving care.

When institutionalized patients are able to incorporate parts of their rooms into their personal space, it increases their self-esteem and helps them to maintain a sense of identity. This feeling of security is evidenced when a patient asks, "Close my door, please." Freedom from worry about personal space allows the patient to trust the nurse and fosters a therapeutic relationship. When invasions of personal space are necessary while performing a procedure, you can minimize the impact by explaining why a procedure is needed. Conversation at such times reinforces their feelings that they are human beings worthy of respect and not just objects being worked on. Advocating for patient personal space needs is an aspect of the nursing role. This is done by communicating the patients' preferences to other members of the health team and including them in the care plan.

Home is not quite home when the home health nurse, infusion nurse, or other aides invade personal space. Some modification of "take-charge" behavior is required when giving care in a patient's home.

Cultural Barriers

Cross-cultural communication is further discussed in Chapter 7. Every interaction encounters a basic challenge of communication when the culture of your patient differs from your own. Barriers include health literacy problems or cultural definitions of the sick role. For example, in some cultures, the sick role is no longer valid after symptoms disappear, so when your patient's diabetes is under control, family members may no longer see the need for a special diet or medication. As we move into a more multicultural society, all healthcare providers need to work to become culturally competent communicators. **Culturally competent communication** is characterized by a willingness to try to understand and respond to your patient's beliefs.

Gender Differences

Gender is defined as the culture's attributions of masculine or feminine. Recently, more attention has been given to gender role, communication barriers, and health inequalities. Research results give mixed findings, though some studies suggest patient perceptions differ according to the nurse's gender. The authors believe gender need not be a factor in developing therapeutic communication with patients. Research does support the need for communications training for all healthcare workers. It takes practice for us to master communication skills.

Organizational System Barriers

Communication barriers inherent in healthcare system agencies are commonly discussed in the professional literature, with frequent interruptions and lack of time cited as leading to errors. Organizational barriers to communication stem from cost containment measures such as higher staff to patient ratios.

Heavy Workload

This is often mentioned as a barrier to communication and to opportunities to engage patients. Lack of time can result from low staff-to-patient ratios or financial pressure for early discharge. In our care for patients with increasingly complex health problems and heavier workloads, we may think we lack the time to spend communicating. Developing quality communication using team rounds may be a solution. This method of reporting at the bedside includes the patient as a team partner in the day's care goals.

Production Expectations

The primary care literature describes agency demand for minimal appointment time with patients. Primary care providers, such as nurse practitioners, are often constrained to focus just on the chief complaint to maximize the number of patients seen, leading to "the 15-minute office visit." These system barriers limit the nurse's ability to develop substantial rapport with patients. Adequate time is essential to develop therapeutic communication to achieve effective care responsive to patient needs. As virtual appointments become the norm, this may change.

Inconsistent Caregivers

Along with workload barriers, another characteristic of organizations that creates communication barriers is lack of consistent nurse assignment and increased use of temporary staff known as agency nurses, casual nurses, or floaters. To overcome system barriers to communication, we need to work as a team to deliver consistent care. Working to develop open communications in our agencies leads to better communication and improved patient safety (AHRQ, 2021).

DEVELOPING AN EVIDENCE-BASED PRACTICE

The Agency for Healthcare Research and Quality (AHRQ, 2019) encourages research that examines attitudes and behaviors of patients as partners in safer care. AHRQ examined studies set in ICUs and pediatric units that enlisted patients in detecting adverse events. Duhn et al. (2020) reviewed 155 papers on patient engagement in safe care; 82 were research studies.

Results

AHRQ found that engaging patients as partners may lead to decreased occurrence of adverse events. Duhn found that patient attitudes about their role vary from passiveness to desire to take action. Those who favored being passive did not feel active role was their responsibility and believed speaking up is challenging authority.

Strength of research evidence: Insufficient data supplied for an independent assessment. More research needed.

Application to Your Clinical Practice

Ask patients to:

1. Take an "active partner" attitude in their healthcare; giving "permission" to participate in avoiding errors.
2. Download AHRQ's "20 Tips to Help Prevent Medical Errors" at https://www.ahrq.gov/questions/resources/20-tips.html.
3. Remind every healthcare worker touching them and their equipment to wash their hands.
4. Have agency staff provide a personalized list of hospital medications, which the patient can check each time someone gives them a medication.
5. Bring a written list of questions to each subsequent healthcare visit.

References

Agency for Healthcare Research and Quality (AHRQ). (2019). *Patient safety primer: patient engagement and safety.* Retrieved from https://psnet.ahrq.gov/primer/patient-engagement-and-safety. (Accessed 26 May 2021).

Duhn, L., Godfrey, C., & Medves, J. (2020). Scoping review of patients' attitudes about their role and behaviors to ensure safe care at the direct care level. *Health Expect, 23*(5), 979–991.

APPLICATIONS

Behaviors described in this chapter can be learned and are fundamental to your nursing role. Many nursing actions recommended here are mandated by the ANA Code of Ethics for Nurses. The actions specified include confidentiality, autonomy, beneficence, veracity, and justice. Mutuality is addressed in the ANA position statement on human rights. Providers with good communication skills have greater professional satisfaction and experience less job-related stress. Studies of patient perceptions generally show a correlation between good nurse communicators and good quality of care. Practice simulation exercises provide you with opportunities to improve your skills. Part of any simulation exercise to strengthen nursing communication is the offering of feedback.

Steps in the Caring Process

Several articles identify four steps to help you communicate C.A.R.E. with your patient:

C = First, *connect* with your patient. *Offer your attention.* Here you introduce your purpose in developing a professional relationship (i.e., meeting his or her health needs). Use the patient's formal name, and avoid terms of endearment, such as "sweetie" or "honey." Show intent to care. Attentiveness is a part of communication skill training that is probably decreased by work-related stress, time constraints, and so forth.

A = The second step is to *appreciate* the patient's situation. Although the healthcare environment is familiar to you, it is a strange and perhaps frightening situation for the patient. Acknowledge your patient's point of view and express concern.

R = The third step is to *respond* to what your patient needs. What are his or her priorities? What are his or her expectations for healthcare?

E = The fourth step is to *empower* the patient to problem-solve with you. The patient gains strength and confidence from interactions with providers, enabling the patient to move toward achievement of goals (see Fig. 11.1).

The ability to become a caring professional is influenced by your previous experiences. A person who has received caring is more likely to be able to offer it to others. Caring should not be confused with caretaking. Although caretaking is a part of caring, it may lack the necessary intentional giving of self. Self-awareness about feelings, attitudes, values, and skills is essential for developing an effective, caring relationship.

Strategies for Empowerment

In the coming years, there will be a highly increased focus on assisting patients to assume more responsibility for their health conditions. We will increasingly teach them new roles and skills to manage their illnesses. We may never fully understand the decisions some patients make, but we support their right to do so. Your method for **empowering** should include the following key strategies:

- *Accept* them as they are by refraining from any negative judgments.
- Assess their level of understanding, *exploring their perceptions and feelings* about their conditions and discussing issues that may interfere with self-care.
- Establish mutual goals for healthcare by forming an alliance, *mutually deciding* about their care.
- Find out how much information they want to know.
- Reinforce *autonomy,* for example, by allowing them to choose the content in the teaching plan.
- *Offer information* in an environment that enables them to use it.
- Make sure your patients *actively participate* in their care plans.
- Encourage networking with a support group and the use of mHealth Apps (see Chapter 26).
- Clarify with them that they hold the major *responsibility* for both the healthcare decisions they make and their consequences.

Application of Empathy to Levels of Nursing Actions

Nursing actions that facilitate empathy can be classified into three major skills: (1) recognition and classification of requests, (2) attending behaviors, and (3) empathetic responses.

Processing Requests

Two types of requests are for information and action. These requests do not involve interpersonal concerns and are easier to manage. Another form of request is for understanding involvement, which entails the patient's need for empathetic understanding.

Attending Behaviors

Attending behaviors facilitate empathy and include an attentive, open posture; responding to verbal and nonverbal cues through appropriate gestures and facial expressions; using eye contact; and allowing patient self-expression. Verbally acknowledging nonverbal cues shows you are attending, as does offering time and attention, showing interest in the patient's issues, offering helpful information, and clarifying problem areas. These responses encourage patients to participate in their own healing. Preverbal children require adaptations such as soothing vocal tone and comforting touch as shown with the baby in Fig. 11.2.

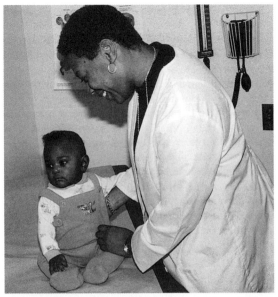

Figure 11.2 Infants lack verbal communication skills. The nurse's comforting touch and pleasant vocal tone help overcome this barrier. (Courtesy Adam Boggs.)

Make Empathetic Responses

You communicate **empathy** when you show your patients that you understand how they are feeling. This helps them identify emotions that are not readily observable and connect them with the current situation. For example, observing nonverbal cues, such as a worried facial expression, and verbalizing this reaction with an empathetic comment, such as "I understand that this is very difficult for you," validate what they are feeling and tell them you understand them. Using the actions listed in Table 11.2, the nurse applies attending behaviors and nursing actions to express empathy. Verbal prompts, such as "Hmm," "Uh-huh," "I see," "Tell me more," and "Go on," facilitate expression of feelings. The nurse uses open-ended questions to validate perceptions. Using informing behaviors from this table enlarges the database by providing new information and gives feedback to your patient. Remember, demonstrating empathy as a communication behavior has been shown to positively affect the outcome of your care.

Reduction of Barriers in Nurse–Patient Relationships

Recognition of barriers is the first step in eliminating them and thus enhancing the therapeutic process. Practice with exercises in this chapter should increase your recognition of possible barriers. Findings from many studies have emphasized the crucial importance of honesty, cultural sensitivity, and caring, especially in listening actively to

TABLE 11.2   Levels of Nursing Communication Behavior

Level	Category	Nursing Communication Behavior
1. Process	Gathers data	Becomes aware of goals and patient care plan
	Accepts	Uses patient's correct name
		Maintains eye contact
		Adopts open posture
2. Act	Listens	Responds to cues
		Nods head
		Smiles
		Encourages responses
		Uses therapeutic silence
	Clarifies	Asks open-ended questions
		Restates the problem
		Validates perceptions
		Acknowledges confusion
	Informs	Provides honest, complete answers
		Assesses patient's knowledge
		Confronts conflict
		Summarizes teaching points
3. Reflect	Analyzes	Identifies unknown emotions
		Interprets underlying meanings
		Evaluates outcomes
		Communicates with team to revise care plan

BOX 11.3   Tips to Reduce Relationship Barriers

- Establish trust.
- Demonstrate caring and empathy.
- Empower your patient.
- Recognize and reduce anxiety.
- Maintain appropriate personal distance.
- Practice cultural sensitivity, and work to be bilingual.
- Use therapeutic relationship-building activities such as active listening.
- Avoid medical jargon.

suggestions and complaints from the patient and family. Refer to Box 11.3 for a summary of strategies to reduce communication barriers in nurse–patient relationships.

Respect for Personal Space

We need to assess a patient's personal space needs. Assessment includes cultural and developmental factors that affect perceptions of space and reactions to intrusions. In some situations, if you need to increase your patient's sense of personal space, you can decrease direct eye contact or position your body at an angle. Examples might be when bathing, changing dressings, etc. At the same time, it is important for you to talk gently during such procedures and to elicit feedback, if appropriate.

There is a discrepancy between the minimum amount of space an individual needs and the amount of space hospitals are able to provide in multiple-occupancy rooms. Actions to ensure private space and show respect include the following:

- closing the door to the room to allow rest;
- providing privacy when disturbing matters are to be discussed;
- explaining procedures before implementation;
- entering another person's personal space with warning (e.g., knocking or calling the patient's name) and, preferably, waiting for permission to enter;
- providing an identified space for personal belongings and treating them with care;
- encouraging the inclusion of personal and familiar objects on the nightstand;
- decreasing direct eye contact during hands-on care;
- minimizing bodily exposure during care;
- using only the necessary number of people during any procedure; and
- using touch appropriately.

SUMMARY

This chapter focuses on essential concepts that act as bridges in constructing a meaningful, effective nurse–patient relationship, including caring, empowerment, trust, empathy, mutuality, and confidentiality. Respect for the patient as a unique person is a basic component of each concept.

Caring is described as a commitment by the nurse that involves profound respect and concern for the unique humanity of every patient and a willingness to confirm their personhood.

Empowerment is assisting patients to take charge of their own health.

Trust represents an individual's emotional reliance on the consistency and continuity of experience. The patient perceives the nurse as trustworthy, a safe person with whom to share difficult feelings about health-related needs.

Empathy is the ability to accurately perceive another person's feelings and to convey their meaning to the patient. Nursing behaviors that facilitate the development of empathy are accepting, listening, clarifying and informing, and analyzing. Each of these behaviors implicitly recognizes the patient as a unique individual worthy of being listened to and respected.

Mutuality is characterized by reciprocity in setting goals and collaborating in methods. To foster mutuality within the relationship, nurses need to remain aware of their own feelings, attitudes, and beliefs.

Barriers described include anxiety, stereotyping, over-familiarity, and personal space violations. Organizational system demands, such as a heavy workload, limit time for nurse–patient communication. Solutions focus on open communication among all team members caring for the patient.

ETHICAL DILEMMA: What Would You Do?

There are limits to your professional responsibility to maintain confidentiality. Any information that, if withheld, might endanger the life or physical and emotional safety of the patient or others needs to be communicated to the health team or appropriate people immediately. Consider the teen who confides his plan to shoot classmates. Can you breach confidentiality in this case? Consider what you would do when you notice genital warts (from sexually transmitted human papilloma virus) on a 5-year-old child, but who shows no other signs of sexual abuse?

DISCUSSION QUESTIONS

1. How would you teach a nurse to apply the strategies for anxiety reduction and destressing provided in Box 11.2?
2. Reflect on which behaviors in Simulation Exercise 11.4 demonstrated empathy. Could you add the phrase, "That must have been difficult," to what the nurse role-player said?
3. Contrast stereotypes you have heard about in a health-care setting. Discuss them in a group.
4. Analyze how proxemics changes in different situations. What is your own preferred space distance? To what do you attribute this preference? Under what circumstances do your needs for personal space change?

REFERENCES

Agency for Healthcare Research and Quality (AHRQ). (2021). *TeamSTEPPS*. www.ahrq.gov/teamstepps/index.html. [Accessed 25 May 2021].

American Nurses Association (ANA). (2010). *Nursing's social policy statement: The essence of the profession.* Silver Spring, MD: ANA.

American Nurses Association (ANA). (2015). *The code of ethics for nurses with interpretive statements.* Silver Spring, MD: ANA. Retrieved from http://nursingworld.org/practice-policy/nursing-excellence/ethics//Code-of-Ethics-for-Nurses/. [Accessed 21 June 2021].

Erikson, E. (1963). *Childhood and society* (2nd ed.). New York: Norton.

Levetown, M., & American Academy of Pediatrics Committee on Bioethics (2008). Communicating with children and families: From everyday interactions to skill in conveying distressing information. *Pediatrics, 121*(5), e1441–e1460.

Rogers, C. (1961). *On becoming a person.* Boston: Houghton-Mifflin.

World Health Organization (WHO). (n.d.). Patient participation in decisions. Retrieved from www.who.int/.

Wune, G., Ayalew, Y., Hailu, A., & Gebretensaye, T. (2020). Nurses to patients communication and barriers perceived by nurses at Tikur Anbessa specialized hospital, Addis Ababa, Ethiopia 2018. *International Journal of Africa Nursing Sciences, 12*, e100197.

12

Communicating With Families

OBJECTIVES

At the end of the chapter, the reader will be able to:
1. Define family and identify its components.
2. Apply family-centered concepts to the care of the family in clinical settings, using standardized family assessment tools.
3. Apply the nursing process to the care of families in clinical and community settings.
4. Plan nursing interventions for families in the intensive care unit (ICU) versus families in the community.

The purpose of this chapter is to describe family-centered relationships and communication strategies that nurses can use to support family integrity in healthcare settings. Chapter 12 identifies family theory frameworks and ways to maximize productive communication with family members. Practical assessment and intervention strategies address family issues that affect a patient's recovery and support self-management of chronic health conditions or peaceful death in clinical practice.

BASIC CONCEPTS

Definition of Family

Nurses have an ethical and moral obligation to involve families in their patient's healthcare (Shajani & Snell, 2019). The term *family* can have several definitions, particularly in

today's society. The legal definition describes the family as individuals related through marriage, blood ties, adoption, or guardianship. As a biological unit, *family* describes the genetic connections among people. The US Census Bureau defines family as a group of two people or more (one of whom is the householder) related by birth, marriage, or adoption and residing together; all such people (including related subfamily members) are considered as members of one family. A household consists of all people who occupy a housing unit regardless of relationship. There no longer exists a typical American family, rather many variation. As healthcare providers, it is most appropriate to use Sanjani & Snell's definition that a family is who they say they are (Shajani & Snell, 2019). Identified family members may or may not be blood related. Strong emotional ties and durability of membership characterize family relationships

---

CASE STUDY: **Joey Getz Overdoses**

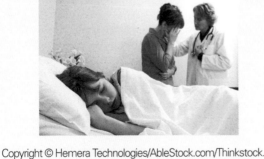

Copyright © Hemera Technologies/AbleStock.com/Thinkstock.

Joey is 8 years old and is assigned to your pediatric unit. He is semiconscious due to an overdose of Ritalin.

Parents are Joan Gardner and Ron Getz, who are separated but share legal custody. Nurse Diane Mann comforts Ms Gardner and demonstrates acceptance by allowing her to vent her grief and anger toward Mrs Gardner, the grandmother, for leaving the medication where Joey could reach it. Ms Gardner agrees to be the primary contact person, obtaining daily reports which she will share with the paternal side of the family. She agrees to text Mr Getz twice a day if he stays away while she stays at the bedside. However, her mother (Joey's grandmother) sneaks Mr Getz into the hospital while Ms Gardner goes home for a quick shower and change of clothes. What would you do?

160

TABLE 12.1 Needs of Families With Critically Ill Patient

Need	Behavior	Suggested Intervention
Open communication	Nursing staff inundated with phone calls/texts requesting information on patient	Have family designate ONE person to contact staff and share information with other family. Call contact to notify of any changes in patient condition.
Understanding	Low health literacy, so understanding is incomplete	Frequent explanation in simple terms; family conferences with team. Allow hope. Support whatever decision family makes.
Need for proximity	Many family members gathering in ICU waiting room	Open visiting, one person at a time at bedside so nurses can do work.
Family in crisis	Demands for prognosis versus not really wanting to know	Assess family structure and functioning: who is the decision-maker? What support resources are available? Recognize family is stressed. Demonstrate caring. Allow questions, giving honest answers.
Decision-making	Confusion	Involve family in plan of care. Allow simple direct care such as giving ice chips. Begin discharge transition plan early so caretakers can learn role.

sometimes positively and sometimes with conflict as in the case of Joey Getz.

During times of crisis, such as a seriously ill family member, family members react to the situation and one another with a wide range of reactions. Each family member responds in unique ways. Communication, even when reactive, should maintain the integrity of the family. Nurses play a central role not only in care of the critically ill but also as support providers to the patient's family (Edwards, 2010).

Understanding the family as a system is relevant in today's healthcare environment, as the family is an essential part of the healthcare team. Families have a profound influence on ill family members as advisors, caretakers, supporters, and sometimes irritants. Patients who are very young, very old, and those requiring assistance with self-management of chronic illness are particularly dependent on their families.

Support from the healthcare team during times of stress and crisis is necessary to provide information and empowerment to successfully adapt. Both resources and supports are essential for family empowerment. Resources and supports include beliefs, past experiences, help-giving and receiving practices, strengths, and capabilities; and they are pieces of information that help explain patient and family responses to health disruptions. Conducting a family assessment is essential to (1) assure that the needs of the family are met, (2) uncover any gaps in the family plan of action, and (3) offer multiple supports and resources to the family. Table 12.1 lists needs of families when a member is critically ill.

Theoretical Frameworks

Theoretical frameworks are used to provide a means for understanding relationships among essential concepts. Numerous theoretical frameworks exist that can be used to understand family composition. Remember the concept that stress occurs when a person or family encounters a situation that exceeds their ability to adapt or cope.

General Systems Theory

Hans Seyle's General Systems Theory was discussed in Chapter 1. A system interacts with other systems in the environment. An interactional process occurs when inputs are introduced into the system in the form of information, energy, and resources. Within each system, the information is processed internally as the system actively processes and interprets its meaning (*throughput*). The *output* refers to the result or product that leaves the system. Each system is separated from its environment by boundaries that control the exchange of information, energy, and resources into and out of the system. Evaluations of the output and feedback loops from the environment inform the system of changes needed to achieve effective outputs. See Fig. 12.1 diagram of systems theory.

Von Bertalanffy's Theory

Ludwig von Bertalanffy's (1968) general systems theory provides a conceptual foundation for family system models. Systems perspective is used to analyze how the family

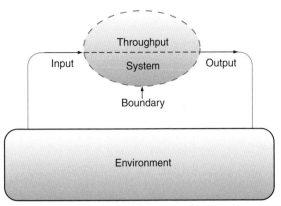

Figure 12.1 Systems model: interaction with the environment.

functions as a whole. In this viewpoint, the sum of the whole is greater than the total of its parts, with each part reciprocally influencing its function. If one part of the system changes or fails, it affects the functioning of the whole. A clock is a useful metaphor. It displays time correctly, but only if all parts work together. If any part of the clock breaks down, the clock no longer tells accurate time.

A family is part of the larger society. The family creates a balance between change and stability (homeostasis). A change in one member affects all.

Bowen's Systems Theory

Murray Bowen's (1978) family systems theory conceptualizes the family as an interactive emotional unit. Family members assume reciprocal family roles, develop automatic communication patterns, and react to one another in predictable, connected ways, particularly when family anxiety is high. Once anxiety heightens within the system, an emotional process gets activated, and dysfunctional communication patterns can emerge. For example, if one person is overly responsible, another family member may become less likely to assume normal responsibility. Until one family member is willing to challenge the dysfunction of an emotional system by refusing to play their reactive part, the negative emotional energy fueling a family's dysfunctional communication pattern persists.

Bowen developed eight interlocking concepts to explain his theoretical construct of the family system (Bowen Center for the Study of the Family, n.d.): Differentiation of self; multigenerational transmission of behaviors and roles; nuclear family emotional relationship patterns; triangle strategies to bring in a third member to decrease anxiety; family projection of positive or negative feelings onto one member (scapegoat); sibling position; emotional cutoff to avoid uncomfortable issues; and societal emotional climate internalized into the family.

The Calgary Family Assessment and Family Interaction Models

First published by Wright and Leahey and now by Shajani and Snell (2019), these models give an organizing frameworks for nurses to understand families. The Calgary model looks at structure, development, and function patterns within the family.

Structure. Who is part of the family unit? Have there been losses, especially recent deaths or divorces? To what extent does the family rely on larger systems to help meet needs? Examples include friends and neighbors, school or work systems, churches, or social services. According to Sajani and Snell, in today's world, the Internet can be a larger system relationship. Many rely on texting or virtual communication platforms such as Facetime for support. Internet resources can provide information and validation, but they can also be a source of misinformation.

Development. This model examines the developmental cycle and family tasks associated with its developmental cycle, such as childrearing. These cycles are influenced by past and present events and future expectations. For example, the family welcoming a new child is faced with adjustments that differ greatly from those adjustments a family with an ill elder faces.

Instrumental and Expressive Functions. The instrumental aspect of function includes all the activities involved in daily living. This is an important area of consideration if the patient's condition adds new demands on what is an already busy family. The expressive functioning includes all the communication within the family. What types of emotion are discussed? Who expresses feelings? Are there coalitions of some family members? What is the balance of power? Who makes decisions? Who shuts down discussion? Does the family think they are functioning well? What needs for help and support can they tap into? Considering all this, the nurse needs to know who will participate in problem-solving regarding the patient.

Use of the Calgary Family Intervention model changes the focus from the parts to assessing the family as a whole. Examine the domains of family function: cognitive, affective, and behavioral. The Calgary model focuses on strengths rather than dysfunctions. Nursing interventions focus on sustaining or improving family function. Nurses can offer suggestions but cannot change the ways in which families choose to function.

Family Legacies

Families tend to pass traditions and rituals down across the generations. This can serve as an affirming phenomena. Shared family traditions strengthen family bonds. What rituals does your family have? Helping families gain clarity can be an asset in healthcare.

APPLICATIONS

Family-Centered Care

Family-centered care allows healthcare providers to have a uniform understanding of the patient and family's knowledge, preferences, and values as the basis for shared decision-making. This provides consistent information to all involved in the patient's care and allows the family to identify any barriers that might arise with the care plan. Family members are involved in decision-making ranging from treatment options to end-of-life issues. Family plays an advocacy role by monitoring care and insisting on quality. It helps nursing staff if one family member is identified as the contact person who then spreads the news to all other family members.

The nurses in family-centered care are to
- understand the impact of a medical crisis on family functioning, dynamics, and health;
- communicate clearly, frequently with family members/contact person;
- appreciate and respond empathetically to the emotional intensity of the experience for the family; and
- determine the appropriate level of family involvement.

Orientation

Nurse–family relationships depend on reciprocal interactions. Nurses begin offering information during the preadmission interview or as soon as the patient is admitted. An information packet can contain maps to restrooms, cafeteria, parking options, nearby lodging, and information about

---

BOX 12.1   Indicators for Family Assessment

- Initial diagnosis of a serious physical or psychiatric illness or injury in a family member, especially if it alters family roles
- Family involvement and understanding needed to support the recovery of the patient
- Deterioration of the family member's condition
- Illness in a child, adolescent, or cognitively impaired adult
- Discharge
- Death
- Health problem defined by the family as a family issue
- Indicators of threat to relationships such as abuse, neglect, or anticipated loss of family member

---

BOX 12.2   Examples of Therapeutic Questions to Ask Family Members

- How does the family view the current health crisis?
- What is each family member's most immediate concern?
- Has anyone else in the family experienced a similar problem?
- Who in the family is best at encouraging the patient to comply with their treatment?
- What information do you still need to understand the prognosis of this disease?
- Are there any other recent changes or sources of stress in the family that make the current situation worse?
- How has the family handled problems to date?
- If there were one question you could have answered now, what would it be?
- How can we best help you and your family?

---

how to contact staff or physicians. Information about the best ways to navigate the healthcare system is helpful.

The initial family encounter sets the tone for the relationship. How nurses interact with each family member may be as important as what they choose to say. Begin with formal introductions, and explain the purpose of gathering assessment data. Even this early in the relationship, you should listen carefully for family expectations and general anxiety or expressed concerns about the patient, which may be revealed more through behavior than through words.

Ask the family and patient what information they most need. The words are not as important as is the climate the nurse seeks to create. When interacting, nurses must be aware of legal or professional restrictions governing what information can be released without violating the patient's right to privacy. In the United States, under the Health Insurance Portability and Accountability Act (HIPAA), family members receive information only with permission of the patient or designee. This means you as a nurse cannot give out information over the telephone or to visitors without specific patient permission.

Assessment

It cannot be overemphasized that family dynamics affect communication. Health disruption becomes a family event. Use verbal and nonverbal skills described in the book to gather information from family members, especially active listening. Box 12.1 lists suggestions for family assessment and intervention. Assessing current family coping strategies is crucial. Determining the association/relationship of the family member to the patient is an initial step nurses can take in establishing a relationship. You might say, "I would like to hear what you think is the impact of your child's illness on the entire family." This statement not only guides your assessment but also reminds the family that each family member is of concern to the healthcare team. Knowledge of a family's past medical experiences, concurrent family stressors, and family expectations for treatment are essential pieces of family assessment data. Box 12.2 lists suggestions for questions.

Our communication should be sensitive to family dynamics, cultural beliefs, and religious sensitivities. Nonsupportive family responses have been associated with negative patient outcomes. Simulation Exercise 12.1 allows you to analyze positive and negative family responses. Family participation in the assessment process enhances the therapeutic relationship and completeness of the data. It is important to inquire about the family's cultural identity, rituals, values, level of family involvement, decision-making, spiritual beliefs, and traditional behaviors as they relate to the healthcare of the patient. Family members can suffer from ICU stress syndrome with significant symptoms such as anxiety and depression (Petrinec & Martin, 2018). Up to 75% of families reported depression in one Canadian study (Charles et al., 2017).

Intervention

Problem Identification. Based on assessment data, identify any problems with family communication and function that might interfere with your patient's treatment. Some problems identified might stem from unexpressed fear or anger or uncertainty. These may be dealt with by the nursing staff, but significant problems require referral to experts in family dynamics.

SIMULATION EXERCISE 12.1   Positive and Negative Family Interactions

Purpose
To examine the effects of functional versus dysfunctional communication.

Procedure
Answer the following questions in a brief essay:
1. Recall a situation in dealing with a patient's family that you felt was a positive experience. What characteristics of that interaction made you feel this way?
2. Recall a situation in dealing with a patient's family that you felt was a negative experience. What characteristics of that interaction made you feel this way?

Reflective Discussion Analysis
Compare experiences, both positive and negative. What did you see as the most striking differences? In what ways were your responses similar or dissimilar from those of your peers? What do you see as the implications of this exercise for enhancing family communication in your nursing practice?

Interventive Questioning. Questions focus on family interrelationships and the effect a serious health alteration has on individual family members and the equilibrium of the family system. The nurse uses information the family provides as the basis for additional questions.

Planning

The more the family can become involved in the planning process, the greater the likelihood of success. The development of appropriate nursing actions should be based on mutually established goals. For the bedside nurse, these goals are often short term, focusing on improving awareness of areas to improve communication. Planning for discharge begins with admission. Development of nursing actions should be based on mutual goals. For the bedside direct care nurse, such goals may be relatively short term. The nurse must be alert for cues that indicate potential problems in family communication and function. Some problems related to family function may require referral to a social worker, family therapist, or other member of the healthcare team. In other instances, it may be appropriate for the nurse to provide assistance to the family. Health-related communication issues can involve: unexpressed fears or anger management of uncertainty, or finding common ground for shared decision-making.

Resources are available to help ensure family engagement. The Agency for Healthcare Research and Quality (AHRQ) has developed the Guide to Patient and Family Engagement in Hospital Quality and Safety. This document has a multidisciplinary focus with four specific strategies:
Strategy 1: Working with patients and families as advisors
Strategy 2: Communicating to improve quality
Strategy 3: Nurse bedside shift report
Strategy 4: IDEAL discharge planning (AHRQ, 2013)

Try Simulation Exercise 12.2 for experience in developing family-centered care planning. AHRQ has developed "A Guide to Patient Engagement in Hospital Quality and Safety." Content for the healthcare team includes the following:
- Working with family as advisors
- Communicating to improve quality
- Using the bedside shift report
- IDEAL discharge planning

Family Meetings. Ideally, all family members and the entire healthcare team should meet in one or more sit-down sessions. This not only facilitates communication but also allows development of a comprehensive, clearly understood plan for care. As already noted, change in one family role causes family reorganization in new ways of functioning. For example, the debilitating illness of the breadwinner necessitates both financial and role reorganizations. The team may find a need for community referrals so they can begin early.

Family Inclusive Bedside Rounds. The Society for Critical Care Medicine as well as others advocates including a family member in rounds to improve communication, improve satisfaction, and encourage engagement, empowering family (Halm, 2020). Simulation Exercise 12.3 gives practice assessing family coping strengths. Reflect on the Spence case study.

Case Study: Mrs Alice Spence and Mr Mike Spence Express their Concerns

Mrs Spence, Daughter: It is difficult for me to find a balance between caring for my mother and also caring for my children and husband. I have also had to learn a lot about the professional and support resources that are available in the community.

Mr Spence: For me, the biggest challenge has been convincing my wife that I can take over for a while, for her to get some rest. I worry that she will become exhausted.

Mrs Diane Under, Mother: I have appreciated all the help that they give me. My biggest concern is to not become too much of a burden on them. I want to be as independent as possible, but sometimes I wonder about moving to a palliative care setting or a hospice.

SIMULATION EXERCISE 12.2   Developing a Family Nursing Care Plan

Purpose

To practice skills needed with difficult family patterns.

Procedure

Read the case study, and think of how you could interact appropriately with this family.

Mr Monroe, age 43 years, was chairing a board meeting of his large, successful manufacturing corporation when he developed shortness of breath, dizziness, and a crushing, viselike pain in his chest. An ambulance was called, and he was taken to the medical center. Subsequently, he was admitted to the coronary unit with a diagnosis of an impending myocardial infarction (MI).

Mr Monroe is married with three children: Steve, age 14; Sean, age 12; and Lisa, age 10. He is the president and majority stockholder of his company. He has no history of cardiovascular problems, although his father died at the age of 38 of a massive coronary occlusion. His oldest brother died at the age of 42 from the same condition, and his other brother, still living, became a semi-invalid after suffering two heart attacks, one at the age of 44 and the other at 47.

Mr Monroe is tall, slim, suntanned, and very athletic. He swims daily; jogs every morning for 30 min; plays golf regularly; and is an avid sailor, having participated in every yacht regatta and usually winning. He is very health conscious and has had annual physical checkups. He watches his diet and quit smoking to avoid possible damage to his heart. He has been determined to avoid dying young or becoming an invalid like his brother.

When he was admitted to the coronary care unit, he was conscious. Although in a great deal of pain, he seemed determined to control his own fate. While in the unit, he was an exceedingly difficult patient, a trial to the nursing staff and his physician. He constantly watched and listened to everything going on around him and demanded complete explanations about any procedure, equipment,

or medication he received. He would sleep in brief naps and only when he was totally exhausted. Despite his obvious tension and anxiety, his condition stabilized. The damage to his heart was considered minimal, and his prognosis was good. As the pain diminished, he began asking when he could go home and when he could go back to work. He was impatient to be moved to a private room so that he could conduct some of his business by telephone.

When Mrs Monroe visited, she approached the nursing staff with questions regarding Mr Monroe's condition, usually asking the same question several times in different ways. She also asked why she was not being "told everything."

Interactions between Mr Monroe and Mrs Monroe were noted by the staff as Mr Monroe telling Mrs Monroe all the things she needed to do. Little intimate contact was noted.

Mr Monroe denied having any anxiety or concerns about his condition, although his behavior contradicted his denial. Mrs Monroe would agree with her husband's assessment when questioned in his company.

Reflective Discussion Analysis

1. What questions would you ask the patient and family to obtain data regarding their adaptation to crisis?
2. What family nursing diagnosis would apply with this case study?
3. What nursing interventions are appropriate to interact with this patient and his family?
4. What other members of the healthcare team should be involved with this family situation?
5. How would you plan to transmit the information to the family?
6. What outcomes and measures would you use to determine success or failure of the nursing care plan?

Developed by Conrad, J. University of Maryland School of Nursing, Baltimore, MD.

Meaningful involvement in the patient's care differs not only from family to family but also among individual family members (Ylvén & Granlund, 2009). Individual family members have different perspectives. Hearing each family member's perspective helps the family and nurse develop a unified understanding of significant treatment goals and implications for family involvement.

Although treatment plans should be tailored around personal patient goals, acknowledging family needs, values, and priorities enhances compliance, especially if they are

different. Shared decision-making and the development of realistic, achievable goals make it easier for everyone concerned to accomplish them with a sense of ownership and self-efficacy about the process. Taking small achievable steps is preferred to attempting giant steps that misjudge what the family can realistically do.

Implementation

Nurses can only offer interventions; it is up to the family to accept them. Shoring up family coping can involve

SIMULATION EXERCISE 12.3 Assessing Family Coping Strategies

Purpose

To broaden awareness of coping strategies among families.

Procedure

Each student is to recall a time when his or her family experienced a significant health crisis and how they coped. (Alternative strategy: Pick a health crisis you observed with a family in clinical practice.) Respond to the following questions:

1. Did the crisis cause a readjustment in roles?
2. Did it create tension and conflict, or did it catalyze members into turning to one another for support? Look at the behavior of individual members.
3. What would have helped your family in this crisis? Write a descriptive summary about this experience.

Reflective Discussion Analysis

Each student shares his or her experience. Discuss the differences in how families respond to crisis. Compile a listing of coping strategies and helpful interventions on the board. Discuss the nurse's role in support of the family.

BOX 12.3 Caring for Family Needs in the Intensive Care Unit

Families of critically ill patients need to do the following:
- Have frequent, clear communication with staff daily and when there is a change in condition.
- Feel there is hope, without receiving unrealistic comments.
- Feel that hospital personnel care about the patient.
- Have open, brief visiting hours.
- Have a waiting room near the patient.
- Feel supported by staff who recognize their increased stress level.
- Have the contact person called at home about changes in the patient's condition.
- Know the prognosis.
- Have questions answered honestly.
- Know specific facts about the patient's prognosis.
- Have explanations given in understandable terms.

encouraging both emotion-focused strategies and problem-focused strategies. Actively seeking outside support from family friends, church, community agencies, etc., is helpful. One goal should be to encourage primary caretakers to invest in their own well-being. Suggested nursing actions to promote positive change in family functioning when caring for families with a patient in ICU are listed in Box 12.3.

Case Study: Francis Chin

Frances Chin, 48 years, is diagnosed with breast cancer. When she sees her oncologist, Mrs Chin reports that she is feeling fine, eating, and able to function in much the same way as before receiving chemotherapy. Mr Chin's perception differs. He reports that her appetite has declined such that she only eats a few spoonfuls of food and she spends much of the day in bed. What Frances is reporting is true. When she is up, she enjoys doing what she did previously, although at a slower pace, and she does eat at every meal. Frances is communicating her need to feel normal, which is important to support. What her husband adds is also true. Her husband's input allows Frances to receive the treatment she needs to stimulate her appetite and give her more energy.

Meeting the Needs of Families of Critically Ill Patients

Incorporating Family Strengths

Otto (1963) introduced the concept of family strengths as a resources that families can use to make their lives more satisfying and fulfilling when healthcare changes are required as happens with patients suffering from serious illness or injury. Viewing the family as having strengths to cope with a problem rather than being a problem is a healing strategy. While each family's experience with illness varies, commonalities exist. The nurse should share strategies that families in similar situations have found effective. Family-centered relationships are key dimensions of quality care in the ICU.

Giving Commendations

Commendations involve expressing recognition of capabilities, skills, and competencies. Commendations are particularly effective when the family seems dispirited or confused about an illness or accident. More than a simple compliment, commendations should reflect patterns of behavior observed in the family unit over time. Differentiate between a commendation such as "Your family is showing much courage in living with your wife's cancer for 5 years." and a compliment like "Your son is so gentle despite feeling so ill." Situations may seem extremely dire, but by identifying even one positive factor, a family may feel empowered to push through the difficult situation.

Informational Support

Helping a family become aware of information and how to access it empowers families. By showing interest in

---

BOX 12.4   Tips for Helping Families Cope

- Encourage the telling of illness narratives.
- Commend family and individual strengths.
- Offer information.
- Validate or normalize emotional responses.
- Encourage family support.
- Support family members as caregivers.
- Encourage respite.
- Initiate end-of-life discussion, if necessary.

---

the coping strategies that have and have not worked, the nurse can help the family recognize progress in their ability to cope with a difficult situation. Refer to Box 12.4 for tips on helping families cope with member's condition.

Teaching Family Members. You can offer family members support related to talking with extended family, children, and others about the patient's illness. You can help family members prepare questions for meeting with physicians and other health professionals. Encouraging family members to write down key points to be addressed with other family members and physicians can be helpful. Written instructions should also be provided upon discharge. The use of the "teach-back" method can be used with families and individual patients.

End-of-Life. If the patient is more seriously ill, and is receptive, the nurse should see this as an opportunity to provide information regarding end-of-life decision-making. Decisions regarding end-of-life care are best carried out when families are not in a crisis mode. Thus, you can engage with families in discussions about the cultural, ethical, and physical implications of using or discontinuing life support systems. This is nursing's special niche, as these conversations are rarely one-time events, and nurses can provide informal opportunities for discussing them during care provision.

Proximity to the Patient. The need to remain near the patient is a priority for many family members of patients in the ICU. Although the family may appear to hover too closely, it is usually an attempt to rally around the patient in critical trouble. *Viewed from this perspective, nurses can be more empathetic.* Visitation policies may need to be adjusted based on the availability of family members and patient needs. Many recommend open visitation with brief visits at the bedside. When families visit loved ones in the ICU, the nurse should acknowledge them and provide any updated information that is available.

Caretaker Burden. Families can be a primary support to patients, but they usually need encouragement and concrete suggestions for maximum effect and satisfaction. Family members feel helpless to reverse the course of the patient's condition and appreciate opportunities to help their loved one. Suggesting actions that family members can take at the bedside include doing range-of-motion exercises, holding the patient's hand, positioning pillows, and providing mouth care or ice chips. Talking with and reading to the patient, even if the person is unresponsive, can be meaningful for both the family and patient. Helping families balance the need to be present with the patient's needs to conserve energy and have some alone time to rest or regroup is important. Family members also need time apart from their loved one for the same reasons.

Nurses can role-model communication with patients, using simple caring words and touch. Multiple studies show half of patients and half of families suffer emotional distress during the hospitalization and for at least a year postdischarge.

Breaking Bad News to Families

It is usually the physician who delivers life-threatening critical information to patients and families. It is often the nurse at the bedside who ensures adequate patient and family understanding of information that has been provided. Additionally, nurses often notify patients and family members of significant changes in patient status, such as poor wound healing, transfers, a need for further testing, or deterioration in status. First, alert the family that bad news is coming. Be factual and concrete. Make a list of information you want to cover. Use of the SBAR format is helpful. Sometimes, this occurs over the telephone, which further complicates the communication process. In each instance, well-planned communication can facilitate positive coping and adaptation. Present some background information. Allow for a period of silence to show respect for the individual and to allow the person to process the information. In follow-up, the nurse should ask if the person understands the information that has been presented and ask for questions. The interaction should close with a summary of the treatment plan and when further communication can be expected.

Evaluation

Evaluation should include determining the effectiveness of nursing interventions. Use self-reflection. Direct care bedside nurses may not see long-term benefits from family interactions due to the episodic nature of contemporary healthcare. It is important to provide closure to interactions in any setting. You can accomplish this task by summarizing the interaction, asking the family if they have any questions, and providing information regarding follow-up. Bereaved families have reported that the support received from nurses played an important role in how they were able to cope. No matter how brief family interactions are, your impact may be substantial.

Referrals. Family caregivers should receive a written copy of the discharge plan, as should the primary physician. Include a verbal summary of the information gained to date and medications and support care referrals as well as contact telephone numbers.

Family-Centered Relationships in the Community

More than half of all adult US citizens are affected by at least one chronic disease (Centers for Disease Control and Prevention CDC 2021). A chronic disease is defined as one lasting more than 1 year, which requires medical care and limits a person's activities. Four modifiable risk factors (physical activity, obesity, smoking, and alcohol consumption) contribute substantially to the financial and emotional burden associated with chronic disease. Community-based nurses have many opportunities to teach individuals to self-manage their disease. A major portion of your interactions should focus on encouraging families to adopt a healthy lifestyle to decrease the incidence of disease and illness. For community-dwelling individuals, the concept of patient-centered care focuses on empowering individuals to not only self-manage chronic diseases but also make appropriate lifestyle modifications with the intent of either preventing disease or minimizing the effects of disease. Nurses in clinics and community-based centers should be responsive to cues from caregivers indicating deficient knowledge. Nurses can offer suggestions about how to respond to these changes and offer support to the family caregiver as they emerge. Helping family members access services, support groups, and natural support networks at each stage of their loved one's illness empowers family members because they feel they are helping in a tangible way.

A significant change in health status can exacerbate previously unresolved relationship issues, which may need advanced intervention, in addition to the specific healthcare issues. When individual family members are experiencing a transition, for example, ending or entering a relationship or a job change, they may not be as available to provide support and can experience unnecessary guilt. Nurses need to consider the broader family responsibilities people have as an important part of the context of healthcare in providing holistic care to a family.

Supporting the Caregiver

Family caregivers are common as more people live with chronic illness on a daily basis; the level of assistance required varies on a person-by-person basis. Healthy family members have concurrent demands on their time from their own nuclear families, work, church, and community responsibilities. Remember that your words can either strengthen or weaken a family's confidence in their ability to care for an ill family member. Focus initially on issues that are manageable within the context of home caregiving. This provides a sense of empowerment. Many families will need information about additional home care services, community resources, and options needed to meet the practical, financial, and emotional demands of caring for a chronically ill family member. There are support groups available for family caregivers of patients with chronic illnesses. These are extremely helpful supports for family members. Not only can they provide practical ideas, but the support of being able to talk about your feelings, and finding that you are not alone, is healing for family members and indirectly beneficial for patients (Vranceanu et al., 2020).

Validating and Normalizing Emotions

Families can experience many conflicting emotions when placed in the position of providing protracted care for a loved one. Compassion, protectiveness, and caring can be intermingled with feelings of helplessness and being trapped. Major role reversals can stimulate anger and resentment for both patient and family caregiver. Some caregivers find themselves mourning for their loved one, even though the person is still alive, wishing it could all end, but feeling guilt about having such thoughts. These emotions are normal responses to abnormal circumstances. Listening to the family caregiver's feelings and struggles without judgment can be the most healing intervention you can provide. Nurses can normalize negative feelings by offering insights about common feelings associated with chronic illness. Family members may need guidance and permission to get respite and recharge their commitment by attending to their own needs. Support groups can provide families with emotional and practical support and a critical expressive outlet.

Pitfalls to Avoid

While we, as nurses, strive to be effective in all communication, there are times that our communication efforts are less than ideal. Shajani and Snell (2019) identify common errors that occur in family nursing.
1. Failing to assess coping abilities.
2. Failing to create context for change. This happens when we fail to establish a therapeutic environment for open discussion of family concerns. Another example would be a plan of care that would not be effective in light of

the family situation (resources, distance, health state). To avoid this pitfall, the nurse should be respectful of each family member and acknowledge the difficulty of the situation.

3. Underestimating the health literacy of members.
4. Taking sides. To minimize the risk of taking sides, the nurse should use questioning skills that help family members develop insight into the depth and scope of the problem. The use of circular questions, as discussed earlier, can be helpful.
5. Giving too much advice prematurely. We are very busy but need to resist the temptation to provide more information than the family can process at one time.
6. Letting family become too dependent or too attached. That is why you have boundaries and why you prepare the family early for termination.

Using Technology to Enhance Family Communication

Most community-dwelling individuals use electronic communication devices on a daily basis, whether via a cellular phone or the Internet. Nurses communicating with family members must adhere to federal regulations as outlined in HIPAA which applies to all modes of communication and must be considered when communicating with family members in an electronic format.

During the recent pandemic, nurse encouraged isolated patients to cyber chat with family members frequently. Caring Bridge (caringbridge.org) is an organization that offers free personalized websites for individuals undergoing serious health concerns. Online support groups are prevalent. Technology is discussed in Chapter 26.

▮ SUMMARY

This chapter provides an overview of family communication and the complex dynamics inherent in family relationships. Families have a structure, defined as the way in which members are organized. Family function refers to the roles people take in their families, and family process describes the communication that takes place within the family. Family-centered care is developed through a combination of strategies designed to gather information in a systematic, efficient manner starting with the genogram, ecomap, and timeline. Therapeutic questions and giving commendations are interventions nurses can use with families. Families with critically ill members need continuous updated information and the freedom to be with their family member as often as possible. Involving the family in the care of the patient is important. Nursing interventions are aimed at strengthening family functioning and supporting family coping during hospitalization and in the community.

> **ETHICAL DILEMMA: What Would You Do?**
>
> Terry Connors is a 90-year-old woman living alone in a two-story house. She has two daughters, Maria and Maggie. Maria lives 90 miles away, but works two jobs because her husband has been laid off for 9 months. Her other daughter, Maggie, lives in another state. So far, Terry has been able to live by herself, but within the past 2 weeks, she fell down a few stairs in her house and she has trouble hearing the telephone. Terry has very poor vision, walks with a cane, and relies on her neighbors for assistance several times a week. Maria and her husband visit every 2 weeks to bring groceries. Both Maria and Maggie worry about her and would like to see her in a nursing home. Terry will not consider this option. As the nurse working with this family, how would you address your ethical responsibilities to Terry, Maria, and Maggie?

DISCUSSION QUESTIONS

1. Identify family communication situations (e.g., end of life, family discord) that you believe would be professionally challenging. Describe strategies that you, as a nurse, could use to be prepared to better manage those situations.
2. How would you personally feel as a nurse delivering bad news to a family?

REFERENCES

Agency for Healthcare Research and Quality (AHRQ). (2013). *Guide to patient and family engagement in hospital quality and safety*. Retrieved from http://www.ahrq.gov/professionals/systems/hospital/engagingfamilies/guide.html. [Accessed 23 June 2021].

von Bertalanffy, L. (1968). *General systems theory*. New York: George Braziller.

Bowen, M. (1978). *Family therapy in clinical practice*. Northvale, NJ: Jason Aronson.

Bowen Center for the Study of the Family. (n.d.). *Societal emotional process*. Retrieved from https://www.thebowencenter.org/societal-emotional-process?rq=emotional%20process. [Accessed 23 June 2021].

Centers for Disease Control and Prevention (CDC). (2021). *National center for chronic disease prevention and health promotion*. Retrieved from https://www.cdc.gov/chronicdisease/index.htm. [Accessed 23 June 2021].

Charles, L., Brémault-Phillips, S., Parmar, J., Johnson, M., & Sacrey, L. A. (2017). Understanding how to support family caregivers of seniors with complex needs. *Canadian Geriatrics*, *20*(2), 75–84.

Edwards, M. (2010). How to break bad news and avoid common difficulties. *Nursing and Residential Care, 12*(10), 495–497.

Halm, M. A. (2020). Can structured communication affect the patient-family experience? *American Journal of Critical Care, 29*(4), 320–324.

Otto, H. A. (1963). Criteria for assessing family strength. *Family Process, 2*(2), 329–338.

Petrinec, A. B., & Martin, B. R. (2018). Post-intensive care syndrome symptoms and health-related quality of life in family decision-makers of critically ill patients. *Palliative & Supportive Care, 16*(6), 719–724.

Shajani, Z., & Snell, D. (2019). *Wright & Leahey's nurses and families: A guide to family assessment and intervention* (7th ed.). Philadelphia: F.A. Davis.

Vranceanu, A. M., Bannon, S., Mace, R., et al. (2020). Feasibility and efficacy of a resiliency intervention for the prevention of chronic emotional distress among survivor-caregiver dyads admitted to the neuroscience intensive care unit. *JAMA Network Open, 3*(10), e2020807.

Ylvén, R., & Granlund, M. (2009). Identifying and building on family strength: A thematic analysis. *Infants and Young Children, 22*(4), 253–263.

13

Resolving Conflicts Between Nurse and Patient

OBJECTIVES

At the end of the chapter, the reader will be able to:

1. Define conflict and contrast the functional with the dysfunctional role of conflict in a therapeutic relationship.
2. Analyze personal styles of response to conflict situations and discriminate among passive, assertive, and aggressive responses to conflict situations.

3. Synthesize characteristics of assertive communication strategies with promotion of conflict resolution of your nurse–patient relationships, including strategies to deescalate workplace violence.
4. Evaluate findings from research studies that can be applied to communicating with patients holding differing values.

Our goal is to fully partner with our patients so that they are active participants in the management of their care (Agency for Healthcare Research and Quality [AHRQ], n.d.). As discussed in the first chapter, patient-centered care is one of the six Quality and Safety Education for Nurses competency standards (QSEN, n.d.). According to QSEN, one desired "Attitude" is that we respect our patient as a central, core member of the health team. However, even when nurse–patient goals are mutual, our values or viewpoints may differ. Collaboration is our focus but, as in all interactions among human beings, some disagreements are inevitable.

Conflict is a natural part of human relationships. We all have times when we experience negative feelings about a situation or person, but in nursing this can compromise patient safety. When this occurs, direct communication is needed. This chapter emphasizes the dynamics of conflict and the problem-solving skills needed for successful resolution between you and your patients. Effective nurse–patient communication is critical. Open communication is a key factor in avoiding threatening situations. When conflict occurs, knowing how to respond calmly allows you to use feelings as a positive force. Some patients approach their initial encounter with a nurse with verbal hostility or

even physical aggression, as when we admit an intoxicated patient to the emergency department. Maintaining safety for self and patient is paramount. To listen and to respond creatively to intense emotion when your first impulse is to withdraw or to retaliate demands a high level of skill, empathy, and self-control. Skills include acknowledging another's feelings, identifying clearly the problem issue, and working toward a mutual solution (Byrne, 2013). Many of these skills can also be applied to the workplace conflicts discussed in Chapters 22 and 23.

BASIC CONCEPTS

Definition

Conflict is defined as disagreement arising from differences in attitudes, values, or needs in which the actions of one party frustrate the ability of the other to achieve his or her expected goals. This results in stress or tension. Conflict serves as a warning that something in the relationship needs closer attention. Conflict is not necessarily a negative; it can become a positive force, leading to growth in relationships (Sherman, 2020). Conflict resolution is a learned process and an expected nurse competency (QSEN, n.d.).

Nature of Conflict

All conflicts have certain things in common: (1) a concrete *content problem issue* and (2) relationship or *process issues*, which involves our emotional response to the situation. It is immaterial whether the issue makes realistic sense to you. It feels real to your patient and needs to be dealt with. Unresolved, such issues will interfere with your and your patient's success in meeting goals. Most people experience conflict as discomfort. Previous experiences with conflict situations, the importance of the issue, and possible consequences all play a role in the intensity of our reactions. For example, a patient may have great difficulty asking questions of the physician regarding treatment or prognosis but experience no problem asking similar questions of the nurse or family. The reasons for the discrepancy in comfort level may relate to previous experiences. Alternatively, it may have little to do with the actual persons involved. Rather, the patient may be responding to anticipated fears about the type of information the physician might give.

Causes of Conflict

Poor communication is a main cause of conflict. Psychological causes of conflict include differences in values or personality and multiple demands causing high levels of stress. If your nursing care does not fit in with your patient's cultural belief system, conflict can result. Recognize that our culture has moved toward greater incivility in mainstream society. This is reflected within the healthcare system. According to The Joint Commission (TJC), miscommunication is most often the cause of conflict between nurse and patient. Sometimes nurses act in such a way as leads to anger in a patient of visitor as reflected in Box 13.1. Can you add to this list? According to the National Institute of Occupational Safety and Health (NIOSH), causes of conflict include bullying by colleagues. Bullying behavior has been shown to escalate to violence (Lewis-Pierre et al., 2019).

Workplace Violence

A safe work environment is a prerequisite for providing good-quality care (AACN, 2019). Violence in the workplace

> ### BOX 13.1 Behaviors of a Nurse That Create Anger in Others
>
> - Violating one's personal space
> - Speaking in a threatening tone
> - Providing unsolicited advice
> - Judging, blaming, criticizing, or conveying ideas that try to create guilt
> - Offering reassurances that are not realistic
> - Communicating using "gloss it over" positive comments
> - Speaking in a way that shows you do not understand your patient's point of view
> - Exerting too much pressure to make a person change his or her unhealthy behavior
> - Portraying self as an infallible "I know best" expert
> - Using an authoritarian, sarcastic, or accusing tone
> - Using "hot button" words that have heavy emotional connotations
> - Failing to provide health information in a timely manner to stressed individuals

is defined as an expression of anger by others manifested as threats or attacks either physical or psychological. Behaviors include negative dysfunctional aggression expressed as verbal abuse, derogatory speech, harassment, bullying, pushing, hitting, or even attacks with weapons. Violence is classified as an occupational hazard. Globally, nurses are at higher risk owing to their direct contact with distressed people (International Council of Nurses [ICN], 2019). At the same time, the incidence of violence is greatly underreported (Hartley et al., 2019).

Conflict can escalate to violent threats or actions. Education about situational awareness about cues to prevent violence needs to occur in basic nursing curriculum (O'Keeffe et al., 2021). Nurses need to be aware that the stressful nature of illness can aggravate factors that lead to violent behavior on the part of patients or their family members. Reflect on the case of Mr Dixon:

CASE STUDY: Mr Dixon Is Angry

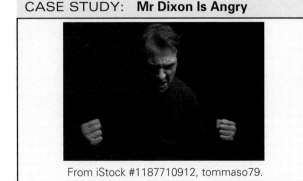

From iStock #1187710912, tommaso79.

Experienced staff nurse Elaine Kaye RN works in a busy emergency department where access to the treatment rooms is blocked by a locked security door. Staff do not wear necklaces or neck chains, nor do they carry implements, but Ms Kaye does wear an ID badge (per the US Department of Labor Occupational Safety and Health Administration [OSHA] recommendations). While Dr Hughes is treating Vonny, age 12, who appears to be suffering from convulsions related to

Continued

CASE STUDY: **Mr Dixon Is Angry—cont'd**

overdosing on methylphenidate (Ritalin), Ms Kaye notices that Mr Dixon is becoming increasingly agitated in the waiting room.

Mr D: "Why aren't you people doing more?"

Nurse Kaye (in a low tone of voice): "My name is Ms Kaye and I am helping with your son. I'll be keeping you up to date with information as soon as we know anything. I know this is a stressful ..."

Mr D (interrupting in a louder voice): "I demand to know why you people won't tell me what is going on."

Ms Kaye: "I see that you are really upset and feeling angry. Let's move over here to the conference area for privacy."

Mr D: "You guys are no good."

Ms Kaye: "I want to understand your point of view. You ..."

Mr D throws a chair.

Ms Kaye: "This is an upsetting time for you, but violence is not acceptable. Please calm down and we will sit down. Let's both take a deep breath, and then you can explain to me what you need ..."

Incidence of Violence

According to WHO, workplace violence is a global problem. Statistics show that violence against healthcare workers is increasing in every country and in every healthcare setting (World Health Organization [WHO], n.d.). Nurses and social workers are at three times greater risk for experiencing violence in the workplace than are other professionals. The highest risk exists in emergency departments, psychiatric settings, and nursing homes (Occupational Safety and Health Administration [OSHA], n.d.). Approximately 80% of nurses will experience violence, often physical violence, at some time during their careers (The Joint Commission [TJC], 2018). TJC's *Sentinel Event Alert*, Issue 45 (2019), addresses prevention, specifying controlling access to healthcare agencies and advocating staff education. TJC notes that communication failures were inherent in 53% of reported acts of violence. Violence against healthcare workers ranges from threats to assaults to murder, yet it is estimated that about 80% of these occurrences remain unreported. TJC's *Sentinel Alert* 59 (2018) lists both management and nurse interventions to decrease violence.

Organizational Policies and Practices

Most of the needed changes are at the organizational level. Organizations lose more money coping with the resultant harm to staff such as time off, decreased efficiency, job loss than they would reasonably spend on deterrence. Of first importance is collecting accurate data of reported incidents, rather than ignoring their occurrence. Staff need to be encouraged to report every incident without punitive outcome.

The CDC recommendations for *environmental management* include secure locked treatment/clinical areas, exits locked against outside entry, provision of two clear exits for staff, screening for weapons brought in by patients or visitors via metal detectors, entrances guarded by security details or CC TV cameras, securing possible onsite weapons such as furniture, decor items, fire extinguishers, and fixtures. They also suggest comfortable waiting areas, temperature controlled and noise controlled.

Staff Management
Preevent: Preventive Interventions

Training in conflict deescalation includes talking "down" individuals in stressed situations, offering to notify visitor of status of treatment for patient, to talk about what they want so as to avoid acting-out behaviors, with patients being alert to cognitive impairment with known high risks such as alcohol intoxication or drug use. Have a secure lock-up for patient possessions which the nurse has thoroughly searched for weapons.

Maintain situational awareness, especially cues that patient or visitor is getting frustrated or angry. CDC calls for a change in the attitudes of staff who believe that "violence is part of the job." Reporting every incident of physical or significant verbal abuse is needed to compile data about risk.

Event: Active Interventions

Clear communications about antiviolence policies and containment measures. TJC suggests uses of a code word to summon assistance, use of an alarm or panic button, exit to a secure area such as a locked staff room. Notify security if they have not already responded, or community police if necessary. Unfortunately, in today's world, preparation for an "active shooter" scenario is also to be considered.

Postevent

Debriefing immediately following incident is recommended. Report to designated personnel in violence prevention position, so risk assessment and change can occur to prevent another staff from having similar problems. Lack of a report = no data = no problem.

Outcomes

Adverse outcomes for nurses include increased stress, job dissatisfaction, somatic illness, emotional trauma, increased absenteeism, posttraumatic stress disorder, self-medication abuse, and death. In addition to physical harm to the worker, *Healthy People 2030* (U.S. Department of Health and Human Services, n.d.) and other sources have identified problems for the health system, such as increased agency costs due to lost work days, job turnover, and occasionally litigation. Nurses educated in violence prevention and management will be better prepared.

Strategies to prevent escalation of violent behavior are discussed in the "Applications" section of this chapter. Additional suggestions for physical and organizational safeguards are available from the Occupational Safety and Health Administration (www.osha.gov).

Stage of Anger

- Mild: Feels some tension, irritability. Acts argumentative, sarcastic, or is difficult to please
- Moderate: Observably angry behaviors such as motor agitation and loud voice
- Severe: Shows acting-out behaviors, cursing, using violent gestures but is not yet out of control
- Rage: Behaving in an out-of-control manner, physically aggressive toward others or self

Goal: Work for Conflict Resolution

Unresolved nurse–patient conflict impedes the quality and safety of patient care. It not only undermines your therapeutic relationship but can also result in your emotional exhaustion, leading to **burnout**. Energy is transferred to conflict issues instead of being used to build the relationship.

As nurses, our goal is to collaborate with patients to maximize their health. To accomplish this, we need to communicate clearly to prevent or reduce levels of conflict. We know that resolving a long-standing conflict is a gradual process in which we may have to revisit the issue several times to fully resolve it.

Conflict Resolution Principles

It goes without saying that professionals always demonstrate respect for patients. Gender and cultural factors that influence responses are described elsewhere. Fig. 13.1 lists some principles of conflict resolution. These may also be applied to conflicts with colleagues.

Understand Your Own Personal Responses to Conflict

Conflicts between nurse and patient are not uncommon. First gain a clear understanding of your own personal responses, since conflict creates anxiety that may prevent

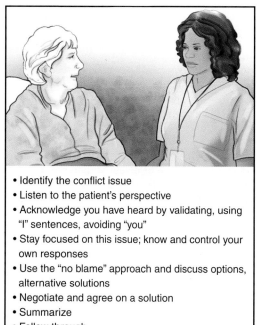

- Identify the conflict issue
- Listen to the patient's perspective
- Acknowledge you have heard by validating, using "I" sentences, avoiding "you"
- Stay focused on this issue; know and control your own responses
- Use the "no blame" approach and discuss options, alternative solutions
- Negotiate and agree on a solution
- Summarize
- Follow through

Figure 13.1 Principles of conflict resolution.

you from behaving in an effective, assertive manner. No one is equally effective in all situations. Completing Simulation Exercise 13.1 may help you identify your personal responses.

Recognize your own "triggers" or "hot buttons." What words or patient actions trigger an immediate emotional response in you? These could include having someone yelling at you or speaking to you in an angry tone of voice. Once you recognize the triggers, you can better control your own responses. It is imperative that you focus on the current issue. Put aside history. Listing prior problems will raise emotions and prevent resolution. Identify *available options*. Rather than immediately trying to solve the problem, look at the range of possible options. Create a list of these options and work with the other party to evaluate the feasibility of each option. By working together, you shift expectations from adversarial conflict to an expectation of a win-win outcome. After discussing possible solutions, select the best one to resolve the conflict. Evaluate the outcome based on fair, objective criteria.

Know the Context

Second, understand the context or the circumstances in which the situation occurs. Most interpersonal conflicts involve some threat to one's sense of control or self-esteem. Nurses have been shown to respond to the stress of not having enough time to complete their work by imposing

SIMULATION EXERCISE 13.1 Personal Responses to Conflict

Purpose
To increase awareness of how students respond in conflict situations and the elements in situations (e.g., people, status, age, previous experience, lack of experience, or place) that contribute to their sense of discomfort.

Procedure
Break the class up into small groups of two. You may do this as homework or create an Internet discussion room. Think of a conflict situation that could be handled in different ways.

The following feelings are common correlates of interpersonal conflict situations that many people say they experienced in conflict situations that they have not handled well.

Anger	Competitiveness	Humiliation
Annoyance	Defensiveness	Inferiority
Antagonism	Devaluation	Intimidation
Anxiousness	Embarrassment	Manipulation
Bitterness	Frustration	Resentment

Although these feelings are generally not ones we are especially proud of, they are a part of the human experience. By acknowledging their existence within ourselves, we usually have more choice about how we will handle them.

Reflective Discussion Analysis
Construct different responses and then explain how the different responses might lead to different outcomes.

more controls on their patients, who then often react by becoming more difficult. Patients who feel listened to and respected are generally receptive.

Situations that may cause nurses to become frustrated or angry include working with patients who dismiss what they say or who ask for more personal information than nurses feel comfortable sharing, patients who sexually harass or target a nurse in a personal attack, or family members who make demands that nurses are unable to fulfill.

Develop an Effective Conflict Management Style

Five distinct *styles of response* to conflict have been documented. In the past, nurses were found to commonly use avoidance or accommodation when they were faced with a conflict situation. Many felt that any conflict was destructive and needed to be suppressed. Current thinking holds that conflict can be healthy and can lead to growth when, with conflict resolution training, we develop a collaborative problem-solving approach.

Avoidance is a common response to conflict. Nurses using avoidance distance themselves from their patients or provide less support. Sometimes an experience makes you so uncomfortable that you want to avoid the situation or person at all costs, so you withdraw. This style is appropriate when the cost of addressing the conflict is higher than the benefit of resolution. Sometimes you just have to "pick your battles," focusing your energy on the most important issues. However, use of avoidance postpones the conflict, leads to future problems, and damages your relationship with your client, making it an *I lose, you lose* situation.

Accommodation is another common response. We surrender our own needs in a desire to smooth over the conflict. This response is cooperative but nonassertive. Sometimes this involves a quick compromise or giving false reassurance. By giving in to others, we maintain peace but do not actually deal with the issue, so it will likely resurface in the future. It is appropriate only when the issue is more important to the other person. This is an *I lose, you win* situation. Harmony results. Good will may be earned that can be used in the future (McElhaney, 1996).

Competition is a response style characterized by domination. You exercise power to gain your own goals at the expense of the other person. It is characterized by aggression and lack of compromise. Authority may be used to suppress the conflict in a dictatorial manner. This leads to increased stress. It is an effective style only when there is a need for a quick decision, but leads to problems in the long term, making it an *I win now but then lose and you lose* situation.

Compromise is a solution still commonly found to be employed by nurses. By compromising, each party gives a little and gains a little. It is effective only when both parties hold equal power. Depending on the specific work environment and the issue in dispute, it can be a good solution, but since neither party is completely satisfied, it can eventually become an *I lose, you lose* situation.

Collaboration is a solution-oriented response in which we work together cooperatively to solve problems. To manage the conflict, we commit to finding a mutually agreeable solution. This involves directly confronting the issue, acknowledging our feelings, and using open communication. Steps for productive confrontation include identifying concerns of each party, clarifying assumptions, communicating honestly to identify the real issue, and working collaboratively to find a solution that satisfies everyone. Collaboration is considered to be the most effective style for genuine resolution. This is an *I win, you win* situation.

Structure Your Response

In mastering assertive responses, it may be helpful initially to use these steps:

1. Express empathy: "I understand that_____";
   "I hear you saying _____." *Example:* "I understand that things are difficult at home."
2. Describe your feelings or the situation: "I feel that _____"; "This situation seems to me to _____." *Example:* "But your 8-year-old daughter has expressed a lot of anxiety, saying, 'I can't learn to give my own insulin shots.'"
3. State expectations: "I want_____"; "What is required by the situation is _____." *Example:* "It is necessary for you to be here tomorrow when the diabetic teaching nurse comes so you can learn how to give injections and your daughter can, too, with your support."
4. List consequences: "If you do this, then _____ will happen" (state positive outcome); "If you don't do this, then _____ will happen" (state negative outcome). *Example:* "If you get here on time, we can be finished and get her discharged in time for her birthday on Friday." Focus on the present.
5. The focus should always be on the present. Focus only on the present issue. The past cannot be changed, so "stay in the moment."
6. Limit your discussion to *one topic issue* at a time to enhance the chance of success. Usually, it is impossible to resolve a conflict that is multidimensional with a single solution. By breaking the problem down into simple steps, you will allow enough time for a clear understanding. You might paraphrase the patient's words, reflecting the meaning back to the him or her to validate its accuracy. Once the issues have been delineated clearly, the steps needed for resolution may appear quite simple.

Being assertive in the face of an emotionally charged situation demands thought, energy, and commitment. Assertiveness also requires the use of common sense, self-awareness, knowledge, tact, humor, respect, and a sense of perspective. Although there is no guarantee that the use of assertive behaviors will produce the desired interpersonal goals, the chances of a successful outcome are increased because the information flow is optimally honest, direct, and firm. Often the use of assertiveness brings about changes in ways that could not have been anticipated. Changes occur because the nurse offers a new resource in the form of objective feedback with no strings attached.

Use "I" Statements

Statements that begin with "You …" sound accusatory. When statements point a finger or imply judgment, most people respond defensively. "We" statements should be used only when you actually mean to look at an issue collaboratively. Use of "I" statements is one of the most effective conflict management strategies you can use. Assertive statements that begin with "I" suggest that the person speaking accepts full responsibility for his or her own feelings and position in relation to the conflict. "I" statements feel clumsy at first and take a little practice to use. The following is one suggested format:

"I feel_____ (use a name to claim the emotion you feel)

when_____ (describe the behavior nonjudgmentally)

because_____ (describe the tangible effects of the behavior)."

Make Clear Statements

Statements rather than questions set the stage for assertive responses to conflict. When you do use a question, "how" questions are best because they are neutral, seek more information, and imply a collaborative effort. Avoid "why" questions as they put other people on the defensive, asking them to explain their behavior. Use a strong, firm, tactful manner, and state the situation clearly. Consider the case of Mr Gow.

Case Study: Mr Gow's Inappropriate Behavior

Mr Gow is a 35-year-old executive who has been hospitalized with a myocardial infarction. He has been acting seductively toward some of the young nurses but he seems to be giving Miss O'Hara an especially hard time.

Mr Gow: Come on in, honey, I've been waiting for you. (reaching toward her)

Nurse O'Hara (using appropriate facial expression and eye contact, and replying in a firm, clear voice): Mr Gow, I would rather you called me Miss O'Hara. I do not want to be touched.

Mr G.: Aw, come on now, honey. I don't get to have much fun around here. What's the difference what I call you?

Nurse O'Hara: I feel that it does make a difference, and I would like you to call me Miss O'Hara.

Mr G.: Oh, you're no fun at all. Why do you have to be so serious?

Nurse O'Hara: Mr Gow, you're right. I am serious about being respected. I would prefer that you call me Miss O'Hara. I would like to work with you; however, it might be important to explore the ways in which this hospitalization is hampering you so you harass young nurses.

Discussion. In this interaction, the nurse's position is defined several times, using successively stronger statements before the shift is made to refocus on Mr Gow's behavior. Notice that the nurse labeled the behavior, not the patient, as unacceptable. Persistence is essential when initial attempts at assertiveness appear too limited.

Use Moderate Pitch and Vocal Tone

The strength of a forceful assertive statement depends on the nature of the conflict situation as well as the degree of confrontation needed to resolve the conflict successfully. Starting with the least amount of assertiveness required to meet the demands of the situation conserves energy and does not place you in an "overkill" bind. It is not necessary to use all your resources at one time or to express your ideas too strongly. We sometimes lose effectiveness by becoming too long-winded. Long explanations detract from the spoken message. Get to the main point quickly, saying what is necessary in the simplest, most concrete way possible. This cuts down on the possibility of misinterpretation.

Pitch and tone of voice contribute to another person's interpretation of the meaning of your assertive message. A soft, hesitant, passive presentation can undermine an assertive message. The same is true if a harsh, hostile, aggressive tone is used. To pitch an assertive message, try a firm but moderate presentation to effectively convey your message by doing Simulation Exercise 13.2.

Outcome: Positive Growth

Traditionally, conflict was viewed as a destructive force to be eliminated. Actually, conflicts that are successfully resolved lead to stronger relationships. The critical factor is the willingness to explore and resolve it mutually. Appropriately handled, conflict can provide an important opportunity for growth. Practice to develop conflict management skills is essential and effective.

Outcome: Dysfunction, Such as Unresolved Conflict

As mentioned, unresolved conflicts tend to resurface later, impeding your ability to give quality care. If the emotional aspect of the conflict is expressed too strongly, the nurse can feel attacked.

Nature of Assertive Behavior

Assertive behavior is defined as setting goals; acting on those goals in a clear, consistent manner; and

---

> ### SIMULATION EXERCISE 13.2   Pitching the Assertive Message
>
> **Purpose**
> To increase awareness of how the meaning of a verbal message can be significantly altered by changing one's tone of voice.
>
> **Procedure**
> Break class up into groups of five. Write on a slip of paper one of the following five vocal pitches: whisper, soft tone with hesitant delivery, moderate tone and firm delivery, loud tone with agitated delivery, and screaming. Have each person in turn pick one of five pieces of paper and demonstrate that tone while the others in the group try to identify in which tone the assertive message is being delivered.
>
> **Reflective Discussion Analysis**
> Using information learned from the text to support your answer, justify how tone can affect perceptions of a message's content.

taking responsibility for the consequences of those actions. Assertive communication is conveying this objective in a direct manner, without anger or frustration. The assertive nurse is able to stand up for his or her personal rights and the rights of others.

Components of assertive communication include the ability (1) to say no, (2) to ask for what you want, (3) to appropriately express both positive and negative thoughts and feelings, and (4) to initiate, continue, and terminate the interaction. This honest expression of yourself does not violate the needs of others but does demonstrate self-respect rather than deference to the demands of others. Conflict creates anxiety, which may prevent you from behaving assertively. Assertive behaviors range from making a direct, honest statement about your beliefs to taking a very strong, confrontational stand about what will and will not be tolerated. Assertive responses contain "I" statements that take responsibility. This behavior is in contrast with **aggressive behavior**, which has a goal of dominating while suppressing the other person's rights. Aggressive responses often consist of "you" statements that fix blame on the other person. Box 13.2 lists characteristics of assertive behavior. Remember that assertiveness is a learned behavior and assertive responses need to be practiced! Starting with the least amount of assertiveness required to meet the demands of the situation conserves energy and does not place the nurse into the bind of overkill. It is not necessary to use all of your resources at one time or to express ideas strongly when this type of response is not needed. You

BOX 13.2 Characteristics Associated With the Development of Assertive Behavior

- Express your own position, using "I" statements.
- Make clear statements.
- Speak in a firm tone, using moderate pitch.
- Assume responsibility for personal feelings and wants.
- Make sure verbal and nonverbal messages are congruent.
- Address only issues related to the present conflict.
- Structure responses so as to be tactful and show awareness of the client's frame of reference.
- Understand that undesired behaviors, not feelings, attitudes, and motivations, are the focus for change.

can sometimes lose your effectiveness by becoming long-winded in your explanation when only a simple statement of rights or intentions is needed. Getting to the main point quickly and saying what is necessary in the simplest, most concrete way cuts down on the possibility of misinterpretation. This approach increases the probability that the communication will be received constructively.

Nonassertive behavior in a professional nurse is related to lower levels of autonomy. Continued patterns of non-assertive responses have a negative influence on you and on the standard of care you provide. Try a firm assertive response with moderate presentation to convey your message when you practice Simulation Exercise 13.3.

Safety

It is your responsibility to maintain your own safety and that of patients. Mindfully be aware. Team STEPPS suggests the use of "situation monitoring" to recognize emergent conflicts. When you are confronted by an angry patient or family member, use your skills to defuse the situation, addressing their concerns. If anger enters the *rage stage*, leave and get help. Do not stay in a dangerous situation. It cannot be overemphasized that if you feel in danger, LEAVE! Each agency should have a resource team to call for intervention assistance. Don't be a hero, CALL FOR HELP!

DEVELOPING AN EVIDENCE-BASED PRACTICE

It is well documented that conflict in the workplace occurs more in healthcare than elsewhere (WHO, 2021). Some units such as emergency departments and psychiatric units are documented to have higher incidence of violence against staff by patients or family. The need for nursing interventions is evident; especially training in conflict management and deescalation strategies. Spelten et al. (2020) for the Cochrane Library database evaluated seven studies of nursing homes describing programs and workplace practices that reduce patient aggression. Agencies such as TJC, CDC/NIOSH, and OSHA have published extensively on this topic.

Results

According to Spelten, interventions such as playing music, using humor, or using patient's personal towels during bathing were weakly found to decrease aggression. Their analysis of 209 emergency department staff found no successful interventions. But these results are contradicted by earlier studies showing deescalation training and unit-specific prevention plan development decreases or prevents increases in patient violence (Arnetz, 2017).

Strength of evidence: Low (Spelten) to moderate (Arnetz).

Application to Your Clinical Practice

Staff management including training in conflict deescalation, situational awareness especially cues that patient or visitor is getting frustrated or angry. CDC calls for a change in the attitudes of staff who believe that "violence is part of the job" (CDC, 2020). Reporting every incident of physical or significant verbal abuse is needed to compile data about risk. Nurses have reported they tend not to report when the think "the patient didn't mean it" or when they feel they will be faulted by the employer.

References

Arnetz, J. E., Hamblin, L., Russell, J., et al. (2017). Preventing patient-to-worker violence in hospitals: Outcomes of a randomized controlled study. *Journal of Occupational and Environmental Medicine. 59*(1), 18–27.

Centers for Disease Control and Prevention (CDC), The National Institute for Occupational Safety and Health (NIOSH). (2020). *Occupational violence: Workplace violence prevention for nurses.* Retrieved from: https://www.cdc.gov/niosh/topics/violence/training_nurses.html. (Accessed 17 June 2021).

Spelten, E., Thomas, B., O'Meara, P. F., Maguire, B. J., FitzGerald, D., & Begg, S. J. (2020). Programmes, policies and work practices that reduce aggression by patients towards healthcare workers. *Cochrane.* Retrieved from: www.cochrane.org/CD012662/programs-policies-and-work-practices-reduce-aggression-patient-to-wards-healthcare workers/. (Accessed 26 May 2021).

World Health Organization (WHO). (2021). Violence prevention alliance. Definition and typology of violence. Retrieved from: https://www.who.int/violenceprevention/approach/definition/en/. (Accessed 17 June 2021).

SIMULATION EXERCISE 13.3   Assertive Responses

Purpose
To increase awareness of assertiveness.

Procedure
Role-play the following scenario:
   You are working full time, raising a family, and taking 12 credits of nursing classes. The teacher asks you to be a student representative on a faculty committee. You say the following:
1. "I don't think I'm the best one. Why don't you ask Karen? If she can't, I guess I can."
2. "Gee, I'd like to, but I don't know. I probably could if it doesn't take too much time."
3. "I do want students to have some input to this committee, but I am not sure I have enough time. Let me think about it and let you know in class tomorrow."

Reflective Discussion Analysis
1. Critique the options, describing how they could be altered.
2. Select the most assertive response. Defend your choice using the text.

APPLICATIONS

It is essential to recognize the potential for conflict. And Team STEPPS reminds us to use situation monitoring, continually scanning our environment to understand what is going on around us. Practicing the following strategies can help you to improve your conflict resolution skills. By doing so we demonstrate that we are developing the QSEN attitude of continuously improving our own communication and conflict resolution skills.

Preventing Conflict

In addition to managing your own responses to patient provocations, model behavior by adopting a professional, "calm" demeanor and low tone of voice. Use conflict prevention strategies: Signal your readiness to listen with attending behaviors such as good body position, eye contact, and a receptive facial expression. Give your undivided attention to a patient or visitor whom you identify as potentially becoming aggressive. Multiple studies show that nurses' anticommunication attitudes act as a barrier. Increasing your positive appreciation of your patient does facilitate communication. As nurses, we hold the belief that all patients have value as human beings. Try some of the strategies described in this chapter to help prevent or resolve conflict.

Assessing the Presence of Conflict in the Nurse–Patient Relationship

To get resolution, you need to acknowledge the presence of conflict. Often the awareness of our own feelings of discomfort is an initial clue. Evidence of the presence of conflict may be *overt*, that is, observable in the patient's behavior and expressed verbally. For example, a patient might criticize you. No one likes to be criticized, and a natural response might be anger, rationalization, or blaming others. But as a professional nurse, you recognize your response, recognize the conflict, and work toward resolution so that constructive changes can take place.

More often, conflict is *covert* and not so clear-cut. The conflict issues are hidden. Your patient talks about one issue, but talking does not seem to help and the issue does not get resolved. He or she continues to be angry or anxious. Subtle behavioral manifestations of covert conflict might include a reduced effort by your patient to engage in self-care; frequent misinterpretation of your words; and behaviors that are out of character for your patient, such as excessive anger. For example, your patient might become unusually demanding, have a seemingly insatiable need for your attention, or be unable to tolerate reasonable delays in having his or her needs met. Such problems may represent anxiety stemming from conflicting feelings. Behaviors are often negatively affected by feelings of pain, loss, helplessness, frustration, or fear. As nurses, we affect the behavior of our patients through our actions. This can lead to positive or negative outcomes. See Simulation Exercise 13.4 for practice in defining conflict issues.

Sometimes the feelings themselves become the major issue, so that valid parts of the original conflict issue are hidden; consequently, conflict escalates. Consider how to respond to Ms Dentoni's case.

Case Study: Mrs Dentoni Is Upset

Mrs Dentoni is scheduled for surgery at 8 am tomorrow. As the student nurse assigned to care for her, you have been told that she was admitted to the hospital 3 h ago and that she has been examined by the house resident. The anesthesia department has been notified of her arrival. Her blood work and urine have been sent to the laboratory. As you enter her room and introduce yourself, you notice that Mrs Dentoni is sitting on the edge of the bed and appears tense and angry.

Mrs D.: I wish people would just leave me alone. Nobody has come in and told me about my surgery tomorrow. I don't know what I'm supposed to do—just lie around here and rot, I guess.

SIMULATION EXERCISE 13.4 Defining Conflict Issues: Case Analyses

Purpose
To help organize information and define the problem in interpersonal conflict situations.

Procedure
In each conflict situation, look for specific behaviors (including words, tone, posture, and facial expression); feeling impressions (including words, tone, intensity, and facial expression); and need (expressed verbally or through actions).

Identify the behaviors, your impressions of the behaviors, and needs that the client is expressing in the following situations. Suggest an appropriate nursing action. Situation 1 is completed as a guide.

Situation 1
Mrs Patel, a patient from India, does not speak much English. Her baby was just delivered by cesarean section, and it is expected that Mrs Patel will remain in the hospital for at least 4 days. Her husband tells the nurse that Mrs Patel wants to breastfeed, but she has decided to wait until she goes home to begin because she will be more comfortable there and she wants privacy. The nurse knows that breastfeeding will be more successful if it is initiated soon after birth.

Behaviors: The client's husband states that his wife wants to breastfeed but does not wish to start before going home. Mrs Patel is not initiating breastfeeding in the hospital.

Your impression of behaviors: Indirectly, she is expressing physical discomfort, possible insecurity, and awkwardness about breastfeeding. She may also be acting in accordance with cultural norms of her country or family.

Underlying needs: Safety and security. Mrs Patel probably will not be motivated to attempt breastfeeding until she feels safe and secure in her home environment.

Suggested nursing action: Provide family support and guarantee total privacy for feeding.

Situation 2
Mrs Moore is brought back to the unit from surgery after a radical mastectomy. The doctor's orders call for her to ambulate, cough, and deep breathe and to use her arm as much as possible in self-care activities. Mrs Moore asks the nurse in a very annoyed tone, "Why do I have to do this? You can see that it is difficult for me. Why can't you help me?"

At this point, you can probably sense the presence of conflicting feelings, but it is unclear whether this patient's emotions relate to anxiety about the surgery or to anger about some real or imagined invasion of privacy because of the necessary laboratory tests and physical examination. Your patient might also be annoyed by you or by a lack of information from the surgeon. She may feel the need to know that hospital personnel see her as a person and care about her feelings. Before you can respond empathetically to the patient's feelings, they will have to be decoded.

Nurse Tom (in a concerned tone of voice): You seem really upset. It's rough being in the hospital, isn't it?

Notice that the reply is nonjudgmental and tentative and does not suggest specific feelings beyond those the patient has shared. There is an implicit request for her to validate your perception of her feelings and to link the feelings with a concrete issue. You process verbal as well as nonverbal cues. Concern is expressed through your tone of voice and words. The content focus relates to the patient's predominant feeling tone, because this is the part of the conflict that is shared with you. It is important to maintain a nonanxious, relaxed presence.

Preliminary Techniques for Conflict Resolution
Remember that your goal is to *deescalate* the conflict. We need to be modeling respect. Use the strategies for conflict resolution described in this section. Mastery takes practice. Although this seems like a lot of information, an incident can occur in only a few minutes. Stay calm. Use *The 3 Ps of Crisis Deescalation:*

- *Position* (face patient but remain closer to the exit, making eye contact only 60% of the time)
- *Posture* (relax your stance with uncrossed arms; rotate and relax your shoulders)
- *Proximity* (stay 1.5–3 feet away)

Reaching a common understanding of the problem in a direct, tactful manner is the first step in conflict resolution, moving you toward a goal of reaching a resolution acceptable to both parties. Try to understand the patient's viewpoint. The case featuring Mr Pyle illustrates this idea.

Case Study: Mr Pyle Feels Hopeless
Mr Pyle is an 80-year-old bachelor who lives alone. He has always been considered a proud and stately gentleman. He has a sister, 84 years old, who lives in Florida. His only other living relatives, a nephew and his wife, also live in another state. Mr Pyle recently

changed his will so that it excludes his relatives, and he refuses to eat. When his neighbor brings in food, he eats it, but he will not fix anything for himself. He tells his neighbor that he wants to die and that he reads in the paper about a man who was able to die in 60 days by not eating. As the visiting nurse assigned to his area, you have been asked to make a home visit and assess the situation.

The issue in this case example is not one of food intake alone. Any attempt to talk about why it is important for him to eat or expressing your point of view in this conflict immediately on arriving is not likely to be successful. Mr Pyle's behavior suggests that he feels that there is little to be gained by living any longer. His actions suggest further that he feels lonely and may be angry with his relatives. Once you correctly ascertain his needs and identify the specific issues, you may be able to help Mr Pyle resolve his intrapersonal conflict. His wish to die may not be absolute or final because he eats when food is prepared by his neighbor and he has not yet taken a deliberate, aggressive move to end his life. Each of these factors needs to be assessed and validated with him before an accurate nursing diagnosis can be made.

Time the Encounter

Timing is a determinant of success. Know specifically the behavior you wish to have the patient change. Make sure that they are capable physically and emotionally of changing the behavior. Select a time when you both can discuss the matter privately and use neutral ground, if possible. Select a time when the patient is most likely to be receptive.

Timing is also important if an individual is very angry. The key to assertive behavior is choice. Sometimes it is better to allow someone to let off some "emotional steam" before engaging in conversation. In this case, the assertive thing to do is to choose silence accompanied by a calm, relaxed body posture. These nonverbal actions convey acceptance of feeling and a desire to understand. Validating the anger and reframing the conflict are useful steps. Comments such as "I'm sorry you are feeling so upset" recognize the significance of the emotion being expressed without getting into the cause.

Put Situation Into Perspective

Do not play the blame game. Put the issue into perspective. How urgent is it to resolve this issue? How important is the issue? Will the issue be significant in a year? In 10 years? Will there be a significant situational change with resolution?

This is another way of saying "pick your battles." Not every situation is worth expending your time and energy. Remind yourself that anger may be caused by a problem in communicating; patients who are frustrated may become angry when they cannot make staff understand.

Use Therapeutic Communication Skills

Particularly useful is *active listening.* Really trying to understand what the patient is upset about requires more skill than just listening to his or her words. Listening closely to what they are saying may help you understand their point of view. This understanding may decrease the stress. Repeat what the patient said to make sure communication is crystal clear.

APPLYING THE CONFLICT RESOLUTION PROCESS

Mastery of the steps in conflict resolution takes practice. Although this seems like a lot of information, an incident can occur in only minutes. Stay calm, use moderate tone of voice, and avoid becoming defensive. Use assertive communication skills. Be clear and direct in conveying your thoughts, avoiding expressing your frustration or anger. Try following the "*POPPA*" acronym as in Table 13.1.

Prepare for the Encounter
Goal

Your goal is to deescalate the conflict situation. Careful preparation often makes the difference between success and not asserting yourself when necessary. Mentally visualize yourself responding assertively.

Own Your Contribution

In addition to recognizing your own contribution to the conflict, you may be at odds with the values of your client. Not everyone holds the same views as you. It is not wrong to have ambivalent feelings about caring for a certain patient, but acknowledge this to yourself. A useful strategy is using "I" statements. When you begin with "You …" this is perceived as an accusation, escalating conflict. Another strategy is to "take a break." This is a brief cooling off period until anger subsides. Do reengage with the discussion, not avoiding, which still is a common nurse response. Communicate with the correct person, do not take out your anger on others.

Manage Your Feelings

You may feel anxious or angry, but you need to recognize this. You should see this discomfort as a signal that you need to deal with the situation. Part of an initial assessment

TABLE 13.1	**Nursing Communication Interventions in Conflict Situations: Use the P.O.P.P.A. Steps**	
P	Prepare	• Identify the issue in conflict. • Prepare to use communication skills such as active listening to determine patient's point of view. • Manage own anxiety (deep breathing, guided imagery). • Focus only on current issue.
O	Organize	• Arrange for privacy. • Analyze why behavior is a problem, put into perspective. • Identify barriers to resolution.
P	Proceed with interventions	• Work with the entire health team so all use the same uniform approach to the patient's demands. • Clarify expectations. • Ask for behavioral change. • Show respect. • Develop a mutual plan, set goals.
P	Possibilities for resolution	• Restate the problem issue to be clear. • Explore alternative solutions, options with outcomes. • Verbalize incentives versus withdrawal of privileges to modify unacceptable behavior.
A	Agree on solution	• Agree on best solution. • Acknowledge solution by restating. • Promote trust by providing feedback.

of an interpersonal conflict includes recognition of the nurse's intrapersonal contribution to the conflict as well as that of the patient. Most people feel some physical response. If so, use an immediate destressing strategy of taking three deep breaths. Controlling your own natural emotional response to upsetting behavior may be one key factor in managing conflict. Use some immediate destressing behaviors. Conflict produces anxiety and creates feelings of helplessness. It is not wrong to have ambivalent feelings about taking care of people with different lifestyles and values; however, you must acknowledge this to yourself. Confronting the behavior now should keep you from losing control later as the problem escalates. Most people experience some variation of a physical response when taking interpersonal risks. A useful strategy for managing your own anger is to vent to a friend using "I" statements as long as this does not become a complaining, whining session. Another strategy to manage your own anger is to "take a break." A cooling-off period, doing something else for a few minutes or hours until your anger subsides, is acceptable. Take care that you reengage, however, so that this does not become just an avoidance response style. Communicate with the correct person; do not take out your frustration on someone else.

Focus Only on the Issue

You are going to discuss the one issue involved. Try saying, "I would like to talk something over with you before the end of shift/before I go." Before you actually enter the patient's room, do the following:

- Cool off. Wait until you can speak in a calm, friendly tone.
- Take a few deep breaths. Inhale deeply and count "1-2-3" to yourself. Hold your breath for a count of 2 and exhale, counting again to 3 slowly.
- Fortify yourself with positive statements (e.g., "I have a right to respect."). Anticipation is usually far worse than the reality.
- Defuse your own anxiety or anger before confronting the patient.
- Focus discussion on one issue.

Organize Information
Get Background Information

Plan your approach for a time and place conducive to collaborative discussion. Do not respond in the heat of the moment. Organizing your information and validating the appropriateness of your intervention with another knowledgeable person who is not directly involved is useful. Sometimes it is wise to rehearse out loud what you are going to say. Remember to adhere to the principle of focusing on the conflict issue. Avoid bringing up the past. There will obviously be situations in which such a thorough assessment is not possible, but each of these variables affects the success of the confrontation. For example, a patient with dementia who makes a pass at a nurse may simply be expressing a need for affection in much the same way that a small child does; this behavior needs a caring response rather than a reprimand. A 30-year-old patient with all his cognitive faculties who makes a similar pass needs a more confrontational response. Readiness is vital. The behavior may need to be confronted, but the manner in which the confrontation is approached and the amount of preparation or groundwork that has been done beforehand may affect the outcome.

Proceed With the Intervention

If you wish to be successful, you must consider not only what is important to you in the discussion but what is important to the other person. Bear in mind the other person's viewpoint.

Name the Conflict Issue

Clearly identify the issue in conflict. For communication to be effective, it must be carefully thought out in terms of certain basic questions, such as the following:

*   *Purpose.* What is the purpose or objective of this information? What is the central idea, the one most important statement to be made?
*   *Organization.* What are the major points to be shared, and in what order?
*   *Content.* Is the information to be shared complete? Does it convey who, what, where, when, why, and how?
*   *Word choice.* Has careful consideration been given to the choice of words?

Metacommunication

Make sure verbal and nonverbal communication is congruent. Maintain an open stance and omit any gestures that might be interpreted as criticism, such as rolling your eyes or sighing heavily. Avoid mixed messages.

Feelings

Acknowledge the feelings associated with conflict, because it is emotions that escalate conflict.

Request a Behavior Change

Avoid blaming. This would only make your patient feel defensive or angry. Clearly *request that he or she changes* the behavior. Rather than just stating your position, try to use some objective criterion to examine the situation. Saying, "I understand your need to …. , but the hospital has a policy intended to protect all our patients" might help you talk about the situation without escalating into anger. Psychiatric units have known rules against verbal abuse, violence such as throwing objects, violence against others, and so on. You can restate these "rules" together with their known violation outcomes (medication, seclusion, manual restraint), in a calm but firm voice.

Find Options

Mutually generate some options for resolution. Focus on ways to resolve the problem by listing possible options. You are familiar with the "fight-or-flight" response to stress: Many people can respond to conflict only by either fighting or avoiding the problem. But brainstorming possible options and discussing pros and cons can turn the "fight" response into a more mutual "seeking a solution" mode of operations. Set mutual goals. Every member of the healthcare team needs to be "on the same page," presenting a similar approach to this patient.

For longer-term behavioral problems consider the use of a written contract, spelling out alternative behaviors, unacceptable ones, and their consequences.

Possibilities for Resolution

By brainstorming possibilities and talking about the pros and cons of each, you turn the oppositional discussion into a mutual search for success. Encourage behavior change by stating the outcomes, the positive consequences of changing, or the negative implications for failing to change. Evaluate the degree to which the interpersonal conflict has been resolved. Sometimes a conflict cannot be resolved in a short time, but the willingness to persevere is a good indicator of a potentially successful outcome. Accepting small goals is useful when the attainment of large goal is not possible. Your goal is open communication, with frequent **feedback** leading to successful problem-solving.

For a patient, perhaps the strongest indicator of conflict resolution is the degree to which he or she is actively engaged in activities aimed at accomplishing tasks associated with the treatment goals. Here are some questions that you, as the nurse, might want to address if modifications are necessary:

*   What is the best way to establish an environment that is conducive to conflict resolution? What else needs to be considered?
*   What self-care behaviors can be expected if these changes are made? These need to be stated in ways that are measurable.

Agree to a Solution

Discuss the options and mutually agree to try the best one. Everyone on the healthcare team needs to agree with the plan and agrees to use a similar approach to the patient.

State the Solution

Restate the mutually agreed solution. Begin applying this intervention, testing its success to determine whether this is a true solution to the conflict. Consider how to manage the case of Mr Plotsky.

Case Study: Mr Plotsky's Acting-Out Behavior

Mr Plotsky, age 29, has been employed for 6 years as a construction worker. About 4 weeks ago, while operating a forklift, he was struck by a train, leaving him paraplegic. After 2 weeks in intensive care, he was transferred to a neurological unit. When staff members attempt to provide physical care, such as changing his position or getting him up in a chair, Mr Plotsky throws things, curses angrily, and sometimes spits at the nurses. Staff members become very upset; several nurses have requested assignment changes. Some staff members try bribing him with food to encourage good behavior; others threaten to apply restraints. The manager schedules a behavioral consultation meeting with a psychiatric nurse or clinical specialist. The immediate goal of this staff conference is to bring staff feelings out into the open and facilitate increased awareness of the staff's behavioral responses when confronted with Mr Plotsky's behavior. The outcome goal is to use a problem-solving approach to develop a behavioral care plan so that all staff members respond to Mr Plotsky in a consistent manner.

DEALING WITH VIOLENCE

In the anger management process, nurses use behaviors to avoid violent patient behavior. Often a person displaying anger is really trying (ineffectively) to deal with their fear.

Recognize Signs of Anger

You can expect to encounter patients who express anger. This may take the form of refusal to comply with the treatment plan, withdrawal from any positive interaction with you, or the exhibition of hostile behaviors. Hostility may be verbalized, as when a patient curses at you or even becomes physically violent. When you are dealing with a difficult patient, ask yourself what he or she is gaining from the violent behavior. Some people have not learned how to communicate successfully, so they revert to behavior that has gained them something in the past. For example, as children, they may have gotten needed attention only when they acted out in a negative way or when they pouted or sulked. Ask yourself whether a patient who is behaving in a difficult way is being rewarded by becoming the focus of staff attention. Does such an individual only need to learn a more effective way of communicating? Remind yourself that usually a patient's feelings center on their disease or treatment and are not a reflection of their feeling about you. Do not take a patient's frustration or anger personally!

Nonverbal clues to anger include grimacing, clenching one's jaws or fists, turning away, and refusing to maintain eye contact. Verbal cues may, of course, include the use of an angry tone of voice, but they may also be disguised as witty sarcasm or as condescending or insulting remarks. To become comfortable in dealing with anger, the nurse must first become aware of his or her own reactions and learn not to feel threatened or respond in anger.

Maintain Self-control

Once you identify that a patient in a conflict situation may be so angry that they could be at risk for acting-out or violent behavior, your initial step is to maintain your self-control—to "keep your cool." Remember, you are modeling self-control! Early recognition is the key to preventing escalation. Illness generates feelings of powerlessness where your patients may feel they have little control. Anger is more powerful, so by focusing on their anger, they can feel more in control. This coping mechanism may work for them temporarily, but when you are the target, it can be difficult. Understanding this dynamic may help you to not take their behavior personally.

To maintain the situation, you attempt to reduce strong emotion to a workable level by providing a neutral, accepting, interpersonal environment. Within this context, you can acknowledge their emotion as a necessary component of adaptation to life. You convey acceptance of the individual's legitimate right to have feelings. Say, "I'm not surprised that you are angry about …" or simply stating, "I'm sorry you are hurting so much." Such statements acknowledge your patients' uncomfortable emotions, convey an attitude of acceptance, and encourage them to express themselves. Once a feeling can be put into words, it becomes manageable because it has concrete boundaries. Remember, there is a continuum:

Anxiety → Anger → Aggression

Talk About It Briefly

The use of "I" statements is one of the most effective conflict management strategies. Another strategy in defusing a strong emotion is to talk the emotion through. Unlike complaining, the purpose of talking the emotion through is to help the person bring the feeling up to a verbal level, which helps him or her to gain control. Verbalization helps the individual to connect with the personal feelings surrounding the incident.

Use Tension-Reducing Actions and Therapeutic Communication Skills

Identify Options. Rather than jumping to immediately try to find solutions, look at the range of possible options. By conveying mutuality, the expectation shifts from adversarial conflict to an expectation of a "win-win" outcome.

Listen. Sometimes the most effective action is simply to listen and avoid any "put-down" type of comment. Active listening in a conflict situation involves concentrating on what the other person is upset about. Listening can be so powerful that it alone may reduce feelings of anxiety and frustration.

Deescalate. Your only goal is to lower the individual's level of rage and to protect them and yourself. Always leave yourself a clear exit.

- *Approach.* In an acute situation you **deescalate** and contain. If you are in danger of mortal harm, leave! Using "calming interventions" is recommended if there is no weapon.
- *Actions.* Table 13.2 lists some useful strategies for coping with angry, potentially violent individuals. Remember, your goal is to defuse the threat of violence if possible and to protect yourself and others from harm. Do not try for a rational discussion, just focus on calming interactions.
- Be aware that escalating conflict can be a threat not only to your patient but also to you. In no case is violence acceptable. Limits must be set. Failing this, you must remove yourself from a potentially harmful situation. Starcher (1999) describes the behavior of Sam,

TABLE 13.2   Five Steps for Nursing Behaviors With an Angry Patient to Avoid Violence

Step	Nurse	Angry Patient or Family Member
1. Control self	Appear calm, relax, and take two deep breaths. Remember to talk in low tone, monotone. Focus only on defusing anger or potential for violence. Remove any necklaces, cords around neck (risk of being strangled). Do not respond to insults to self or team; do not become defensive. Avoid arguing, saying no, or hurrying.	Assess for unusually stressed individual and potential for violence. Does the patient appear out of control? If so, **leave**! Remember, showing your anxiety will increase the patient's anxiety and anger. Reasoning with an enraged individual is impossible; **focus on deescalation.** Devote only 3–5 min in attempting to deescalate! (If it takes longer, it is not working.) Skip to the last step!
2. Nonthreatening body posture	Never touch an angry person; respect his or her personal space. Relax facial muscles; do not smile. Assume a neutral position, hands down by your side, one foot in front of the other in a relaxed posture. Stay at same eye level; try to get the patient to sit. If standing, do not position yourself face to face; be at an angle (so you can sidestep). Never turn your back. If standing, stay four times farther away than usual: Do not "crowd" the patient. Do not gesture; never point finger. Always be closest to the door (so you can escape if necessary).	Allow the patient to move around or pace (movement can help control stress). Allow the patient to break eye contact; avoid a constant stare. Monitor the patient's body position; watch for escalation in gestures.

Continued

TABLE 13.2	Five Steps for Nursing Behaviors With an Angry Patient to Avoid Violence—cont'd	
Step	**Nurse**	**Angry Patient or Family Member**
3. Verbal deescalation	Be nonconfrontational, nonjudgmental.	Allow the patient to ventilate some of his or her anger and discuss the problem.
	Use the communication skills such as active listening and paraphrasing.	Help the patient identify his or her own anger (e.g., "I notice you are clenching your fists and talking more loudly than usual. These are things people do when angry. Help me to understand").
	Introduce yourself; call the patient by name while making occasional eye contact.	
	Communicate clearly and simply.	
	Respond in a low, calm, gentle tone of voice; do not raise your voice.	
	Be empathetic.	
	Be neutral; avoid being defensive. Do not argue.	Help the patient identify the source of his or her anger.
	Always be respectful.	Have the patient use a relaxation technique such as deep breathing.
	Do not dismiss any concern but always answer a request for information.	Give the patient permission to feel angry, but set limits on acting-out and violent behavior (e.g., "It's okay to feel angry about ... but not okay to act on it" or "It's natural to feel angry about ... but throwing things isn't okay ...").
	Appeal to the patient's cognitive rather than emotional self in trying to identify the underlying problem.	
	Help the patient verbalize his or her anger.	
	Offer to work with the patient to help him or her deal with the issue.	
	Answer selectively, ignore generalized ranting comments, and focus on just giving the information requested.	Support the patient's attempts to control his or her feelings.
	Set limits (empathize with the patient's underlying feelings but not with his or her behavior). State clearly that violence is **not** acceptable.	The patient needs to know the consequences of his or her continued acting-out behavior.
	Give the patient options for alternative behavior (e.g., "Let's take a break and have a [paper] cup of water").	
	If the patient has a weapon, ask permission to move; do *not* be a hero.	
4. Containment	Be aware of backup resources (orderlies, call to security, etc.).	Implement agency violence code.
	You can choose to leave.	Allow or ask the patient to leave.
	Use physical restraints if necessary.	Represent containment as a policy of the institution, not "I will restrain you."
	Place patient in seclusion or locked isolation room in psychiatric setting.	
	Use enforced chemical restraint (medication).	For some patients with brain damage or mental illness, it is appropriate to remove them from the source of their irritation to a calm environment, such as a lock room, to give them a sort of a time-out.
	Report all threats.	
	Do not allow contagion from family member upset to spread to patient.	
5. Debrief immediately: analyze and report	Reflect on the incident. What can be done to prevent a recurrence? Can you identify the trigger? Sometimes too long a wait, too little information, or even an insensitive or hostile comment from staff can be a trigger.	After calming down, the patient needs assistance to reflect on alternative ways of behaving and to plan for the future. Activate the patient's support system.

an emotionally disturbed patient who was admitted to a geriatric unit. Sam's behavior ranged from bullying or pushing other patients to noncompliance with his treatment. Staff tried setting clear limits and identifying specific negative outcomes, including restraints and medication, without success. Eventual successful interventions included a consistent response by all staff members and using written patient contracts for each of his unacceptable behaviors. Outcomes were specifically stated for both negative behaviors (restrictions) and positive acceptable behaviors (rewards with his favorite activities).

Employ Physical Activity. Physical activity can reduce tension. For example, taking a walk can help control anxiety and defuse an emotionally tense situation.

Try Relaxation Techniques. Some relaxation exercises can be quickly taught, such as deep breathing. Nurses frequently find the use of humor to be helpful. Humor can also be used as a means of reducing tension. To paraphrase a famous advice columnist, two of the most important words in a relationship are "I apologize." And this columnist recommended making amends immediately when you have made a mistake, because "it is easier to eat crow while it is still warm." Is this advice easier to take (we will not say *swallow*) because it comes with a chuckle? Humor serves as an immediate tension reliever.

Containment

A priority is to maintain a safe environment for yourself and all agency patients. Many hospitals and psychiatric units have a "code word" that is used to summon trained help. Isolation in a locked room is standard in many psychiatric facilities, as is the use of restraints and pharmaceutical tranquilizers. Sometimes maintaining safety necessitates summoning agency resources, such as a critical incident response team, security, or the community police. An additional strategy for helping nurse–patient problem interactions is the *staff-focused consultation.* Consider the following situation. Students are particularly prone to feeling rebuffed when they first encounter negative feedback from a patient. Support from staff, instructors, and peers, coupled with efforts to understand the underlying reasons for the patient's feelings, can help you to resist the trap of avoiding the relationship. To develop these ideas further, practice.

Evaluation: Immediate Debriefing

The final strategy is to do an evaluation of the effectiveness of responses. What was the trigger? Sometimes it was something simple, such as having had to wait too long to get information or hearing an insensitive or even hostile comment from a staff person. Your goal is to apply insight toward preventing future occurrences. It is not the responsibility of any nurse to help a patient resolve all conflict. Long-standing conflicts require more expertise to resolve. In such cases, refer them to the appropriate resource.

Each step in the process may need to be taken more than once and refined or revised as circumstances dictate.

Analysis. Postincident analysis may offer insight into how to prevent the next situation (Fig. 13.2). Some patients have mental problems, are truly confused, or have dementia. The AHRQ recommends that clinicians assess their patients' level of cognitive functioning.

Reporting. It has been estimated that a significant number of incidents go unreported; some say up to 80%. This is an international problem for nurses, and ICN urges you to report all incidents of abuse or violence.

Recap of Conflict Communication Skills

1. **Be assertive.** Assertive communication means you convey objectives with directness but not with anger or frustration.
2. **Demonstrate respect.** Responsible, assertive statements are made in ways that do not violate the rights of others or diminish their standing. They are conveyed by a relaxed, attentive posture and a calm, friendly tone of voice. Statements should be accompanied by the use of appropriate eye contact.
3. **Use "I" statements.** Assertive statements that begin with "I" suggest that you accept full responsibility for your feelings and position in relation to the presence of conflict.
4. **Make clear statements.** Statements, rather than questions, set the stage for assertive responses to conflict.
5. **Use proper pitch and tone.** Pitch and tone of voice contribute to another person's interpretation of the meaning of your assertive message. A firm but moderate presentation is often as effective as content in conveying the message.

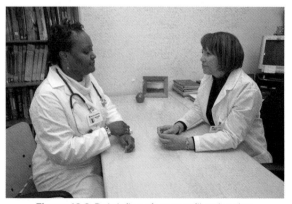

Figure 13.2 Debriefing after a conflict situation.

Strategies to Use in Clinical Encounters With Demanding, Difficult Patients

Every nurse encounters patients who seem overly demanding of the nurse's limited time and resources. Although this may reflect a personality characteristic, most often it is a sign of the patient's anxiety. Reflect on behaviors that increase anger in others and how to avoid these triggers. Conversely, ignoring inappropriate behavior does not make it go away. For example, in the case of Mr Gow, discussed earlier, he is making inappropriate sexual suggestions. The nurse could have ineffectively responded by ignoring his verbal comments or by avoiding him. Instead, she responded assertively in a "no nonsense" professional manner. How would you handle such a situation? Usually, we tend to label people as "difficult to deal with" when our normal way of dealing with them has failed. Remember, we cannot change another's personality, but we can change the way we react to them.

Help the patient express anger in an acceptable manner. Help patients own their angry feelings by getting them to verbalize things that make them angry. Acknowledging their anger may prevent an expression of abusive ranting.

Defuse Hostility. Avoid responding to a patient's anger by getting angry yourself. Verbal attacks follow certain rules, that is, the abusive person expects you to react in specific ways. Usually people will respond by becoming aggressive and attacking back or by becoming defensive and intimidated.

Use Communication Skills. Use empathy in your communication. An angry person needs to have you acknowledge both the issue and his or her feelings about that issue. Only then can they begin to interact in a meaningful way. Deliberately begin to lower your voice and speak more slowly. When we get upset, we tend to speak quickly and use a higher tone of voice. If you do the opposite, the person may begin to mimic you and thus calm down.

Realistically Analyze the Current Situation That Is Disturbing the Patient.

- Be assertive in setting limits. If the behavior persists, you need to assert limits, saying, for example, "Jim, I want to help you sort this out, but if you continue to curse at me and raise your voice, I'm going to have to leave. Which do you want?" Another response might be, "Yelling at me isn't going to get this worked out. I will not argue with you. Come back when you can talk calmly and I will try to help you."
- Help your patients to develop a plan to deal with the situation (e.g., use techniques such as role-playing to help them express anger appropriately, using "I" statements such as, "I feel angry" rather than "You make me

angry"). Bringing behavior up to a verbal level should help alleviate the need for acting out and other destructive behaviors.

Prevent Escalation of Conflict. In nurse–patient confrontations, the recognition of "trigger" factors, which often lead to escalation, may help in prevention. Do assess whether the person is intoxicated, disoriented, or whether there may be substance abuse. Using respectful patient-centered care approaches can help to prevent any escalation in interpersonal conflict. Hurt feelings or misunderstandings can quickly grow into a conflict. Keep the focus on the individual's *behavior* rather than on the person. If eye contact seems confrontational, then break eye contact. If the person is acting out by throwing or hitting, set limits.

Defusing Potential Conflicts When You Are Providing Home Healthcare

Recognizing potential situations lending themselves to conflict is, of course, an important initial step. Caregivers have been shown to experience conflict through incompatible pressures suffered between caregiver demands and demands from their other roles, such as parenting their children or maintaining employment. In addition to this interrole conflict, caregivers suffer pressures when a nurse comes into the home to participate in the care of an ill relative. A Canadian study of home health nurses and family caregivers of elderly relatives identified four evolving stages in the nurse–caregiver relationship. The initial stage is "worker–helper," with the nurse providing care to the ill patient and the family helping. Next comes "worker–worker," when the nurse begins teaching the needed care skills to family members. Third is "nurse as manager; family as worker," as the family members learn needed care skills. The final stage, "nurse as nurse for family caregiver," occurs as the family member becomes exhausted. A source of conflict for nurses was the dual expectation of the family that the nurse would provide not only care for the identified patient but also relief for the exhausted primary caregiver. When the nurse operated as manager and treated the caregiver as worker, the discrepancy in expectations and values resulted in increased tension in the relationship. Discussion of role expectations is essential. Because of the high cost of providing direct care to the chronically ill, home health nurses may be expected to quickly shift to teaching the necessary skills to the family members. Although this shift in responsibility may result in a reduction of expensive professional time, it should not compromise your commitment to the family.

SUMMARY

Conflict represents a struggle between two opposing thoughts, feelings, or needs. This chapter focuses on conflict between nurse and patient or family. All conflicts have certain things in common: a concrete content problem issue and relationship issues arising from the process of expressing the conflict. Generally, conflicts stimulate feelings of emotional discomfort. Strategies to defuse strong emotion were highlighted. Most interpersonal conflicts involve some threat, either to one's sense of power to control an interpersonal situation or to ways of thinking about the self. Giving up ineffective behavior patterns in conflict situations is difficult, because such patterns are generally perceived to be safer because they are familiar.

Behavioral responses to conflict situations fall into five styles. In the past, nurses most commonly chose avoidance. However, this chapter describes other strategies (e.g., assertion) that have been more successfully used by nurses to manage patient–nurse conflicts. Assertive behaviors range from making a simple statement, directly and honestly, about one's beliefs, to taking a very strong, confrontational stand about what will and will not be tolerated.

The principles of conflict management were described. To apply conflict management principles, you need to identify your own conflictive feelings or reactions. In conflict between nurse and patient, you need to think through the possible causes of the conflict as well as your own feelings before making a response. To resolve conflict, you need to use "I" statements and respond assertively. This chapter discussed workplace violence and strategies to maintain or restore a safe environment.

ETHICAL DILEMMA: What Would You Do?

You are caring for Kim, born at the gestational age of 24 weeks in a rural hospital and transferred this morning to your neonatal intensive care unit. Today her father arrives on the unit. Seeing you taking a blood sample from one of the many intravenous lines attached to Kim, he yells at you to "Stop poking at her! What are you trying to prove by keeping her alive? Turn off those machines." This is both a communication problem and an ethics problem. How do you respond to his anger?

DISCUSSION QUESTIONS

1. Describe how the tone and pitch effect a conflict situation.
2. Using the knowledge gained in the chapter, design a response where you deescalate a conflict.

REFERENCES

Agency for Healthcare Research and Quality (AHRQ). (n.d.). [Website]. www.ahrq.gov. [Accessed 26 May 2021].

American Association of Critical-Care Nurses (AACN). (2019). *AACN position statement: Preventing violence against healthcare workers*. Retrieved from: https://www.aacn.org/policy-and-advocacy/aacn-position-statement-preventing-violence/. [Accessed 17 June 2021].

Byrne, J. (2013). *Conflict resolution in 6 easy steps*. [Video]. Retrieved from: https://www.youtube.com/watch?v=DSGy5yvC0hM. [Accessed 17 June 2021].

Hartley, D., Ridenour, M., & Wassell, J. T. (2019). Workplace violence prevention for nurses. *American Journal of Nursing, 119*(9), 19–20.

International Council of Nurses (ICN). (2019). *Healthcare under attack! International Council of Nurses condemns violence against healthcare workers*. Retrieved from: https://www.icn.ch/news/healthcare-under-attack-international-council-nurses-condemns-violence-against-healthcare. [Accessed 17 June 2021].

Lewis-Pierre, L., Anglade, D., Saber, D., Gattamorta, K. A., & Piehl, D. (2019). Evaluating horizontal violence and bullying in the nursing workforce of an oncology academic medical center. *Journal of Nursing Management, 27*(5), 1005–1010.

McElhaney, R. (1996). Conflict management in nursing administration. *Nursing Management, 27*(3), 49–50.

Occupational Safety and Health Administration (OSHA). Washington, DC: U.S. Department of Labor. [Website]. www.osha.gov/.

O'Keeffe, V. O., Boyd, C., Phillips, C., & Oppert, M. (2021). Creating safety in care: Student nurses' perspectives. *Applied Ergonomics, 90*, 103248.

Quality and Safety Education for Nurses (QSEN). (n.d.). [Website]. www.qsen.org.

Sherman, R. O. (2020). *Promoting a leadership mindset*. EmergingRNLeader.com. [Website]. Available at: https://www.emergingrnleader.com/promoting-a-leadership-mindset/. [Accessed 26 May 2021].

Starcher, S. (1999). Sam was an emotional terrorist—and he victimized everyone within earshot. *Nursing, 29*(2), 40–41.

The Joint Commission (TJC). (2018). *Sentinel event alert 59: Physical and verbal violence against health care workers*. Available at: https://www.jointcommission.org/resources/patient-safety-topics/sentinel-event/sentinel-event-alert-newsletters/. [Accessed 26 May 2021].

The Joint Commission (TJC). (2019). *Sentinel event alert 45: Preventing violence in the health care setting*. Available at: https://www.jointcommission.org/resources/patient-safety-topics/sentinel-event/sentinel-event-alert-newsletters/. [Accessed 26 May 2021].

U.S. Department of Health and Human Services. (n.d.). Healthy people 2030. [website]. Available at: https://health.gov/healthypeople/. [Accessed 26 May 2021].

World Health Organization (WHO). (n.d.). *Violence and injury prevention: Violence against health workers*. [Website]. Available at: http://who.int/violence_injury_prevention/violence/workplace/en/. [Accessed 26 May 2021].

14

Communication Strategies for Health Promotion and Disease Prevention

OBJECTIVES

At the end of the chapter, the reader will be able to:

1. Define concepts related to health promotion and disease prevention.
2. Identify national agendas for health promotion and disease prevention.
3. Apply conceptual frameworks to health promotion actions.
4. Analyze evidence for health promotion and disease prevention strategies for individuals.
5. Evaluate health promotion and disease prevention strategies at the community level.

Health promotion can refer to international level policy issues or to policies within a community that raise awareness of healthy lifestyle behaviors (RHIhub, 2018). It can also be applied to individual nurse–patient interventions and communications, which will be the focus of this chapter.

An overarching goal of *Healthy People 2030* is promotion of quality of life and healthy development and behaviors across all stages of life (U.S. Dept. of Health & Human Services, 2020). This chapter focuses on concepts affecting nursing roles in achieving specific health promotion and disease prevention. Underlying barriers are also explored. Underlying causes of health problems are increasingly recognized as a matter of concern. However, many nurses underutilize opportunities to provide our patients with health promotion concepts (Iriarte-Roteta et al., 2020).

BASIC CONCEPTS

Definitions

Health is the ability to function and to experience well-being. Factors such as genetics, environment, economics, and societal conditions influence our health status, as do factors such as healthcare availability and our educational level. Health is considered by many to be a fundamental human right (United Nations, 2021).

Health promotion is defined as the process in which a person takes control of their own health.

Well-being is personal satisfaction in six dimensions: intellectual, physical, emotional, social, occupational, and health.

Health promotion activities are lifestyle activities that promote optimum health. Fig. 14.1 lists critical elements of health and well-being. Activities include the following:

- Health education
- Supplying preventive health services
- Advocating for health promotion
- Safeguarding the environment
- Providing community-based education at schools and workplaces
- Media outreach in all forms including blogs
  Consider the case of Bele Chase.

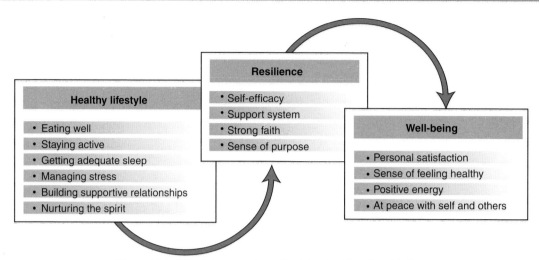

Figure 14.1 Critical elements for maintaining health and well-being.

CASE STUDY: Bele Chase Fears Vaccination

From James Gathany, Centers for Disease Control and Prevention [CDC], 2009.

Mrs Chase, age 70, tells you she spent a year in lockdown during the recent pandemic and really wanted to be able to visit her grandchildren. However, she now fears flying and exposing herself to possible disease. Diane Gibb, FNP, is her longtime nurse practitioner with an established trusting relationship. She explains the efficacy of immunization and recommends the procedure, explaining dosage and possible mild side effects. Diane tells Ms Gibb that she herself has been immunized and would recommend it to her mother for her protection.

Theoretical Concepts in Health Promotion

While experts stress the need to look beyond individual patients to promote community and corporate policies, nurses primarily deal with helping patients change unhealthy behaviors. Pender's health promotion model, Prochaska's transtheoretical model, Bandura's social learning theory, and the disease prevention epidemiological models are useful frameworks to guide health promotion strategies and help us understand the individual's choices in health behavior.

Pender's Health Promotion Model

Nurses use Nola Pender's health promotion model to understand what motivates people to engage in specific health behaviors (Pender et al., 2011). As shown in Fig. 14.2, this focuses on three areas: characteristics and experiences of individuals; their behavior-specific cognition and affect; and behavioral outcomes. In Pender's view, health is a dynamic process affected by personal factors, social support systems, and situational variables. The patient's belief about the degree to which they believe their actions can affect health outcomes needs to be considered, a concept known as **self-efficacy**. Perceived barriers to action have an impact of the patient's willingness to try to change their health-related behaviors.

Nurses can help patients modify unhealthy behaviors, but their capacity to change depends on what they believe about their illness, the seriousness if it, and their belief in the extent to which their own actions can produce positive outcomes. Nurses assess the degree of value patients place on their good health. Simulation Exercise 14.1 provides practice applying Pender's model. Pender's model identifies perceived benefits, barriers, and ability to take action related to health and well-being as important components of people's health decision-making.

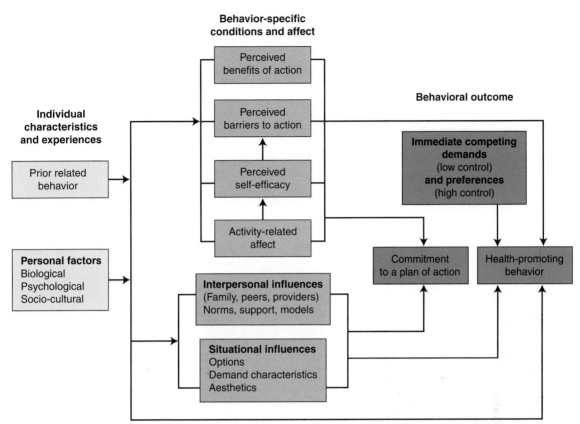

Figure 14.2 Pender's revised health promotion model. From Pender, N., Murdaugh, C., & Parsons, M. (2011). *Health promotion in nursing practice* (6th ed., p. 45). Upper Saddle River, NJ: Prentice Hall.

SIMULATION EXERCISE 14.1   Motivational Interviewing Using Pender's Model

Purpose

To help students understand the value of the health promotion model in assessing and promoting healthy lifestyles (Fig. 14.2).

Procedure

1. Using the health promotion model as a guide, interview a person in the community about his or her perception of a common health problem (e.g., heart disease, high cholesterol, osteoporosis, breast or prostate cancer, obesity, or diabetes).
2. Record the person's answers in written diagram form following Pender's model of health promotion. Identify the behavior-specific cognitions and affect action that would best fit the person's situation.

3. Share your findings with your classmates, either in a small group of four to six students with a scribe to share common themes with the larger class or in the general class.

Reflective Discussion Analysis

1. Were you surprised by anything the patient said, his or her perception of the problem, or interpretation of its meaning?
2. As you compare your findings with other classmates, do common themes emerge?
3. How could you use the information you obtained from this exercise in future healthcare situations?

TABLE 14.1   Prochaska's Stages of Change With Suggested Approaches and Sample Statements Applied to Alcoholism

Stage	Characteristic Behaviors	Suggested Approach	Sample Statement
Precontemplation	Patient does not think there is a problem; is not considering the possibility of change.	Raise doubt; give informational feedback to raise awareness of a problem and health risks.	"Your lab tests show liver damage. These tests can be predictive of serious health problems and premature death."
Contemplation	Patient thinks there may be a problem; is thinking about change; goes back and forth between concern and unconcern.	Tip the balance; allow open discussion of pros and cons of changing behavior; build motivation for change; help patient justify a positive commitment.	"It sounds as though you think you may have a drinking problem but are not sure you are an alcoholic. What would your life be like without alcohol?"
Preparation	Patient decides there is a problem and is willing to make a change: "I guess I do need to stop drinking."	Help the patient choose the best course of action for resolving the problem.	"What kinds of changes will you need to make to stop drinking? Most people find Alcoholics anonymous (AA) helpful as a support. Have you heard of them?"
Action	Patient engages in concrete actions to effect needed change.	Help the patient take active steps to resolve health problem; review progress; give feedback.	"I am impressed that you went to two AA meetings this week and have not had a drink either. What has this been like for you?"
Maintenance	Patient perseveres with positive behavioral change.	Help the patient identify and use strategies to sustain progress; point out positive changes; accept temporary setbacks and use steps in preparation phase if needed.	"It's hard to let go of old habits, but you have been abstinent for 3 months now, and your liver tests are significantly improved."

Prochaska's Transtheoretical Model for Change

This model is also called the Stages of Change Model. It is a decision-making model developed in the 1970s exploring the individual's motivational readiness to intentionally change their behaviors and health habits (Prochaska & Norcross, 2013). Stages of readiness range from lack of acknowledgment of the problem to the taking of constructive actions to correct unhealthy behaviors. It employs cognitive and affective processes. By the last stage, the person has no desire to return to their former (unhealthy) behavior. Small changes are rewarded to reinforce the new behavior. Table 14.1 presents Prochaska's model with suggested approaches for each stage and corresponding sample statements. Simulation Exercise 14.2 provides an opportunity to work with Prochaska's transtheoretical model.

Bandura's Social Learning Theory

Albert Bandura's (1997) social learning theory proposes that humans observe and then copy a new behavior in a reciprocal interaction. According to Bandura, a person does not learn a new behavior by simply trying it out. Instead, they replicate the actions of others who serve as models. A big contribution to the study of health promotion is the concept of self-efficacy. *Self-efficacy* is defined as a personal belief in one's ability to execute the actions required to achieve a goal. It represents a powerful mediator of behavior and behavioral change. Self-efficacy and motivation are reciprocal processes. Increased self-efficacy strengthens motivation, which, in turn, increases an individual's capacity to complete the learning task.

Bandura considers learning to be a social process. He identified three sets of motivators: physical motivators,

SIMULATION EXERCISE 14.2 Assessing Readiness Using Prochaska's Model

Purpose

To identify elements in teaching that can promote readiness, using Prochaska's model.

Procedure

Identify as many specific answers as possible to the following questions:

1. Patrick drinks four to six beers every evening. Last year he lost his job. He has a troubled marriage and few friends. Patrick does not consider himself an alcoholic and blames his chaotic marriage for his need to drink. There is a strong family history of alcoholism. What kinds of information might help Patrick want to learn more about his condition?

2. Lily has just learned she has breast cancer. Although there is a good chance that surgery and chemotherapy will help her, she is scared to commit to the process and has even talked about taking her life. What kinds of health teaching strategies and information might help Lily become ready to learn about her condition?

3. Shawn has just been diagnosed as having epilepsy. He is ashamed to tell his friends and teachers about his condition. Shawn is considering breaking up with his girlfriend because of his newly diagnosed illness. How would you use health teaching to help Shawn cope more effectively with his illness?

social incentives, and cognitive motivators. *Physical motivators* can be internal, such as memory of previous discomfort or a symptom that the patient cannot ignore. *Social incentives*, such as praise and encouragement, increase self-esteem and give the patient reason to continue learning. *Cognitive motivators* are thought processes associated with change.

As a nurse, you might combine aspects of these theories, relating them to something your patient values to move the change process along toward achieving the desired outcome, such as in the Francis Cox case.

Case Study: Francis Cox and Louise Kelly, RN

Louise Kelly, RN, has a meeting with her patient Mr Cox, age 47, who is diagnosed with chronic obstructive pulmonary disease (COPD). Ms Kelly expresses concern that Mr Cox continues to smoke, further damaging his lungs. "I notice you are having more difficulty breathing. If you stopped smoking it would preserve the healthy lung tissue areas (physical motivator) and maybe you wouldn't have as much trouble breathing. I bet your grandson would appreciate it if you were able to take him fishing as you said (social motivator)."

Discussion: The intent of this intervention was to help remind the patient about possible outcome of changing his smoking (unhealthy) behavior. If Mr Cox notices he is coughing less after giving up cigarettes, this perception could act as another internal motivator to maintain abstinence.

Disease Prevention Epidemiological Framework

There are several disease prevention frameworks concerned with risk and protective factors associated with specific diseases. Nurse can use case finding to identify risk factors in individuals, families, or communities. The goal is to prevent or delay the onset of disease or to manage progression to disability. Health promotion and disease prevention, with special attention to the underlying causes of a health problem, is increasingly recognized as a reimbursable, essential component of comprehensive healthcare. Regular health screenings can identify emerging treatable health problems such as osteoporosis, high blood pressure, or glaucoma.

1. **Primary disease prevention**—Intervention targets modifiable risk factors with suggestions for a healthier lifestyle. For example, promoting exercise and healthier diet to prevent onset of diseases such as diabetes. What other preventive advice have you heard? Were any communication strategies promoting this message any better than others? Fig. 14.3 depicts American National Prevention Strategies.

2. **Secondary disease prevention**—The focus is on early disease detection through regular screening. Early diagnosis allows implementation of treatment to hopefully prevent or modify the progression of a disease.

3. **Tertiary disease prevention**—These strategies minimize the damaging effects of a disease or injury once it occurs. The goal is to help patients achieve best quality of life possible. Simulation Exercise 14.3 provides an opportunity to develop your health profile and examine risk factors in your life.

Protective factors are defined as circumstances, resources, and personal characteristics that delay the emergence of chronic disease or lessen its impact. Although protective factors do not guarantee a life free of serious illness or early death, they play a significant role in helping patients improve their health and quality of life. Examples of protective factors include developing a healthy lifestyle, getting

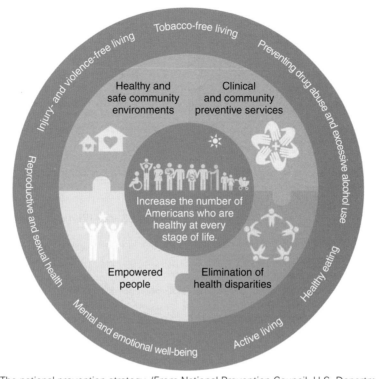

Figure 14.3 The national prevention strategy. (From National Prevention Council, U.S. Department of Health and Human Services, Office of the Surgeon General. (2011). *National prevention strategy.* Washington, DC: U.S. Department of Health and Human Services, Office of the Surgeon General.)

daily exercise, eating a healthy diet, having annual medical checkups, increasing the number of available support systems, obtaining health insurance, and so on. Health education, social marketing, and screening services help people to become aware of health risk factors.

Global and National Health Promotion Agendas

The World Health Organization's (WHO) global agenda is guided by a series of reports including The Ottawa Charter for Health Promotion (WHO, 1986), The Jakarta Declaration of the fourth International Conference on Health Promotion (WHO, 1997), and the Shanghai Declaration on Promoting Health in the "2030 Agenda for Sustainable Development" (WHO, 2018).

Social Determinants of Health

Societal and community systems interacting with personal factors impact health over time. Individuals incorporate norms and values from social networks often without conscious reflection. Economic factors and political policies affect the availability.

Social, economic, religious, and political factors affecting health promotion and disease prevention are embedded

at the level of the community as well as the larger society. They have a significant effect on health and well-being. Although each person enters the world with a distinct set of constitutional factors (size, gender, intellect, and personality), each grows up within social and community networks and, over time, incorporates the social values of those networks. One's environment interacts with personal factors to influence, enhance, or limit one's health behaviors. Larger social community systems create roles and expectations that further shape and modify the individual's health behaviors (Gray, 2017).

Health Disparities

Health disparities describes fundamental differences in adverse health outcomes and lost opportunities to achieve optimal health and well-being as it relates to demographics, income, education, and access. It is essential that nurses not just understand that health inequities exist, but also understand their causes (McFarland & MacDonald, 2019). Nationally, disparities account for significant variations in life expectancy, positive health outcomes, and the incidence of chronic disease and disability.

SIMULATION EXERCISE 14.3 Developing a Health Profile

Purpose
To help students understand the relationship between lifestyle health assessment factors and related health goals from a personal perspective.

Procedure
Out-of-class assignment: Develop a personal health profile in which you
1. Assess your own personal risk factors related to each of the following:
   a. Family risk factors (diabetes, cardiac, cancer, osteoporosis)
   b. Diet and nutrition
   c. Exercise habits
   d. Weight
   e. Alcohol and drug use
   f. Safe sex practices
   g. Perceived level of stress
   h. Health screening tests: cholesterol, blood pressure, blood sugar
2. Identify unhealthy behaviors or risk factors
3. Develop a personalized action plan to identify strategies to address areas that need strengthening
4. Identify any barriers that might prevent you from achieving your personal goals

Reflective Discussion Analysis
1. In small groups, discuss findings that you feel comfortable sharing with others.
2. Get input from others about ways to achieve health-related goals.
3. In the larger group, discuss how doing this exercise can inform your practice related to lifestyle changes and health promotion.

Causes
Social determinants associated with health disparities include lack of adequate health insurance, social isolation, cultural factors, access and availability of services, finances, lack of knowledge or education, food or job security, language barriers, health literacy, and poverty. Social determinants critically affect health, morbidity, and mortality. The elimination of health disparities is a primary objective of our nation's public health agenda and a central focus of the National Center for Minority Health and Health Disparities within the National Institutes of Health.

Nurse Role
Except for our function educating patients, we nurses seem to have a lack of clarity about what constitutes our responsibility in social policies that underpin health disparities. Broadly our mission could include action to
- achieve health equity, eliminate disparities, and improve the health of all groups;
- create social and physical environments that promote good health for all;
- promote healthy development and healthy behaviors across every stage of life.

Topic areas proposed to achieve these goals identify the population focus of attention. Objectives are organized in three categories—interventions, determinants, and outcomes. *Healthy People 2030* reinforces the importance of social determinants as critical antecedents that influence health and well-being.

Case Study: Mary Noland
Mary Nolan knows that walking will help diminish her risk for developing osteoporosis, but the threat of potentially having this problem in her 60s is not sufficient to motivate her to take action in her 40s. Mary does not feel any signs or symptoms of the disorder, and it is easier to maintain a sedentary lifestyle. To create the most appropriate learning conditions and types of teaching strategies, the nurse will have to understand Mary's value system and other factors that influence Mary's readiness to learn. To remain healthy, Mary will have to effect positive change in her health habits.

Disease Prevention
Disease prevention frameworks are concerned with identifying modifiable risk and protective factors associated with specific diseases and mental disorders. Nurses can use strategies in health counseling such as those suggested in Box 14.1. The goals of prevention emphasize managing and/or

---

DEVELOPING AN EVIDENCE-BASED PRACTICE

Obesity, especially in children, has tripled in the last 50 years. Obesity adversely affects health and increases healthcare utilization (Bomberg, 2021). Obesity is usually measured by body mass index (BMI). Brown and associates at Cochrane Database have done a meta-analysis of 110 studies examining interventions to prevent obesity. Most studies reduced dietary intake of sugar. The World Health Organization (WHO) developed a concept called "health tax" encouraging countries to pass legislation taxing consumer items with high sugar

DEVELOPING AN EVIDENCE-BASED PRACTICE-cont'd

content such as soft drinks as well as taxing alcohol and tobacco. When two British studies modeled potential effects of a 20% tax on sugar sweetened drinks, they predicted obesity would decrease by 1.3% (Briggs, 2013; Scheelbeck, 2019).

Results

Brown's analysis showed study evidence which determined that controlled diet with increased physical exercise resulted in less obesity than in control groups without such interventions. The WHO website lists many countries assessing "health taxes" resulting in increased government revenue and decreased consumer consumption. However, they do not list supporting evidence, nor do they discuss countries where such taxes failed. Anecdotally, we know New York City was unable to sustain such a tax in the face of citizen complaints. Whether health taxes on sugar products affect long-term health is unknown.

Strength of Research Evidence: Low

Application to Your Clinical Practice

1. Health promotion interventions: Evidence lends some support to attempting interventions to reduce sugar consumption, especially if combined with increases in physical activity.
2. Advocacy: In the area of community health promotion, nurses through their professional organization could lobby for changes, such as eliminating sugar soft drinks from school vending machines, or provision of health food options.

References

Bomberg, E. M., Addo, O. Y., Sarafoglou, K., & Miller, B. S. (2021). Adjusting for pubertal status reduces overweight and obesity prevalence in the United States. *The Journal of Pediatrics, 231*, 200–206.e1.

Briggs, A. D. M., Mytton, O. T., Kehlbacher, A., Tiffin, R., Rayner, M., & Scarborough, P. (2013). Overall and income specific effect on prevalence of overweight and obesity of 20% sugar sweetened drink tax in UK: Econometric and comparative risk assessment modeling study. *British Medical Journal, 347*, f6189.

Scheelbeek, P. F. D., Cornelsen, L., Marteau, T. M., Jebb, S. A., & Smith, R. D. (2019). Potential impact on prevalence of obesity in the UK of a 20% price increase in high sugar snacks: Modelling study. *British Medical Journal, 366*, l4786.

World Health Organization (WHO). (2019). *Health taxes: A primer.* Geneva, Switzerland: WHO. Retrieved from https://www.who.int/publications/i/item/WHO-UHC-HGF-Policy-brief-19.7. (Accessed 28 May 2021).

BOX 14.1   Strategies in Health Promotion and Counseling

- Incorporate the patient's preferences.
- Fully inform patients of the purposes and expected outcomes of interventions and when to expect these effects.
- Suggest small changes and baby steps rather than large ones.
- Be specific.
- Add new behaviors rather than eliminating established behaviors whenever possible.
- Link new behaviors to old behaviors.
- Obtain explicit commitments from the patient; ask patients to state exactly how they plan to achieve goals (what, when, and how often—start with "How will you begin?")
- Refer patients to appropriate community resources that are accessible and convenient.
- Use a combination of strategies to achieve outcomes tailored to individual needs.
- Monitor progress through follow-up contact.

Modified from Agency for Healthcare Research and Quality (AHRQ). (2002). *Guide to clinical preventive services: Report of the U.S. Preventive Services Task Force* (2nd ed., pp xxvii–lxxx). New York: International Medical Publishing. Retrieved from www.ahrq.gov/.

preventing the risk of future disease, disability, and premature death. Three tiers of prevention—primary, secondary, and tertiary—offer a continuum of disease prevention focus.

APPLICATIONS

Providing Health Education for Health Promotion

Health promotion strategies should be a part of everyday nursing care. Education and coaching can be introduced informally as you provide care. To succeed, nurses must become aware of the individual needs of each patient, take time to develop a personalized teaching plan, and access materials to supplement their teaching. Some suggest that this should be a priority (Bennett et al., 2020; Pueyo-Garrigues et al., 2019). Communication for patient education is discussed in Chapter 15.

Community-based interventions can be formally presented through patient education, screening programs, and social media. Choosing topics of interest to high-risk populations might include screening for disease common among certain population groups. Nurses can be influential in helping communities to create supportive health environments. For example, nurses can serve on health-related community advisory committees and provide relevant discussions regarding care and funding. The provision of health fairs for area schools or community groups is another avenue nurses can use to support health promotion and disease prevention at the community level.

Common examples of general health promotion include developing a healthy lifestyle, good nutrition, regular physical activity, adequate sleep patterns, and stress reduction. But in addition to these desired outcomes, engaging in meaningful health promotion activities supports the development of patient autonomy, personal competence, and social relatedness.

Formal and informal instruction can focus on condition-specific topics. A wide variety of topics lend themselves to a health promotion focus. A sampling includes the following:

- Alcohol, nicotine, and other types of drug abuse prevention, including the DARE anti–drug use program presented in elementary schools
- Prevention, screening, and early detection of common chronic diseases such as human immunodeficiency virus (HIV), diabetes, cancer, heart disease, osteoporosis, and associated disorders
- The fall prevention strategies, especially for older adults
- Stress reduction for informal caregivers and organizational work sites
- Healthy dietary practices
- Regular exercise habits
- Developing effective support systems

Motivational Interviewing

MI is "theoretically congruent" with the transtheoretical model of behavior change. A motivational intervention encompasses a patient's values, beliefs, and preferences incorporated into relevant functional abilities and learned skills. Motivation is seen as a state of readiness rather than a personality trait. An overarching goal of individuals who need to improve their health is to develop a better health-related quality of life. To achieve this goal, people must want to change behaviors that compromise their health.

Treatment for many chronic diseases such as cancer, heart disease, asthma, diabetes, and arthritis often requires significant ongoing lifestyle changes. Patients are charged with taking a much more active role in designing and implementing the sometimes significant lifestyle changes that are required to live a purpose-filled life while coping with chronic illness. MI is a useful strategy in dealing with ambivalent patients who must make significant lifestyle changes.

The person must believe that success is "achievable" with his/her personal efforts and/or resources. The decision to change, the choice of goals, and the commitment to developing new behaviors is always under the patient's control.

Readiness to change can be influenced. Nurses can better understand and influence a patient's deeper perception of a problem through Socratic questioning. This type of questioning allows nurses to point to discrepancies between a patient's goals or values and his or her current behaviors without argument or direct confrontation. MI helps patients address resistance and ambivalence about making health-related lifestyle changes in a nonjudgmental environment. Therapeutic strategies center on resolving problem behaviors, increasing committed collaboration, and joint decision-making.

Case Study: Mr White Wants to Be Discharged

Mr White: "I'm ready to go home now. I know once I get home, that I'll be able to get along without help. I've lived there all my life and I know my way around."

Nurse Brook: "I know that you think you can manage yourself at home. But most people need some rehabilitation after a stroke to help them regain their strength. If you go home now without the rehabilitation, you may be shortchanging yourself by not taking the time to develop the skills you need to be independent at home. Is that something important to you?"

MI is an intervention in which the nurse uses empathetic exploration to help a patient become aware of discrepancies in their behavior that are hurting their health and well-being. This exploration is coupled with teaching them new skills to achieve more healthy life goals.

Negotiating behavior change is conceptualized as a shared endeavor in which both patient and provider examine the patient's potential and willingness to change destructive health behaviors. When motivational strategies match an individual's readiness to change, this match increases the likelihood of positive intentional behavioral lifestyle changes.

There are two phases of MI. The first phase focuses on mutually exploring and resolving ambivalence to change as a collaborative endeavor. This is accomplished through weighing the pros and cons of the current situations and the actions one would have to take to make change possible. With the patient in charge of determining change activities, the second phase emphasizes strengthening and supporting the patient's commitment to change based on the patient's choice and capacity for change.

A good starting point is a simple introductory question, such as, "I wonder if you could tell me what you do to keep yourself healthy?" This type of question helps you to see what the patient values or even if he or she thinks about taking a personal role in achieving and maintaining healthy behaviors. It also provides an opportunity to assess for possible issues that actually may be counterproductive, as in the Janet Chico case.

Case Study: Janet Chico

Janet is a 77-year-old woman with osteoporosis. She is health conscious and walks regularly to build bone strength. She wears a weighted vest to increase her workout strength and recently upped this weight to 15 pounds without consulting her physician. This change caused pain, and Janet was advised to decrease the weight. In this case, the concept of bone strengthening was appropriate, but its application had become inappropriate.

When a patient begins to tell you about his or her personal health habits, you can reflect on the relevant details and ask for clarification. The purpose of the dialog is to deepen the patient's understanding. Use empathy in your responses. For example, "It sounds like you have been having a tough time and not getting a lot of support."

Open-ended questions allow patients the greatest freedom to respond. Asking a patient if he regularly exercises may yield a one-sentence answer. Inviting the same patient to describe his activity and exercise during a typical day and what makes it easier or harder for him to exercise can provide stronger data. Potential concerns and inconsistency with values, preferences, or goals are more readily identified.

Patient and family perspectives on disease and treatment are not necessarily the same as those of their healthcare providers. For example, you may think that an emaciated or an obese woman would be worried about her weight and would want to modify it because she values the way she looks. On the other hand, her culture or family values and traditions may be in conflict with making significant behavioral changes. Until the patient can understand a health-related value for making a change, she will not put serious effort into doing so. This level of data allows nurses to tailor interventions based on the patient's readiness to change and the availability of a support system.

As patients progress to the contemplative stage, nurses provide coaching guidance, information, and practical support to help them consider different choices and potential solutions. The pros and cons of each possible choice are explored. Empathy for the challenges faced by the patient and affirming the patient's reflection process encourages patients to consider alternative options and to choose the most viable among them. A critical component of MI is acceptance of the patient's right to make the final decision and the need for the clinician to honor the patient's right to do so.

In the preparation stage, your role is to help patients establish realistic goals and develop a plan for achieving them. Goals should be realistic, patient-centered, and achievable. For example, the goal of losing 10 pounds in 3 months sounds more doable than a goal to simply losing weight (too vague) or losing 75 pounds (potentially overwhelming). Incremental goals build a sense of confidence, as the patient sequentially meets them.

Personalizing goals and treatment plans for your patients is critical. Each patient has a unique life situation, support system, and way of coping with problems. Unhealthy habits are cumulative and hard to break. Work with patients to monitor their progress, offering suggestions, revising goals or plans when needed, and reminding patients of progress made. It is useful to help patients proactively identify potential obstacles and to anticipate the next steps. You can offer additional suggestions, empathize or commend patient efforts, and revisit actions from the preparation stage if goals need revision. For example, you could say, "You have really worked hard to master your exercises" or "I'm really impressed that you were able to avoid eating sweets this week." Availability to help patients solve problems or rethink plans, if needed, is also key.

Empowerment Strategies

We distinguish between empowerment as a *goal* in having control over the determinants of one's quality of life and as a *process* in which one has control over problem formulation, decision-making, and the actions one takes to achieve relevant health goals. Patient empowerment takes place through clinician-initiated patient-centered care approaches *and* through actions patients take on their own initiative.

As a process strategy, empowering people to take the initiative with their own health and well-being supports a person's ability to maintain his or her role as a functioning adult and facilitates the self-management of chronic disorders, as in the Yon case.

Case Study: Mrs Yon's Poststroke Status

Mrs Yon had a stroke a month ago. She began learning how to dress herself. At first, she took an hour to complete this task, but with guidance and practice, she eventually dressed herself in less time. Her home health nurse could have done it for her in only a few minutes but realized Mrs Yon needed to do it herself.

Empowerment Through Social Support

Empowerment implies a gathering of power. Social support from friends and family is an important empowerment resource in health promotion activities. *Social support* describes a person's "integration within a social network," and "the perceived availability of support" when it is needed. The interested support of significant others can strengthen a person's resolve, provide input for innovative solutions, and nurture the development of self-efficacy.

Health-related support groups in the community are available for a wide variety of diagnoses, providing relevant information, direct assistance, referral to appropriate resources, and the opportunity to simply interact with others experiencing similar challenges. For example, the Alzheimer's Association (for Alzheimer disease and related disorders) holds regularly scheduled support groups in most major locations to assist family members. Community-based cancer support groups provide valuable information and support for many common cancer diagnoses. Educational and referral supports enable patients and families to learn the skills they need to effectively manage chronic conditions and to live healthy lives.

Health Promotion as a Population Concept

Community is defined as a group of citizens that have either a geographic, population-based, or self-defined relationship and whose health may be improved by a health promotion approach. The community offers a natural social system with special significance for facilitating health promotion activities, particularly for people who are economically or socially disadvantaged. It is difficult to change attitudes and lifestyles to promote health when a patient's social or economic environment does not support prevention efforts.

Successful community-based health promotion activities start with a community analysis of health issues identified by the community. Consciousness raising is critical, as engagement and buy-in of the community in which the activity is to take place is essential. The active participation of individuals, communities, and systems means a stronger and more authentic commitment to the establishment of the realistic regulatory, organizational, and sociopolitical supports that will be needed to achieve targeted health outcomes. Box 14.2 presents health promotion strategies useful at the community level as well as with our individual patients.

Community empowerment seeks to enhance a community's ability to identify, mobilize, and address the issues that it faces to improve the overall health of the community.

BOX 14.2 Guiding Principles for Community Engagement

Before starting a community engagement effort
- Be clear about the purposes or goals of the engagement effort and the populations and/or communities you want to engage.
- Become knowledgeable about the community's culture, economic conditions, political and power structures, norms and values, demographic trends, history, and experience with the efforts by outside groups to engage it in various programs. Learn about the community's perceptions of those initiating the engagement activities.

For *engagement to occur*, it is necessary to
- Go to the community, establish relationships, build trust, work with the formal and informal leadership, and seek commitment from community organizations and leaders to create processes for mobilizing the community.
- Remember and accept that collective self-determination is the responsibility and right of all people who are in a community. No external entity should assume it can bestow to a community the power to act in its own self-interest.

For *engagement to succeed*,
- Partnering with the community is necessary to create change and improve health.
- All aspects of community engagement must recognize and respect the diversity of the community. Awareness of the various cultures of a community and other factors of diversity must be paramount in designing and implementing community engagement approaches.
- Community engagement can be sustained only by identifying and mobilizing community assets and strengths and by developing the community's capacity and resources to make decisions and take action.
- Organizations that wish to engage a community as well as individuals seeking to effect change must be prepared to release control of actions or interventions to the community and be flexible enough to meet the changing needs of the community.
- Community collaboration requires long-term commitment by the engaging organization and its partners.

From Clinical and Translational Science Awards (CTSA) Consortium and Community Engagement Key Function Committee Task Force on the Principles of Community Engagement (2011). *Principles of community engagement* (2nd ed., pp. 46–52). NIH Publication No. 11–7782. Washington, DC: National Academies Press. Retrieved from http://www.atsdr.cdc.gov/communityengagement/pdf/PCE_Report_508_FINAL.pdf.

This type of empowerment is fueled by *both* public policy and targeted education. Successful health promotion programs require individuals, groups, and organizations to act as active agents in shaping health practices and policies that have meaning to a target population. Specific interventions are designed to engage those people who are most involved as active participants in a common environmental concern related to health. Proactive social and political action to enhance health services can augment educational efforts to ensure program viability.

Health promotion activists recognize the community as their principal voice in promoting health and well-being. Health promotion represents a multidisciplinary approach, also inclusive of health education, public health, and environmental health. Health promotion strategies are relevant in clinics, schools, communities, and parishes; they can be introduced during many aspects of routine care in hospitals.

PRECEDE–PROCEED Model

The PRECEDE–PROCEED model is a community education structural framework for designing, implementing, and evaluating community-based health promotion. Developed by Green and Kreuter (2005), this model consists of two components. The PRECEDE dimension refers to the assessment and planning components of the program. The acronym PRECEDE stands for the predisposing, reinforcing, and enabling factors contributing to the educational/organizational diagnosis, which are directly addressed in the proceed component. Behavioral factors that can affect the success of the PRECEDE–PROCEED model are presented in Table 14.2.

Nurses also determine population needs and establish evaluation methods in the PRECEDE phase. Evaluation is a continuous process that begins when the program is implemented and is exercised throughout the educational experience. Sufficient resources, knowledge about target populations, and leadership training are part of an essential infrastructure needed to support health promotion approaches in the community.

A sustainable educational model needs political, managerial, and administrative supports for full implementation of a community-based approach to health promotion and disease prevention. Green later added the PROCEED component (policy, regulatory, organizational constructs in educational and environmental development). This component considers critical environmental and cost variables such as budget, personnel, and critical organizational relationships as part of the implementation phase. Having resources in place and assessing their sustainability is important in successful health promotion programs, although it is not always thought through in the planning

TABLE 14.2	PRECEDE–PROCEED Model: Examples of PRECEDE Diagnostic Behavioral Factors
Factors	**Examples**
Predisposing factors	Previous experience, knowledge, beliefs, and values that can affect the teaching process (e.g., culture and prior learning)
Enabling factors	Environmental factors that facilitate or present obstacles to change (e.g., transportation, scheduling, and availability of follow-up)
Reinforcing factors	Perceived positive or negative effects of adopting the new learned behaviors, including social support (e.g., family support, risk for recurrence, and avoidance of a health risk)

phase. Components of the PRECEDE–PROCEED model are presented in Table 14.3.

As with all types of education and counseling, learners need to be actively engaged in goal setting and developing action plans that have meaning to them. The healthcare system is complex and requires a new level of patient decision-making.

Choosing the right strategies requires special attention to the learner's readiness, capabilities, and skills. Box 14.1 presents strategies in health promotion counseling. Evaluation of health promotion activities is essential. In addition to evaluating immediate program effects, longitudinal evaluation of the impact of health promotion activities on morbidity, mortality, and quality of life is desirable. Keep in mind that what constitutes quality of life is a subjective reality for each patient and may differ from person to person.

Health Promotion Models for Community Empowerment

Community empowerment strategies are used to help identify and address environmental and social issues needed to improve the overall health of the community. This strategy is sometimes referred to as "capacity building." Community-focused empowerment strategies build on the personal strengths, community resources, and problem-solving capabilities already existing among individuals

TABLE 14.3   PRECEDE–PROCEED Model Definitions

Phase	Definition
PRECEDE Components	
1. Social diagnosis	People's perceptions of their own health needs and quality of life
2. Epidemiological diagnosis	Determination of the extent, distribution, and causes of a health problem in the target population
3. Behavioral and environmental diagnosis	Determination of specific health-related actions likely to affect a (behavioral) problem; systematic assessment of factors in the environment likely to influence health and quality-of-life (environmental) outcomes
4. Educational and organizational diagnosis	Assessment of all factors that must be changed to initiate or sustain desired behavioral changes and outcomes
5. Administrative and policy diagnosis	Analysis of organizational policies, resources, and circumstances relevant to the development of the health program
PROCEED Components	
6. Implementation	Conversion of program objectives into actions taken at the organizational level
7. Process evaluation	Assessment of materials, personnel performance, quality of practice or services offered, and activity experiences
8. Impact evaluation	Assessment of program effects of intermediate objectives inclusive of all changes as a result of the training
9. Outcome evaluation	Assessment of the teaching program on the ultimate objectives related to changes in health, well-being, and quality of life

Adapted from Green, L., & Kreuter, M. (2021). *Health program planning: An educational and ecological approach* (5th ed.). New York: McGraw-Hill.

and within communities that can be used to address potential and actual health problems. Capacity building requires the inclusion of informal and formal community leaders as valued stakeholders. Networking, partnering, and creating joint ventures with indigenous and local religious organizations is a powerful consensus-building strategy that communities can use for effective health education planning and implementation. Box 14.2 outlines a process for engaging the community in health promotion activities.

Case Study: Jonathan Jones

Jonathan is a 14-year-old adolescent recently discharged from a mental health unit. This was his fourth admission over an 18-month period. Mrs Jones assumed responsibility for seeing that he took his medications as directed and knew the names of his medications and faithfully monitored his taking of them. But Jonathan's behavior began to deteriorate again. At one of Jonathan's follow-up visits, the nurse asked him to show her the meds he was on, and how he was taking them. It turned out that Jonathan's mother could not read, got the meds mixed up, and was administering the daily med three times a day and the thrice daily medication once daily.

Developmental Level

Developmental level affects both teaching strategies and the delivery of content. You will have patients at all levels of the learning spectrum with regard to their social, emotional, and cognitive development.

Developmental learning capability is not necessarily age-related; it is easily influenced by culture and stress. Social and emotional development does not always parallel cognitive maturity or literacy. Mirroring the patient's communication style and framing messages to reflect cultural characteristics help improve comprehension and understanding. Parents and other family members can provide information about their child's immediate life experiences and suggest commonly used words to be incorporated into the nurse's health teaching.

Avoid information overload and giving vague or conflicting health information to older adults, particularly if there is any evidence of cognitive processing issues. For example, it is better to say, "Take the white pill when you get up and before you eat your breakfast" than it is to say, "You need to take this medication on an empty stomach." Written plus oral instructions reinforce messages. Another issue for older adults is that they often have multiple medications, some of which may look alike.

Incorporating Cultural Understandings

Cultural understandings add to the complexity of health promotion strategies in healthcare. Values, norms, and beliefs are an integral part of a person's self; they influence individual and community lifestyles and health perceptions. Respecting a patient's cultural values increases a patient's trust of individual care providers. Eliciting and integrating explanatory information regarding health and illness into health teaching promotes better understanding *and* greater acceptance of health promotion and disease prevention recommendations. Cultural sensitivity includes knowledge of the preferred communication styles of different cultural groups.

Nurses participate routinely in community health promotion and disease prevention activities. They have an ethical and legal responsibility to maintain the expertise and interpersonal sensitivity required to promote effective patient learning.

█ SUMMARY

This chapter focuses on communication strategies nurses can use to help people increase understanding of how they can increase health promotion activities. National and global agendas over the past decade reinforce the importance of developing public health policies to create supportive health environments. Specific attention to reducing health disparities, negative social determinants through strengthened community action for health, and increased access for all is advocated. Optimal health and well-being are considered the desired outcomes of health promotion activities.

Health promotion frameworks were presented. Pender's health belief model identifies perceptions of benefits, barriers, and ability to take action related to health and well-being as components of the individual's willingness to engage in health promotion activities.

Prochaska's transtheoretical model is used to explore a person's readiness to intentionally change his or her health habits.

Bandura's social learning theory explores the role of self-efficacy in empowering patients to use health promotion and disease prevention recommendations to take better care of their health. The epidemiological model was used to demonstrate that health promotion can occur at any level of health status.

Community-based interventions are critical in addressing broader causal influences on health, referred to as social determinants.

ETHICAL DILEMMA: What Would You Do?

Jack Marks is a 16-year-old adolescent who comes to the clinic complaining of symptoms of a sexually transmitted disease (STD). He receives antibiotics, and you give him information about safe sex and preventing STDs. Two months later, he returns to the clinic with similar symptoms. It is clear that Jack has not followed instructions and has no intention of doing so. He tells you he is a regular jock and just cannot get used to the idea of condoms. He says he cannot tell you the names of his partners—there are just too many of them. What are your ethical responsibilities as his nurse in caring for Jack? What are the implications of your potential decisions?

DISCUSSION QUESTIONS

1. In what ways are the concepts of health literacy and functional health literacy different and alike and why is this important?
2. Why are health promotion and disease prevention strategies receiving so much emphasis in contemporary healthcare?
3. How would you implement Pender's model to enhance personal responsibility for health promotion and disease prevention practices?
4. Discuss how you could use MI as a tool for helping patients to learn self-management strategies.

REFERENCES

Bandura, A. (1997). *Self-Efficacy: The exercise of control.* New York: W. H. Freeman.

Bennett, W. L., Pitts, S., Aboumatar, H., et al. (2020). *Strategies for patient, family, and caregiver engagement.* Technical Brief #36, AHRQ Pub. No. 20-EHC017. Rockville, MD: AHRQ.

Green, L., & Kreuter, M. W. (2005). *Health program planning: An educational and ecological approach* (4th ed.). New York: McGraw-Hill.

Grey, M. (2017). Lifestyle determinants of health: Isn't it all about genetics and environment? *Nursing Outlook, 65*(5), 501–505.

Iriarte-Roteta, A., Lopez-Dicastillo, O., Mujika, A., et al. (2020). Nurses' role in health promotion and prevention: A crucial interpretive synthesis. *Journal of Clinical Nursing, 29*(21–22), 3937–3949.

McFarland, A., & MacDonald, E. (2019). Role of the nurse in identifying and addressing health inequalities. *Nursing Standard, 34*(4), 37–42.

Pender, N., Murdaugh, C., & Parsons, M. (2011). *Health promotion in nursing practice* (6th ed.). Upper Saddle River, NJ: Prentice Hall.

Prochaska, J., & Norcross, J. (2013). *The transtheoretical model in systems of psychotherapy: A transtheoretical analysis* (8th ed.). Stamford, CT: Cengage Learning.

Pueyo-Garrigues, M., Whitehead, D., Pardavila-Belio, M. I., Canga-Armayor, A., Pueyo-Garrigues, S., & Canga-Armayor, N. (2019). Health education: A rogerian concept analysis. *International Journal of Nursing Studies, 94*, 131–138.

Rural Health Information Hub (RHIhub). (2018). *Defining health promotion and disease prevention.* Retrieved from www.ruralhealthinfo.org/toolkits/health-promotion/1/definition#[tilden]text=Typical-activities-for-health-promotion/. [Accessed 27 May 2021].

U.S. Department of Health and Human Services (DHHS). (2020). *Healthy people 2030.* Retrieved from https://health.gov/healthypeople.

World Health Organization (WHO). (1986). *Ottawa charter for health promotion: First international conference on health promotion.* Retrieved from http://www.who.int/healthpromotion/conferences/previous/ottawa/en/. [Accessed 27 May 2021].

World Health Organization (WHO). (1997). *The Jakarta declaration on leading health promotion into the 21st century.* Geneva, Switzerland: WHO. Retrieved from https://www.who.int/publications/i/item/WHO-HPR-HEP-4ICHP-BR-97.4. [Accessed 28 May 2021].

World Health Organization (WHO). (2018). *Promoting health: Guide to national implementation of the Shanghai declaration.* Geneva, Switzerland: WHO. Retrieved from https://www.who.int/healthpromotion/publications/guide-national-implementation-shanghai-declaration/en/. [Accessed 28 May 2021].

Communication in Health Teaching and Coaching

Saretha R. Lavarnway

OBJECTIVES

Upon the completion of this chapter, the reader will be able to:

1. Describe the principles of patient-centered health education.
2. Discuss theoretical frameworks used in patient-centered health teaching.
3. Apply various teaching methods and coaching strategies to case situations.
4. Create a health education scenario, which evaluates effectiveness of using printed educational materials to increase patient health literacy.

This chapter examines evidence-based patient education communication strategies in healthcare. Nurses are legally and ethically charged with providing relevant health-related education to patients, family, caregivers, and the community across clinical settings (Baur, 2011). This chapter describes selected theories of teaching and learning as an evidence-based foundation for effective health teaching and coaching of patients needed to self-manage their chronic illness, and work effectively with community resources to maximize their health, and well-being (Deek et al., 2016).

BASIC CONCEPTS

Definitions

Patient Education

Patient education represents a focused form of instructional communication. Its purpose and design are to provide patients and families with the specific knowledge, life skills, and practical and emotional support needed to

- cope with diagnosed health disruptions;
- self-manage and minimize the effects of chronic disorders;
- make effective health-related decisions;
- slow or prevent disease progression; and
- promote patient's attainment of a high quality of life.

Personal Health Literacy

Personal **health literacy** is the degree to which a patient has the ability to understand, communicate, and use information to make healthcare decisions. Health literacy is associated with a person's cognitive function and can be affected by a person's culture, ethnicity, education level, age, socioeconomic status, English proficiency, or learning disabilities (Halm, 2021).

Shared Decision-Making

Shared decision-making is a process in which healthcare professionals work together with patients to use evidence-based data to access treatment options, risks involved, and possible outcomes to make the best health choices for individuals. When the process of shared decision-making is utilized with patients and families, health outcomes are better, patient experiences and satisfaction levels improve, and costs are lower (Heath, 2017).

Theory

Health teaching related to chronic conditions extends beyond simple medical and clinical data. Each teaching situation requires an individualized teaching approach and "learner buy-in" to ensure successful outcomes. Assessment of a patient's readiness to learn and learning style are important details in developing tailored nursing approaches with patients and families. Studies confirm that communicating evidence-based data using appropriate tools decreases patient stress, frustration, and confusion while increasing patient compliance to health plans (Happ, 2021).

Professional standards specify health teaching and health promotion as required components of professional nursing practice (Standard 5B) (American Nurses Association [ANA], 2004). Medicare also identifies health teaching as a skilled nursing intervention for reimbursement purposes.

CASE STUDY: Mrs Kelly Needs to Learn About Taking Her Medicines

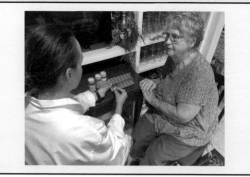

Mrs Kelly is 80 years old and lives alone. She has trouble reading directions on her prescription bottles. Her home health nurse, Olga Pavlov, RN, is using a combination of demonstration and teach-back techniques with a color-coded pill box with separate compartments for each day of the week and morning and evening doses as shown in this photograph.

Documentation of patient-specific education provided to patients about treatment options in a language the patient can fully understand is required for informed consent. Although the informed consent document is the physician's responsibility, nurses play an important role in providing appropriate pre- and follow-up health teaching, particularly with patients having limited mental or literacy capacity and with surrogate decision-makers (Menendez, 2013).

Science of Teaching

Andragogy refers to the "art and science of helping adults learn" (Knowles et al., 2011). Adult learners tend to be self-directed, action-oriented, and practical. They want to see the usefulness of what they are learning. Generally adults favor a problem-focused approach to learning. They want to be directly engaged in developing the skills needed to master immediate life problems. The adult learner expects the nurse to inquire about previous life experience and to incorporate this knowledge into a jointly agreed upon health plan. See Fig. 15.1 on methods of engaging patients and increasing health literacy.

Bastable (2019) describes learning approaches in older adulthood as *geragogy*. In normal aging, a person's knowledge changes, and asking about the particular life experiences of older adults is essential for successful health teaching. It can be much harder for an older adult to adapt to new ways of managing his or her health. Others may have significant mobility or sensory deficits that interfere with ease in learning formats. These impairments can make performing self-management skills challenging.

Older patients may need a slower pace, as many are likely to be cautious about trying new self-management strategies. Simple accommodations such as cueing, brighter lighting, and enlarged print can facilitate learning. Encouragement and positive reinforcement also improve motivation, self-efficacy, and performance. More communities are making community-based efforts to provide free or low-cost exercise and stress management programs for older adults. Specific targeted classes on fall prevention and bone strengthening are available in many communities.

Pedagogy describes the processes used to help children learn. Children need direct health education, but they come to the learning experience with far less life experience that can be tapped as resources for learning. They pass through cognitive and psychosocial stages, which dictate different teaching formats for successful participation.

A key difference between pedagogy and andragogy is the need to provide the child learner with additional direct guidance and structure in learning content. Parent participation is critical to successful education with school-aged children. It provides both oversight management guidance and essential emotional support (Kelo et al., 2013).

Bandura's Social Cognitive Model

Bandura's social cognitive model links successful behavioral changes to a person's perception that he or she has the capability to carry out the actions (self-efficacy) required to meet identified goals or expected outcomes within his or her unique social context. If people think they have the skills or can easily learn them, they tend to be more confident and are more likely to succeed.

Health teaching is a dynamic interactive process. A patient's knowledge about the reasons for using the skill and the steps involved provides a stronger foundation in the cognitive domain. For example, health teaching for a person with a recent diagnosis of diabetes might include knowledge of the disease; the roles of diet, exercise, and insulin in diabetic control; and guidance about how to identify trouble signs requiring immediate attention. Concrete information—provided through verbal discussions, images and line drawings, written instructions, and Web data—can help to explain the steps needed to achieve negotiated health goals. Paying attention to the emotional impact of a diabetes diagnosis allows patients to work through emotional issues that potentially could compromise compliance with essential

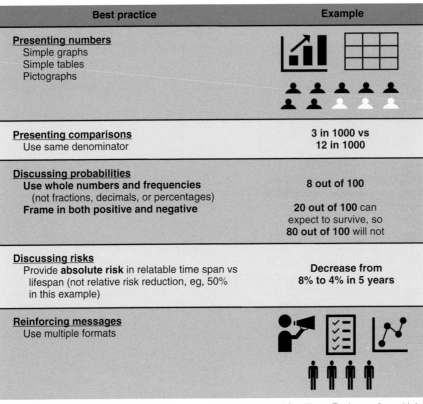

Best practice	Example
Presenting numbers Simple graphs Simple tables Pictographs	
Presenting comparisons Use same denominator	3 in 1000 vs 12 in 1000
Discussing probabilities **Use whole numbers and frequencies** (not fractions, decimals, or percentages) **Frame in both positive and negative**	8 out of 100 **20 out of 100** can expect to survive, so **80 out of 100** will not
Discussing risks Provide **absolute risk** in relatable time span vs lifespan (not relative risk reduction, eg, 50% in this example)	**Decrease from 8% to 4% in 5 years**
Reinforcing messages Use multiple formats	

Figure 15.1 Best practices to improve numeracy among patients and families. (Redrawn from Halm, M. A. (2021). When stakes are high and stress soars: Addressing health literacy. *American Journal of Critical Care, 30*(4), 326–330.)

treatment. Emotions are a powerful backdrop for self-efficacy and motivation.

The Bloom Taxonomy: Classifying Behavioral Objectives

Objectives are essentially guides to action related to achieving goals. Nurses use the Bloom taxonomy as a guide to writing behavioral objectives in healthcare. The utility of the taxonomy originally described by Bloom and associates is that it provides a common language about learning goals to facilitate communication across persons and subject matter. The Bloom taxonomy identifies a hierarchy of learning objectives ranging from simple to the most complex. These objectives were revised in the 21st century to represent verbs rather than nouns. The revised Bloom taxonomy consists of the following:

- Remembering: recognizing, recalling information and facts
- Understanding: interpreting, explaining, or constructing meaning

- Applying: carrying out or executing a procedure, using information in a new way
- Analyzing: considering individual components of the whole and how they relate to each other and the whole
- Evaluating: making judgments, critiquing, prioritizing, selecting, verifying
- Creating: putting material together into a coherent whole, reorganizing material into a new pattern, creating something new (Anderson & Krathwohl, 2000)

Behavioral objectives begin with the phrase "the patient will," followed by step-by-step achievable, measurable patient behaviors toward treatment goals. Ideally, there should be an objective for each significant component of the teaching session. An example of leveled objectives, applied to patient teaching for diabetes, is presented in Fig. 15.2.

Patient Literacy and Education

Patient's health literacy can be improved through the provision of information, effective communication, and structured education (Nutbeam et al., 2018). The teaching–learning process

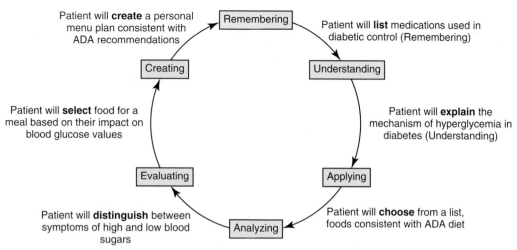

Figure 15.2 Leveled objectives using Bloom's revised taxonomy. (Text adapted from Krau, S. D. (2011). Creating educational objectives for patient education using the new Bloom's taxonomy. *Nursing Clinics of North America, 46*(3), 299–312.)

is designed to empower patients with the conceptual understandings and skills they need to self-manage their health and quality of life. Patient-centered education should start with and incorporate the patient's perspective across all activities. Health teaching and coaching approaches should be built on give-and-take relationships between healthcare professionals and patients, which in turn are based on the sharing of knowledge and the understanding of perspectives. Healthcare providers must first ascertain an individual's personal history and cultural perspective. Then they should consider the individual's health literacy, Internet access, and media exposure. All of this together will help create a patient-centered framework for positive communication. Tailoring interventions begin with listening for hidden emotional cues. Accommodating individual differences into teaching plans whenever possible shows respect for patient preferences.

APPLICATIONS

There are three major types of learning styles: visual, auditory, and kinesthetic. The visual learner will learn best by reading or viewing web-based material and graphic images rather than listening to explanations. Auditory learners need to hear the information and appreciate discussion rather than strictly depending on visual material. Kinesthetic learners learn best with demonstration and hands-on practice. Therefore, a wide variety of communication strategies should be used to convey health information. Positive and accurate communication between healthcare providers and patients will improve health literacy levels. For example, studies show that using printed educational materials such as brochures improves the quality of healthcare (Mbanda et al., 2021).

DEVELOPING AN EVIDENCE-BASED PRACTICE

Purpose

The goal of Halm's (2021) study was to provide a comprehensive understanding of the impact on healthcare from low health literacy rates and to determine how low health literacy levels could be improved. The literature review included searching for keywords such as health literacy, critical care, family communication, and education.

Results

Up to 53% of adult caregivers have low health literacy. However, research also determined that incorporating web-based educational tools with visual aids and brochures allowed participants to more easily understand materials.

Strength of Research Evidence: Moderate.

Application to Your Clinical Practice
1. Assess literacy level in each patient and caretaker.
2. Use vocabulary level at patient's level of understanding, choosing simple words as necessary.
3. Accompany all teaching with learning aides such as brochures.

Reference

Halm, M. A. (2021). When stakes are high and stress soars: Addressing health literacy in the critical care environment. *American Journal of Critical Care, 30*(4), 326–330).

BOX 15.1   Patient-Centered Verbal Communication Skills

- Make appropriate eye contact
- Speak slowly with shorter sentences (<8 words)
- Use culturally appropriate vocabulary and metaphors
- Use active listening skills
- Chunk small amounts of information and then use teach-back to confirm understanding of information
- Prioritize information to keep the patient from being overwhelmed
- Allow for wait time so that information can be absorbed and understood
- Ask "What questions do you have?" instead of "Do you have any questions?"

If the goal is to increase health literacy, then information should be communicated both verbally and in written form. See Box 15.1 for suggested strategies for patient centered verbal communication.

Plain language is defined as a major instructional strategy for making written information easier to understand, especially for individuals with lower literacy capabilities, English as a second language, and older adults. Low literacy is related to but not the same as low health literacy; medical vocabulary can be daunting for many people. Therefore, health providers also need access to easy to understand written materials and resources that can be provided to patients. It is estimated that one-third to one-half of adults have low health literacy. Incorporating visual aids such as pictures or brochures can improve health literacy (Fig. 15.3). For example, 95% of family members reported that a brochure helped them understand information (Halm, 2021). See Box 15.2 for effective strategies for written communication.

There are many factors that contribute to low health literacy, including situational stress and anxiety. Patients or family members in a critical care situation have increased levels of stress and increased levels of frustration and misunderstanding. Patients, especially when they are in crisis mode, do not always ask questions. Anxiety limits cognitive skills even in the best of us, and medical vocabulary can be daunting.

Communicating with patients that are nonverbal, such as due to the intubation of a ventilator, becomes even more challenging. Healthcare providers must assess the patient's cognitive ability and motor function. For example, if there is cognitive function but low motor ability, healthcare providers could use items such as picture boards. If the patient has low cognitive ability and motor function, then healthcare providers could use simple yes or no cards or gestures for communication (Happ, 2021).

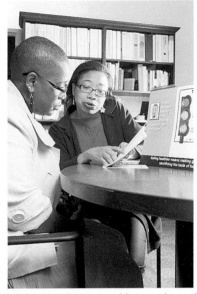

Figure 15.3 A health educator teaching a patient using written material accompanied by a graphic chart.

BOX 15.2   Strategies for Written Communication

- Words should be at a fifth-grade reading level
- Use a large font (font size 14, Arial script)
- Have clear headings and pictures that explain the text
- Translate materials as needed for English as a second language families

---

Case Study: Mr Winston Overdoses on Coumadin

"Everything was happening so fast and everybody was so busy," and that is why Mitch Winston, 66 years old and suffering from atrial fibrillation, did not ask his doctor to clarify the complex and potentially dangerous medication regimen that had been prescribed for him on leaving the hospital emergency department. When he returned to the emergency department via ambulance, bleeding internally from an overdose of warfarin (Coumadin), his doctor was surprised to learn that Mitch had not understood the verbal instructions he had received and that he had ignored the written instructions and orders for follow-up visits that the doctor had provided. In fact, Mitch had never retrieved these from his wallet. Despite their importance, they were useless pieces of paper, as Mitch cannot read.

TABLE 15.1　Core Constructs of Health Literacy With Application Examples

Basic literacy or comprehension	• Reading various text such as appointment cards • Interpreting medical tests, dosages instructions, and side effects • Understanding what is read, including brochures, medication labels, informed consent documents, and insurance documents
Interactive and participatory literacy (able to participate in two-way interactions	• Provision of appropriate and usable information • Comprehension and ability to act on information • Remembering and acting on information
Critical literacy	• Ability to weigh critical scientific facts • Capacity to assess competing treatment options

Patients with limited literacy struggle harder to understand and usually need more time to process information. They tend to decode messages one word at a time and may not grasp the whole message. To facilitate understanding, use fewer rather than more words to explain a concept and allow extra time to practice psychomotor skills with ongoing feedback. Learning goals should be simple and stated in words familiar to the learner. Provide only essential basic information in a sequential format and avoid information overload. Using open-ended questions and other listening responses can help you clarify your information for the patient. Some patients have adequate literacy skills but a limited background or lack of interest in medical matters. This makes it difficult for a patient to understand medical terminology and complex medical explanations. The advice to keep information simple and straightforward applies to all health education situations. See Table 15.1 for core constructs of health literacy with application examples.

Developing Individualized Teaching Plans

Since nurses are identified as key providers of patient education across clinical settings, it is especially important for us to incorporate health literacy strategies in all aspects of care. Evidence suggests that when healthcare providers and patients work together to make data-driven,

informed decisions, then there is more patient engagement in their personalized health plan. This philosophy of shared decision-making is not new to the nursing field but is often underused. Healthcare providers are responsible for quality of health teaching even though only the patient can ensure the outcome. Effective teaching plans provide patients and families with new or reorganized knowledge, skills, and attitudes based on scientific evidence and personally tailored to patient needs, resources, preferences, and values.

Shared Decision-Making

Shared decision-making can be defined as the gathering and evaluation of data, the exchange of information about treatment options, and the creation of an agreed upon health plan (Godolphin, 2009). In addition to understanding the treatment options, patients might need help navigating the healthcare system, which can be challenging for those with a low health literacy. Forms can be confusing or instructions misunderstood (AHRQ, 2021). It can be a time-consuming process, and the communication skills associated with the shared decision-making process can be difficult to learn and require practice. If healthcare providers are going to implement a shared decision-making process, then they will need to take the time necessary to help patients and their families understand the options available as well as the cost of those options.

As patients assume stronger collaborative responsibility for the self-management of their conditions, coaching becomes a major nursing strategy in health education and the promotion of health literacy. The nurse acts not only as an information provider but also as a guide, resource, and knowledgeable emotional support. As guides, nurses coach patients on actions they can take to improve their health. They offer suggestions on modifications as their condition changes. As information providers, they help patients become more aware of why, what, and how they can learn to take better care of themselves. As resource supports, nurses help patients connect with appropriate community social and health supports to promote health and well-being while preventing the emergence of chronic disorders and disability. Nurses act as a knowledge source and emotional support, encouraging positive learning efforts by helping patients minimize the impact of temporary setbacks and never giving up on them. For example, helping patients to anticipate actual and potential effects of a medication or treatment reduces anxiety and the incidence of errors.

Components of Patient Education

Patient-centered education should start with and incorporate the patient's perspective across all activities.

BOX 15.3 Questions to Assess Learning Needs

- What does the patient already know about his or her condition or treatment?
- In what ways is the patient affected by the condition?
- In what ways are those persons intimately involved with the patient affected by the patient's condition?
- What does the patient identify as his or her most important need?
- What goals would the patient like to achieve?
- To what extent is the patent willing to take personal responsibility for achieving goals?
- What resources are available for the patient and the family?
- What are the barriers or difficulties to accomplishing goals?

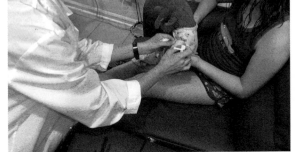

Figure 15.4 Nurse teaches diabetic child to inject insulin using favorite stuffed bear as developmentally appropriate model.

Effective health teaching tailors interventions to be compatible with patient values, goals, and resources available. Self-management strategies are designed to optimize chronic disease management for patients and families in the home and community. The focus is on skill enhancement, with full patient engagement in clinical decision-making and consistent self-management activities. Strategies start with obtaining an active provider/patient collaborative commitment to setting realistic, achievable health goals. The next step is to mutually identify specific learning outcomes with the patient and incorporate the support of essential others in the coaching process. This is followed by developing specific action plans to meet learning outcomes and evaluating their effectiveness. Consider including family members in the process to ensure a comprehensive understanding of the patient's needs and goals. See Box 15.3 for questions to help in assessing needs.

Case Study: Jack's Snacks

Jack Cominski needs help to manage his Diabetes. Jack "knows" that following his diabetic diet is essential to control his diabetes. He can tell you everything there is to know about the relationship of diet to diabetic control. Although he follows his diet at home, he eats snack foods at work and insists on extra helpings at dinner, especially when he is stressed. He says he does not mind taking extra insulin and that it is his choice to do so. Jack's problem with compliance lies in the affective domain; he resents having a lifelong condition that limits his food selections.

Motivational interviewing might be useful in working with this patient to look at his health picture from a broader perspective. This strategy would allow him to explore his ambivalence and frustration at dietary restrictions imposed by his health condition. Use questions such as "What has been the hardest thing for you?" or "What do you think needs to happen to make changes?" Without such a discussion, his behavior is unlikely to change. The cognitive domain consists of the knowledge base for the self-management skill and an understanding of the nature and dimensions of the underlying medical and psychological issues associated with the patient's diagnosis.

Developmental Factors

The patient's developmental learning factors significantly influence his or her ability to learn (Bastable, 2019). Children at different levels of cognitive development need health teaching that is specifically tailored to their developmental level. For example, children who cannot think abstractly will not understand a conceptual explanation of what is happening to them. Instead, they need simple, concrete explanations and examples. Refer to Fig. 15.4 that shows a nurse using a stuffed animal to teach a diabetic child how to give insulin injections.

Increasing health literacy in children is important because their health literacy will be carried into adulthood (Ozturk & Ayaz-Alkaya, 2020). Recommended teaching strategies for patient learners at different developmental levels are presented in Table 15.2. See Fig. 15.5 for the nurse's role in supporting patients.

TABLE 15.2 Recommended Teaching Strategies at Different Development Levels

Preschool	Allow child to touch and play with safe equipment Relate teaching to a child's immediate experience Use a child's vocabulary whenever possible Involve parents in teaching
School Age	Give factual information in simple, concrete terms and items Focus teaching on developing competency Use simple drawings and models to emphasize points Answer questions honestly and factually
Adolescent	Use metaphors and analogies in teaching Give choices and multiple perspectives Incorporate the patient's norm group values and personal identity issues in the teaching strategies
Adult	Involve patient as an active partner in the learning process Encourage self-directed learning Keep content and strategies relevant and practical Incorporate previous life experiences into teaching
Older Adult	Involve patient as an active partner in the learning process Keep content and strategies relevant and practical Incorporate previous life experiences into teaching Accommodate for sensory and dexterity deficits Use short, frequent learning sessions (<30 minutes)

Adaptations for Cognitive Processing Deficits

Learners with memory deficits, lack of insight, poor judgment, and limited problem-solving abilities require accommodations. Special needs learners respond best when the content is presented in a consistent, concrete, and patient manner, with clear and frequent cues to action. Patience and the repetition of key ideas are essential. Illustrated materials can result in greater comprehension and recall, but they should be simple, without distracting details (Friedman et al., 2011). If the deficit is more than minimal, it may be helpful to include significant others in the teaching session, as this may increase the chance of following through with instructions.

Family Involvement

Constructive family involvement is an essential component of successful self-management. The Joint Commission's standards (2014) require evidence of direct education provided to the family as well as the patient. Health teaching similar to that provided to fully functional patients is required of anyone actively involved in the patient's care as a primary caregiver or reliable supportive influence. Information and anticipatory guidance about what to expect when the patient goes home, and early warning signs of complications or potential problems, should also be given to family members. Knowing when to seek professional assistance and resource support is critical. Examples of appropriate goals for family teaching relate to empowerment of family members in using equipment, understanding what is happening to their loved one, and promoting direct involvement in therapeutic care. Note changes in the level of support from primary caregivers, as this circumstance can affect a patient's willingness or ability to learn. When these supports are no longer available through death, incapacity, or for other reasons, the patient may lack not only motivation but also the skills to cope with complex health problems.

Case Study: Teaching an Adolescent

"I am a high school student and the name of my nurse was Nadine. She was the first person who clearly explained what a bladder augmentation entailed. She described different tubes I'd have and the purpose of each. When I returned from surgery, she helped me cope with my body image by teaching me how to use my bladder and by being a compassionate listener."

Case Study: Preparing a Diabetic Teaching Plan for Mr Flanigan

Edward Flanigan, an 82-year-old recently widowed man, has severe diabetes. There is no evidence of memory problems, but there are significant emotional components to his current healthcare needs. All his life, his wife pampered him and did everything for him, from meal preparation to monitoring his diabetes. Since her death, Edward has taken no interest in controlling his diabetes. He does not follow his prescribed diabetic diet and is not consistent in taking his medication. Predictably, his diabetes has become increasingly unstable. His family worries about him, but he is unwilling to consider leaving his home of 42 years. To enhance Edward's learning readiness, how could Edward's teaching plan related to diabetic self-care management skills be individualized?

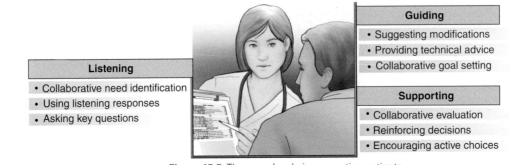

Figure 15.5 The nurse's role in supporting patients.

BOX 15.4   Suggested Format for Teaching Care Plans

- Identify patient's needs and preferences
- Identify goals (no more than three or four)
- Write a summary statement of the outcomes you and the patient want to achieve
- State two or three specific measurable behavioral objectives related to goal achievement
- Identify materials, handouts, charts, diagrams, and other resources needed to achieve patient success
- Use teach-back method to evaluate patient understanding

BOX 15.5   Guidelines for Developing Effective Goals and Objectives

- Link goals to the nursing diagnosis
- Make goals action oriented
- Make goals specific and measurable
- Define objectives as behavior outcomes
- Set a specific time frame for achievement
- Show a logical progression with established priorities
- Review periodically and modify goals as needed

Creating a Successful Teaching Plan

Teaching plans provide a guide for choosing and sequencing content and for identifying the best approach. Box 15.4 provides a sample format for developing a relevant teaching plan.

Setting realistic collaborative goals with patients with periodic reviews not only helps motivate patients but also serves as a benchmark for evaluating changes. Establish goals with your patient rather than for your patient. Clear step-by-step learning goals that the patient agrees to are more likely to be met.

Developing Measurable Objectives

Objectives help organize content and identify logical action steps. Box 15.5 provides guidelines for developing effective health teaching goals and objectives. Collaboratively developed objectives should describe an immediate action step-by-step plan for goal achievement based on the patient's most pressing clinical issues (Edwards, 2013). Each action step should build on the previous one for maximum effectiveness.

Objectives should be achievable within the allotted time frame. To determine whether an objective is achievable, consider the patient's level of experience, educational level, resources, skills, and motivation. This information helps ensure that the objectives are defined in specific measurable behavioral terms. Objectives also should directly relate to medical and nursing diagnoses and support the overall health outcome. Simulation Exercise 15.1 provides practice with the development of goals.

Evaluation and Documentation
Teach-Three and Teach-Back

Teach-back method is a simple, effective means of checking patient comprehension of care concepts, and executing self-management skills postdischarge (Klingbeil & Gibson, 2018). Patients are initially taught up to three key actions, knowledge concepts, and care skills related to self-management of their health condition. This information should be delivered in small chunks of data or skill demonstrations using terminology that the patient can easily understand. The first step in the process is to determine what the patient knows about their medical condition. Listen to questions, explain the patient's condition in terms that he or she can understand, and teach-back or "show me" is a participatory evaluation method used to confirm a patient's understanding of and/or ability to execute self-management skills through demonstration or explanation of major points. It involves having the patient explain relevant information and treatment instructions in his or her own words (Weatherspoon et al., 2015). Teach-back

SIMULATION EXERCISE 15.1 Developing Goals

Purpose
To provide practical experience with developing teaching goals.

Procedure
Establish a nursing diagnosis related to health literacy and teaching a goal that supports the diagnosis in each of the following situation:
1. Maria is a 22-year-old single woman. She is in the clinic for the first time because of cramping. She is 7 months pregnant but has had no prenatal care.
2. Shantel is an overweight middle-aged parent. She desperately wants to lose weight. However, she finds it difficult to resist snacks, especially when her kids are eating chips. She wants a plan to help her lose weight.

Reflective Discussion Analysis
1. What factors did you have to consider in developing a goal for each patient?
2. How does understanding a person's motivation help you develop personalized goals?

SIMULATION EXERCISE 15.2 Teach-Back

Purpose
To help students understand the teach-back process.

Procedure
Break into small groups. Each student will take a turn being the nurse and the patient. Using one medication that your patient is on, role-play the teach-back process for a patient receiving the medication for the first time.

Reflective Discussion Analysis
1. Reflect on the role-play simulations and discuss what each person did well as the nurse. What would you have changed to improve the teach-back?
2. What did you learn about the importance of the teach-back method?

offers nurses valuable data about areas of skill learning needing additional attention. Start with a statement such as, "I just want to be sure that I have explained everything you need to know. Can you tell me, in your own words, how you will determine that your blood sugar is low, and what you will do if it is?" Encourage the patient to ask questions. If the content is complex, consider using teach-back after each segment, before moving on to the next concept. Redo instruction if needed. Document your use of teach-back and the patient's response. Simulation Exercise 15.2 provides practice with the teach-back process.

Documenting Health Teaching

The Joint Commission (2014) requires written documentation of all patient health teaching. Notes about the initial assessment should be succinct but comprehensive and objective. Teaching content should be linked to assessment data, including patient preferences, previous knowledge, and values. Included in the documentation are the teaching actions, the patient response, and any clinical issues or barriers to compliance. If family members are involved, you should identify their role, content provided, and teaching outcomes in your documentation. Accurate documentation promotes continuity of care and prevents duplication of teaching efforts. Ask patients to keep a self-report log and share it with you as needed.

Giving Feedback

Feedback is of central importance in successful health coaching. Giving immediate feedback is important with learning psychomotor tasks. To appreciate its significance in learning new skills, consider the effect on your performance if you never received feedback from your instructor. For maximum effectiveness, give feedback as soon as possible after the learning event or observation. Consider the impact on the patient. Encourage patient reflection by asking open-ended questions such as, "How did you feel about doing your treatment by yourself?" "Is there anything you would do differently next time?"

Indirect feedback—provided through nodding, smiling, and sharing information about the process and experiences of others—also reinforces learning. When providing feedback, keep it participatory and simple. Focus only on behaviors that can be changed. Include strengths as well as areas needing improvement. Simulation Exercise 15.3 provides practice with giving feedback.

Group Presentations

On some occasions, increasing health literacy can be done in a group setting. Group settings allow individuals to hear other people's perspectives and questions. Create a presentation that focuses on a few key points. Make sure the information is accurate and easy to understand. Logical organization of the material being presented is essential. Providing specific examples helps the audience process the information being provided. Repeating key points in a summary helps to reinforce learning. Be sure to anticipate possible questions and to praise people for their questions.

SUMMARY

This chapter describes the theoretical frameworks of health teaching, patient-centered teaching of health literacy, and the implementation of a health plan. Health teaching consists of three categories: information gathering, sharing of information, and the development of an agreed upon health plan. Patient learning needs help mold individual health plans. Several teaching strategies such as coaching, visual aids, and shared decision-making are described in the chapter. Using methods such as teach-back ensures the patient's understanding of the health plan.

The Joint Commission requires documentation of patient education. The patient's record becomes a communication tool that documents areas that have been taught as well as addressing areas that need future teaching sessions.

SIMULATION EXERCISE 15.3   Feedback

Purpose
To give students perspective and experience in giving usable feedback.

Procedure
Break into small groups. One group member creates a sketch of some aspect of your current learning that you find difficult such as writing papers, speaking in front of people, group projects, time management, etc. Each member of the group should provide usable feedback for coping with the situation.

Reflective Discussion Analysis
1. What were your thoughts and feels about the feedback you heard in regard to resolving the situation presented to the group?
2. What were your thoughts and feels about providing usable feedback?
3. Reflect about the ease of providing feedback. In what situations might it be more difficult to provide feedback?

NEXT-GENERATION NCLEX® EXAMINATION-STYLE CASE STUDY

Patient Instructional Needs
Sara, a 17-year-old emancipated minor, has presented at a community-based free clinic requesting medical treatment of a foot wound. Sara's physical confirmed the presence of a 2-inch laceration on her left foot that is reddened, edematous, and producing purulent drainage. The primary care provider determines the wound is infected and will require medical interventions including laceration cleansing, dressing, and antibiotic therapy.

During her history interview, Sara stated she left her home 2 years ago after years of being physically and emotionally abused by her parents, who were both seriously abusing drugs. She moved in with extended family and went to school while working to support herself financially. When she was eventually awarded legal emancipation by the court 7 months ago, she moved to the city and joined a group of teenagers who reside in a local park. Sara volunteered that she is a diagnosed asthmatic but ran out of medication 3 weeks ago and does not know where to get more. When asked, Sara expressed in interest in being vaccinated but stated, "I'm just not sure about getting the COVID shot."

Complete the following sentences by choosing from the list of options.

The nurse would first provide verbal and written information to _____(1)_____ to ____(2)_____.

Options for 1	Options for 2
Discuss the benefits and safety of the COVID-19 vaccine options	Manage existing health needs
Explain the options for immediate treatment of laceration	Provide for environmental safety
Review options for securing prescribed medication	Secure informed consent to treat
Present community housing resource options	Minimize risk of contracting a communicable disease

ETHICAL DILEMMA: What Would You Do?

Louisa is a low-literacy patient at the mental health clinic who wants a refill of her medication. She states that she has reduced her medication to every other day rather than every day because she thinks it "works better for her." She does not want to lower her dose. She also tells the nurse that she gave several of her extra pills to her brother because he ran out of his pills. Although she listens politely to the nurse's concerns, Louisa tells her that she thinks her current regimen is appropriate for her. She sees nothing wrong with sharing her meds with her brother as he is on the same medication. If you were the nurse, how would you respond to this patient?

DISCUSSION QUESTIONS

1. Discuss what is meant by the following statement: "Patient education is essential to safe, ethical and clinical practice."
2. What specific strategies would you use to help low health literacy patients learn essential information?
3. As patients want to become more involved in their health, how is the process of shared decision-making a crucial aspect of the nursing profession?

REFERENCES

Agency for Healthcare Research and Quality (AHRQ). (2021). *Health literacy improvement tools.* Retrieved from https://www.ahrq.gov/health-literacy/improve/index.html. [Accessed 17 September 2021].

American Nurses Association (ANA). (2004). *Nursing: Scope and standards of practice.* Washington, D.C.: ANA.

Anderson, L. W., & Krathwohl, D. R. (Eds.). (2000). *A taxonomy for learning, teaching, and assessing: A revision of Bloom's taxonomy of educational objectives.* New York: Pearson.

Bastable, S. B. (2019). *Nurse as educator: Principles of teaching and learning for nursing practice* (5th ed.). Sudbury: MA: Jones & Bartlett.

Baur, C. (2011). Calling the nation to act: Implementing the national action plan to improve health literacy. *Nursing Outlook, 59*(2), 63–69.

Deek, H., Hamilton, S., Brown, N., et al. (2016). Family-centered approaches to healthcare interventions in chronic diseases in adults: A quantitative systematic review. *Journal of Advanced Nursing, 72*(5), 968–979.

Edwards, A. L. (2013). Asthma action plans and self-management: Beyond the traffic light. *Nursing Clinics of North America, 48*(1), 47–51.

Friedman, A. J., Cosby, R., Boyko, S., Hatton-Bauer, J., & Turnbull, G. (2011). Effective teaching strategies and methods of delivery for patient education: A systematic review and practice guideline recommendations. *Journal of Cancer Education, 26*(1), 12–21.

Godolphin, W. (2009). Shared decision-making. *Healthcare Quarterly, 12 Spec No Patient,* e186–e190.

Halm, M. A. (2021). When stakes are high and stress soars: Addressing health literacy in the critical care environment. *American Journal of Critical Care, 30*(4), 326–330.

Happ, M. B. (2021). Giving voice: Nurse-patient communication in the intensive care unit. *American Journal of Critical Care, 30*(4), 256–265.

Heath, S. (2017). *3 best practices for shared decision-making in healthcare.* Patient Engagement HIT. Retrieved from: https://patientengagementhit.com/news/3-best-practices-for-shared-decision-making-in-healthcare. [Accessed 6 August 2021].

Kelo, M., Eriksson, E., & Eriksson, I. (2013). Pilot educational program to enhance empowering patient education of school-age children with diabetes. *Journal of Diabetes and Metabolic Disorders, 12*(1), 16.

Klingbeil, C., & Gibson, C. (2018). The teach-back project: A system-wide evidence based practice implementation. *Journal of Pediatric Nursing, 42,* 81–85.

Knowles, M. S., Holton, E. F., & Swanson, R. A. (2011). *The adult learner: The definitive classic in adult education and human resource development* (7th ed.). Oxford, UK: Butterworth-Heinemann.

Mbanda, N., Dada, S., Bastable, K., Gimbler-Berglund, I., & Schlosser, R. W. (2021). A scoping review of the use of visual aids in health education materials for persons with low-literacy levels. *Patient Education and Counseling, 104*(5), 998–1017.

Menendez, J. B. (2013). Informed consent: Essential legal and ethical principles for nurses. *JONA's Healthcare Law, Ethics, and Regulation, 15*(4), 140–146.

Nutbeam, D., McGill, B., & Premkumar, P. (2018). Improving health literacy in community populations: A review of progress. *Health Promotion International, 33*(5), 901–911.

Ozturk, F. O., & Ayaz-Alkaya, S. (2020). Health literacy and health promotion behaviors of adolescents in Turkey. *Journal of Pediatric Nursing, 54,* e31–e35.

The Joint Commission. (2014). *Health literacy and The Joint Commission (HLOL #139).* [Podcast]. Available at: https://www.jointcommission.org/resources/news-and-multimedia/podcasts/health-equity/health-literacy-and-the-joint-commission/. [Accessed 17 September 2021].

Weatherspoon, D. J., Horowitz, A. M., Kleinman, D. V., & Wang, M. Q. (2015). The use of recommended communication techniques by Maryland family physicians and pediatricians. *PLoS One, 10*(4), e0119855.

16

Communication With Patients Who Are in Stressful Situations

At the end of the chapter, the reader will be able to:
1. Define stress and describe theoretical models.
2. Discuss concepts related to coping with stress.

3. Discuss stress assessment strategies.
4. Apply stress reduction strategies to simulated cases in which nurses could help patients manage stressful situations.

Stress is both a cause and a consequence of illness and injury. Everyone feels stress at some time but normally it is time limited, lasting less than 6 weeks. When stress is chronic, it can cause either physical or psychological harm (APA, 2020).

When a person is admitted to the hospital, that person enters a new and usually unfamiliar world. This circumstance, in itself, represents a stressful situation. This chapter will discuss biological and psychosocial models of stress reactions and the types of coping mechanisms used to deal with stress. This chapter focuses on helping patients develop coping strategies to reduce the impact of stress reactions in healthcare. It identifies communication strategies nurses can use to help patients and families reduce stress levels.

Nurses and other primary providers of care, especially those working in highly acute nursing situations, are especially vulnerable to stress and burnout. Chapter 27 will discuss intrapersonal communication and strategies nurses can use to self-manage stress.

BASIC CONCEPTS

Definition

A **stressor** is any demand, situation, internal stimulus, or circumstance that threatens the individual. Selye (1950) defined stress as a nonspecific response of the body to any demand made upon it, regardless of whether it is caused by a pleasant or unpleasant situation. As stress levels increase, both physical and psychological responses are triggered. A stress response is a common reaction to serious illness that affects quality of life for all family members as well as the patient's ability to function.

Stress represents a natural physiological, psychological, and spiritual response to the presence of a stressor. A stress reaction differs from a crisis situation. Unlike crisis, stress responses are usually less dramatic. Internal stressors such as pregnancy, fever, menopause, or emotions originate within the body. External stressors—such as social or work stressors, accidents, debt, and exams—start outside the self. Strengthening a patient's capacity to cope effectively with stress has important implications for clinical outcomes as well as the patient's motivation and capacity to perform self-management. A stress assessment should be incorporated as part of the complex data needed to support a person's ability to adapt to chronic illness.

Crisis represents an extreme acute stressor situation for which coping mechanisms fail and the person is unable to function normally. By definition, a crisis situation is usually resolved within 6 weeks.

Incidence

Stress is a common part of life, a universal experience. The stress response is commonly present in most healthcare situations. According to the American Psychological Society, 77% of people with stress report developing physical symptoms (Hunt, 2019). We each develop different coping mechanisms. Stress represents a personal experience.

CASE STUDY: **Michael Johns Has Parkinson's Disease**

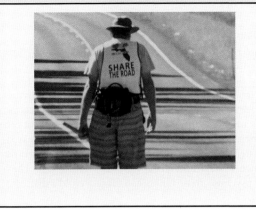

Michael has been diagnosed with Parkinson's disease, a degenerative condition for which there is no known cure. Medication is available for management of tremors. Knowing that the disease will eventually rob him of physical self-care abilities, and that he will increasingly experience cognitive dysfunction, is very stressful. He vows to fight. His physician tells him exercise is a best practice to postpone dysfunction, so he walks daily and plays tennis three to four times each week. His nurse wife works on helping him with cognitive aids, such as making lists, doing crossword puzzles, and marking "to do" items on his calendar.

What is stressful for one person may not be for another. Stress can develop over time or can strike without warning. Stressors can affect many people at the same time—for example, war, hurricane, earthquake or severe flood damage, community shootings in schools, or terrorist attacks can be cumulative, continuous, or just minor hassles. Consider the case of Mr Johns.

Etiology

Personal stress can be related to a major life change (marriage, divorce, death, moving to a new area, becoming a parent, graduating from college, starting a new job) or an illness or injury. A new diagnosis, loss of social ties, premature death, and potential damage from adjuvant therapy are common health-related stressors. Some of the more common personal sources of stress are identified in Box 16.1.

Symptoms of Stress
Patient
Somatic symptoms vary but can include gastrointestinal upsets, headaches, changes in weight, and many more reflecting the increased release of cortisol. Psychological symptoms may include sleep disturbances, worry, anxiety, increased irritability, etc.

Family
In healthcare situations, sources of emotional stress include watching a loved one steadily decline physically or mentally, concern about finances, uncertainty about the future, balancing other family responsibilities with patient care, and coping with personal frustration.

Stressors likely to stimulate an intense stress response are those where a person has limited control over the

---

BOX 16.1 Examples of Personal Sources of Stress

Physical Stressors
- Acute or chronic illness
- Trauma or injury
- Pain
- Insomnia
- Mental disorder

Psychological Stressors
- Loss of job or job security
- Loss of a significant person or pet
- Significant change in residence, relationship, work
- Personal finances
- Work relationships
- High-stress work environment
- Caretaking (frail elderly, children)
- Significant change or loss of role

Spiritual Stressors
- Loss of purpose
- Loss of hope
- Questioning of values or meaning

---

situation, the situation is ambiguous, or aspects of the current situation resemble past unresolved stressful events.

Intensity
The intensity and duration of stress vary according to the circumstances, level of social support, and the person's emotional state. Significant or prolonged stress can increase the impact of a current stressful situation.

Mentally ill patients have a double set of chronic stressors. Some stem from their mental disorder, which lowers a patient's threshold for stress and diminishes a person's capacity to act effectively to reduce the stress.

Levels of Stress

Mild

Selye used the term *eustress* to describe a mild level of stress, which is a positive response with protective and adaptive functions. Mild stress heightens awareness and can motivate people to master challenges and develop new skills. Coping skills learned in mastering a stressful situation help people cope better with other life circumstances as well.

Severe

Distress, defined as a negative stress level, creates a level of anxiety exceeding a person's normal coping abilities. Distress diminishes performance and quality of life. High stress levels interfere with a person's ability to function. Severe, chronic stress weakens the immune system, thereby contributing to the development of stress-related illnesses.

Acute

Stress can create a very intense form of anxiety, which is disabling for the person experiencing it. Once the situation is resolved, homeostasis is reestablished. Untreated, severe mental stress reactions associated with traumatic events can develop into posttraumatic stress disorder, a clinical syndrome requiring psychiatric intervention.

Chronic

While stress can be a lifesaving response, the accumulation of many stressors, termed chronic stress, is harmful. It is implicated in the development and exacerbation of cardiac conditions, migraine, and digestive disorders. Stress and coping contribute various psychological symptoms.

Variation in Stress Responses

Although stress is a universal occurrence, it is a subjective personal experience. People have different tolerance levels for stress. Some people are extremely sensitive to any stressor. Others are laid back and appear less disturbed by unexpected stressful circumstances.

More than mild stress reduces the efficiency of cognitive functions and clouds perceptual acuity. Secondary stressors, such as insomnia caused by worry and financial issues, can heighten the impact of primary stressors on a person's personal life and routines. The level of social and resource support that a person receives when stressed can reduce the impact of a stressor.

Gender

Some researchers have suggested that men and women respond to stress differently, that men respond with patterns of "fight or flight," whereas women use a "tend and befriend" approach. Women use nurturing activities to reduce stress and promote safety for self and others as priority interventions. They seek social support from others, particularly from other women. Children express stress through behavior, usually corresponding with their developmental stage and family patterns. Acting-out behaviors and psychosomatic illness can mask a child's distress.

THEORETICAL MODELS OF STRESS

Systemic Physiological Response

Walter Cannon (1932) described stress as a systemic physiological response to a perceived threat. It occurs in a similar way regardless of the stressor. Cannon believed that when people feel physically well, emotionally centered, and personally secure, they are in a state of dynamic equilibrium, or **homeostasis**. Stress disturbs homeostasis. Physiologically, the hypothalamus and sympathetic nervous system set in motion an immediate hormonal cascade designed to mobilize the body's energy resources to cope with acute stress. The autonomic nervous system and sympathetic nervous subsystem signal nerve endings and the adrenal medulla. Adrenaline and noradrenalin release enhances muscle strength, increases heart rate, and releases sugars and fats to increase available energy to prepare for "fight or flight" (NIH, 2020).

The "fight" response refers to a person's inclination to take action against a threat. This response is used if the threat appears to be resolvable. People use a flight response if they perceive that the threat cannot be overcome through personal effort.

General Adaptation Syndrome

Hans Selye (1950) described stress as a physiological whole-body response to stress, evidenced primarily through the endocrine and autonomic nervous systems. Referred to as the *general adaptation syndrome*, this causes the same physiological responses described earlier, occurring regardless of whether a stressor is psychological or physical.

Selye described a three-stage progressive pattern of nonspecific physiological responses: alarm, resistance, and exhaustion. The "*alarm* stage" is similar to Cannon's acute stress response. If the stressor is not resolved in the initial alarm stage, a second level adaptive phase, *"resistance stage"* occurs as the body tries to accommodate for the stressor. In the resistance stage, overt alarm symptoms subside as the immune system helps the body to adapt to the demands of the stressor. If the body fails to adapt or is unable to resist the continued stress, it leads to an *"exhaustion stage."* At this point, the person becomes higher risk for a stress-related illness, or mental disorder. The longer the physiological stress response remains elevated, the greater is the negative impact on the person.

Allostasis

Huber and others describe the human organism as being in a state of physical homeostasis. **Allostasis** is this theory of stress response. It describes how the human organism maintains physiological homeostasis through changing circumstances. The brain serves as a primary mediator between the current exposure, internal regulation of bodily processes, and health outcomes.

Allostatic accommodation is the physiological process through which the brain tries to find a new homeostasis, using a range of adaptive functioning. The interaction between stressors and physical responses is ongoing, such that individuals become more or less susceptible to the negative consequences of stress over time. Inclusion of genetic risk factors, early life events, and adaptive lifestyle behaviors offers a way to understand the interaction between stressful events and physiological adaptation processes (McEwen, 2012). Fig. 16.1 identifies the relationships in the model.

Stress hormones protect the body against short-term acute stress (allostasis). Stress mediators, such as social support, can provide protective effects. When slight or moderate levels of stressor exposure are encountered and social support is available, coping with stress can actually work to strengthen well-being and quality of life.

Complex or prolonged stress levels are more problematic. According to McEwen (2007), early life experiences with stress can have a cumulative wear and tear on the brain and body. If a stressor presents continued challenges or coping responses are ineffective, there is "wear and tear" on the body, which can have a damaging effect. McEwen terms this phenomenon *allostatic load.* The allostatic load can be negligible, severe, or protracted enough to result in significant illness or death if untreated.

Psychosocial Frameworks
Critical Life Events

Holmes and Rahe (1967) consider stressful life events—such as marriage, divorce, death, and losing a job—as stimuli

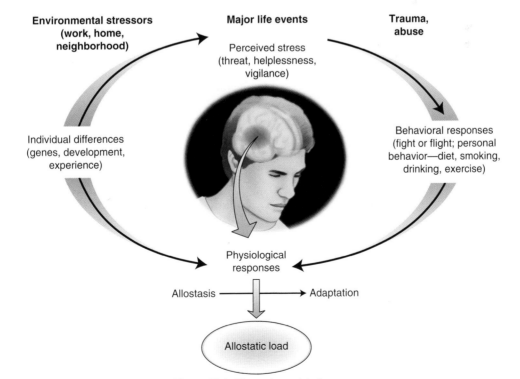

Figure 16.1 Allostasis model of stress.

sufficient to disrupt homeostasis and thus create stress. The Holmes and Rahe scale assigns each life event a weighted numeric score reflecting its potential impact. Stressors requiring a significant change in the person's lifestyle have greater impact, as do the number of cumulative stresses on the scale.

Transactional Model of Stress

Lazarus and Folkman's (1984) transactional appraisal model of stress is widely used in healthcare. Basically this is a psychological model; it considers stress as a two-way interactive process involving both the stressor and the individual's interpretive response to the stressor. According to the transactional model of stress and coping, when stress occurs, the stressor creates a significant adaptive demand requiring a response from the individual.

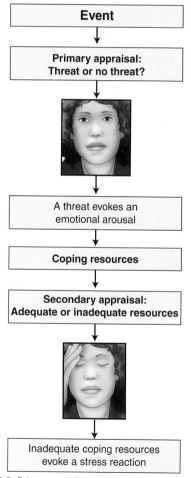

Figure 16.2 Primary and secondary appraisal in stress reactions.

It is not the objective stressor that accounts for how a person responds to a stressor. Rather, primary response mediators are as follows: (1) primary appraisal refers to a person's interpretation of the severity of a stressor, and (2) secondary appraisal describes a person's perception of his or her personal ability to resolve the stressful situation (Fig. 16.2).

This transactional model helps explain individual differences in personal responses to stressors that objectively could be thought of as having the same stress value. There are two forms of appraisal. A primary appraisal examines the strength of a person's belief about the potential harm that a stressor holds for a person. The stronger the perceived threat to self-integrity, the greater the stress response. The secondary appraisal considers a person's perception of personal coping skills and availability of appropriate social environmental resources to reduce a stressor's impact. Both appraisals are required to determine whether a stressor will be considered to be a harmful threat or challenge. People experience stress if they appraise the stressor to be threatening and/or feel incapable of meeting the stressor's demands with available resources.

COPING

Coping is defined as the constantly changing cognitive and behavioral efforts to manage specific external or internal demands that are appraised as taxing or exceeding the resources of the person. The classical definition of coping is any response to external life strains that serves to prevent, avoid, or control emotional distress. They identify three purposes of coping strategies:
- To change the stressful situation (problem-focused)
- To change the meaning of the stressor (meaning-focused)
- To help the person relax enough to take the stress in stride (emotion-focused)

Cultural Impact on Coping Strategies

Culture plays a role in determining a person's stress and coping behaviors by
1. shaping the types of stressors a person is likely to experience;
2. influencing the patient's appraisal of stress;
3. affecting the choice of coping strategies; and
4. providing different resources and institutional mechanism as coping options.

People learn coping strategies from their parents, peers, and life experiences. Those with varied life opportunities and supportive people in their lives have an advantage over those who lack opportunity and/or support systems.

SIMULATION EXERCISE 16.1   Examining Own Personal Coping Strategies

Purpose
To help students identify the wide range of adaptive and maladaptive coping strategies.

Procedure
1. Identify all of the ways in which you handle stressful situations.
2. List three personal strategies that you have used successfully in coping with stress.
3. List one personal coping strategy that did not work and identify your perceptions of the reasons it was inadequate or insufficient to reduce your stress level.
4. List on a chalkboard or flip chart the different coping strategies identified by students.

Reflective Discussion Analysis
1. What common themes did you find in the ways people handle stress?
2. Were you surprised at the number and variety of ways in which people handle stress?
3. What new coping strategy might you use to reduce your stress level?
4. Are there any circumstances that increase or decrease your automatic reactions to stress?

People who have been overprotected or were repeatedly exposed to danger without support generally lack adequate coping skills. Simulation Exercise 16.1 is intended to help identify common personal coping strategies.

Types of Coping

Appraisal theory describes coping as a process by which a person makes cognitive and behavioral efforts to manage psychological stress. Two types of coping, an approach problem focused style and an emotion focused style, are the most commonly used coping strategies.

Problem-focused coping strategies tend to be purposeful active, task-oriented methods to reduce stress. Examples include confronting a problem directly, negotiating for a different solution, seeking social support, constructive problem-solving, and taking action. In general, problem-focused coping strategies have been found to be the most effective in reducing stress. For example, studies have shown that adolescents using problem-solving strategies to control their diabetes demonstrate better diabetic control

and experience a higher quality of life than those who do not.

Emotion-focused coping strategies act in a different way to minimize the influence of stress in the patient's mind. These strategies can be effective when the stressor is perceived as an overwhelming irreversible situation or a person needs respite from overthinking about a stressful situation. Emotion-focused coping strategies—such as meditation, yoga, or spirituality—are constructive when a person deliberately chooses to "let go" of negative feelings associated with an unmanageable stressor and employ other strategies.

Most people use both types of coping strategies, with the choice of strategy dependent on the nature of the stressor and a person's typical coping style. Awareness of personal and external resources adds options. Individuals who believe that they have options are generally better able to cope with stress. Common personal coping assets, referred to as "resource options," include health, energy, problem-solving skills, the amount and availability of social supports, and other material resources to cope effectively with the stressor.

Meaning-focused coping strategies help to reframe the meaning or significance of the stressor so that it loses its power as an overwhelming challenge and becomes a challenge in need of a change in focus level. The stressor may still exist, but the greater calmness that the behavioral focused coping strategy provides can realign its impact.

Defensive Coping Strategies

Although some forms of coping yield positive results to reduce stress, others are negative influences. Rumination, denial, anger, excessive anxiety, use of drugs, or alcohol can increase the effects of stressors and further add to distress. **Ego defense mechanisms** are defined as a coping style that people use to protect the self from full awareness of challenging conflict situations. They are designed to protect the ego from anxiety and loss of self-esteem by denying, avoiding, or projecting responsibility for a challenging conflict to an external source.

Ego defense mechanisms can be temporarily adaptive by minimizing the threat of a potentially overwhelming stressor. Persistent use of the ego defense mechanisms presented in Table 16.1 is considered pathological. As a primary stress reducer, defense mechanisms are ineffective because avoidant behavior typically delays action and compromises trust in relationships. Some defense mechanisms—humor, anticipation, affiliation (asking for help), and sublimation—can be adaptive. Reflect on the Lopez case.

TABLE 16.1   Ego Defense Mechanisms

Ego Defense Mechanism	Clinical Example
Regression: Returning to an earlier, more primitive form of behavior in the face of a threat to self-esteem	Julie was completely toilet-trained by 2 years of age. When her younger brother was born, she began wetting her pants and wanting a pacifier at night.
Repression: Unconscious forgetting of parts or all of an experience	Elizabeth has just lost her job. Her friends would not know from her behavior that she has any anxiety about it. She continues to spend money as if she were still getting a paycheck.
Denial: Unconscious refusal to allow painful facts, feelings, or perceptions into awareness	Bill Marshall has had a massive heart attack. His physician advises him to exercise in moderation with caution. Bill continues to jog 6 miles a day.
Rationalization: Offering a plausible excuse or explanation for unacceptable behavior	Ann Marie tells her friends she is not an alcoholic, even though she has blackouts, because she drinks only on weekends and when she is not working.
Projection: Attributing unacceptable feelings, facts, behaviors, or attitudes to others; usually expressed as blame	Ruby just received a critical performance evaluation from her supervisor. She tells her friends that her supervisor does not like her.
Displacement: Redirecting feelings onto an object or person considered less of a threat than the original object or person	Mrs. Jones took Mary to the doctor for bronchitis. She is not satisfied with the doctor's explanation and feels he was condescending, but she says nothing. When she gets to the receptionist's desk to make the next appointment, she yells at her for not having the prescription ready and taking too much time to set the appointment.
Intellectualization: Unconscious focusing on only the intellectual and not the emotional aspects of a situation or circumstance	Johnnie has been badly hurt in a car accident. There is reason to believe he will not survive surgery. His father, waiting for his son to return to the intensive care unit, asks the nurse many questions about the equipment, and philosophizes about the meaning of life and death.
Reaction formation: Unconscious assumption of traits that are the opposite of undesirable behaviors	John has a strong family history of alcoholism on both sides. He abstains from liquor and is known in the community as an advocate of prohibition.
Sublimation: Redirecting socially unacceptable unconscious thoughts and feelings into socially approved outlets	Bob has a lot of aggressive tendencies. He decided to become a butcher and thoroughly enjoys his work.
Undoing: Verbal expression or actions representing one feeling, followed by expression of the direct opposite	Barbara criticizes her subordinate, Carol, before a large group of people. Later, she sees Carol on the street and tells her how important she is to the organization.

Case Study: Lynn Lopez and Weight Loss

Lynn was diagnosed as having high cholesterol and was advised to lose weight. She sees no purpose in going on a diet because "it's all in the genes." Both her parents had high cholesterol and died of heart problems. Lynn claims that there is nothing she can do about it, even though her physician advised her differently. Her defensive interpretation prevents her from taking actions needed to reduce her risk for cardiovascular disease. Motivational interviewing offers guidelines for gently casting doubt, providing new information, and introducing problem-solving to resistant patients. Her nurse inquires about Lynn's personal health goals and provides her with information about the link between diet, exercise, and heart disease. Linking information to Lynn's stated life goals provides her with a different frame of reference.

Resilience

Resilience is a physiologic and psychologic phenomenon. It is linked to well-being and burnout prevention. It is defined as the ability of individuals who are exposed to highly disruptive stressors to remain relatively stable and functional and cope successfully with stress (Henshall et al., 2020). Resilience is a fluid process ebbing and flowing, changing with one's circumstances (Taylor et al., 2020). Resilience explains why some people seem to weather stress and adversity more easily than others and are able to grow from the experience. Through development of a strong internal sense of control and a positive attitude, patients can develop the skills needed to override their stress and move forward despite stressful life events.

Characteristics of resilience include empowerment and creativity. Resilient people develop coping mechanisms that allow them to see a situation as it is, to focus on what can be changed, and to accept what cannot be altered. Helping patients develop clear goals, shape relevant problem-solving skills, and take baby steps toward identified goals is a means of improving personal resilience. A person develops resiliency through practice, social support, and learning self-efficacy strategies. Examples of relevant strategies include developing an organized way of coping with challenges and cultivating a meaningful support system. A strong faith and sense of purpose are other factors associated with resilience.

Hardiness

Hardiness is considered as a protective factor that can minimize the effects of stress. The concept of **hardiness** consists of three basic elements:

- *Challenge*—looking at stressors and characterizing the need for change as an opportunity for personal growth
- *Commitment*—developing a sense of purpose and a strong involvement in directing one's life
- *Taking control*—the belief that one can help to influence one's life's outcomes

Resilience and hardiness act as protective factors that influence a person's ability to view stress events as ultimately being manageable.

Maladaptive Coping

Using some coping strategies on a short-term basis enables individuals to manage stress. But when their usual cooping fails, they may employ harmful strategies such as use of street drugs, alcohol, or uncontrolled anger. Even denial, while useful in the short-term protection of a patient from the full awareness of the stressor, it can eventually hinder them from actually dealing with their illness and can lead to other health problems.

Health Organization Imperative

Organizations

Rapid changes in healthcare systems impact our working environment. The National Academies Press released a major report in 2019 advocating six specific steps healthcare organizations need to take. Changes center now on new technology and effects of regulating agencies. But in the future, societal changes and evolving healthcare models may radically affect our nursing practice. Some changes are not always compatible with our professional values (National Academies, 2019). This can become stressful for physicians and nurses. Organizational factors can be contributors to burnout. Employing organizations have a responsibility to build strategies to help staff cope with difficult experiences in the workplace (Taylor, 2020). Fostering a culture of collegiality, establishing manageable workloads, and involving employees in decision-making have been advocated (IHI, 2020).

Nurses

Some agencies have established mentorship or residency programs for new nurses. Nurse managers have instituted debriefing sessions immediately following difficult clinical experiences, especially deaths of multiple patients (Kelly et al., 2020). Additional training and frequent supportive conversations have been suggested when there is a pattern of poor staff communication. Nurses who are female, younger, and assigned to demanding medical units have been shown to be more vulnerable with the high demands placed upon them. They need support (Molina-Praena et al., 2018). Such strategies have helped reduce staff turnover. For organizations, this is a motivator, since it costs the organization up to a hundred thousand dollars to recruit and train a replacement nurse.

APPLICATIONS

Communication

Since stress is universal, it is something you have in common, perhaps to a lesser degree. When the patient of a family is highly stressed, it is important to communicate frequently. Use a calm manor and vocal tone. It takes practice to cultivate a positive attitude. When you observe nonverbal cues to stress, try to help the patient give voice to their feelings, moving up to a level that gives more control. Try saying "This must be difficult for you; can you tell me what worries you the most?"

Stress Assessment

Stress is an unwelcome part of most illnesses and injury. It is rarely a personal choice. People experience and cope with stress in different and sometimes unexpected ways. Nurses can be instrumental in helping patients cope with stress effectively so that their anxiety does not dominate

DEVELOPING AN EVIDENCE-BASED PRACTICE

Resilience has been called a personality characteristic that serves as a buffer for people coping with severe stress. Currently a number of studies are examining resilience levels and outcomes, while some are examining the effects of *resiliency training programs* on outcomes for patients or healthcare staff that are designed to build resilience and psychological strength. Dombrowsky's 2021 study examined the effects of resilience on postoperative outcomes for 73 patients having shoulder arthroplasty. Komachi (2018) and Chen (2021) studied the resilience of family members. Kim's 2019 analysis of 17 studies actually examined the effects of resiliency training programs on patients with chronic diseases.

Results

Studies show a correlation between higher resilience and lower occurrence of adverse conditions. Dombrowsky found greater resilience correlated with less post-op pain, better range of motion, and greater patient perception of normalcy. Chen found that low resiliency correlated with higher stress (PTSD) and also found that family social support acts as a mediator of adverse outcomes. In Kim's meta-analysis, attending a resiliency training program resulted in less depression and stress for patients with chronic disease. These findings are supported by Henshall's (2020) examination of effects of resiliency training programs.

Strength of research evidence: Low due to variability in definition of resiliency, the length of resiliency training interventions, and the lack of long-term follow-up.

Application to Your Clinical Practice

1. Since there is some evidence that increasing patient resiliency results in better health outcomes, nurses may want to teach patients some resiliency and stress reduction techniques.
2. Since family support is associated with higher patient resiliency, nurses may advocate for increasing family presence at the patient's bedside.

References

Chen, J. J., Wang, Q. L., Li, H. P., Zhang, T., Zhang, S. S., & Zhou, M. K. (2021). Family resilience, perceived social support, and individual resilience in cancer couples: Analysis using the actor-partner interdependence mediation model. *The European Journal of Oncology Nursing, 52*, 101932.

Dombrowsky, A. R., Kirchner, G., Isbell, J., et al. (2021). Resilience correlates with patient reported outcomes after reverse total shoulder arthroplasty. *Orthopaedics & Traumatology: Surgery & Research, 107*(1), 102777.

Henshall, C., Davey, Z., & Jackson, D. (2020). Nursing resilience interventions—A way forward in challenging healthcare territories. *Journal of Clinical Nursing, 29*(19–20), 3597–3599.

Kim, G. M., Lim, J. Y., Kim, E. J., & Park, S. M. (2019). Resilience of patients with chronic diseases: A systematic review. *Health & Social Care in the Community, 27*(4), 797–807.

Komachi, M. H., & Kamibeppu, K. (2018). Association between resilience, acute stress symptoms and characteristics of family members of patients at early admission to the intensive care unit. *Mental Health & Prevention, 9*, 34–41.

---

their health experience and they are able to function effectively. The stress of receiving care in an intensive care unit may be high for both patient and family members so they may eventually experience symptoms commonly associated with PTSD, such as anxiety and depression (Komachi & Kamibeppu, 2018). Factors that influence the impact of stress are identified in Box 16.2.

Addressing stress issues and teaching patient-related coping strategies enhance clinical outcomes and recovery potential. An initial assessment should include the patient's

- perception of current stressors;
- perception of the stressor causing the greatest stress;
- insight about the value or meaning attached to the stressor;
- identification of usual coping strategies used to manage stressful situations;

BOX 16.2   Factors That Influence the Impact of Stress

- Magnitude and demands of the stressor on self and others
- Multiple stressors occurring at the same time
- Suddenness or unpredictability of a stressful situation
- Accumulation of stressors and duration of the stress demand
- Level of social support available to the patient and family
- Previous trauma, which can activate unresolved fears
- Presence of an associated mental disorder
- Developmental level of the patient
- Normal attitude and outlook
- Knowledge, expectations, and realistic picture

- assessment of linked issues such as developmental stage, culture, family ways of coping, and level of support; and
- religious and spiritual beliefs and activities.

Assess Coping Mechanisms

Assess patient's past coping mechanisms by asking "What do you do to relieve your stress?" or "Who do you rely on when you feel very stressed?"

Ask open-ended questions about changes in daily routines, new roles, and responsibilities. Explore the patient's and family's current understanding of diagnosis and treatment options. Pay close attention to cultural values.

Prevention of Stress

Experts cite the four A's to relieve stress: avoid, alter, accept, and adapt. You can teach patients to avoid stress by planning ahead to take control of their surroundings. The classic example concerns heavy traffic. It that is a stressor, leave earlier or use an alternate route. If work demands are increasing, prioritize what needs to be done, say "no" when asked to take on extra jobs, and manage time by setting limits on how long to devote to a task. Accept that some things are beyond their control and cannot be changed. Reframe problems, look at things from another point of view, and cultivate a positive attitude.

Sources of Stress in Healthcare

Goal. As nurses, we should try to reduce patient stress when possible. Be open to letting them vent their feelings. Name the feelings as you observe them. Try saying "You seem to really be struggling right now. How can I help?" All health disruptions create a sense of vulnerability. Health-related stressors for patients and families include fear of death, uncertainty about diagnosis, clinical outcomes, changes in roles, disruption of family life, and financial concerns. Hospital-related sources of stress include physical discomfort, strange noises and lights, unfamiliar people asking personal questions, and strange equipment. Simulation Exercise 16.2 provides practice with helping patients handle stressful situations.

Identify the Stressor. A patient-centered approach pays attention to the *type* of stress a patient is experiencing. When stress presents as anxiety, the nurse might suggest problem-solving techniques. However, if the stress is related to a significant loss, the nurse would want to focus on the loss and work with the patient from a grief perspective. Box 16.3, developed by a nursing student, provides an assessment and intervention tool that you can use to organize assessment data and plan interventions.

SIMULATION EXERCISE 16.2 Impact of Stress: Relationships Between Anger and Anxiety

Purpose

To help students appreciate the links between anger and anxiety and understand how anger is triggered.

Procedure

1. Think of a time when you were really angry. It need not be a significant event, or one that would necessarily make anyone else angry.
2. Identify your thoughts, feelings, and behavior in separate columns of a table you construct. For example, what were the thoughts that went through your head when you were feeling this anger? What were your physical and emotional responses to this experience? Write down words or phrases to express what you were feeling at the time. How did you respond when you were angry?
3. Identify what was going on with you before experiencing the anger. Sometimes it is not the event itself but your feelings before the incident that make the event the straw that breaks the camel's back.
4. Identify underlying threats to your self-concept in the situation (e.g., you were not treated with respect, your opinion was discounted, you lost status, you were rejected, you feared the unknown).

Reflective Discussion Analysis

1. In what ways were your answers similar to and different from those of your classmates?
2. What role did anxiety and threat to your self-concept play in the development of the anger response? What percentage of your anger related to the actual event and to your self-concept?
3. In what ways did you see anger as a multidetermined behavioral response to threats to your self-concept?
4. Did this exercise change any of your ideas about how you might handle your feelings and behavior in a similar situation?
5. What are the common threads in the events that made people in your group angry?
6. In what ways could experiential knowledge of the close association between anger and anxiety be helpful in your nursing practice?

Behavioral Observations

Stress behaviors are sometimes hard to understand or accept. Distress often presents through behavior rather than through words. For example, anxiety can present in

BOX 16.3   Assessment and Intervention Tool

Assessment

A. Perception of stressors
  1. Major stress area or health concern
  2. Present circumstances related to usual pattern
  3. Experienced similar problem? How was it handled?
  4. Anticipation of future consequences
  5. Expectations of self
  6. Expectations of caregivers
B. Intrapersonal factors
  1. Physical (mobility, body function)
  2. Psychosociocultural (attitudes, values, coping patterns)
  3. Developmental (age, factors related to present situation)
  4. Spiritual belief system (hope and sustaining factors)
C. Interpersonal factors
  1. Resources and relationship of family or significant others as they relate to or influence interpersonal factors
D. Environmental factors
  1. Resources and relationships of community as they relate to or influence interpersonal factors

Prevention as Intervention

A. Primary
  1. Classify stressor
  2. Provide information to maintain or strengthen strengths
  3. Support positive coping mechanisms
  4. Educate patient and family
B. Secondary
  1. Mobilize resources
  2. Motivate, educate, involve patient in healthcare goals
  3. Facilitate appropriate interventions; refer to external resources as needed
  4. Provide information on primary prevention or intervention as needed
C. Tertiary
  1. Attain/maintain wellness
  2. Educate or reeducate as needed
  3. Coordinate resources
  4. Provide information about primary and secondary interventions

Unpublished, Developed by Conrad, J. (1993). Baltimore, MD: University of Maryland School of Nursing.

the form of heart palpations, shortness of breath, sweating, and muscle tension. Other physical and mental symptoms of stress include the following:

- Significant changes in eating or sleeping habits
- Headaches, gastric problems, muscular tension, aches and pains, tightness in the throat
- Restlessness and irritability
- Inability to cope with normal everyday concerns and obligations
- Inability to concentrate

Processing Strong Feelings

When strong stress feelings get bottled up in the patient, constructive problem-solving ceases. Often nurses can tell that patients are stressed from their body language, even when they deny strong feelings. Some patients say they are okay when they are not. Helpful statements include "This must be very difficult for you to absorb" or "Can you tell me what you are experiencing?" Your immediate goal is to help patients step back and take a second look at their situation from a broader perspective. A calm accepting presence and willingness to listen to the patient's story allow nurses and patients to develop a shared understanding of a stressful event. You can help a patient normalize stressful feelings such as, "I think I'm losing my mind," with a statement such as, "What you are feeling is not unusual; although it feels that way, you are having a normal response to a sudden, overwhelming situation. Can you tell me what worries you the most?" Notice in both probes, the nurse acknowledges the legitimacy of feelings as a normal response to an abnormal situation. Once the patient begins to calm down, it becomes possible to look at the situation more realistically.

Anger and Hostility

Anger and hostility are common stress responses associated with feeling helpless or psychologically threatened. Patients (and/or families) become hostile when they feel threatened about what is happening or feel they have little control in a situation. Anxiety usually exists as the underpinning of anger. What hostile patients or families need most, despite their hostile behavior, is understanding and caring.

Carefully listening to a patient's concerns goes a long way toward neutralizing anger and hostility. The patient feels heard, even if the issues cannot be fully resolved to the patient's satisfaction. Set limits if necessary, but do so with a calm attitude and empathetic matter-of-fact manner. If patient and/or family expectations are unrealistic, or cannot be met in the current situation, alternative explanations and suggestions can be introduced.

Use an open, nonthreatening stance and a calm attitude. Use an informal conversational format. Being patient and willing to listen is important. Your patient's reactions will serve as a guide as to how much and how quickly the information can be gathered.

Contemporary healthcare environments with advanced technology, shorter stays, and multiple caregivers are complex and anxiety producing. Sources of stress for families can include fear of death, uncertain outcome, emotional turmoil, financial concerns, role changes, disruption of routines, and unfamiliar hospital environments. Families look to nurses for support and direction. Regular communication and providing updated information about a family member's condition is a key component of stress reduction. Statements such as "Most people would feel anxious in this situation" or "It would be hard for anyone to have all the answers in a situation like this" can normalize difficult situations. Or "Seeing your husband like this must be a terrible shock. I suspect you might be wondering how you are going to cope with his care at home." This type of statement normalizes feelings and introduces subjects that are difficult but necessary to talk about. Nurses can help families process complex information and address specific concerns. Topics should focus on what will happen next, how to explain the illness to others, or what the patient or family is experiencing related to the stressor. Table 16.2 identifies interventions to decrease family stress.

Social Support as a Resource to Cope With Stress

Social support is defined as the emotional comfort, advice, and instrumental assistance that a person receives from other people in their social network. Social support is an essential buffer against stress. Families can be a major support for patients in managing health-related distress. The concept has three distinct functions in helping patients reduce stress levels: validation, emotional support, and correction of distorted thinking. Social support refers to both the perceived availability of help and support actually received.

Support Network

A person's social networks are drawn from family, friends, church, work, social groups, or school. Being able to contact family and friends when you need help reduces stress. Not only does sharing with others reduce stress by "externalizing" negative emotions, but family, friends, and support groups can provide a sounding board, practical assistance, and tangible encouragement. Seeking help can empower both seeker and provider of emotional support.

Community Support

Community resources include support groups, social services, and other public health agencies that provide practical support, as well as social contacts. Nurses need to be aware of community support services, including support groups such as AA, Parkinson's support groups, diabetes support groups, and so on. Large numbers of support groups are available on the Internet. Many meet using platforms such as "Zoom."

Spiritual Support

Belief in a personal god or higher power provides patients with a personal resource. Multiple studies reveal that spiritual interventions can help prevent and improve physical illnesses, and have helped patient cope with chronic pain and death. Some people rely on faith to facilitate their acceptance of a reality that cannot be changed. Assessing spiritual needs and offering to arrange a chaplain visit is a nursing consideration.

Assessing Impact of Stress on Family Relationships

Stress Issues for Children

Health disruptions create special stress for children; they lack the words and life experience to sort out the meaning of illness, either their own or that of a significant family member. Children express their stress through behavior. Signs of distress, such as academic decline, gastric distress, and headaches, can alert the nurse to unvoiced stress. In the hospital, children may withdraw, demonstrate clinging behaviors, or have frequent meltdowns. Uncertainty creates stress for both parents and children. Communicating information frequently helps parents. Children need to have their questions answered simply and honestly, consistent with their developmental stage. Small children can be encouraged to express their stress feelings through drawings or play.

Stress Issues for Older Adults

Stress issues for older adults often relate to multiple health challenges and an increased potential for loss of important interpersonal supports and independent living during this phase of life. Worry about finances is common. Stress management strategies for older adults from a health promotion perspective include maintaining an active social life and a healthy lifestyle, and engagement in hobbies of volunteer work not only reduces stress but also improves quality of life.

Education for Stress Reduction

Information is an essential stress reducer. Relevant information can range from providing basic data about visiting

TABLE 16.2   Nursing Interventions to Decrease Family Anxiety

Recommendation	Specific Actions
Identify a family spokesperson and support persons involved in decision-making.	Choose a person the family and patient trusts; establish mechanisms for contact.
Identify a primary nursing contact for the family.	If possible, choose the nurse most in contact with the patient. Meet with the family within 24 hours of admission to explain roles of each healthcare team member. Provide contact number to family spokesperson.
Discuss family access to the patient.	Arrange for visitation based on unit protocols, patient condition and needs, and family preferences. Educate the family about visiting hours, how to reach the hospitalist, when rounds occur. Involve family in patient care whenever possible and desired.
Call the family about any changes in patient condition or treatment.	Inform family of changes as they occur. Provide frequent status reports. Allow time for questions.
Provide complete data in easily understandable terms.	Ask questions about what the patient and family understand about the patient's condition, how they are coping, and what they fear. Check for misunderstandings and incomplete information. Provide information based on family needs. Respect cultural and personal desire for level of information disclosure.
Actively involve the patient and family in all clinical decisions.	Hold formal care conferences for important care decisions. Take into account and respect patient preferences as well as spiritual and cultural attitudes. Allow time for questions. Strive for consensus in decisions.
Connect family with support services.	Provide information about support groups, hospital-based social, spiritual, medicare, hospice, home care, and other care services as needed.
Ensure collaborative rapport and support among healthcare team members.	Maintain clear communication among healthcare team members. Avoid conflicting messages to the family. Provide opportunities for staff to decompress and discuss difficult situations and feelings.

hours, the timing of tests and procedures, plans for discharge, or contact phone numbers, to complex facts about the patient's condition or treatment. Information sharing should begin with orienting patients and families to the healthcare situation or unit. Types of information patients and families find helpful during a hospital stay include the following:

- What stress coping activity has worked for you in the past?
- What will happen during tests or surgery?
- Who is likely to interview the patient, and why?
- How can the patient best cooperate or assist in their treatment process?

In stressful situations, the perceptual field narrows. Information and directions given in the first 48 hours of an admission should be repeated, usually more than once, because this is the time of high stress. The same is true when there is a change in treatment plans or prognosis. A calm approach and repetition help patients in stressful situations relax enough to hear new information. Providing simple written instructions, particularly about medications, that can be discussed at the time and then left with the patient or family enhances understanding. Allow time to answer questions and provide the patient's family with the health provider's contact numbers to call if other issues arise.

Developing Realistic Goals

Without command over controllable parts of life, most people feel helpless and stressed. Relevant goals for stress reduction should relate to assessment data, for example, patient-identified needs, strengths, resources, barriers, and goal achievement priorities. Treatment goals and objectives should build on past successful coping efforts and preferences. Choosing personal responses to stress is empowering and has a ripple effect on patient self-efficacy around other health issues.

Coping mechanisms such as negotiation, specific actions, seeking advice, and rearranging priorities can significantly diminish stress through direct action. Once stressors are named, nurses can use health teaching formats and coaching that help patients to

- develop a realistic plan to offset stress;
- deal directly with obstacles as they emerge;
- evaluate action steps; and
- make needed modifications in the plan and essential lifestyle adjustments.
  Consider the Hamilton case.

Case Study: Sam Hamilton Is Diagnosed With Cancer

Sam Hamilton received a diagnosis of stomach cancer on a routine physical examination. His way of coping (problem-focused) included obtaining as much information on the disease as possible. He researched treatment options and sought advice from physician friends as to which surgeons had the most experience with this type of surgery. As he shared his diagnosis with friends and colleagues, he found several men who had successfully survived without a cancer recurrence. Sam used the time between diagnosis and surgery to finish projects and delegate work responsibilities. He attended a support group with his wife and was able to obtain valuable advice on handling his emotional responses to what would happen. When the time came for his surgery, Sam's actions before surgery reduced his stress.

Priority Setting

Patients do not always know where to start. Priority setting helps reduce hesitation and offers a stepwise framework for resolving stress. You can help patients determine which task elements are critical and achievable, and which can be addressed later. Break objective tasks into smaller manageable progressive segments. The most important tasks should be scheduled during times when the patient or family has the most energy, and freedom from interruption.

The next step is to help patients identify the concrete tasks needed to achieve treatment goals, including the people involved, necessary contacts, amount of time each task will take, and specific hours or days for each task.

Some tasks are more important than others in reducing stressful situations and not everything can be handled at once. A helpful suggestion might be, "Let's see what you need to do right now and what can wait a little while." Tasks that someone else can do and those that are not essential to the achievement of goals should be delegated or ignored for the moment.

Anticipatory Guidance

Fear of the unknown intensifies the impact of a stressor. **Anticipatory guidance** is a proactive strategy to help patients cope effectively with stressful situations. The term refers to the process of sharing information about a circumstance, concern, or situation before it occurs. Knowing what lies ahead often prevents the development of a crisis. In framing a response, you might reflect on the following:

- What type of information would be most helpful to this patient at this particular time, given what the patient has told me?
- How would I feel if I was in this person's position?
- What would I want to know that might bring me comfort in this situation?

Providing anticipatory guidance can put needless worry to rest. You can prepare your patients for a procedure, beginning with a simple statement, "You've never had this procedure before. Let me explain how it works." When you are providing anticipatory guidance, do not offer more than what the situation dictates. Encourage the patient to expand on suggestions rather than outlining a full plan. The growth in patient ability to set priorities, develop a plan with personal meaning, and establish benchmarks to measure progress stimulates self-confidence and decreases stress.

Anticipatory guidance should relate only to behaviors that can be changed. Stress-related questions about uncertainties do not qualify, for example, "If I take this chemotherapy, will I be cured, or am I going to die anyway?" The reality is that there may be no single answer. It helps to ask the patient what prompted the question and to have a good idea of the patient's level of knowledge before answering. Honest communication is essential, but sensitivity to the patient's experience is also critical.

Promoting a Healthy Lifestyle

Encouraging a healthy lifestyle is an essential but sometimes overlooks component of stress management strategies. Good health habits improve stress resistance. Eating a healthy diet and avoiding emotional eating give people a sense of control and well-being. Too much caffeine and alcohol can exacerbate stress.

Quality sleep is restorative. Healthy nighttime habits, such as establishing a scheduled bedtime and having a small snack before bedtime, encourage sleep. Regular exercise helps the body release tension, as well as contributes to fitness. Exercise can be accomplished in a social setting, for example, hiking or biking. Certain exercise programs such as yoga or tai chi meditation, deep breathing, and muscle stretching are well-known stress reducers. Organizing time and deliberately choosing activities that energize rather than stress, balancing work with leisure activities, and eliminating unnecessary obligations reduce stress. Table 16.3 gives you the ABCs of burnout prevention.

Cognitive Behavioral Approach to Stress Reduction

Cognitive behavioral approaches have proven useful in addressing stressful negative attributions about oneself, and modifying negative core beliefs. As discussed elsewhere, the cognitive behavioral therapy (CBT) model (Beck & Beck, 2011) helps a patient reframe the meaning of difficult situations. According to Beck, the relationship between a person's thoughts and feelings influences behaviors. Negative thinking causes a person to interpret neutral situations in unrealistic, exaggerated, or negative ways. Helping people through **cognitive restructuring** helps them become aware of and change negative or dysfunctional thoughts, beliefs, and perceptions. One personal example might be doing poorly on a test and cognitively interpreting this as "I am stupid," instead of "I messed up on a test—what can I do so this doesn't happen again?"

Teaching Patients Techniques to Manage Stress

Many of your self-management techniques to decrease your stress covered in Chapter 27 can be taught to patients who can use them on their own, such as follows:

1. *Deep breathing.* Teaching patients to use mind/body exercises to lessen the intensity of a stressor on a person can include immediate activities such as deep abdominal breathing or progressive relaxation. Breathe in through nose for 15 seconds, hold breath for 5 seconds, and breathe out through pursed lips for more than 15 seconds.
2. *Progressive relaxation.* Progressive relaxation is a technique that focuses the patient's attention on conscious control of voluntary skeletal muscles. Alternately tense and relax muscle groups. Davis et al. (2008) provide an excellent step-by-step description of the basic procedure for progressive relaxation.
3. *Guided imagery.* Instruct the patient to imagine a scene, previously experienced as safe, peaceful, or beautiful. Supportive prompts to engage all of senses deepen the imagery experience: see the ocean, feel the breeze, inhale the salty air, for example. Inspirational tapes and music can also be used in connection with guided imagery.
4. *Meditation.* There are many types of meditation. Box 16.4 guides you through a meditation session for stress reduction.

TABLE 16.3   ABCs of Burnout Prevention

Suggested Strategy	
Awareness	Use self-reflection and conversations with others to sort out priorities and identify parts of life out of balance. Recognize and allow feelings.
Balance	Maintain a healthy lifestyle. Balance care of others with self-care and self-renewal needs.
Choice	Differentiate between things you can change and those you cannot. Deliberately make choices that are purpose driven and meaningful.
Detachment	Detach from excessive ego involvement and personal ambition. Share responsibility and credit for care. Use meditation to center self.
Altruistic egoism	Take scheduled time for self, learn to say no, practice meditation, and develop outside interests that enrich the spirit.
Faith	Burnout is a malaise of the spirit. Trust in a higher power or purpose to center yourself when you do not know what will happen next.
Goals	Identify and develop realistic goals in line with your personal strengths. Seek feedback and support.
Hope	Hope is nurtured through conversations with others that lighten the burden and a belief in one's possibilities and personal worth in the greater scheme of things.
Integrity	Recognize that each of us is the only person who can determine the design and application of meaning in our lives.

Data from Arnold, E. (2008). Spirituality in educational and work environments. In V. Carson & H. Koenig (Eds.), *Spiritual dimensions of nursing practice* (revised ed., pp. 386–399). Conshohocken, PA: Templeton Foundation Press.

BOX 16.4 **Meditation Techniques**

1. Choose a private, quiet, calm environment with as few distractions as possible.
2. Get in a comfortable position, preferably a sitting position.
3. To shift the mind from logical, externally oriented thought, use a constant stimulus such as a sound, word, phrase, or object, such as falling water. Eyes are closed. A repetitive sound or word can be used.
4. Pay attention to the rhythm of your breathing: inhale through nose × 15, hold × 5, and exhale through pursed lips × 20.
5. When distracting thoughts occur, blow them away; discard the thought and redirect your attention to the repetition of the word or gazing at the object. Distracting thoughts will occur and do not mean you are performing the techniques incorrectly. Do not worry about how you are doing. Redirect your focus to the constant stimulus and assume a passive attitude.

5. *Biofeedback program.* A referral to an expert who teaches this technique is needed.
6. *Resilience training.* Resilience training focuses on strengthening four areas of function:

    Emotionally focusing on a sense of purpose, as well as cultivating an attitude of acceptance of what cannot be changed

    Cognitively adopting the mindset that this illness can become an opportunity or a time for new learning

    Physically using exercise as a way to relieve stress

    Spiritually renewing faith, placing yourself in a higher power

SUMMARY

This chapter focuses on the stress response in healthcare and supporting patient and family coping with stress through nurse–patient relationships. Stress can negatively impact patient outcomes, level of satisfaction with care, and compliance with treatment. A fundamental goal in the nurse–patient relationship is to empower patients and families with the knowledge, support, and resources they need to cope effectively with stress.

Stress is a part of everyone's life. Mild stress can be beneficial, but greater stress levels can be unhealthy. Concurrent and cumulative stresses increase the response level. Theoretical models address stress as a physiological response, as a stimulus, and as a transaction between person and environment. Factors that influence the development of a stress reaction include the nature of the stressor, personal interpretation of its meaning, number of previous and concurrent stressors, previous experiences with similar stressors, and availability of support systems and personal coping abilities.

People's coping strategies minimize stress. Assessment should focus on stress factors the person is experiencing, the context in which they occur, and identification of coping strategies. Supportive interventions include giving information, opportunities to express their feelings, providing anticipatory guidance, and teaching specific techniques for stress reduction.

ETHICAL DILEMMA: What Would You Do?

The mother of a patient with acquired immunodeficiency syndrome (AIDS) does not know her son's diagnosis because her son does not want to worry her and fears her disapproval if she knew that he is gay. The mother asks the nurse if the family should have an oncology consult because she does not understand why, if her son has leukemia as he says he does, an oncologist is not seeing him. What should the nurse do?

DISCUSSION QUESTIONS

1. What would you identify as tips for self-care to prevent the development of burnout?
2. In what ways does stress manifest itself in your patient's behaviors?
3. What are some of the stress management strategies you have tried or observed that seem to work better than others?

REFERENCES

American Psychological Association (APA). (May 27, 2020). *Stress management for leaders responding to a crisis: Evidence-based techniques to handle stress and effectively lead*, 1–5. Retrieved from www.apa.org/topics/covid-19/stress-management/. [Accessed 27 May 2021].

Beck, J., & Beck, A. T. (2011). *Cognitive behavior therapy: Basics and beyond*. New York, NY: Guilford Press.

Cannon, W. B. (1932). *The wisdom of the body*. New York: Norton.

Davis, M., Eshelman, E., & McKay, M. (2008). *The relaxation and stress reduction workbook*. Oakland CA: New Harbinger Publications, Inc.

Henshall, C., Davey, Z., & Jackson, D. (2020). Nursing resilience interventions—A way forward in challenging healthcare territories. *Journal of Clinical Nursing*, 29(19–20), 3597–3599.

Holmes, T. H., & Rahe, R. H. (1967). The social readjustment rating scale. *Journal of Psychosomatic Research*, 11(2), 213–218.

Hunt, R. (2019). *Conquering stress and anxiety*. Columbia, SC: Self-published.

Institute for Healthcare Improvement (IHI). (2020). *How leaders can promote healthcare workforce well-being*. Boston: IHI. Retrieved from http://www.ihi.org/communities/blogs/how-leaders-can-promote-health-care-workforce-wellbeing. [Accessed 27 May 2021].

Kelly, L. A., Gee, P. M., & Butler, R. J. (2020). Impact of nurse burnout on organizational and position turnover. *Nursing Outlook*, 69(1), 96–102.

Komachi, M. H., & Kamibeppu, K. (2018). Association between resilience, acute stress symptoms and characteristics of family members of patients at early admission to the intensive care unit. *Mental Health & Prevention*, 9, 34–41.

Lazarus, R. S., & Folkman, S. (1984). *Stress, appraisal and coping*. New York: Springer.

McEwen, B. S. (2007). Physiology and neurobiology of stress and adaptation: Central role of the brain. *Physiological Reviews*, 87(3), 873–904.

McEwen, B. S. (2012). Brain on stress: How the social environment gets under the skin. *Proceedings of the National Academy of Sciences of the United States of America*, 109(Suppl. 2), 17180–17185.

Molina-Praena, J., Ramirez-Baena, L., Gómez-Urquiza, J. L., Cañadas, G. R., Del la Fuente, E. I., & Cañadas-De la Fuente, G. A. (2018). Levels of burnout and risk factors in medical area nurses: A meta-analytic study. *International Journal of Environmental Research and Public Health*, 15(12), 2800.

National Academies of Science, Engineering, and Medicine. (2019). *Taking action against clinician burnout: A systems approach to professional well-being*. Washington, DC: The National Academies Press.

National Institute of Mental Health (NIH). (2020). *5 things you should know about stress*. NIH Publication No. 19-MH-8109. Retrieved from https://www.nimh.nih.gov/health/publications/stress/. [Accessed 27 May 2021].

Selye, H. (1950). Stress and the general adaptation syndrome. *British Medical Journal*, 1(4667), 1383–1392.

Taylor, R., Thomas-Gregory, A., & Hofmeyer, A. (2020). Teaching empathy and resilience to undergraduate nursing students: A call to action in the context of Covid-19. *Nurse Education Today*, 94, 104524.

17

Communicating With Patients Experiencing Communication Deficits

OBJECTIVES

At the end of the chapter, the reader will be able to:

1. Describe nursing strategies for communicating with patients experiencing communication deficits secondary to visual, auditory, cognitive, or stimuli-related disabilities or that are treatment related.

2. Discuss a specific communication deficit advocacy issue for nurses.

3. Analyze intervention recommendations from evidence-based databases and apply evidence-based practices to your clinical practice or a simulated case.

Communication is necessary for safe healthcare, but this can be problematic for patients with communication impairments. An inability to communicate leaves patients at risk for unsafe situations and preventable adverse events. Globally, over a billion people have some form of disability (World Health Organization [WHO], 2018a). Access to appropriate healthcare providers occurs less often than in the population as a whole, because people with communication deficits are more likely to forego needed care. For some, the underlying problem is related to physiological impairments making it difficult to communicate their needs. This chapter presents an overview of communication difficulties commonly encountered when caring for patients with communication deficits. Most nurses will be challenged with caring for patients with specialized communication problems. Consider the following case of Sargent Kye Beck.

Changing the patient's position frequently benefits the person physiologically and offers us something to talk about. Recovered patients have reported that our efforts to create a more stimulating environment, to offer reassurance and support, have later been reported to have been meaningful to the patient.

International organizations have affirmed the rights of those with communication problems, among all disabled, to have the highest standard of healthcare. As we strive to meet our Quality and Safety Education for Nurses (QSEN) competency of coordinating patient-centered care, we are also charged with using our skills to communicate their needs to the other members of the healthcare team. In this chapter, we describe strategies for enhancing communication for this population.

BASIC CONCEPTS

Definition

A **communication deficit** is an impairment in the ability to receive, send, process, and comprehend concepts or verbal, nonverbal, and graphic symbol systems, as defined by the American Speech-Language Hearing Association (ASLHA, 1993). These include deficits such as compromised hearing, vision, speech, or language or problems with cognitive

CASE STUDY: Sgt. Kye Beck Is Wounded

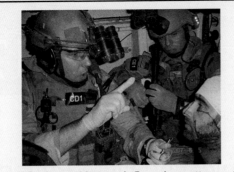

Sgt. Kye Beck, age 26 years, is 5 weeks posttraumatic brain injury and has been a patient in your neurological intensive care unit (ICU) for 2 weeks.

Nurse Sue Nance: Good morning, Kye Beck. I am Sue Nance, your nurse for this fine Sunday morning.

I am going to give you your bath now. The water will feel a little warm to you. After your bath, your wife will be in to see you. She stayed in the waiting room last night because she wanted to be with you. (No answer is necessary if the patient is unable to talk, but the sound of a human voice and attention to his unspoken concerns can be very healing.)

Summary of the strategies this nurse used:
- Called Kye by name
- Introduced self
- Established time (date, time, place would be better)
- Explained procedure before beginning
- Changed his position frequently

processing. They may be congenital or acquired; they range from mild to severe. Severe cognitive and sensory deficits interfere with communication, decrease access to healthcare, and lead to feelings of frustration. In 2001, the World Health Organization (WHO) shifted away from a medical diagnosis model to a functional model, focusing on how people with sensory impairment function in their daily lives or difficulties obtaining healthcare.

Specifically, the patient has a communication difficulty because of impaired functioning of one or more of the five senses or has impaired cognitive processing functioning. Communication deficits can also arise from the kind of sensory deprivation that occurs in some agencies and units, such as ICUs. The degree of difficulty in communicating is an interaction between the patient's type of functional impairment, personal adaptability, and the healthcare environment (i.e., body factors, personal factors, and environmental factors as stated in WHO's model).

Incidence

In America, about 1:4 adults (61 million) adults have some form of disability (Centers for Disease Control and Prevention [CDC], 2020). Globally health conditions related to communication deficits are much more prevalent in developing countries with approximately 15% of the population having some communication disability (WHO, 2021). Many of the physical conditions are preventable or treatable, if only healthcare were accessible. Worldwide, more than a billion people, or 15% of the population, have some form of disability (WHO, 2018). Nearly one in six Americans, nearly

50 million people (U.S. Department of Health and Human Services, 2021), has a sensory or communication deficit.

Goal

Any impairment of patients' abilities to send or receive information from healthcare providers may compromise their health and safety. Our primary goal is to maximize our patient's ability to successfully communicate within the healthcare system. Improving access to care for these people is one of the goals of *Healthy People 2030*. Many of these individuals report delays. When working with patients having communication disabilities, you may need to modify communication strategies presented earlier in this textbook. Assess *every* patient's communication abilities. Two individuals can have the same sensory impairment but not be equally communication disabled. Each person compensates for his or her impairment in different ways.

Evidence shows us that when nurses are unable to understand them, patients with communication disabilities become frustrated, angry, anxious, depressed, or uncertain. Some become so frustrated that they exhibit behavioral problems or even omit needed care. Even when care is accessed, communication deficits interfere with the therapeutic relationship and delivery of optimum care. The patient's deficit is one barrier, but other barriers may include staff's negative attitude or inability to adapt communication.

Legal Mandates

In the legal system, the standard of "effective communication" is based on statutes. Many countries have laws against discrimination similar to the Americans with Disabilities Act (ADA), which prohibit discrimination on the basis of a disability.

Home-Based Healthcare

Visiting patients with communication deficits in their home allows nurses the time to engage in collaborative negotiations for which there may not have been time during acute care management. Home health nurses can build the infrastructure needed to prevent worsening of disability.

TYPES OF DEFICITS

Hearing Loss
Definition
Disabling hearing loss is defined as a loss greater than 40 dB but less than 70 dB. Normal hearing is 20 dB or better in both ears.

Incidence

Hearing loss is a common problem, with approximately 15% of the world's population reporting trouble hearing (National Institute on Deafness and Other Communication Disorders [NIDCD], 2021). Globally, approximately 360 million, or 5%, have disabling hearing loss. By 2050, this figure is expected to double. More than half of hearing loss is preventable. In America, approximately 1:4 (61 million) have a hearing disability (CDC, 2020).

Etiology

Loss can be conductive, sensorineural, or functional. Causes can be genetic, congenital, or acquired, such as due to infections, medication toxicity, or even to exposure to excessive noise, such as that occurs in combat or using ear buds playing music at 85 dB or greater (NIDCD, 2021). Hearing losses, especially in higher ranges, are most often found in older-aged patients, with approximately 50% of those older than 75 years and 80% of those older than 85 years affected.

Nursing

Nurses have both a legal and ethical obligation to provide appropriate care. People who have hearing loss from birth learn American Sign Language (ASL) as their first language. Think of them as folks for whom English is a second language. They may be unable to read health handouts written in English. Title III of the ADA delineates rights of the deaf and applies to communication between deaf clients and medical services.

People's sense of hearing alerts them to changes in the environment so they can respond effectively (Fig. 17.1). The listener hears sounds and words and also a speaker's vocal pitch, loudness, and intricate inflections accompanying the verbalization. Subtle variations can completely change the sense of the communication. Deprived of a primary means

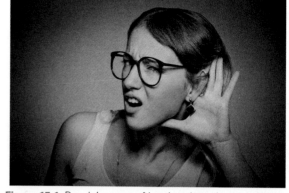

Figure 17.1 People's sense of hearing alerts them to changes in the environment so they can respond effectively. (Copyright © SI photography/iStock/Thinkstock.)

of receiving signals from the environment, patients with hearing loss may try to hide deficits, withdraw from relationships, become depressed, or be less likely to seek information from healthcare providers. Millions could benefit from hearing aids yet have never used them. Nurses teach health promotion when they remind people to avoid noises louder than 85 dB, especially listening to music with ear buds (NIDCD, 2021). The National Institute on Deafness describes other methods that can protect your hearing (CDC, 2020).

Children

Nearly 3 of every 1000 newborns are born deaf or have hearing loss (CDC, 2020). Fortunately, many of these deficits are diagnosed at birth. Newborn hearing is tested in the nursery via auditory brainstem response tests (see the National Institute on Deafness and Other Communication Disorders website at www.nidcd.nih.gov or the American Academy of Pediatrics). Every state has an early detection intervention program.

Older Adults

As we age, we have an increased likelihood for **presbycusis**, or degeneration of ear structures, which is a sensorineural dysfunction that normally occurs with aging (USPSTF, 2021).

Vision Loss
Definition
Humans rely more heavily on vision than do most species. In addition to total loss blindness, visual impairment is defined as vision 20/200 or worse or having less than a 20-degree visual field.

Incidence

Globally, vision problems occur in approximately 285 million people; 180 million are visually disabled, with another 3 million visually impaired (>20/200). The majority of these would be treatable if care were accessible (WHO, 2021). Nearly 5 million Americans are blind or have uncorrectable visual impairments, and this is expected to double by 2050, secondary to our rapidly aging population (Wittenborn & Rein, 2014). The majority of visually impaired are older than 50 years of age.

Etiology

Globally, there are still eye diseases that lead to blindness. Cataracts occur secondary to sun exposure or aging changes in the lens. Other causes include development of glaucoma and diabetic retinopathy.

Children

Children with visual impairments lack access to visual cues, such as the facial expressions that encourage them to develop communication skills. The United States Preventive Services Task Force (USPSTF) recommends testing children younger than 5 years for amblyopia, strabismus, and acuity, but traditional vision screening requires a verbal child and cannot be done reliably until age 3 years.

Older Adults

As we age, the lens of the eye becomes less flexible, making it difficult to accommodate shifts from far to near vision; this is a condition known as **presbyopia**. Macular degeneration has also become a major cause of vision loss in older adults, as do conditions such as cataracts, diabetic retinopathy, or glaucoma (NIH, National Eye Institute, 2019).

Nursing

People who lack vision lose a primary method to decode the meaning of messages. All of the nonverbal cues that accompany speech communication (e.g., facial expression, nodding, and leaning toward the patient) are lost to those who are blind. Even with partial loss, it is important for you to assess whether your patient can read directions, medication labels, and so forth. It is important to remind people to have annual vision exams, especially for older patients to have screening for central vision loss or night vision problems.

Impaired Verbal Communication Secondary to Speech and Language Deficits

Definition

A speech disorder involves impaired articulation, whereas a language disorder is impaired comprehension or use of spoken sounds. Problems can include deficits in talking or reading.

Etiology

Patients who have speech and language deficits resulting from neurological trauma present a different type of communication problem. Normal communication allows people to perceive and interact with the world in an organized

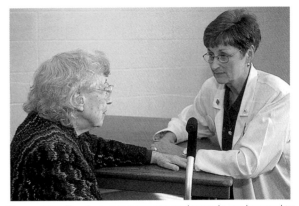

Figure 17.2 Touch, eye movement, and sounds can be used to communicate with patients experiencing aphasia.

and systematic manner. People use language to express self-need and to control environmental events. Language is the system people rely on to represent what they know about the world. Early identification of children with at-risk prelinguistic skills may allow intervention to improve communication competencies. Patients unable to speak, even temporarily because of intubation or ventilator dependency, incur feelings of frustration, anxiety, fear, or even panic.

When the ability to process and express language is disrupted, many areas of functioning are assaulted simultaneously. **Aphasia** is a neurological linguistic deficit, such as that occurs after a stroke. Aphasia can present as primarily an expressive or receptive disorder. The person with **expressive aphasia** can understand what is being said but cannot express thoughts or feelings in words.

Receptive aphasia creates difficulties in receiving and processing written and oral messages. With **global aphasia**, the patient has difficulty with both expressive language and reception of messages. Your patient may have feelings of loss and social isolation imposed by the communication impairment. Although there may be no cognitive impairment, they may need more "think time" for cognitive processing during a conversation. Use of touch may help communicate (Fig. 17.2).

Impaired Cognitive Processing

Definition

In children, this refers to limits on ability to learn and function in everyday life (CDC, 2020). In adults, it may be secondary to traumatic brain injury or infection such as encephalitis. In older adults, it might be associated with degenerative disease or conditions such as Alzheimer's or Parkinson's disease.

Incidence

This is an umbrella category of many varied conditions so statistics are hard to find. Some estimate a quarter of the population develops some cognitive problems, but researchers such as Chen and Liu (2017) found less than 5%. Orgeta et al. (2020) says 60%–80% of people with Parkinson's disease will experience cognitive impairment that impacts their quality of life. About 58% of those with cognitive or intellectual disability have problems with communication. Autism is known to occur in approximately 1:54 children, with boys by far exceeding girls.

Etiology

A multiplicity of causative factors can be involved. With children, the initial sign noted by parents is failure to meet developmental milestones by expected ages. Impaired cognitive processing ability can interfere with the communication process and leads to anxiety and confusion. Understanding involves receiving new information and integrating it meaningfully with prior knowledge. Individuals with impaired processing ability have to work harder and require more time for conceptual integration. The responsibility for assessing ability to understand, to give consent, and to overcome communication difficulties rests with both social services and healthcare workers. You need to continually determine the extent of your patients' understanding and even their ability to understand self-care activities.

Nursing

Interventions vary with type of condition. Assess for use of alternative communication aids. It is suggested that nurses offer information using a variety of strategies including the use of technology. There are many Apps available, check your App Internet store.

Children

Because there is a significant increase in the prevalence of children with developmental disabilities, more nurses will be caring for them both in clinical agencies and in the community. Atypical communication is often the first behavioral clue to cognitive impairment in young children, associated with conditions such as mental retardation, autism, and affective disorders. As these children grow, subtle distortions in communication may exist.

Older Adults

Cognitively impaired older clients may have altered communication pathways. Although most older adults retain their mental acuity, we need to assess risks. For example, memory loss can interfere with ability to correctly take prescribed medications or live independently (Fig. 17.3).

Communication Deficits Associated With Some Mental Disorders

Definition

Patients with serious mental disorders may have a different type of communication deficit resulting from a

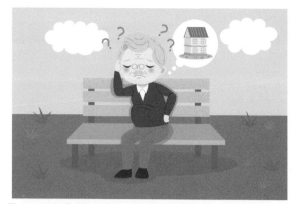

Figure 17.3 Confusion associated with Alzheimer's or Parkinson's disease. (Copyright © KatarzynaBialasiewicz/iStock/Thinkstock.)

malfunctioning of the neurotransmitters that normally transmit and make sense out of messages in the brain.

Incidence

Global incidence is unknown but is estimated as affecting 400 million by the WHO, which has made mental health a part of their 2030 goals (WHO, 2018b). Thirteen million Americans have a serious, debilitating mental illness, as do 20% of children and adolescents (Agency for Healthcare and Quality [AHRQ], 2016). Fifty percent of Americans will be diagnosed with a mental health disorder sometime during their lifetime. Some of these have communication difficulties. In addition to illness-related communication problems, social isolation and impaired coping may accompany your patient's inability to receive or express language signals.

Mental Illness

Communication problems occur with different mental disorders. As an example, some patients with mental disorders can perhaps have intact sensory channels, but they cannot process and respond appropriately to what they hear, see, smell, or touch. In some forms of *schizophrenia*, there are alterations in the biochemical neurotransmitters in the brain, which normally conduct messages between nerve cells and help to orchestrate the person's response to the external environment. Messages have distorted meanings. It is beyond the scope of this text to discuss psychosis. Some patients with mental disorders present with a poverty of speech and limited content. Speech appears blocked, reflecting disturbed patterns of perception, thought, emotions, and motivation. You may notice a lack of vocal inflection and an unchanging facial expression. A "flat affect" makes it difficult for you to truly understand. Illogical thinking processes may manifest in the form of illusions, hallucinations, and delusions. Common words assume new meanings known only to the person experiencing them.

Dementia

An increasing percentage of people, especially older adults, develop **dementia**, including cognitive losses associated with Alzheimer's disease or Parkinson's disease. Globally, more than 24 million people suffer from dementias (Wilfling, 2020). These cognitive losses affect their ability to communicate. Communication skill training is recommended especially for family members and staff employed in extended care facilities. Some communication strategies are listed in Box 17.1. Dementia is discussed in Chapter 19.

Environmental Deprivation as Related to Illness Treatment Such as ICUs

Communication is particularly important in nursing situations characterized by sensory deprivation, physical immobility, limited environmental stimuli, or excessive, constant stimuli. Nurses show sensitivity for patients in bewildering situations, such as emergency departments or ICUs, CCUs, etc. Patients may be frightened, in pain, and unable to communicate easily with others because of intubation or other complications.

Absent Stimulation

Patients, who are immobile, isolated, or intubated, such as in ICUs, often experience absence of stimulation, resulting in gradual decline of cognitive abilities. Patients with normal intellectual capacity can appear dull, uninterested, and lacking in problem-solving abilities if they do not have frequent interpersonal stimulation. Recent studies suggest that this affects family members and patients for up to a year after discharge.

Pain

When assessing pain in patients with communication disabilities, it is difficult to be exact with "yes/no" nodding. Critical care nurses have validated use of a number of pain assessment graphic assessment scales such as FACES. Never assume a nonverbal patient is cognitively impaired.

DEVELOPING AN EVIDENCE-BASED PRACTICE

Delirium in ICUs is associated with poor patient outcome including increased mortality, longer hospitalization, and postdischarge cognitive impairment (Marsh & Alexander, 2021). Parker and colleagues (2021) conducted a qualitative cognitive stimulation study to look at barriers to implementation, even though up to 50% of intensive care patients experience delirium.

Results
Barriers to stimulation for nurses include lack of knowledge, heavy workload, not seeing stimulation as a priority, and the burden of documentation. Barriers for patients included lack of support from family and patient disinterest.
   Strength of research evidence: Moderate. Cognitive stimulation is an evidence-based method for managing delirium.

Application to Your Clinical Practice
In the Parker study, some nurses were unaware of the evidence-based intervention. Work with colleagues to search out evidence-based interventions that improve outcomes for your patients. Work to adapt your communication with critically ill patients, explaining rationale for interventions. Access some of the many databases that summarize research to compile "best practice" guidelines for adapting communication, especially pertinent for those who have communication deficits. Access AHRQ's webpage for Guidelines and Measures at www.guideline.gov/content.aspx?id= 34160&search=best+evidence+statement+ multiple+means for the "best evidence statement" (BESt). They offer suggestions such as using active verbs and short sentences with all patients having communication deficits. Another suggestion is to supplement your oral information with visual aids.

References
Marsh, J., & Alexander, E. (2021). Update on the prevention and treatment of intensive care unit delirium. *AACN Advanced Critical Care, 32*(1), 5–10.
   Parker, A. M., Aldabain, L., Akhlaghi, N., et al. (2021). Cognitive stimulation in an intensive care unit: A qualitative evaluation of barriers to and facilitator of implementation. *Critical Care Nurse, 41*(2), 51–60.

APPLICATIONS

Communication deficits may be developmental or acquired. The emphasis on patient-centered care embodies a need for those with communication deficits to become active participants in their care. Remember many patients do not admit to sensory impairment. Make sure patients with sensory aide such as glasses, hearing aids, and translation/interpretation Apps have their equipment with them easily reachable. In a hospital, all staff need to be aware of the patient's communication disability, perhaps by posting a sign or symbol on the door. Mutual goals involve fostering effective communication with all members of the health team. Nurses with heavy workloads do not always choose to take the time to find alternative communication strategies, sometimes opting just to avoid direct communication, leading to high patient frustration levels. Even when we are aware of a patient's communication deficit, we sometimes lack the ability to communicate effectively. Applying communication accommodation theory, nurses can choose to use strategies in boxes in this chapter. A variety of communication devices are available to assist in communication. Always let your patients know when you cannot understand their communication.

Early Recognition of Communication Deficits

Identification of communication deficit is one aspect of your role. For example, if a 4-year-old child fails to speak at all or uses a noticeably limited vocabulary for his or her age and cannot name objects or follow your directions, would you recognize the need for further assessment? Given this history, you could urge the health team to make a referral for speech and language evaluation.

Assessment of Current Communication Abilities

Are you assessing each patient for communication problems? Do you tailor your plan of care to help meet identified communication needs? Provision of alternative communication methods is a legal requirement. Remember, many patients do not admit to having a sensory deficit.

Communication Strategies

Specific strategies are contained in the accompanying boxes. In general, evidence-based practice suggests you create a quiet environment, allocate more of your time to facilitate communication, take time to listen, ask yes/no questions, observe nonverbal cues, repeat back comments, effectively use communication equipment, assign same staff for care continuity, and encourage family members to be present to assist in communications (see www.AHRQ.gov).

Mobile App Use to Communicate

Handheld devices such as smartphones have downloadable applications (Apps), which provide translation such as picture-to-speech or text-to-speech options. Some nurses expressed concern about their time constraints, device security, and patient conditions/ability to use. On the other hand, they acknowledged mobile Apps could aid in more complex communication than picture boards and could improve communication. A study of American critical care units tested customized recorded messages and words on tablets. All but two subjects reported higher satisfaction with communication and less frustration than those in the control group. Chapter 26 will discuss use of mobile technology for communication.

Patients With Hearing Loss

Assessment of functional hearing ability is recommended for all your patients. Assessment of auditory sensory losses can provide an opportunity for referral. Your assessment should include the age of onset and the severity of the deficit. Hearing loss that occurs after the development of speech means that the patient has access to word symbols and language skills. Deafness in children can cause developmental delays, which may need to be taken into account in planning the most appropriate communication strategies. Clues to hearing loss occur when people appear unresponsive to sound or respond only when the speaker is directly facing them. Ask patients whether they use a hearing aid and whether it is working properly.

Strategies for communicating with patients who have a hearing loss depend on the severity of the deafness. Covering your face with a mask or speaking with an accent may make it impossible for a lip reader to understand you. Communication-assisting equipment should be available. We need to know how to operate auditory amplifiers such as assisted listening devices, hearing aids, and telephone attachments. Often, patients have hearing aids but fail to use them unless family or nurses assist them. For fun, try Simulation Exercises 17.1 and 17.2 that simulate loss of sensory functions. They will help you to understand what it is like to have a sensory deficit. Refer to Box 17.2 to adapt your communication techniques. Consider the case of Timmy Stubbs.

Case Study: Timmy Stubbs Cannot Communicate

Two student nurses were assigned to care for 9-year-old Timmy, who is deaf and does not speak. When they went into his room for assessment, he was alone and appeared anxious. No information was available as to his ability to read lips, the nurses were not sure what reading skills he had, and they did not know sign language. So, instead of using a pad and paper for communication, they decided to role-play taking vital signs by using some funny facial expressions and demonstrating on a doll.

SIMULATION EXERCISE 17.1   Loss of Sensory Function in Geriatric Populations

Purpose

To assist students in getting in touch with the feelings often experienced by older adults, as they lose sensory function. If the younger individual is able to "walk in the older person's shoes," he or she will be more sensitive to the losses and needs created by those losses in the older person.

Procedure

1. The class separates into three groups.
2. Group A: Place cotton balls in your ears. Group B: Cover your eyes with drugstore glasses covered in Vaseline. Group C: Place kernels of hard corn in your shoes to simulate walking with arthritis. A student from group B should be approached by a student from group A. The student from group B is to talk to the student from group A using a whispered voice. The group A student is to verify the message heard with the student who spoke. The student from group B is then to identify the student from group A.
3. The students in group C are expected to make a statement to the others and have that individual retell what they were told.

Reflective Discussion Analysis

1. Explain how the loss you experienced during the activity made you feel. Be sure to describe your comfort level while performing the functions expected of you with your limitation.
2. Evaluate this experience to determine what you think could have been done to make you feel less disabled.
3. Critique and justify how you would feel if "normal" level of functioning was restored, and how you would feel if it was permanent.
4. Construct a response that explains how the knowledge gained from this chapter impacts your future interactions with individuals who have sensory loss.

SIMULATION EXERCISE 17.2   Sensory Loss: Hearing or Vision

Purpose

To help raise consciousness regarding loss of a sensory function.

Procedure

- Pair up with another student. One student should be blindfolded. The other student should guide the "blind" student on a walk around the campus.
- During a 5- to 10-minute walk, the student guide should converse with the "blind" student about the route they are taking.
- Watch the first 2 minutes of a television show with the sound turned off. All students should watch the same show (e.g., the news report or a rerun of a situation comedy).
- In class, students share observations and answer the following questions.

Reflective Discussion Analysis

1. Determine perceptual differences experienced during this exercise. Describe any frustrations experienced and how this made you feel.
2. Evaluate the implications these differences have in working with blind or deaf patients.
3. Appraise what you have learned about yourself from this exercise, and share how you would apply this knowledge to your nursing practice.

Patients With Vision Loss

Vision assessment for impairment is recommended for all patients routinely. Nurses caring for anyone with vision limitations should perform some evaluation and ensure that glasses and other equipment are available to hospitalized patients. Refer to Box 17.2 for strategies of use in caring for those with vision impairments. Use of vocal cues (e.g., speaking as you approach) helps prevent startling. Because the visually impaired cannot see our faces or observe our nonverbal signals, we need to use words to express what they cannot see in the message. It is also helpful to mention your name as you enter the patient's presence. Even people who are partially blind appreciate hearing the name of the person to whom they are speaking. Communication-enhancing equipment for the vision impaired includes electronic magnifier machines, auditory teaching materials, and computer screen readers with voice synthesizers, Braille keypads or cards, and video magnifying machines.

When caring for patients with macular degeneration, remember to stand to their side, an exception to the "face them directly" rule applied with patients with hearing loss. Macular degeneration patients often still have some peripheral vision. Enhanced lighting and use of light filters to reduce glare may help you to communicate with those who have reduced vision.

With blind patients, the use of touch acts as a social reinforcer and can orient them to your presence. However, use of verbal greetings may better alert your patients. Voice

BOX 17.2 Suggestions for Helping the Patient With Sensory Loss

- Assess psychological readiness to communicate.
- Introduce yourself and convey respect, an understanding of patient frustrations, and your willingness to communicate.
- Be concise.
- Always maximize the use of sensory aids, such as communication boards, pictures, sign language, and electronic aids.
- Pick the means of available communication best suited to your patient. Multiple pathways using both audio and visual are standard recommendations.
- Always help patients to use their assistive equipment (adjust hearing aids, glasses, smartphones for texting, etc.).
- Assess the patient's understanding of what was said by having them signal or repeat the message.

- Write important ideas and allow the patient the same option to increase the chances of communication. Always have a writing pad or smartphone available.
- Arrange for a TTY or an amplified telephone handset for those with partial hearing loss, if they do not text.
- If the patient is unable to hear, rely primarily on visual materials.
- Arrange for closed-captioned television.
- Use text messaging, e-mail, and Apps on patient's phone.
- Encourage the patient with hearing loss to verbalize speech, even if the person uses only a few words or the words are difficult to understand at first.
- Use an intermediary, such as a family member who knows sign language, to facilitate communication with deaf patients who sign.

For Hearing-Impaired Patients

- Tap on the floor or table to get the patient's attention via the vibration.
- Communicate in a well-lighted room and face the patient, so they focus their attention, see your facial expression, and watch your lips move.
- Choose a quiet, private place; close doors; and turn off TVs or radios to decrease environmental noise.
- Use facial expressions, hand signals, and gestures that reinforce verbal content, or request a sign language interpreter, perhaps a family member.
- Speak distinctly without exaggerating words or shouting. Partially deaf patients respond best to well-articulated words spoken in a moderate, even tone. Speak only as loudly as you need to.

For Vision-Impaired Patients

- Let the person know when you approach by identifying yourself, use a simple touch, and always indicate when you are leaving.
- Adapt communication to compensate for lack of nonverbal messaging.
- Adapt teaching for low vision by using large print, audio information, or Braille.
- Do not lead or hold the patient's arm when walking; instead, allow the person to take your arm.
- Use touch and close physical proximity while you are with the client; give the person something substantial to touch in your absence.
- Develop and use signals to indicate changes in pace or direction while walking.

tones and pauses that reinforce the verbal content are helpful. They need to be informed when you are leaving the room. Consider the following case of Ms Shu.

Case Study: Ms Tony Shu Is Blind

You can use words to supply additional information to counterbalance the missing visual cues. Ms Shu is a blind, elderly patient who commented to the student nurse Ruth Endel that she felt Ruth was uncomfortable talking with her and perhaps did not like her. Not being able to see Ruth, Ms Shu interpreted the hesitant uneasiness in Ruth's voice as evidence that Ruth did not wish to be with her. Ruth agreed with Ms Shu that she was quite uncomfortable but did not explain further. Had Ms Shu been able to see Ruth's apprehensive body posture, she would have realized that Ruth was quite shy and ill at ease with

any interpersonal relationship. To avoid this serious error in communication, Ruth might have clarified the reasons for her discomfort, and the relationship could have moved forward.

YouTube has several presentations with the latest use of technology to help in communication, such as computers with sensors attached to the person that monitor eye movements and convert impulses into communication. Talking computers are another aid coming into use.

Orientation to Environmental Hazards

When a blind person is being introduced to a new environmental setting, you should orient them by describing the size of the room and the position of the furniture and equipment. When placing your patient's food tray, describe the position of items, perhaps using a clock face analogy (e.g., "Carrots are at 2 o'clock, potatoes at 11 o'clock"). If other people are present, you could name each person. A good communication strategy is to ask the other people in the room to introduce themselves. In this way, he or she gains an appreciation for their voice configurations. You should avoid any tendency to speak with a blind patient in a louder voice than usual or to enunciate words in an exaggerated manner. This may be perceived by some as insensitive to the nature of the handicap. Voice tones should be kept natural.

A blind patient may need guidance in moving around in unfamiliar surroundings. For example, surveyed blind people said they needed assistance getting to and from their bathroom. One way of preserving autonomy is to offer your arm to them instead of taking their arm. Mention steps and changes in movement, as they are about to occur to help them go new places with differences in terrain. Some blind people use wearable navigation systems.

Impaired Verbal Communication Secondary to Speech and Language Deficits

Assessment of speech and language is part of the initial evaluation. Difficulties arise when people are unable to speak (*aphasia*). For these, an assessment of the type of disorder experienced will aid in selecting the most appropriate intervention. Expressive language problems are evidenced in an inability to find words or to associate ideas with accurate word symbols. Some with *expressive aphasia* can find the correct word if given enough time and support. Others have difficulty organizing their words into meaningful sentences or describing a sequence of events. Individuals with receptive communication deficits have trouble following directions, reading information, writing, or relating data to previous knowledge. Even when your patient appears not to understand, you should explain in simple terms what is happening. Using touch, gestures, eye movements, and squeezing of the hand should be attempted. Patients appreciate nurses who take the time to respond to communication attempts.

Refer to Box 17.3 for strategies to use with those having cognitive processing or speech deficits. People who lose both expressive and receptive communication abilities have *global aphasia*. Individuals with these deficits can become frustrated when they are not understood. Struggling to speak causes fatigue. Short, positive sessions are used to communicate. Otherwise, they may become nonverbal as a way of regaining energy and composure. Changes in self-image occasioned by physical changes, the uncertain recovery course and outcome of strokes, shifts in family roles, and the disruption of free-flowing verbal interaction among family members all make the loss of functional communication particularly agonizing. Any language skills that are preserved should be exploited.

> ### BOX 17.3   Strategies to Assist the Patient With Cognitive Processing Deficits or Speech and Language Difficulties
>
> - Speak slowly, using simple sentences; ask yes or no questions.
> - Talk about one thing at a time, or ask one question at a time; do not rush.
> - Give extra time to process and formulate a response; do not interrupt.
> - Avoid prolonged, continuous conversations; instead, use frequent, short talks. Present small amounts of information at a time.
> - When your patient falters in written or oral expression, supply needed compensatory support.
> - Praise efforts to communicate.
> - Provide regular mental stimulation in a nontaxing way.
> - Help patients to focus on the faculties still available to them for communication.
> - Use visual cues; for print materials, use short, bulleted lists.
> - Make referrals so patients can obtain and use AAC devices.

AAC, augmentative and alternative communication.

Alternative means of communication, such as pointing, gesturing, or using pictures, can be used, as well as speech-generating electronic devices. Augmentative and alternative communication (AAC) methods have been found to help nurses better communicate with patients who are unable to speak. AAC options include communication boards, picture cards, and use of picture pain rating scales, but the preferred AAC method for many is use of speech-generating devices. There are several smartphone Apps available that allow the patient to touch a picture on-screen causing a mechanical voice to speak, conveying the intended message.

Communication With Patients Who Have Mental Processing Deficits

Cognitive understanding involves recognition of words and integrating them into schemata of acquired knowledge. Some have difficulty ignoring irrelevant information or have difficulty organizing input meaningfully.

Learning Delays

As a nurse providing care to learning delay (LD) patients, you need to adapt your messages to an understandable level. This is crucial in all communication but especially when you are seeking to gain informed consent for treatment. To what extent should you involve your cognitively impaired patient in decision-making? In communicating about general healthcare, adaptations include simple explanations, touch, and use of familiar objects.

Communication Deficits Associated With Some Mental Disorders

When working with some patients with mental disorders, you will face a formidable challenge in trying to establish a relationship. Those with altered reality discrimination have both verbal and nonverbal communication deficits. Rarely will this person approach you directly. They generally respond to questions, but their answers are likely to be brief, and they do not elaborate without further probes. Although the patient appears to rebuff any social interaction, it is important to keep trying to connect. People with mental disorders such as schizophrenia are easily overwhelmed by the external environment. It has been demonstrated that schizophrenic patients have the same expressive deficits as do those with depression. Keeping in mind that their unresponsiveness to words, failure to make eye contact, unchanging facial expression, and monotonic voice are parts of the disorder and not a commentary on your communication skills helps you to continue to engage.

Nursing

Lack of training and experience is a common barrier in dealing with patients having intellectual disabilities. Recommendation for communication skill development includes roll playing; small group discussions; case study analyses; and even joining Internet "death cafe" discussion sessions. If your patient is hallucinating or using delusions as a primary form of communication, you should neither challenge their validity directly nor enter into a prolonged discussion of illogical thinking. Often you can identify the underlying theme they are trying to convey with the delusional statement. For example, when they say, "Voices are telling me to do …," you might reply, "It sounds as though you feel powerless and afraid at this moment." Listening carefully, using alert posture, nodding to demonstrate active listening, and trying to make sense out of their underlying feelings model effective communication and help you to decode nonsensical messages. Simulation Exercise 17.3 may help you to gain some understanding of communication problems experienced by the person with schizophrenia.

Patients Experiencing Treatment-Related Communication Disabilities

Communication disabilities can stem from sedative medications, mechanical ventilation, isolation in an ICU,

---

SIMULATION EXERCISE 17.3   Schizophrenia Communication Simulation

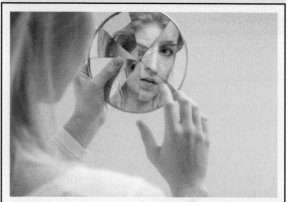

Copyright © KatarzynaBialasiewicz/iStock/Thinkstock.

Purpose

To gain insight into communication deficits encountered by clients with schizophrenia.

Procedure

1. Break class into groups of three (triads) by counting off 1, 2, 3.
2. Person 1 (the nurse) reads a paragraph of rules to the patient and then quizzes him or her afterward about the content.
3. Person 2 (the patient with schizophrenia) listens to everything and tries to answer the nurse's questions correctly to get 100% on the test.
4. Person 3 (representing the mental illness) speaks loudly and continuously in the patient's ear while the nurse is communicating, saying things like "You are so stupid," "You have done bad things," and "It is coming to get you," over and over.

Reflective Discussion Analysis

Determine if any patient has 100% recall after this activity. Critique the simulation. Describe difficulties communicating when the patient is "hearing voices."

Simulation Exercise courtesy Ann Newman, Ph.D., University of North Carolina, Charlotte, NC.

---

or isolation such as that occurs when older adults are in long-term care facilities. A number of studies of communication in intensive care show that patients are very dependent on their nurse to institute communication. Specific recommended skills are listed in Boxes 17.4 and 17.5 and Fig. 17.4. Many items such as mobile devices with text-to-speech apps, computers with gaze-controlled programs, or

BOX 17.4 Strategies for Communicating With Patients With Treatment-Related Communication Deficits Such as That Occur in the Intensive Care Unit

- Encourage your patient to display pictures or a simple object from home.
- Orient them to the environment, time, and place.
- Ask many questions, especially questions the patient can answer with a yes or no.
- Frequently provide information about condition and progress.
- Reassure your patient that cognitive and psychological disturbances are common.
- Give explanations before procedures by providing information about the sounds, sights, and feelings the patient is experiencing.
- Make communication assistive devices available, ranging from paper and pencil or communication cards to computerized communication.
- Always assess whether your communication was successful by having the patient signal back.

BOX 17.5 Situational Factors Affecting Patients in Intensive Care Units

- Anxiety and fear
- Pain
- Altered stimuli—too much or too little, including unusual noises and isolation
- Sleep deprivation
- Unmet physiological needs such as thirst
- Losing track of time
- Multiple life changes
- Multiple care providers
- Immobility
- Frequent diagnostic procedures
- Lack of easily understood information

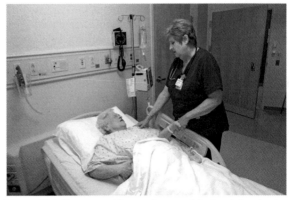

Figure 17.4 Nurse provides environmental stimulation for isolated patient in intensive care unit.

acute. It is not possible to be certain about what level of awareness remains. Good practice suggests you never say anything you would not want them to hear. Always calling them by name; orienting to time, place, and location; explaining all procedures; and using touch are considered best practice. Consider the following case of Mr Lopez.

Case Study: Mr Lou Lopez

Mr Lopez is totally paralyzed and seems unresponsive immediately after a rupture of a blood vessel in his brain. Mrs Lopez thinks he can still blink his eyes. You say: "Mr Lopez, you are in the emergency department of General Hospital. I am your nurse, Kathleen. I need to draw a sample of your blood. Can you feel this? Blink once for yes and twice for no."

For all communication-impaired patients, convey a caring, compassionate attitude, use alternative communication strategies, and give frequent orienting cues, linking events to routines (e.g., saying, "The X-ray technician will take your chest X-ray right after lunch."). When they are unable or unwilling to engage in a dialogue, you should continue to initiate communication in a one-way mode. As professionals, we discourage any use of inappropriate terms. Reflect on Table 17.1 for vocabulary. Can you add to this list? Remember to always focus on the assets our patients have.

Referrals

There are a host of communication specialists available to help patients with communication deficits. As the health team member having the most daily contact with a patient, you may be best positioned to know when they are ready for a referral.

communication boards are useful with ventilator-dependent patients temporarily unable to speak. Better communication leads to psychological improvements such as decreased anxiety and depression.

Lack of Communication Due to Lowered Level of Consciousness

When a patient is not fully alert, it is not uncommon for nurses to speak in his or her presence in ways they would not if they thought the patient could fully understand what is being said, forgetting that hearing can remain

TABLE 17.1   Communicating With People Who Have Sensory Disabilities

Issue	Do's	Don'ts
Limited sensory functions	Emphasize ability not limitations	Avoid disparaging words like mute or restricted
Vocabulary	The person with____ (name the condition)	Terms which suggest the lack of something or suggest stereotypes such as "midget" or "lame" or "slow" or "insane"
Emphasize the type of adaptation needed	"Accessible bathroom" or "handicapped parking"	Decrease use of the word "handicapped" when referring to the patient

Patient Advocacy

Our nurse role also includes acting as an advocate for our patients who have communication disabilities. Too often they are discounted. Medical treatment decisions may be made without seeking input from them. Appropriate communication aids may be withheld while they are hospitalized. In the larger community, we need to advocate for community services designed to foster communication, including referrals to speech and language therapists.

SUMMARY

This chapter discusses the specialized communication needs of patients with communication deficits. Adapting our communication skills and projecting a caring, positive attitude are important in overcoming barriers. Basic issues and applications for communicating with those experiencing sensory loss of hearing and sight are outlined. Sensory stimulation and compensatory channels of communication are needed for patients with sensory deprivation, such as those in ICUs. All workers who come in contact with these patients need to be aware of their communication impairments. We need to learn how to operate and fit equipment such as hearing aids, because hospitalized patients often need help with devices. The mentally ill patient has intact senses, but information processing and language are affected by the disorder. It is important to develop a proactive communication approach with the learning impaired or those who suffer from mental disorders. Patients can experience communication isolation and temporary distortion of reality. They need frequent cues that orient them to time and place, as well as providing sensory stimulation and alternative methods of communication. Evidence shows that we need to be careful not to associate communication disability with intellectual dysfunction. Our skill in adapting communication is important to the patient.

ETHICAL DILEMMA: What Would You Do?

Working in a health department clinic, the nurse—through a Spanish-speaking translator—interviews a 46-year-old married woman about the missing results of her recent breast biopsy for suspected cancer. Because the translator is of the same culture as the patient and holds the same cultural belief that suicide is shameful, he chooses to withhold from the nurse information he obtained about a recent suicide attempt. If this information remains hidden from the nurse and doctor, could this adversely affect the patient? What ethical principle is being violated?

DISCUSSION QUESTIONS

As part of our QSEN patient-centered care expected competencies, evaluate answers for the following situations:

1. You notice your patients on the medical wing at Shangri-La Long-Term Care Facility are rarely out of their rooms and seem withdrawn. Determine what patient-centered interventions might be used to ameliorate stimuli-related communication disabilities.
2. Evaluate opportunities for patient advocacy. Describe one way in which you can advocate for a deficit issue affecting communication.
3. Create a scenario of your first meeting with your confused patient as you begin the 3–11 p.m. shift in General Medical Centers ICU.

REFERENCES

Agency for Healthcare Research and Quality (AHRQ). (2016). *Strategies to improve mental health care for children and adolescents.* Executive Summary. Retrieved from https://effectivehealthcare.ahrq.gov/sites/default/files/related_files/mental-health-children_executive.pdf. [Accessed 17 June 2021].

American Speech-Language-Hearing Association (ASLHA). (1993). *Definitions of communication disorders and variations.* Retrieved from https://www.asha.org/policy/rp1993-00208/. [Accessed 17 June 2021].

Centers for Disease Control and Prevention (CDC). (2020). *Too loud! for too long! Loud noises damage hearing.* Retrieved from www.cdc.gov/vitalsigns/hearingloss/index.html. [Accessed 17 June 2021].

Chen, C. M., & Liu, L. F. (2017). The effect of disability and depression on cognitive function and screening factors. *Archives of Gerontology and Geriatrics, 73,* 154–159.

National Institute on Deafness and Other Communication Disorders (NIDCD). (2021). *Quick statistics about hearing.* Retrieved from https://www.nidcd.nih.gov/health/statistics/quick-statistics-hearing. [Accessed 17 June 2021].

National Institutes of Health (NIH), National Eye Institute. (2019). *Eye health data and statistics.* Retrieved from https://www.nei.nih.gov/learn-about-eye-health/resources-for-health-educators/eye-health-data-and-statistics. [Accessed 17 June 2021].

Orgeta, V., McDonald, K. R., Poliakoff, E., Hindle, J. V., Clare, L., & Leroi, I. (2020). Cognitive training interventions for dementia and mild cognitive impairment in Parkinson's disease. *Cochrane Database of Systematic Reviews, 2*(2), CD011961.

U.S. Department of Health and Human Services. (2021). *Healthy people 2030. Hearing and other sensory or communication disorders.* Retrieved from www.healthypeople.gov/2020/topicsobjectives2020/overview.aspx?topicid=20. [Accessed 17 June 2021].

U.S. Preventive Services Task Force (USPSTF). (2021). *Final recommendation statement: Hearing loss in older adults: Screening.* Retrieved from www.uspreventiveservicestaskforce.org/uspstf/recommendation/hearing-loss-in-older adults-screening/. [Accessed 21 June 2021].

Wilfling, D., Dichter, M. N., Trutschel, D., & Köpke, S. (2020). Nurses' burden caused by sleep disturbances of nursing home residents with dementia: Multicenter cross-sectional study. *BMC Nursing, 19,* 83.

Wittenborn, J. S., & Rein, D. B. (2014). *The future of vision: Forecasting the prevalence and cost of vision problems.* Chicago, IL: NORC at the University of Chicago. Prepared for Prevent Blindness.

World Health Organization (WHO). (2001). *International classification of functioning, disability, and health.* Geneva, Switzerland: WHO.

World Health Organization (WHO). (2018a). *Disability and health.* Geneva, Switzerland: WHO. Retrieved from https://www.who.int/news-room/fact-sheets/detail/disability-and-health. [Accessed 17 June 2021].

World Health Organization (WHO). (2018b). *Mental health atlas 2017.* Geneva, Switzerland: WHO. Retrieved from www.who.int/health-topics/mentalhealth. [Accessed 21 June 2021].

World Health Organization (WHO). (2021). *Deafness and hearing loss.* Geneva, Switzerland: WHO. Retrieved from https://www.who.int/news-room/fact-sheets/detail/deafness-and-hearing-loss. [Accessed 17 June 2021].

FURTHER READING

Machiels, M., Metzelthin, S. F., Hamers, J. P. H., & Zwakhalen, S. M. G. (2017). Interventions to improve communication between people with dementia and nursing staff during daily nursing care: A systematic review. *International Journal of Nursing Studies, 66,* 37–46.

18

Communicating With Children

OBJECTIVES

At the end of the chapter, the reader will be able to:

1. Describe how developmental levels impact the child's ability to communicate and how to modify communication strategies.

2. Describe interpersonal techniques needed to interact with concerned parents of ill children.
3. Apply data from a pediatric website to a case study communicating with a child.

This chapter is designed to help you recognize and apply communication concepts related to the nurse–child–family relationship in pediatric clinical situations. Quality patient–family–centered care has been associated with improved child health outcomes regardless of income or ethnicity, while childhood adversity such as abuse has long-term adverse consequences (Haney, 2020). In mastering the Quality and Safety Education for Nurses (QSEN, n.d.) competency of patient-centered care, effective tools need be cognitively, attitudinally, and developmentally appropriate. For each of these domains, the child's and family's socioeconomic status and cultural background must be considered.

Communicating with children at different age levels requires modifications of the skills learned in previous chapters. By understanding the child's cognitive and functional level, you are able to select the most appropriate communication strategies. Children undergo significant age-related changes in the ability to process cognitive information and in the capacity to interact effectively with the environment. To have an effective therapeutic relationship with a child, you need to understand the feelings and thought processes from the child's perspective and convey honesty, respect, and acceptance of feelings.

Communicating with parents of seriously ill children requires a deliberate effort. Parents need explanations they can understand, need to have established trust with the nurse, and need to feel they have some control over what is happening to their child. This chapter identifies strategies to enhance communication with parents, as well as children.

BASIC CONCEPTS

Definitions

Childhood

The accepted age range for childhood is birth to age 18 years. However, when reporting death statistics, the World Health Organization (WHO) calculates up to age 14 years.

Medical Home

The American Academy of Pediatrics advocates a model of primary care for all children known as a **Medical Home**. It is widely accepted as an effective, consistent care delivery model. According to HRSA's Maternal & Child Health Bureau, however, only half of American children use this model (HRSA, n.d.). One *Healthy People 2030* goal is to increase this number by 5%.

Location

Just as there is a nationwide emphasis on outpatient procedures and home care for adults, the same is true for children. More than 70% of pediatric illness care occurs in ambulatory settings. Inpatient care continues to decline significantly.

Incidence

According to WHO, over 6 million children worldwide, under age 15, died of mostly preventable illnesses in 2018. They predict that another 9.8 million will die by 2030 if current trends continue.

Attitude

Quality-of-care studies indicate that, in all settings, children may receive less than half of "best evidence" interventions.

CASE STUDY: Ty Mull and His Fear of the Physical Exam

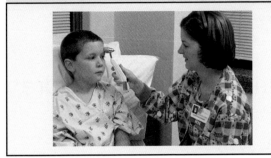

Ty is 5 years old, but due to a bad experience during a prior hospitalization, he is a little fearful of the exam. His nurse, Mary Way. RN, plays a game with him to encourage his cooperation. She pretends to read his thoughts with her thermometer, and then suggest she look in his ear to search for a potato! What other adaptations might she try?

Could this be due to overreliance on healthcare providers' own experience or lack of time to access the latest data and protocols? Major changes in society are mirrored in changing healthcare for children. Involving children in their own healthcare decision-making is a part of QSEN's "patient-centered care." Making the child a (limited) partner might lead to better health outcomes than treating the child as a target for our delivery of care. Do you see this as desirable?

Cognitive Development

Childhood is very different from adulthood. A child has fewer life experiences from which to draw and is still in the process of developing skills needed for reasoning and communicating. Every child's concept of health and illness must be considered within a developmental framework. Erikson's (1963) concepts of ego development and Piaget's (1972) description of the progressive development of the child's cognitive thought processes together form the theoretical basis for the child-centered nursing interventions described in this chapter. Both theorists say that the child's thought processes, ways of perceiving the world, judgments, and emotional responses to life situations are different from those of the adult. Cognitive and psychosocial developments unfold according to an ordered hierarchical scheme, increasing in depth and complexity as the child matures. Reflect on the case of Ty Mull.

Developmentally Appropriate

Piaget's descriptions of stages of cognitive development provide a valuable contribution toward understanding a child's perceptions and communication abilities. Cognitive development and early language development are integrally related. Although current developmental theorists expand on Piaget's theoretical model by recognizing the effects of the parent–child relationship and a stimulating environment on developing communication abilities, his work forms the foundation for the understanding of childhood cognitive development. Piaget observed cognitive development occurring in sequential stages (Table 18.1). The ages are only approximated because Piaget himself was not specific.

Wide individual differences exist in the intellectual functioning of same-age children. Variations also occur across situations, so that the child under stress or in a different environment may process information at a lower level than under normal conditions. Because two children of the same chronological age may have quite different skills as information processors, we need to assess level of functioning. Language alternatives familiar to one child because of certain life experiences may not be useful in providing healthcare and teaching with another. Integrating cognitive and psychosocial developmental approaches into communication with children at different ages enhances effectiveness, as in Terri's case, pictured in Fig. 18.1.

Case Study: Terri Needs Teaching

Terri is 5 years old, admitted for repair of a urinary tract anomaly. Her nurse, Lisa Jax, uses play to do the preop teaching making it a fun time. Lisa uses developmentally appropriate words and avoids medical terms.

Speech Development

Children progress through stages of communication abilities. When an infant uses gestures or cries to get attention to meet a need, this is termed *intentional communication*. This stage continues through age 7 months or so and includes making babbling noises. By 16 months, in the next stage of *symbolic communication,* the child uses single words perhaps combined with gestures in interactions to get what is wanted. With further development, the child enters the *linguistic communication* phase using two words, then increasing until approximately at age 5 when full sentences are used.

Gender Differences in Communication

Some studies show school-age children are more satisfied if their healthcare provider is the same sex. Use of good age-appropriate communication strategies probably outweighs gender as a factor in successful communication with a child, but gender cannot be excluded as a factor affecting communication.

TABLE 18.1 Stages of Cognitive Development

Age	Piaget's Stage	Characteristics	Language Development
Birth to 2 years	Sensorimotor	Infant learns by manipulating objects. At birth, reflexive communication, then moves through six stages to reach actual thinking.	**Presymbolic** Communication largely nonverbal. Vocabulary of more than 4 words by 12 months, increases to >200 words and use of short sentences before age 2 years.
2–6 years	Preoperational	Beginning use of symbolic thinking. Imaginative play. Masters reversibility.	**Symbolic** Actual use of structured grammar and language to communicate. Uses pronouns. Average vocabulary >10,000 words by age 6 years.
7–11 years	Concrete operations	Logical thinking. Masters use of numbers and other concrete ideas such as classification and conservation.	Mastery of passive tense by age 7 years and complex grammatical skills by age 10 years.
12+ years	Formal operations	Abstract thinking. Futuristic; takes a broader, more theoretical perspective.	Near adultlike skills.

Adapted from Piaget, J. (1972). *The child's conception of the world.* Savage, MD: Littlefield, Adams.

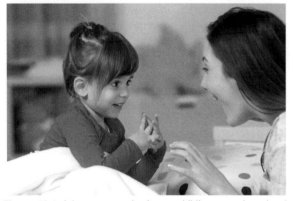

Figure 18.1 Adapt communication to child's appropriate developmental level. (Copyright © AntonioGuillem/iStock/Thinkstock.)

Understanding the Ill Child's Needs

Difficulties arise in adult–child communication, in part because of the child's limited experience in interpreting subtle nuances of facial expression, inflection, and word meanings. When illness and physical or developmental disabilities occur during formative years, situational stressors are added that affect the way children perceive themselves and the environment. Illness may lead to significant alterations in role relationships with family and peers. You need to assess not only the physical care needs of the child but also the impact of the illness on the child's self-esteem and on relationships with family and friends. Responses to hospitalization vary with the individual according to

age. Negative responses may include separation anxiety, night terrors, feeding disturbances, or regression to earlier developmental stage behavior. Things that affect a child's response may include the chronicity of illness, its impact on lifestyle, the child's cognitive understanding of the disease process, and the family's ability to cope with care demands.

Children With Special Healthcare Needs

Some children have chronic physical, developmental, behavioral, or emotional conditions that require health services. In developed countries, one in every five child-rearing households has a child with a chronic health condition (HRSA, n.d.). Many of these children previously would have died but were saved by current technology, leaving some with chronic problems.

Family-Centered Care

In pediatric situations, patient-centered care is really family centered with attention to family diversity and family processes. Evidence documents relationships between such processes and child health outcomes. If the child needs to be hospitalized, this is a *situational crisis* for the child and the entire family. Hospitalization is always stressful. *Prehospitalization preparation* can be done to decrease the child's anxiety. Before elective procedures, many hospitals now offer orientation education tours to youngsters. There are many good books, available in most public libraries, designed to prepare children for their hospitalization.

Child Coping Strategies

Ill children have been shown to successfully develop their own coping strategies. For example, they seek cognitive understanding about their disease or employ distractions such as using electronic devices, television, music, and drawing. Hospitalized children have to contend not only with physical changes but also with possible separation from family and friends, as well as living in a strange, frightening, and probably painful environment. Usually having a family member stay with them helps.

Parent Coping Strategies

Parents are reported to have a strong desire to create a sense of normalcy for their ill child, even to the point of not revealing or discussing a diagnosis has been documented to be very stressful, especially for young parents or those with illness-related perceived financial hardship. Their child's suffering impairs their own coping ability. Nurses are in a position to identify highly stressed parents and intervene to help them cope by the following:

- Providing emotional support. We need to be accessible and caring and demonstrate continuity of care. Expectations for care and information about treatment need to be clearly communicated with consistent team members.
- Involving parents in care decisions.
- Providing needed information. Written literature needs to be used to supplement our teaching.
- Enabling direct care giving by the parent. The extent of responsibility the family assumes for basic care of their hospitalized child needs to be negotiated with staff. Some parents prefer to bathe or feed their child themselves.
- Assisting parents to master procedures needed to care for their child, especially those that will be done in the home.
- Fostering open communication between parents and health team members.

DEVELOPING AN EVIDENCE-BASED PRACTICE

The World Health Organization (WHO) reviewed 63 clinical trials using various modalities for management of chronic pain in children, including medication or psychological interventions. Additional pediatric studies look at use of technology as a nonpharmacologic treatment mode for pain management. For example, studying the use of electronic tablets' (iPads) or wearable devices to download application programs (Apps) to enable self-management of pain, Lau and colleagues found over a thousand Apps by searching App stores (2020). For stress relief, other Apps promote the use of relaxation techniques such as an App titled "Breathe2Relax." Several biofeedback Apps such as "Inner Balance" are also being used on tablets loaned to hospitalized children older than 5 years. Parents and staff are encouraged to coach each child to practice with the Apps to manage their pain.

Results

WHO found studies showed about a 50% reduction in pain intensity with nonpharmacologic interventions. Studies examining use of Internet education or pain management Apps are less available. Few Apps have been peer reviewed. Anecdotal reporting shows unanimous agreement that App use increases parent satisfaction with treatment and teaches children new coping skills. Apps enhance their ability to learn pain management skills. Leemann's study (Leemann et al., 2020) showed use of nonpharmacologic pain relief methods was more important to mothers of end-of-life children than to their fathers. Parents in this Swiss study wanted enough medication to manage their child's pain but to not shorten their life.

Strength of research: WHO finds moderate support for research evidence supporting psychosocial management.

Other studies have lower support due to methodology deficits; lack of peer review of Apps. However, expert consensus including the National Cancer Institute (NIH, 2020) supports the use of nonpharmacological and technology Apps for pain relief in clinical practice.

Application to Your Clinical Practice

1. WHO supports using a biopsychosocial perspective, using a multimodal approach for childhood pain management.
2. There are many evidence-based data websites you can use to aid your pediatric practice. Search your App store. Access CINAHL for application to your practice: which pain assessment scales are available? How much time does it take to use one to assess a child's pain?
3. Consider first approaching the child's mother about alternative pain management.
4. Do support parents in giving medications to manage pain.

References

Lau, N., O'Daffer, A., Colt, S., et al. (2020). Android and iPhone mobile Apps for psychosocial wellness and stress management: Systematic search in App stores and literature review. *JMIR mHealth and uHealth, 8*(5), e17798.

Leemann, T., Bergstraesser, E., Cignacco, E., & Zimmermann, K. (2020). Differing needs of mothers and fathers during their child's end-of-life care: Secondary analysis of the "Pediatric end-of-life care needs" (PELICAN) study. *BMC Palliative Care, 19*(1), 118.

National Institutes of Health, National Cancer Institute (NIH). (2020). *Emotional support for young people with cancer.* Retrieved from https://www.cancer.gov/types/aya/support/. Accessed 23 June 2021.

World Health Organization (WHO). (n.d.). Health top*ics.* Retrieved from www.who.int/health-topics/ [click on health topic desired].

- Parents repeatedly express a desire to be present during team rounds. Bedside rounds not only improve communication, they also assist a parent in coping.

With chronically ill children, the family needs to learn new interactional patterns and coping strategies that take into consideration the meaning of an illness and disability in family life. Caring for a chronically ill child demands considerable resources.

APPLICATIONS

Although children historically have not been the subjects of study, research has contributed to our knowledge of child learning and development. Children are more vulnerable and thus are entitled to extra protection as research subjects. Findings are limited because of overreliance on what parents have told us. Agencies tend to see children as similar, without consideration of differences because of age, gender, race, or culture. To give one example, many of the medicines we use to treat children have been tested only on adults by pharmaceutical companies. Nurses adapt communication, gearing it to the child's developmental level of understanding as illustrated in Fig. 18.2.

Major sources of stress for parents of critically ill children include uncertainty about current condition or prognosis, lack of control, and lack of knowledge about how to best help their hospitalized child or how to deal with their child's response. Although more nursing research is being conducted on effective communication with both parents and their ill children, many of the applications we discuss are based more on experience than on research.

Assessment

Assessing a child's reaction to illness requires knowing the child's normal patterns of communication. Interactions are observed between parent and child. The child's behavioral responses to the entire interpersonal environment (including nurse and peers) are assessed. Are the child's interactions age appropriate? Are behaviors organized, or is the child unable to complete activities? Does the child act out an entire play sequence, or is such play fragmented and disorganized? Do the child's interactions with others suggest imagination and a broad repertoire of relating behaviors, or is communication devoid of possibilities? Because children cannot communicate fully with us, we have a special

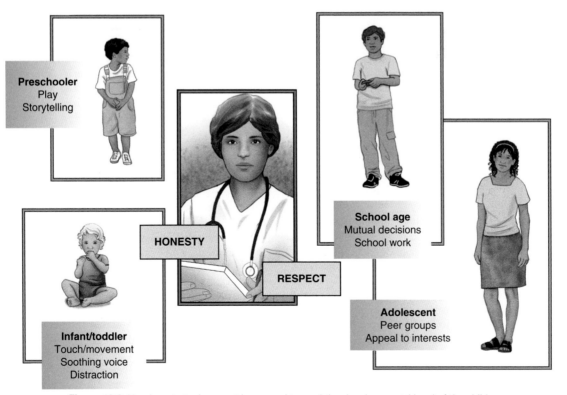

Figure 18.2 Nursing strategies must be geared toward the developmental level of the child.

BOX 18.1   Adapting Communication to Meet the Needs of the Ill Child

- Develop an understanding of age-related norms of development.
- Let the child know you are interested in them; convey respect and authenticity.
- Let the child know how to summon you (call bell, etc.).
- Develop trust through honesty and consistency in meeting the child's needs.
- Use "transitional objects" such as familiar pictures or toys from home.
- Assess:
  - Level of understandings
  - The child's needs in relation to the immediate situation
  - The child's capacity to cope successfully with change
- Observe for nonverbal cues.
- Use *nonverbal* communication:
  - Tactile (soothing strokes)
  - Kinesthetic (rocking)
  - Get down to the child's height; do not tower over him or her
  - Make eye contact and use reassuring facial expressions
  - Interpret the child's nonverbal cues verbally back to him

- Instead of conversation, use some indirect age-appropriate communication techniques (e.g., storytelling, picture drawing, music, and creative writing)
- Use *verbal* communication:
  - Use familiar words
  - Use age-appropriate vocabulary
  - Listen without interrupting
  - Humor and active listening to foster the relationship
  - Use open-ended questions
  - Use "I" statements
  - Help child to clarify his or her ideas and feelings ("Tell me more ..."; "You got scared when ...")
- Respect the child's privacy.
- Accept child's emotions.
- Help child to understand the difference between thoughts and actions.
- Increase coping skills by providing play opportunities; use creative, unstructured play, medical role play, and pantomime.
- Use alternative, supplementary communication devices for children with specialized needs (e.g., sign language and computer-enhanced communication programs).

responsibility to assess for problems. For example, 25% of the world's adults report being physically abused as children, and 20% of girls report having been sexually abused (WHO, 2020). Six million American children are reported victims of neglect, physical abuse, psychological abuse, or even sexual abuse (USDHHS, n.d.). Once baseline data have been collected, you can plan specific communication strategies to meet the specialized needs of the child. An overview of nursing adaptations needed to communicate effectively with children is summarized in Box 18.1.

Regression as a Form of Childhood Communication

A severe illness can cause a child to show behaviors that are reminiscent of an earlier stage of development. A certain amount of regression is normal. Common behaviors in younger children include whining, demanding undue attention, withdrawal, or having toileting "accidents." These behaviors might stem from the powerlessness the child feels in attempting to cope with an overwhelming, frightening environment. Reassuring the parent that this is a common response to the stress of illness can be helpful.

Because children have limited life experience to draw from, they exhibit a narrower range of behaviors in coping with threat. The quiet, overly compliant child who does not complain may be more frightened than the child who screams or cries. This should alert you to the child's emotional distress. You need to obtain detailed information regarding the usual behavioral responses of the family and child. Some behaviors that look regressive may be a typical behavioral response for the child (e.g., the 2-year-old who wants a bedtime bottle). A complete baseline history offers a good counterpoint for assessing the meaning of current behaviors.

Age-Appropriate Communication

An assessment of vocabulary and understanding is essential in fostering communications. Whenever possible, you should communicate using words familiar to the child. Parents are valuable resources in helping to interpret behavioral data. You might assist a child who is having difficulty finding the right words by reframing what he said and repeating it in a slightly different way.

The ill child's peers often have difficulty accepting individual differences created by health deviations. They lack the knowledge and sensitivity to deal with physical changes that they do not understand, as evidenced by "bald" jokes about the child receiving chemotherapy. Children with hidden disorders such as diabetes, some forms of epilepsy, or minimal brain dysfunction seem particularly susceptible to interpersonal distress. For example, it may be difficult for diabetics to regulate their intake of fast foods when all of their friends are able to eat what they want. When peer pressure is at its peak in adolescence, teenagers with newly diagnosed convulsive seizure disorders may find it difficult to tell peers they no longer can ride bicycles or drive cars. Unless the family and nurse provide support, such children have to cope with an indistinct assault to their self-concept alone. Refer to Box 18.2 for a summary of age-appropriate communication strategies.

Communicating With Children With Psychological Behavioral Problems

One out of 10 adolescents and children in our society suffers from a mental illness. These illnesses lead to some level of interactional problems, which may be encountered by nurses in schools, hospitals, clinics, or during home visits to treat physical illnesses. Discussion of nursing interventions with mentally ill children is beyond the scope of this textbook. An

---

BOX 18.2   Key Points in Communicating With Children According to Age Group

Infants
- Nonverbal communication is a primary mode.
- Infants are biologically "wired" to pay close attention to words. In first year, infants are able to distinguish all conversational sounds.
- Infants are bonded to primary caregivers only. Those older than 8 months may display separation anxiety when separated from parent or when approached by strangers.

Use Kinesthetic Communication
- Use stroking, soft touching, and holding.
- Use motion (e.g., rocking) to reassure. Allow freedom of movement and avoid restraining when possible.
- Learn specifically how the primary caregiver provides care in terms of sleeping, bathing, and feeding, and attempt to mimic these approaches.

Hold Close to Adapt to Limited Vision (20/200 to 20/300 at Birth)
- Encourage the infant's caregivers (parents) to use a lot of intimate space interaction (e.g., 8–18 inches). Mimic the same when trust is established.

Talk With Infants
- Talk with infants in normal conversational tones; soothe them with crooning voice tone.

Establish Trust
- Use parents to give care. Arrange for one or both parents to remain within the child's sight.

Shorten Your Stature
- Sit down on chair, stool, or carpet to decrease posture superiority, so as to look less imposing.

Handle Separation Anxiety When Primary Caregiver Is Absent
- Establish rapport with the caregiver (parent) and encourage the caregiver to be with child and reassure child that staff will be there if caregiver is away. At first, keep at least 2 feet between nurse and infant. Talk to

and touch the infant and initially smile often. Provide for kinesthetic approaches; offer self while infant is protesting (e.g., stay with the child; pick the child up and rock or walk; talk to the child about Mommy and Daddy and how much the child cares for them).

1- to 3-Year-Olds
- Child begins to talk around 1 year of age; learns nine new words a day after 18 months.
- By age 2, child begins to use phrases; should be able to respond to "what" and "where" type questions.
- By age 3, child uses and understands sentences.

Adapt to Limited Vocabulary and Verbal Skills
- Make explanations brief and clear. Use the child's own vocabulary words for basic care activities (e.g., use the child's words for defecate [poop, goodies] and urinate [pee-pee, tinkle]). Learn and use self-name of the child.
- Rephrase the child's message in a simple, complete sentence; avoid baby talk. Child should be able to follow two simple directions.

Continue to Use Kinesthetic Communication
- Allow ambulating where possible (e.g., using toddler chairs or walkers). Pull the child in a wagon often if child cannot achieve mobility.

Facilitate Child's Struggle With Issues of Autonomy and Control
- Allow the child some control (e.g., "Do you want a half a glass or a whole glass of milk?").
- Reassure the child if he or she displays some regressive behavior (e.g., if child wets pants, say, "We will get a dry pair of pants and let you find something fun to do.").
- Allow the child to express anger and to protest about his or her care (e.g., "It's okay to cry when you are angry or hurt.").
- Allow the child to sit up or walk as often as possible and as soon as possible after intrusive or hurtful procedures (e.g., "It's all over and we can do something more fun.").

Continued

BOX 18.2   Key Points in Communicating With Children According to Age Group—cont'd

- Use nondirective modes, such as reflecting an aspect of appearance or temperament (e.g., "You smile so often.") or playing with a toy and slowly coming closer to and including the child in play.

Recognize Fear of Bodily Injury
- Show hands (free of hurtful items) and say, "There is nothing to hurt you. I came to play/talk."

Accept Egocentrism and Possible Regression
- Allow child to be self-oriented. Use distraction if another child wants the same item or toy rather than expect the child to share. Some children cope with stress of hospitalization by regressing to an earlier mode of behavior, such as wanting to suck on a bottle, and so forth.

Redirect Behavior to a Verbal Level
- Use a nondirective approach. Sit down and join the parallel play of the child. Reflect messages sent by toddler (nonverbally) in a verbal and nonverbal manner (e.g., "Yes, that toy does lots of interesting and fun things.").

Deal With Separation Anxiety
- Accept protesting when parent(s) leave. Hug, rock the child, and say, "You miss Mommy and Daddy! They miss you, too." Play peek-a-boo games with the child. Make a big deal about saying, "Now I am here."
- Show an interest in one of the child's favorite toys. Say, "I wonder what it does" or the like. If the child responds with actions, reflect them back.

3- to 5-Year-Olds
- Most children at this age can make themselves understood to strangers.
- They speak in sentences but are unable to comprehend abstract ideas.
- Unable to recognize their own anxiety, at this age some will somaticize (i.e., complain only of stomachache, etc.).
- They begin to understand cause-and-effect relationships; should be able to understand, "If you do ..., then we can ..."
- Can follow a series of up to four directions unless anxious about being hurt, and so on.

Use Age-Appropriate, Simple Vocabulary
- Use simple vocabulary; avoid lengthy explanations. Focus on the present, not the distant future; use concrete, meaningful references. For example, say,

"Mommy will be back after you eat your lunch" (instead of "at 1 o'clock").

Behave in a Culturally Sensitive Manner
- In some cultures, a child is unable to tolerate direct eye-to-eye contact, so use some eye contact and attending posture. Sit or stoop, and use a slow, soft tone of voice.

Attempt to Decrease Anxiety About Being Hurt
- Use brief, concrete, simple explanations. Delays and long explanations before a painful procedure increase anxiety.
- Be quick to complete the procedure; give explanations about its purpose afterward. For example, say, "Jimmy, I'm going to give you a shot," and then quickly administer the injection. Then say, "There. All done. It's okay to cry when you hurt. I'd complain too. This medicine will make your tummy feel better." Some experts suggest you create a "safe zone" in the child's bed by doing all painful procedures elsewhere, perhaps in a treatment room.

Use Play Therapy
- Explanations and education can be done using imagination (puppetry, drama with costumes), music, or drawings.
- Allow the child to play with safe equipment used in treatment. Talk about the needed procedure happening to a doll or teddy bear, and state simply how it will occur and be experienced. Use sensory data (e.g., "The teddy bear will hear a buzzing sound.").

Use Distraction and a Sense of Humor
- Tell corny jokes and laugh with the child.

Allow for Child's Continuing Need to Have Control
- Provide for many choices (e.g., "Do you want to get dressed now or after breakfast?").

5- to 10-Year-Olds
- They are developing their ability to comprehend. Can understand sequencing of events if clearly explained: "First this happens ..., then ..."
- They can use written materials to learn.

Facilitate Child to Assume Increased Responsibility for Own Healthcare Practices
- Include the child in concrete explanations about condition, treatment, and protocols.
- Use draw-a-person to identify basic knowledge the child has and build on it.
- Use some of the same words the child uses in giving explanations.

BOX 18.2   Key Points in Communicating With Children According to Age Group—cont'd

- Use sensory information in giving explanations (e.g., "You will smell alcohol in the cast room.").
- Reinforce basic health self-care activities in teaching.

Respect Increased Need for Privacy
- Knock on the door before entering; tell the client when and for what reasons you will need to return to his or her room.

11-Year-Olds and Older
- Have an increased comprehension about possible negative threats to life or body integrity, yet some difficulty in adhering to long-term goals.
- Continue to use mainly concrete rather than abstract thinking.
- They are struggling to establish identity and be independent.

Verbalize Issues in Age-Appropriate Ways
- Talk about treatment protocols that require giving up immediate gratifications for long-term gain. Explore alternative options (e.g., tell a diabetic adolescent who must give up after-school fries with friends that he or she could save two breads and four fats exchanges to have a milkshake). If you use abstract thinking, look for nonverbal cues (e.g., puzzled face) that may indicate lack of understanding; then clarify in more concrete terms. Use humor or street slang, if appropriate.

Remember That Confidentiality May Be an Issue
- Reassure the adolescent about the confidentiality of your discussion, but clearly state the limits of this confidentiality. If, for example, the child should talk of killing himself, be clear that this information needs to be shared with parents and staff.

Foster and Allow a Sense of Independence
- Allow participation in decision-making, such as wearing own clothes. Avoid an authoritarian or judgmental approach.
- Accept behaviors such as regression, but set limits on injurious behavior.
- Encourage responsibility for keeping own appointments, bedtime poutiness, administration of own medications such as insulin and so forth.

Assess Sexual Awareness and Maturation
- Demonstrate a willingness to listen. Provide value-free, accurate information.

Updated from material originally supplied by Joyce Ruth, MSN, University of North Carolina Charlotte, College of Health Sciences.

---

excellent source is available via Web links from the Maternal and Child Health Bureau of the Health Resources and Services Administration (HRSA, www.HRSA.gov).

Communicating With Physically Ill Children in the Hospital and Ambulatory Clinic

Overestimating a child's understanding of information about illness results in confusion, increased anxiety, anger, or sadness. Beyond physiological care, ill children of all ages need support from every member of the health team—support that they normally would receive from parents. The nurse must provide stimulation to talk, listen, and play. Play is their language, especially because children have major difficulties verbalizing their true feelings about the treatment experience. As nurses, we adapt our communication to meet the ill child's needs. Many agencies have play therapists who serve as excellent resources for staff.

Communication With Infants From Birth to 12 Months

Cues to assessment of the preverbal infant include tone of the cry, facial appearance, and body movements. Because the infant uses the senses to receive information, nonverbal communication (e.g., touch) is an important tool for the pediatric nurse. Tone of voice, rocking motion, use of distraction, and a soothing touch can be used in addition to or in conjunction with verbal explanations. Face-to-face position, bending or moving to the child's eye level, maintaining eye contact, and making a reassuring facial expression further help in interactions with infants.

Anticipate developmental behaviors such as "stranger anxiety" in infants between 9 and 18 months of age. Rather than reaching to pick a child up immediately, you might smile and extend a hand toward the child or stroke the child's arm before attempting to hold the child. If the child is able to talk, asking the child's name and pointing out a notable pleasant physical characteristic convey the impression that you see the child as a unique person. To a tiny child, this treatment can be synonymous with caring.

Communication With Children 1–3 Years of Age (Toddlers)

Almost all small children receiving invasive treatment feel some threat to their safety and security, one of Maslow's hierarchies of human needs. This need is exaggerated in toddlers and young children, who cannot articulate their needs or understand why they are ill. To help the child's comprehension, use phrases rather than long sentences and repeat words for emphasis. Because the toddler has a limited vocabulary, you may need to put into words the feelings that the ill child is conveying nonverbally.

Evaluate the Agency Environment

Is it safe? Does it allow for some independence and autonomy? Care in the ambulatory setting is facilitated if a parent or caregiver is present. Agency policies should promote parent–child contact (e.g., unlimited visiting hours, rooming in, or use of CDs, Skype, or podcasts of a parent's voice). Familiar objects make the environment feel safer. Use transitional objects such as a teddy bear, blanket, or favorite toy to remind the alone or frightened child that the security of the parent is still available even when the parent is not physically present. Distraction is a successful strategy with toddlers in ambulatory settings. Use of stuffed animals, windup toys, or "magic" exam lights that blow out "like a birthday candle" can turn fright into delight. The author wears a small toy bear on her stethoscope and asks the child to help listen for a heart sound from the bear, so the child focuses on the toy, making it easier to listen to the child's heart (Fig. 18.3).

Communication With Children 3–5 Years (Preschoolers)

Throughout the preoperational period, young children tend to interpret language in a literal way. For example, the child who is told that he will be "put to sleep" during the operation tomorrow may think it means the same as the action recently taken for a pet dog who was too ill to live. Children do not ask for clarification, so messages can be misunderstood quite easily. Preschool children have limited auditory recall and are unable to process auditory

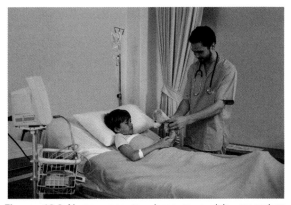

Figure 18.3 Nurse uses toy bear to explain procedure. (Copyright © Wavebreakmedia/iStock/Thinkstock.)

information quickly. They have a short attention span. Verbal communication with the preschool child should be clear, succinct, and easy to understand.

Before the age of 7 years, most children cannot make a clear distinction between fantasy and reality. Everything is "real," and anything strange is perceived as potentially harmful. In the hospital, preschool children need frequent concrete reminders to reinforce reality. Assigning the same caregiver reduces insecurity. Visiting the preschooler at the same time each day and posting family pictures are simple strategies to reduce the child's fears of abandonment. You can link information to activities of daily living. For example, saying, "Your mother will come after you take your nap," rather than "at 2 o'clock" is much more understandable to the preschool child.

Children need to be assessed for misconceptions and troubling problems, preferably using free play and fantasy storytelling exercises. Egocentrism can be a normal developmental process that may prevent children from understanding why they cannot have a drink when they are fasting before a scheduled test. Explanations given a long time beforehand may not be remembered. If something is going to hurt, you should be forthright about it, while at the same time reassuring the child. Simple explanations reduce the child's anxiety. No child should ever be left to figure out what is happening without some type of simple explanation. Reinforce the child's communication by praising the willingness to tell you how he or she feels. Avoid judging or censuring the child who yells such things as, "I hate you," or "You are mean for hurting me." Not being able to recognize or communicate anxiety, the child may just complain of a physical symptom, like a headache or stomachache.

Play as a Communication Strategy

The preschooler lacks a suitable vocabulary to express complex thoughts and feelings. Small children cannot picture what they have never experienced. Play is an effective means by which a puzzling and sometimes painful real world can be approached. Play allows the child to create a concrete experience of something unknown and potentially frightening. By constructing a situation in play, the child is able to put together the components of the situation in ways that promote recognition and make it a concrete reality. When the child can deal with things that are small or inanimate, the child masters situations that might otherwise be overwhelming. Cartoons, pictures, or puppets can be used to demonstrate actions and terminology. Dolls with removable cloth organs help children to understand scheduled operations.

Preschoolers tend to think of their illness, their separation from parents, and any painful treatments as punishment. Play can be used to help children express their feelings about an illness and to role-play coping strategies. Allowing the young child to manipulate syringes and give "shots" to a doll or put a bandage or restraint on a teddy bear's arm allows the child to act out feelings. The child masters fear by becoming "the aggressor." Play can be a major channel for communication. Preschool children develop communication themes through their play and work through conflict situations in their own good time; the process cannot be rushed.

Play materials vary with the age and developmental status of the child. Simple, large toys are used with young children; more intricate playthings are used with older preschoolers. Clay, crayons, and paper become modes of expression for important feelings and thoughts about problems. Play can be your primary tool for assessing preschool children's perceptions about their hospital experience, their anxieties, and their fears. Play can increase their coping ability. Preschoolers love jokes, puns, and riddles—the cornier, the better. Using jokes during the physical assessment, such as "Let me hear your lunch," or "Golly, could that be a potato in your ear?" helps to form the bonds needed for a successful relationship with the preschool child.

Storytelling as a Communication Strategy

A communication strategy often used with young children is the use of story plots. As early as 1986, Gardner described a mutual storytelling technique. You ask the child to help make up a story. If the child is a little reluctant, you may begin, as described in Simulation Exercise 18.1. At the end of the story, the child is asked to indicate what lesson might be learned from the story. If the child seems a little reluctant to give a moral to the story, you might suggest that all stories have something that can be learned from them. Analyze the themes presented by the child, which usually reveal important feelings. Is the story fearful? Are the characters scary or pleasing? The child should be praised for telling the story. The next step in the process is to ask yourself what would be a healthier resolution than the one used by the child, and then suggest an alternative ending. In your version of the story, the characters and other details remain the same initially, but the story contains a more positive solution or suggests alternative answers to problems. The object of mutual storytelling is to offer the child an opportunity to explore different alternatives in a neutral communication process with a helping person.

Communication With Children 6–11 Years (School Age)

As children move into concrete operational thinking, they begin to internalize the reasons for illness: illness is caused by germs, or you have cavities because you ate too much

---

SIMULATION EXERCISE 18.1 Using a Mutual Storytelling Technique

Purpose

To give practical experience with the mutual storytelling technique.

Procedure

1. Use the mutual storytelling process described in the text with a 5- to 8-year-old child in your neighborhood.
2. Write down the story the child told. Read the story this child told, and suggest alternative endings.
3. Analyze commonalities.

Reflective Discussion Analysis

1. Explain any surprises from the child's story.
2. Describe what you learned about the child when using this technique?
3. Determine any difficulties in engaging the child and explain what techniques you would use next time.
4. After listening to all scenarios, draw conclusions to determine what were the most effective and least effective techniques.

Sample Answer

Nurse: Once upon a time in a land far away, there lived a ...
Child: Dragon.
Nurse: A dragon who ate ...
Child: Carrots.
Nurse: The dragon ate carrots and slept ...
Child: In a cave.
Nurse: One day he left the cave to go out and find many sweet carrots to eat, but as he walked along he ran into a ...
Child: Bike.
Nurse: He was afraid of the bike and so he ...
Child: Kicked it and ran away.
Nurse: After he ran away, is there any more to the story?
Child (upset): He got hit with a stick.
Nurse: What is the message to this story? What does it tell us?
Child: About running away not to be punished.

---

candy or did not brush your teeth. In later childhood, most children become better able to work with you verbally. It is still important to prepare responses carefully and to anticipate problems, but the child is capable of expressing feelings and venting frustration more directly through words. Use Simulation Exercise 18.2 to reformulate medical technology into age-appropriate expressions.

SIMULATION EXERCISE 18.2 Age-Appropriate Medical Terminology

Purpose
To help students think of terminology appropriate to use with young clients.

Procedure
This can be fun if the instructor quickly asks students, going around the room.
  Reformulate the following expressions using words a child can understand:

Anesthesia	Inflammation	NPO
Cardiac catheterization	Injection	Operating room
Disease	Intake and output	Sedation
Dressings	Isolation	Urine specimen
Enema	IV needle	Vital signs
Infection	Nausea	Hydration

Reflective Discussion Analysis
Higher-level vocabulary words can be difficult for some children. Try explaining the meaning of the aforementioned words.
  IV, intravenous; *NPO*, nothing by mouth.

or story. Written or digital materials such as in Cary's case can assist you in understanding hidden thoughts or emotions.

Case Study: Cary Is Not Talking With Assigned Student Nurse
Ashley, a second-year student nurse, becomes frustrated during the course of her conversation with her assigned child, 11-year-old Cary, admitted 5 days ago to the psychiatric unit. Despite a genuine desire to engage him in a therapeutic alliance, he will not talk. Attempts to get to know him on a verbal level seemed to increase rather than decrease his anxiety. Ashley correctly infers that despite his age, this preadolescent needs a more tangible approach. Knowing that he likes cars, Ashley brought in an automotive magazine. Together, they looked at the magazine; the publication soon became their special vehicle for communication, bridging the gap between inner reality and Cary's ability to express himself verbally in a meaningful way. Feelings about cars gradually generalized to verbal expressions about other situations, and Cary began describing his attitudes about himself. When Ashley left the unit, he asked to keep the magazine and frequently spoke of her with fondness. This simple recognition of his awkwardness in verbal communication and use of another tool to facilitate the relationship had a positive effect.

Assessment of the child's cognitive level of understanding continues to be essential. Search for concrete examples to which the child can relate rather than giving abstract examples. If children are to learn from a model, they must see the model performing the skill to be learned. School-age children thrive on explanations of how their bodies work and enjoy understanding the scientific rationales for their treatment. Ask questions directly to the child, consulting the parent for validation.

Using Audiovisual AIDS or Hobbies as a Communication Strategy

Audiovisual aids and reading material geared to the child's level of understanding may supplement verbal explanations and diagrams. Details about what the child will hear, see, smell, and feel are important. For the younger school-age child, expressive art can be a useful method to convey feelings and to open up communication. The older school-age child or adolescent might best convey feelings by blogging or posting on social media or writing a poem

Mutuality in Decision-Making

Children of this age need to be involved in discussions of their illness and in planning for their care. Explanations giving the rationale for care are useful. Involving the child in decision-making may decrease fears about the illness, the treatment, or the effect on family life. Videos and written materials may be useful in involving the child in the management phase of care.

Communication With Children Older Than 11 Years of Age (Adolescents)

An understanding of adolescent developmental principles is essential in working with teens. Adolescence is the time when we clinicians encourage a shift in responsibility for health-related decisions from parent to the teen. Even teens enjoying good health are forced to deal with new health issues such as acne, menstrual problems, or sexual activity. The adolescent vacillates between childhood and adulthood and is emotionally vulnerable. The ambivalence of the adolescent period may be normally expressed through withdrawal, rebellion, lost motivation, and rapid mood changes. A teen may look adultlike but in illness especially may be unable to communicate easily with care providers. Identity issues become more difficult to resolve when the normal opportunities for physical independence, privacy, and social contacts are compromised by illness or handicap. All adolescents have questions about their developing body and sexuality. Ill teens have the same longings, but problems may be greater because the natural outlets for their expression with peers are curtailed by the disorder or by hospitalization. Use of peer groups, adolescent lounges (separate from the small children's playroom), and smartphones, as well as provisions for wearing one's own clothes, fixing one's hair, or attending hospital school, may help teenagers to adjust to hospitalization. When the developmental identity crisis becomes too uncomfortable, adolescents may project their fury and frustration onto family or staff. Identifying rage as a normal response to a difficult situation can be reassuring.

Assessment of the adolescent should occur in a private setting. Attention to the comfort and space of an adolescent will have a tremendous impact on the quality of the interaction. To the teenager, the nurse represents an authority figure. The need for compassion, concern, and respect is perhaps greater during adolescence than at any other time in the life span. Often lacking the verbal skills of adults, yet wishing to appear in control, adolescents do well with direct questions. Innocuous questions are used first to allow the teenager enough space to check the validity of his or her reactions to the nurse. In caring for a teen in an ambulatory office or clinic, conduct part of the history interview without the parent present. If the parent will not leave the examination room, this can be done while walking the teen down to the laboratory. Questions about substance use or sexual activity demand confidentiality.

To assess a teen's cognitive level, find out about the teen's ability to make long-term plans. An easy way to do this is the "three wishes question." Ask the teen to name three things he or she would expect to have in 5 years. Answers can be analyzed for factors such as concreteness, realism, and goal-directness.

Some teens lack sufficient experience to recognize that life has ups and downs and that things will eventually be better. Suicide is the second leading cause of death in teenagers, and many experts think that the actual rate is greater because many deaths from the number one cause, motor vehicle accidents, may actually be attributed to this cause. Be aware of danger signs such as apathy, persistent depression, or self-destructive behavior. When faced with a tragedy, teens tend to mourn in doses with wide mood swings. Grieving teens may need periods of privacy but also need the opportunity for relief through distracting activities, music, and games. In communicating with an ill adolescent, remember to listen. When teens ask direct questions, they are ready to hear the answer. Answer directly and honestly.

Dealing With Care Problems
Pain Management

The literature reflects major concern that pain in children is underestimated and inadequately relieved. Care providers have a long history of dismissing pain in children (Sisk et al., 2020). Lack of adequate pain relief may, in part, be due to fears of oversedating a child but more likely is due to the child's limited capacity to communicate the nature of their discomfort.

Assessment. We need to adapt our **pain assessment scales** to be age appropriate. A major transition in pediatric pain management is the shift from the pharmacological intervention model to a biopsychosocial model, which gives us many more intervention strategies to be used instead of or in conjunction with medication. The Wong-Baker FACES scale is often used as pictured in Chapter 21, Fig. 21.1. The Cumulative Index to Nursing and Allied Health (CINAHL) website has compiled "Evidence-Based Care Sheets" you can access. For example, they have summarized the best evidence to list strategies for *pediatric pain assessment.* They describe research results showing that three-quarters of the children admitted to emergency departments are in pain but that only half of these children receive analgesics. This may be because emergency department nurses are not all using age-appropriate visual pain scales to assess the child's pain, even though data show self-reporting is the most reliable tool in children older than age 4 years.

Symptoms of Pain. Infants indicate pain with physiological changes (e.g., diaphoresis, pallor, increased heart rate, increased respirations, and decreased oxygen saturation). With toddlers or preschoolers, we use one of the many child-based assessment scales, such as smiley faces or poker chips. We also need to instigate protocols for preventing pain associated with treatment. Examples include use of local anesthetics for effective reduction of the pain associated with venipuncture. Effective nonpharmacological interventions for pain include nonnutritive sucking/pacifiers, rocking, physical contact, and swaddling. Use Simulation Exercise 18.3 to develop your own approach to caring for children in pain.

SIMULATION EXERCISE 18.3 **Pediatric Nursing Procedures**

Purpose
To give practice in preparing for painful procedures.

Procedure
Timmy, age 4, is going to have a bone marrow aspiration. (The insertion of a large needle into the hip is a painful procedure.) Answer the following questions:
1. Create a dialog between nurse and young patient that will help to prepare them for a painful procedure.
2. If this is a frequently repeated procedure, how can you make him feel safe before and after the procedure?
3. How soon in advance should you prepare him?

Reflective Discussion Analysis
In a group critically examine the responses of others. Try to reach consensus on the best practices for pain intervention.

SIMULATION EXERCISE 18.4 **Preparing Children for Treatment Procedures**

Purpose
To help students apply developmental concepts to age-appropriate nursing interventions.

Procedure
Students divide into four small groups and role-play interventions in the following situation. As a large group, each small group spokesperson writes the intervention on the board under the label for the age group.

Situation
Jamie is scheduled to go to the surgical suite later today to have a central infusion catheter inserted for hyperalimentation. This is Jamie's first procedure on the first day of this first hospitalization experience.

Reflective Discussion Analysis
Group focuses on comparing and contrasting interventions across the various age spans to determine age-appropriate nursing interventions.
1. How does each intervention differ according to the age of the child? (Describe age-appropriate interventions for preschooler, school-age child, and adolescent.)
2. What concept themes are common across the age spans? (education components; assessing initial level of knowledge; assessing ability to comprehend information, readiness to receive information; adapting information to cognitive level of child)
3. What formats might be best used for each age group? (Role-play with tools such as dolls, pictures, comic books, educational pamphlets, and peer group sessions.)

Treatment of Pain. We have already discussed alternatives to pharmacologic treatment, such as bundling infants, use of distraction in preschoolers, and teaching relaxation exercises such as abdominal breathing or use of Apps for school agers.

Anxiety

Illness is often an unanticipated event. Uncertainty and even anxiety should be expected when both treatment and outcome are unknown. Young children react to unexpected stimuli, to painful procedures, and even to the presence of strangers with fear. Older children fear separation from parents but also may fear injury, loss of body function, or even a sense of shame for being perceived by friends as different. Many children with chronic health problems experience tension between balancing the restrictions of their treatment regime and their own desires for normal activities. Think of the diabetic teen who goes to a friend's birthday party and is urged to eat cake! Simulation Exercise 18.4 helps to develop age-appropriate explanations that may reduce anxiety.

Acting-Out Behaviors

Behavior problems present a special challenge to the nurse. Clear communication of expectations, treatment protocols, and rules is of value. As much as possible, adolescents should be allowed to act on their own behalf in making choices. At the same time, limits need to be set on **acting-out behavior**. Limits define the boundaries of acceptable behaviors in a relationship. Initially determined by the parents or the nurse, limits can be developed mutually as an important part of the relationship as the child matures. Determining consequences has a positive value in that it provides the child with a model for handling frustrating situations in a more adult manner.

Once the conflict is resolved and the child has accepted the consequences of his or her behavior, he or she should be given an opportunity to discuss attitudes and feelings that led up to the need for limits, as well as reaction to the limits set. Serious symptoms such as substance abuse require specialist interventions.

Although communication about limits is necessary for the survival of the relationship, it needs to be balanced with time for interaction that is pleasant and positive.

Sometimes with children who need limits set on a regular basis, discussion of the restrictions is the only conversation that takes place between nurse and child. When this is noted, nurses might ask themselves what feelings the child might be expressing through their actions. Putting into words the feelings that are being acted out helps children to trust the nurse's competence and concern. Usually it is necessary for the entire staff to share this responsibility. Box 18.3 presents ideas for setting limits.

Children With Special Needs

The Maternal and Child Health Bureau's national survey of children's health (HRSA, 2020) revealed that 13.2% (8 million) children have a current diagnosis of some behavioral problem. Since nurses are caring for these children when they require treatment for other illnesses, we will briefly mention some communication issues.

Autism Spectrum Disorder

Autism is among the most common neurodevelopmental disorders. Neurodevelopmental disorders including autism, Asperger syndrome, and pervasive developmental disorder affect the child's ability to communicate and socialize. Problems may be exacerbated during a hospitalization. Treatment target ways to improve communication and reduce anxiety triggering events such as bright lights, loud noises, and exposure to many staff (AHRQ, 2011; Whippey et al., 2019). Often these children have communication difficulties, requiring alternative/augmented communication devices, with assistance from speech–language pathologists. IPad Apps or speech-generating devices are useful (DeCarlo et al., 2019).

Hyperactive Disorders

To learn, children need to be able to focus. This is difficult for hyperactive children who manifest fidgeting and inattention. They are often treated with medications such as Ritalin and more structured environments. Some have language deficits, but DSM-5 diagnoses are difficult (Redmond, 2020). Communication strategies include controlling distractions, utilizing parents, and using specific directions.

Mental Health Problems

Half of all alterations in mental health status occur by age 14, yet often remain undiagnosed. Depression in adolescents is one of the leading causes of disability. Suicide is the second leading cause of death in teens aged 15–24 years (Jiang et al., 2015). Adolescents are known for risk-taking behaviors. Older adolescent males are especially susceptible for harm from violence. Nurses need to assess for mental health issues and make referrals (Kessler et al., 2007). Not asking is not helpful.

Helpful Strategies When Communicating With Children

Adapting communication strategies presented earlier in this book to interactions with children requires some imagination and creativity. Working with children is rewarding, hard work that sometimes must be evaluated indirectly. For example, George was the primary care nurse who had worked very hard with a 13-year-old girl over a 6-month period while the girl was on a bone marrow transplant unit. He felt bad when, at discharge, the girl stated, "I never want to see any of you people again." However, just before leaving, the nurse found her sobbing on her bed. No words were spoken, but the child threw her arms around George and clung to him for comfort. For this nurse, the child's expression of grief was an acknowledgment of the meaning of the relationship. Children, even those who can use words, often communicate through behavior rather than verbally when under stress.

BOX 18.3   Guidelines for Developing Workable Limit-Setting Plan

1. Have the child describe his or her behavior.
   Key: Evaluate realistically.
2. Encourage the child to assess behavior. Is it helpful for others and him or her?
   Key: Evaluate realistically.
3. Encourage the child to develop an alternative plan for governing behavior.
   Key: Set reasonable goals.
4. Have the child sign a statement about his or her plan.
   Key: Commit to goals.
5. Consequences for unacceptable behavior are logical and fit the situation.
   Key: Consequences are known.
6. At the end of the appropriate time period, have the child assess his or her performance.
   Key: Evaluate realistically.
7. Consequences are applied in a matter-of-fact manner, without lengthy discussion.
   Key: Consequences immediately follow the transgression.
8. Provide positive reinforcement for those aspects of performance that were successful.
   Key: Evaluate realistically.
9. Encourage the child to make a positive statement about his or her performance.
   Key: Teach self-praise.

Active Listening

The process of active listening takes initially from watching the behaviors of children as they play and interact with their environments. As a child's vocabulary increases, listening begins to approximate the communication process that occurs between adults, but the perceptual world of the child is concrete; therefore, the nurse's communication should be at the child's developmental level.

Authenticity and Veracity

Sometimes adults ignore children's feelings or else deceive them about procedures, illness, or hospitalization in the mistaken belief that they will be overwhelmed by the truth. Just the opposite is true. Children can cope with most stressors as long as they are presented in a manner they can understand and given enough time and support from the environment to cope. Teens rate honesty, attention to pain, and respect as the three most important factors in their quality of care. You should never allow any individual, even a parent, to threaten a child. For example, a few parents have been heard to say, "You be good or I'll have the nurse give you a shot." It is appropriate to interrupt this parent.

Convey Respect

It is easy for adults to impose their own wishes on a child. Respecting a child's right to feel and to express feelings appropriately is important. Providing truthful answers is a hallmark of respect. When interacting with the older child, using the concept of mutuality will promote respect and should foster more positive and lasting healthcare outcomes. Confidentiality needs to be maintained unless the nurse judges that revealing information is necessary to prevent harm to the child or adolescent. In such cases, the child needs to be advised of the disclosure.

Communication Alternatives

Alternative communication strategies for preverbal children can include art therapy or play therapy (with Child Life Staff). Today's kids are amazingly computer savvy, so some agencies use computer-assisted instructional programs explaining lab tests, diagnoses, or virtual classrooms. Other alternative methods of communication include picture boards or sign language.

Providing Anticipatory Guidance to the Child

The nursing profession advocates education for children, as do pediatricians. The American Academy of Pediatrics has published suggestions for giving caretakers health promotion information at appropriate ages. There is an increased focus on the role a child can assume in being responsible for his or her own healthcare. It is never too early to begin. For example, written handouts for incorporating violence prevention can be incorporated into well-child visits. A shift in placing responsibility for good health practices onto the individual is in line with recommendations in *Healthy People 2030*.

End-of-Life Care for Children

Children are supposed to live into adulthood in the natural order, but pediatric nurses care for children facing end-of-life issues. They also deal with parents who may feel guilt, grief, helplessness, and demands on their time by other family members. Referrals to palliative care should be a priority (Sisk et al., 2020). The following interventions are supportive to children with life limiting conditions:

- Continuing to communicate and interact with friends and family members
- Informing the child of everything that is going on in words they can understand
- Providing support, maybe joining a support/play group
- Determining the ill child's preferences

Suggestions for parents include the following:

- Encouraging them to maintain as normal a family life as possible
- Seeking respite in care of the ill child
- Encouraging periods of quality time spent with siblings
- Offering emotional support for parents and providing them with timely, frequent information

Grief

Children do not experience grief in the same way adults do. They may not have the words nor the experience to verbalize their grief. They may demonstrate some acting-out behaviors: anger, withdrawal, or fear. Preschoolers and young elementary age children probably do not understand the permanence of death. The National Cancer Institute identifies common concerns children have when a loved one dies: did they cause this death to happen? Is it going to happen to me? Who will take care of me now?

Forming Healthcare Partnerships With Parents

Having an ill child is stressful for parents. Evidence shows that loss of the ability to act as the child's parent, to alleviate their child's pain, and to offer comfort is more stressful than factors connected with the illness, including coping with uncertainty over the outcome. Studies point to a lack of needed information and support from professionals as being a top stressor. It is essential that we work in partnership with families, especially if we assess risk factors that endanger the child. Most parents want to participate

BOX 18.4 Guidelines for Communicating With Parents

- Present complex information in informational chunks.
- Repeat information and allow plenty of time for questions.
- Keep parents continually informed of progress and changes in condition.
- Involve parents in determining goals; anticipate possible reactions and difficulties.
- Discuss problems with parents directly and honestly.
- Explore all alternative options with parents.
- Share knowledge of community supports; help parents to role-play responses to others.
- Acknowledge the impact of the illness on finances; on emotions; and especially on the family, including siblings.
- Use other staff for support in personally coping with the emotional drain created by working with very ill children and their parents.

in their child's care during acute hospitalizations but need information, advice, and clarification as to their role (i.e., what is okay to do). They need to feel valued but not pressured into doing tasks they are uncomfortable with or do not want to do. Parents often have questions about discussing their child's illness or disability with others. Telling siblings and friends the truth is important. For one thing, it provides a role model for the siblings to follow in answering the curious questions of their friends. It is frustrating when parents are critical of the nurse's interventions. See Box 18.4 for guidelines in communicating with parents. The nurse may be tempted to become defensive or to dismiss the comments of the parent as irrational. However, a more helpful response would be to place oneself in the parents' shoes and to consider the possible issues. Asking the parents what information they have or might need, simply listening in a nondefensive way, and allowing the parents to vent some of their frustrations may help to get at underlying feelings. Use of listening strategies is helpful. Sometimes a listening response that acknowledges the legitimacy of the parent's feeling is helpful: "I'm sorry that you feel so bad," or "It must be difficult for you to see your child in such pain." These simple comments acknowledge the very real anguish parents experience in healthcare situations having few palatable options. If possible, parental venting of feeling should occur in a private setting out of hearing range from the child. It is very upsetting to children to experience splitting in the parent–nurse relationship.

Communicating With Parents of Special Healthcare Needs Children

Many children have a chronic health condition requiring additional services. Caring for these children requires parental time and alters family communication patterns. Studies show these families have less time for communication. Nurses need to provide care and information about the child's condition and time for discussions about balancing family needs with care for this child and suggest strategies for moving the child toward future independence. Refer parents to community resources. We need to recognize that as the child reaches developmental milestones, this can be a time of increased family stress, requiring additional support from us.

Community

Partnering with the family can be the best method you have to address the complex healthcare needs of children. Parents are the central figures in care planning, especially for chronically ill children. We need to help provide information about which community agencies, networks, and professionals will be mobilized to provide care to their child. For example, school nurses often act as case managers by communicating about the child's needs among parent, care providers, teachers, and other resource personnel. By law in the United States, children with special needs in the educational system are required to have an Individualized Education Program. A part of this may be the health plan for children who need medical intervention or treatment during school.

Anticipatory Guidance in the Community. Because the parents usually assume responsibility for the child's care after they leave the hospital, it is essential to encourage active involvement from the very beginning of treatment. Parents may also need facts about normal development and milestones to expect, as well as information about prevention of illness.

Community Support Groups. Community groups have organized to assist families. Often, information about the groups' meeting times can be obtained from healthcare providers, from the national or local organization, or the Internet. For parents who cannot travel to meetings, Internet support groups are available.

Nurse as Advocate for Children in the Community. Because children cannot communicate their needs to policy makers, we need to broaden our advocacy to fight for better child health at local and national levels. Children's access to healthcare is affected by their neighborhood, the level of their parent's education, their insurance status, and problems with referrals. Poverty is associated with poorer child health status, lack of a regular care provider, lack of dental care, and a myriad of other health problems. Part of our advocacy role is to become actively involved in improving access to care and to focus public attention on pediatric health problems. For example, *Healthy People 2030* has designated obesity and physical activity as priorities for action, stating that only 1 in 10 American youth meet national guidelines for exercise (1 h per day). Child obesity is causing a huge increase in related health problems such as diabetes.

SUMMARY

Communicating with ill children requires modification of standard communication skills to suit the children's developmental stage. Children's ability to understand and communicate with you is largely influenced by their cognitive understanding, vocabulary level, and their limited life experiences. We need to develop an understanding of feelings and thought processes from the child's perspective, and our adaptation of communication should reflect these understandings. Various strategies for communicating with children of different ages are suggested. Parents of ill children are under considerable stress. We need to form a trusting relationship and offer open, full communication. A marvelous characteristic of children is how well they respond to caregivers who make an effort to understand their needs and take the time to relate to them.

ETHICAL DILEMMA: What Would You Do?

You are caring for Mika Soon, a 15-year-old adolescent. She has confided to you that she is being treated for chlamydia. Her mother approaches you privately and demands to know if Mika has told you if she is sexually active with her boyfriend. Because Mika is a minor and Mrs Soon is paying for this clinic visit, are you obligated to tell her the truth?

DISCUSSION QUESTIONS

1. Using the case in the ethical dilemma, describe any interventions you would use with this single mother.
2. Evaluate your pain assessment: how does it differ for an infant and a 5-year-old? Use text to support your answer.

REFERENCES

Agency for Healthcare and Research (AHRQ). (2011). *Comparative effectiveness of interventions for adolescents and young adults with autism spectrum disorders*. Retrieved from https://effectivehealthcare.ahrq.gov/products/autism-adolescents/research-protocol. [Accessed 24 June 2021].

DeCarlo, J., Bean, A., Lyle, S., & Cargill, L. P. M. (2019). The relationship between operational competency, buy-in, and augmentative and alternative communication use in school-age children with autism. *American Journal of Speech-Language Pathology, 28*(2), 469–484.

Erikson, E. H. (1963). *Childhood and society*. New York: Norton.

Haney, S. B. (2020). *Child adversity and the medical home*. American Academy of Pediatrics Journals Blog [website]. Retrieved from https://www.aappublications.org/news/2020/09/16/child-adversity-medical-home-pediatrics. [Accessed 23 June 2021].

Health Resources and Services Administration (HRSA). (2020). *Maternal & child health*. National Survey of Children's Health. Retrieved from https://mchb.hrsa.gov/data/national-surveys. [Accessed 23 June 2021].

Health Resources and Services Administration (HRSA). (n.d.). *Maternal and Child Health Bureau*. Retrieved from https://mchb.hrsa.gov/.

Jiang, C., Mitran, A., Miniño, A., & Ni, H. (2015). *Racial and gender disparities in suicide among young adults aged 18–24: United States, 2009–2013*. Centers for Disease Control and Prevention, National Center for Health Statistics. Retrieved from www.cdc.gov/nchs/data/hestat/suicide/racial_and_gender_2009_2013.htm. [Accessed 24 June 2021].

Kessler, R. C., Angermeyer, M., Anthony, J. C., et al. (2007). Lifetime prevalence and age-of-onset distributions of mental disorders in the World Health Organization's world mental health survey initiative. *World Psychiatry, 6*(3), 168–176.

Leemann, T., Bergstraesser, E., Cignacco, E., & Zimmermann, K. (2020). Differing needs of mothers and fathers during their child's end-of-life care: Secondary analysis of the "Paediatric end-of-life care needs" (PELICAN) study. *BMC Palliative Care, 19*(1), 118.

Piaget, J. (1972). *The child's conception of the world*. Savage, MD: Littlefield: Adams.

Quality and Safety Education for Nurses (QSEN). Retrieved from www.qsen.org/competencies.

Redmond, S. M. (2020). Clinical intersections among idiopathic language disorder, social (pragmatic) communication disorder, and attention-deficit/hyperactivity disorder. *Journal of Speech, Language, and Hearing Research, 63*(10), 3263–3276.

Sisk, B. A., Feudtner, C., Bluebond-Langner, M., Sourkes, B., Hinds, P. S., & Wolfe, J. (2020). Response to suffering of the seriously ill child: A history of palliative care for children. *Pediatrics, 145*(1), e20191741.

U.S. Department of Health and Human Services (USDHHS). (n.d.). *Healthy people 2030. Increase the proportion of children and adolescents who receive care in a medical home-MICH-19*. Retrieved from https://health.gov/healthypeople/objectives-and-data/browse-objectives/health-care/increase-proportion-children-and-adolescents-who-receive-care-medical-home-mich-19. [Accessed 23 June 2021].

Whippey, A., Bernstein, L. M., O'Rourke, D., & Reddy, D. (2019). Enhanced perioperative management of children with autism: A pilot study. *Canadian Journal of Anaesthesia, 66*(10), 1184–1193.

World Health Organization (WHO). (2020). *Global Health Estimates 2019: Deaths by cause, age, sex, by country and by region, 2000–2019*. Geneva, Switzerland: WHO.

19

Communicating With Older Adults

At the end of the chapter, the reader will be able to:

1. Discuss supportive self-management care strategies with older adults as applied to nurse–elder communication.

2. Differentiate concepts of normal aging from dementias and other pathological conditions in older adults.
3. Apply communication adaptations to cases of older adults with sensory or cognitive impairments.

Older adults are the fastest growing segment of the US population. By 2060, people over 65 years will constitute 25% of the population. This is a quadruple increase over the last century (USDHHS, 2020). The minority older adult population is expected to increase by 555% by 2060. Once-fatal diseases have been replaced with chronic diseases as the major cause of disability and death as people live longer. These disorders require coordinated, long-term care and attention, but the current healthcare system has yet to catch up with needs.

This chapter addresses features of the aging process, identifies selected theory frameworks, and discusses how nurses can effectively communicate with older adults to promote their health and well-being. The chapter concludes with discussion of dementia and related communication strategies nurses can use with cognitively impaired patients.

BASIC CONCEPTS

Aging and Age-Related Changes

Definition

Aging represents a universal life process of advancing through the life cycle. Age 65 has commonly been identified as the marker for late adulthood. We tend to break-down older adulthood into three age cohorts: young old, mid-old, and oldest-old. There is so much variation in physical, psychological, and social abilities that attaching age limits to these terms is not useful. Aging

is accompanied by changes in appearance, mobility, energy levels, immunity, sensory, and organ function. It often takes longer to recover from illness or injury. Ultimately, decreases in abilities may interfere with the person's ability to live independently.

Illness Incidence

According to Agency for Healthcare Research and Quality (AHRQ), 98% of older adults have at least two chronic diseases (Butler et al., 2020).

Successful Aging

Definition

Successful aging is the ability to ameliorate or adapt to age-related changes without compromising one's sense of self. The terms older adult, senior, or elder are used interchangeably.

Goal

Our mutual goal is to maintain quality of life and autonomy; to prevent or reduce major functional losses and to maximize wellness. Most seniors would prefer to age in place, remaining in their own home. Referrals to community-based services can help keep seniors engaged. How the aging process influences one's life reflects each person's genetic makeup, personality, motivation, life experiences, level of support, environmental and cultural factors, and engagement with health promotion activities. Nurses can empower older adults by helping them accommodate to changes.

Successful aging is the ability to adapt flexibly to age-related changes without relinquishing the central components of self-definition. Limitations are to some extent preventable, reversible, or at least manageable through careful self-management health strategies. Developing the resilience to prevent and/or to effectively self-manage chronic conditions is key to leading a meaningful life as an older adult. Refer to Box 19.1.

Psychologically, changes in role responsibilities, and even the meaning of life, can force a reevaluation of how older adults choose to spend their time. As people age, role responsibilities and expectations change; some are desired and embraced. Becoming a grandparent can be an ongoing experience of joy and satisfaction. There is more free time to renew and enjoy friendships, to travel, and to do meaningful volunteer work contributing to the lives of others. Other age-related changes are not chosen. Limitations in mobility and function, loss of social supports through death or retirement, and significant changes in income can be stressful. Reflect on the case of Mr Hay.

CASE STUDY: **Pat Hay Volunteers**

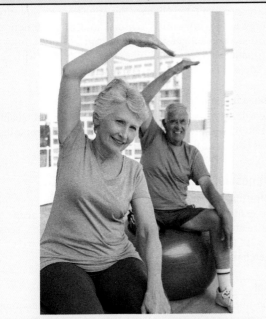

Before he retired, Mr Hay was a highly paid lawyer, well respected, and very busy. Now retired, he volunteers at his area public library to help young people and immigrants learn English. He does this twice a week and derives a great deal of pleasure from his new work. He also joined a yoga class that meets three times a week. In retirement, his own life has become enriched.

BOX 19.1   **Fundamental Older Adult Rights**

Older adults need to be able to:

- Live in safe and appropriate living environments.
- Establish and maintain meaningful relationships and social networks.
- Have equal access to health care, legal and social services consistent with their needs.
- Have the right to make decisions about their care and quality of life.
- Have their rights, autonomy, and assets protected.
- Have appropriate information to make reasoned decisions.
- Have their personal, cultural, and spiritual values, beliefs, and preferences respected.
- Participate in all aspects of their care plan, including care decisions, to the fullest extent possible.
- Expect confidentiality of all communication and clinical records related to their care.
- Be involved in advocacy and the formulation of policies that directly impact their health and well-being.

Healthcare Communication

Older adults are the largest consumers of health services. Aggregated chronic diseases, such as cancer, macular degeneration, glaucoma, cognitive disorders, cardiac and circulatory problems, diabetes, stroke, and degenerative bone loss, occur with greater frequency as people live longer. Debilitation problems associated with aging include falls, urinary incontinence, pressure ulcers, functional decline, and delirium. Normal physiologic changes associated with aging can make it harder for elders to hear, to see, or to understand the complexities of the healthcare system, yet their need for services increases. A shift in focus from illness care to wellness promotion is partly due to legislation such as the Affordable Care Act and Medicare, which provide reimbursement for screening and services such as mammograms.

Table 19.1 lists some bridges and barriers involved in communicating with seniors.

Barriers to Treatment

There are language, health literacy, cultural, and socioeconomic barriers to delivering care. Financial challenges are exacerbated by providers limiting the number of Medicare patients. Decreased mobility can impede a senior from traveling to obtain healthcare.

TABLE 19.1 Nurse and Older Adult Communication

Bridges to Foster Communication	Barriers Which Interfere With Communication
Nonverbal • Congruent with words • Head nods • Positive facial expression, smile • Maintains eye contact	• Looks away, glances at clock • Negative facial expression, frown • Rolls eyes
Proximics • Sits face to face or side by side • Sits at same level	• Speaks from too far away • Looms over, looking down on
Attentive Behaviors • Uses active listening, leans slightly forward	• Appears hurried, no time to listen
Haptics • Touches hand, strokes hand • Hugs (if senior is willing)	
Verbal Tone • Moderate, calm	• Use demeaning tone, monotonous • Talks too rapidly • Talks overly loud, slowly • Uses "elder peak" talking down as if to a child
Understandable • Uses common vocabulary, verifies if understood • Speech is clear	• Lots of medical words, jargon
Respectful • Conveys worthiness, value	

Ageism

This is described as discrimination against older adults. Older adults can experience discrimination in accessing healthcare or choosing treatment options.

Health Promotion

Nurses are in a position to work with patients on strategies to prevent falls, which is a major cause of death and disability in the elderly. Having knowledge of community resources as a basis to recommend community-based strengthening programs such as Tai Chi, bone builders, and other exercise and general fitness classes for older adults is also helpful.

Nurses need to be prepared to perform nursing functions in both acute and community-based healthcare settings Use Simulation Exercise 19.1 to reflect on what it is like to be old!

Theoretical Models of Aging and Care

The Transition Healthcare Model

The transitional model is designed to provide continuity of care as the older adult moves from one healthcare agency to another. It is a version of the case management model in which a nurse or social worker is assigned to be the coordinator of healthcare for an older adult. A prime example is discharge from hospital to community, either to their own home or to an extended care facility. Transition nurses provide assessments, ensure adequate follow-up care and coordinate communication among many providers. They verify the need for medications to avoid polypharmacy, help with referrals to support agencies, physical therapy, verify follow-up appointments, etc. They provide health education, particularly about potential risks based on evidence. For example, *Healthy People 2030* states that one in three seniors fall every year, so the nurse assesses for hazards such as loose scatter rugs, poor lighting, or need for handrail grips.

Erikson's Ego Development Model

Erikson's model addresses stage development in later adulthood (Erikson, 1980). Ego integrity becomes the dominant. **Ego integrity** describes acceptance of one's one and only life cycle as something that had to be and that by necessity permits no substitutions. Ego integrity develops

---

SIMULATION EXERCISE 19.1   **What Will It Be Like to Be Old?**

Purpose
To stimulate personal awareness and feelings about the aging process.

Procedure
Think about and write down the answers to the following questions about your own aging process:

- What do you think will be important to you when you are 65 years of age?
- Prepare a list of the traits, qualities, and attributes you hope you will have when you are this age?
- What do you think will be different for you in terms of physical, emotional, spiritual, and social perceptions and activities?
- How would you like people to treat you when you are an older adult?

Reflective Discussion Analysis
In groups of three to four students, share your thoughts. Have one person act as a scribe and write down common themes. Students should ask questions about anything they do not understand.

- In what ways did doing this exercise give you some insight into what the issues of aging might be for your age group?
- In what ways might the issues be different for people in your age group and for people currently classified as older adults?
- How could you use this exercise to better understand the needs of older adults in the hospital, long-term setting, or home?

---

through self-reflection and dialogue with others about the meaning of one's life. Nurses can help frame the older adult's illness story with recognition of social supports and patterns of psychosocial responses in ways that help them reflect on the personal meaning of life. Nursing strategies encouraging life review and reminiscence groups facilitate the process. *Ego despair* describes the failure of a person to accept one's life as appropriate and meaningful. Left unresolved, despair leads to feelings of emotional desolation and bitterness.

Wisdom is the virtue associated with this stage of ego development. It is a form of "knowing" about the meaning and conduct of life, and being willing to share one's wisdom with others. *Practical wisdom* emphasizes good judgment and the capacity to resolve complex human problems in

the real world. *Transcendent wisdom* focuses on self-knowledge, which allows a person to transcend subjectivity, bias, and self-centeredness in relation to an issue. Wisdom allows older adults to share their understanding of life with those who will follow.

Quality of Life Functionality Framework

An older adult's quality of life correlates with their functional capacity to meet personal independence needs. Nurses can use this framework to assess patients across a continuum of functioning, from high functioning to frail older adults. This framework emphasizes interventions that focus on stimulating cognitive reasoning and activities essential to self-management. Activities include self-care, mobility, relationships with others, and engagement with life tasks.

Maslow's Hierarchy of Needs Theory

Maslow's (1954) hierarchy of needs helps nurses prioritize nursing actions, beginning with basic survival needs. Physiological integrity, followed by safety and security, emerge as the most basic critical issues for older patients. They need to be addressed first. For example, Touhy and Jett (2015) note that an agitated patient with dementia looking for a toilet and not being able to find it will not respond to a nurse's comfort or redirection strategies until the toileting need is met. Love and belonging needs in older adults are challenged by increased losses associated with death of important people. Esteem needs, especially those associated with meaningful purpose, and independence remain important issues in later life. Self-actualization occurs more often in middle-aged and older adults.

Elder Abuse

A major threat to the well-being of older adults is passive neglect or even abuse. Active neglect is deliberate while passive neglect occurs when seniors lack needed supervision or essential supports to perform activities of daily living. Elder abuse is difficult to identify. In Burnes et al. (2019) study, only about 15% of cases were reported to authorities. Impaired elders might not even realize what is happening let alone be capable of reporting or taking other actions to stop abuse. If nurses recognize abuse, they are legally obligated to report it to social or legal service agencies.

Mental Health Issues

Older adult brains undergo some minor changes. These may affect memory, but generally cognitive powers remain intact even into very old age. Exceptions are dementia or disease-related cognitive processing problems. Signs of mental problems include the following:

- Changes in eating or sleeping habits
- Substance abuse
- Social isolation, withdrawing from relationships or activities formerly enjoyed
- Chronic feelings of depression, sadness, hopelessness
- Having thoughts of self-harm

Social Isolation

Pathologic social isolation is a lack of connectedness associated with decreased life expectancy (National Academies of Sciences, 2020). Reportedly, social isolation occurs in 25% of elders, while approximately 43% of seniors report feeling lonely. Nurses have a role in identification and mitigation. Box 19.1 identifies fundamental rights of older adults.

APPLICATIONS

Communication Strategies

Nurses adapt communication strategies to successfully assess and care for elders. Remember to affirm dignity by avoiding "elderspeak," which is defined as speaking down to a senior, talking to them as if they were a child. New situations can be temporarily confusing, requiring a little more patience. Give them time to process questions. Problems communicating with seniors having sensory dysfunction are covered in Chapter 17.

Nursing Goals

Goals focus on health promotion, disease prevention, and efficacy with self-management of chronic disorders. Self-management may require active partnership by the patient

---

DEVELOPING AN EVIDENCE-BASED PRACTICE

Disability in older adults can be mediated by healthy lifestyle behaviors such as weight control and exercise, especially balance exercises. Since approximately 30% of seniors fall every year, it is important to focus on prevention (Healthy People 2030). Resnick (2020) lists contributing factors such as poor lighting, slippery surfaces, poor balance, and an overly sedentary lifestyle.

Meneguci et al. (2021) investigated the relationship between sedentary behavior and functionality in 419 adults over age 60. Liu-Ambrose et al. (2019) examined the effects on fall occurrences after attending a fall prevention program focusing on improving strength and balance, while Burton and colleagues' 2018 study identified factors predicting falls as a history of falling, physical inactivity, balance difficulties, and mobility issues.

Results

Lower levels of physical activity were found to correlate with falls. Participation in a fall prevention program was significantly correlated with fewer falls. This is supported by statistics from The Center for Healthy Living, which found a 40% reduction in falls after participation in the Otago Exercise Program to improve strength and balance (NCOA, 2020).

Strength of research evidence: Moderate. Research findings are supported by clinician expertise.

Application to Your Clinical Practice

Causes of falls in older adults are multifactorial, so no one intervention is going to make a major impact. These studies do suggest the following clinical interventions:

1. Assess all frail elderly for fall risk.
2. Recommend attending a strength and balance exercise program (three times/week).
3. Refer patients with a history of falls to a fall prevention program.
4. Teach seniors safety measures, such as wearing supportive shoes (no flip-flops, mules), avoiding slippery surfaces, controlling weight.

References

Burton, E., Lewin, G., O'Connell, H., & Hill, K. D. (2018). Falls prevention in community care: 10 years on. *Clinical Interventions in Aging, 13,* 261–269.

National Council on Aging (NCOA). (2020). *Evidence-based program: Otago exercise program.* Center for Healthy Aging. Retrieved from www.ncoa.org/article/evidence-based-program-otago-exercise-program/. Accessed 25 June 2021.

Liu-Ambrose, T., Davis, J. C., Best, J. R., et al. (2019). Effect of a home-based exercise program on subsequent falls among community-dwelling high-risk older adults after a fall: A randomized clinical trial. *JAMA, 321*(21), 2092–2100.

Meneguci, C. A. G., Meneguci, J., Sasaki, J. E., Tribess, S., & Virtuoso Júnior, J. S. (2021). Physical activity, sedentary behavior and functionality in older adults: A cross-sectional path analysis. *PLoS One, 16*(1), e0246275.

Resnick, B. (2020). Falls: Do we know anything more than we did 40 years ago? *Geriatric Nursing, 41*(2), 67–68.

BOX 19.2 Communication Guidelines for Assessment Interviews

1. Establish rapport.
2. Use open-ended questions first, followed by focused questions.
3. Ask one question at a time.
4. Elicit patient perspectives first.
5. Elicit family perspectives, if indicated.
6. Invite ideas and feelings about diagnosis and treatment.
7. Acknowledge feelings and emotions.
8. Communicate a willingness to help.
9. Provide information in small segments.
10. Summarize the problem or condition discussed in the interview.
11. Validate with the patient and/or family for accuracy.
12. Provide contact information for further questions or concerns.

SIMULATION EXERCISE 19.2 The Story of Aging

Purpose
To promote an understanding of what older adults think.

Procedure
1. Interview (10–15 minutes) someone in your family or acquaintance who is over 65 years.
2. Ask, what was different growing up then versus now? What values were most important? What advice would they give you about how to achieve satisfaction?

Reflective Discussion Analysis
1. Were you surprised at any of the answers older adults gave you?
2. What are some common themes you and your classmates found that related to values and the type of advice older adults gave each of you?
3. What implications do the findings from this exercise have for your future nursing practice?

---

and family in collaboration with healthcare professionals to achieve optimal health in seniors.

Assessment

Communication

Guidelines for communication in assessment interviews are found in Box 19.2. Heightened anxiety can be true for any patient, but it is even more so for the elderly with multiple comorbidities. Older adults are aware of stereotypes associated with aging and may be reluctant to expose themselves as inadequate in a new situation, so they wait and see how their comments will be received. Older adults may stumble over questions when unusually stressed because of anxiety or needing more processing time. Should this occur, the presence of family members can be helpful in giving the healthcare team a verbal picture of the patient's pre-illness state and normalizing care situations for the patient. Simulation Exercise 19.2 on the story of aging provides a glimpse into your awareness of what it is like to be old.

Older adults tend to be more responsive when time is taken to establish a supportive environment before conducting a formal assessment. Sensitive issues such as loneliness, abuse and neglect, caregiver burden, fears about death or frailty, memory loss, incontinence, alcohol abuse, and sexual dysfunction will only be discussed within a trustworthy relationship. Continuity of care with one primary caregiver, when possible, helps foster the development of a comfortable nurse–patient relationship.

Assessing for Cognitive Changes

Appraisal of serious cognitive changes is a critical assessment with older adults, because it has such a significant effect on a person's ability to perform activities of daily living (ADLs). Performing a mental status assessment early in the interview helps with an accurate diagnosis. The Mini-Mental State Examination (Folstein et al., 1975) measures several dimensions of cognition (e.g., orientation, memory, abstraction, and language). An abnormal score (<26) suggests dementia and the need for further evaluation of cognition. Guides for mental status assessment are presented in Box 19.3.

Assessment of Functional Status

The ability to perform ADLs and instrumental activities of daily livings (IADLs) is an essential competency for older adults, especially for those who live alone.

Functional status refers to a broad range of purposeful abilities related to physical health maintenance, role performance, cognitive or intellectual abilities, social activities, and level of emotional functioning. Impaired functional status is a determinant of an older adult's ability to live independently. Functional status rather than chronological age should be a stronger indicator of disability-related needs in older adults, as functional impairment is not associated solely with age. A chronically ill 50-year-old with no support system may have more disabling symptoms of

BOX 19.3   Guide for Mental Status Assessment of Older Adults

- Select a standardized test such as the Mini-Mental State Examination.
- Administer the test in a quiet, nondistracting environment at a time when the patient is not anxious, agitated, or tired.
- Make sure the patient has eyeglasses and/or hearing aids, if needed, before testing.
- Ask easier questions first and provide frequent reassurance that the patient is doing well with the testing.
- Determine the patient's level of formal education. If the patient never learned to spell, it will be impossible to spell "world" backward. Saying the days of the week backward is a good alternative.
- Document your findings clearly in the patient's record, including the patient's response to the testing process, so that future comparisons can be made.

aging than a healthy, active 75-year-old with a strong social support system in place.

Evaluation of functional abilities helps determine the type and level of care an older adult requires. Essential ADLs refer to six areas of essential function: toileting, feeding, dressing, grooming, bathing, and ambulation.

Assessing Pain in Older Adults

Pain is a common concern of older adults, related to an increased number of chronic and acute medical conditions. Moderate, episodic pain associated with chronic disorders of aging occurs more frequently than not and needs to be assessed and addressed. Ask your patient:

- What is the specific nature of your pain (aching, burning, acute, stabbing)?
- Tell me under what circumstances the pain begins (trigger).
- Can you identify patterns of changes in intensity?
- What location (deep, superficial, localized, radiating)?
- How does this pain affect your daily activities?

Chronic pain is defined as pain that persists for 3 months or more. Persistent pain probably occurs in more than 50% of the elderly, but is not a "normal" product of aging. Pain limits an older adult's functional ability and compromises well-being. Pain in the older adult is often underreported because people equate pain with being a natural part of the aging process. In a study by Macieira et al. (2020) of hospitalized adults over age 85, those with cognitive impairment were less likely to receive nursing interventions including

medications to reduce pain. Once identified, reducing pain to improve function should be every nurse's treatment goal.

Medications. Older adults are frequently prescribed opioids such as hydrocodone, meperidine, etc.; however, this has become more controlled as the opioid abuse epidemic spread. Analgesics such as aspirin, Motrin, or Advil are frequently used to self-medicate.

Alternative Methods of Pain Relief. There are a number of interventions other than systemic opioid administration such as local injections into joints or topical creams. Cognitive therapy, guided imagery, and physical therapy can be of help. If pain is severe enough to interfere with daily activities or with sleep, consider a referral to a pain management specialist.

Drug Abuse. Prescription drug abuse is a growing public health problems among older adults in the United States, just as it is in the rest of our society. Liberal dispensing of analgesics to older adults for pain relief without full assessment of the nature of the pain can lead to undesired outcomes. But an alternate system where patients can report when their pain interferes with daily functioning, identifying pain levels on a linear scale, can be more of a challenge for the elderly.

Assessment of pain in cognitively impaired patients and in those who cannot communicate verbally is more difficult. It tends to be expressed in behavior instead of words. Behavioral observation of symptoms suggestive of pain includes grimacing, tightened muscles, groaning, crying, agitation, lethargy, and an unwillingness to move.

Assessing Mental Health

Ask about recent losses and changes. Loss is a reoccurring issue for older adults. Many will suffer losses of people, activities, and functions of importance to them during this life stage. Unlike symptoms of depression in younger people, somatization with vague physical complaints is often a presenting sign of depression (Arnold, 2005). Older adults, particularly white males, are at higher risk for suicide. Comments reflecting hopelessness such as "life doesn't hold much for me" or "sometimes I just wish God would take me" should never be taken lightly.

Assessing Level of Support

The *level* of social support people use depends on personal preference, individual, financial, and social resources, plus what older adults have at their disposal and are willing and able to use. Asking questions such as "Can you tell me who visits you?" "Whom have you visited in the last couple of weeks?" or "If you needed immediate help, whom would you call?" are useful ways to introduce the importance of social support as a part of self-management strategies.

Promoting Wellness: Communication Strategies

Education

Nurses can provide information about normal changes associated with aging. Nurses can offer information about contacting community organizations. One example is the Wellness Initiative for Senior Education (WISE). This is a federally supported organization designed to educate seniors about health issues in the aging process and promoting a healthy lifestyle. Common teaching points include healthy diet; limits on foods high in fat or salt; daily exercise; managing stressors; getting sufficient sleep (Mayo Clinic, n.d.). Patients may not be aware of elder care services: transportation, meals on wheels, church-sponsored friendly visitors, and other aging in place initiatives.

Connectedness

Promotion of patient social connectedness is an important dimension of improved health-related quality of life. Nurses can recommend community resources, and whereas older adults can experience negative situational stressors, they also possess a lifetime of strengths. General nursing care for cognitively intact older adult patients in community centers around discussion of supports is related to self-management of chronic illness and promotes healthy lifestyles. Sometimes it is simply a lack of information that prevents older adults from pursuing possible options. Others know of elder support services, but do not know how to access the available resources in their community. With encouragement, older adults may engage in an exercise program, attend senior center activities, or explore a Tai Chi program combining exercise and meditation. Programs such as bone builders and fall prevention classes are often free for elders at local community centers.

Communication as Therapy

Each conversation becomes an opportunity to gain insight into the person, such as what the person values, what aspirations and dreams were fulfilled or unfulfilled, what contributions are valued, and what goals are yet to be attained. Focusing on what a person considers important enhances well-being among older adults and promotes your interpersonal relationship.

Life Review

Life review is a useful intervention with older adult patients. It can occur as an individual sharing. Gentle prompts and relevant questions for clarification are usually sufficient to keep the conversation going. Sharing recollections from youth or early adulthood days with a compassionate listener helps older adults review their life and/or reestablish its meaning. Sometimes, telling the story provides useful reasons for older adults to resolve long-standing conflicts with important people in their lives.

Reminiscence

Reminiscence is an empowerment strategy that reminds older adults of personal strengths and meaningful goals already achieved. Reminiscence groups focus on sharing important life experiences as simple stories. They follow a structured format, with broad category themes decided on beforehand. Examples include special times in childhood or adolescence, child-rearing or work experience, and handling of a crisis. The leader guides the group in telling their stories and asking questions and points out common themes to stimulate further reflections. In the process of remembering critical incidents, patients can reconnect with forgotten moments that held meaning for them, thus giving them a sense of continuity with their current circumstances. Asking simple concrete questions about the older adult's life, where the person grew up, and what was most important to them is a prompt you can use to initiate conversation, or when communication stalls. Notice if the patient's face seems more animated at any point in the conversation. If so, then comment on it, with simple acknowledgment (for example, "It seems like this was a time that was important to you") and ask for more details.

Encouraging Social and Spiritual Supports

Staying engaged with life and stimulating the mind is essential to the health and well-being of older adults. Older adults have the same need for meaningful activity and personal relationships as younger adults. Age-related changes in eyesight, hearing, and mobility make it more difficult to easily socialize with others. Because older adults can lose self-confidence and begin to disengage socially, they may need encouragement to make the additional effort needed to retain social connections. The amount of socialization depends to some extent on inclination and personality factors, but social isolation compromises the health and well-being of older adults. In many cases, providing social support needs to be proactive due to mobility issues.

For people who have lost their "personal" support system for age-related reasons, a connection with a personal God or church community can become an important source of social and spiritual support. Social and spiritual ties share an interdependent link to positive psychological well-being in late adulthood.

Existential awareness of a shortened life span promotes thinking about death and the meaning of life. Spiritual interventions relevant to the care of older adults include instilling hope, prayer, use of spiritual hymns or readings, and talking about the patient's spiritual concerns. Helping patients cope with unfinished business is an important nursing intervention.

Supporting Independence

Independence is something most people take for granted as a younger adult; it becomes a significant issue for older adults and their caregivers.

Nurses need to be sensitive to the often-unexpressed fears of older adults around surrendering their independence. For example, an older adult awaiting discharge from the hospital told his nurse that he had a bedside commode and no stairs in his home. When the nurse visited the home, there was no commode, and the patient's home had a significant number of stairs. The patient told her that he was afraid his nurse would insist he move to a nursing home if he revealed his real circumstances to her. This is not an uncommon fear of the elderly. How could you respond if you were working with this patient? Formal support services in the community, meals on wheels, home health aides, medical alerts, and informal family supports can be critical factors in enabling frail older adults to remain independent. Nurses can help older patients identify and access these supports.

Safety Supports

There is often a delicate balance between the older adult's perceived and actual need for safety in healthcare. Restrictions and supports needed for safety can and should be negotiated, not simply imposed. Interventions to promote quality of life while protecting safety and independence include the following:

- Respecting choices in food selection
- Providing chair risers, walkers, and canes as needed
- Safety modifications in the home (e.g., handrails on stairs, bathtub/shower grip bars, scatter rug removal, night lights); increased frailty may make independent showering a safer option than a bath
- Including older patients in decision-making about healthcare, and giving them the information they need to make responsible choices
- Installing home security and health alarm monitors; giving trusted neighbors or relatives keys and emergency phone numbers
- Providing information about low-cost Tai Chi, and other low-impact exercise programs in the community; informing patients about fall prevention programs for patients with balance

---

BOX 19.4 Teaching Medication Self-Management

Areas of Assessment

- List of current and previously taken medications, herbal and over-the-counter medications
- Medications taken episodically for insomnia, pain, intestinal upsets, colds, and coughs
- Allergies (include exact symptoms)
- Determine if the patient knows what each medication is for, storage, what to do for missed doses, drug interactions, side effects
- Ability to read medication labels or printed instructions
- Motor difficulties with appropriate medication administration
- Expiration dates, brown bag syndrome (having older adult bring all medications in a brown bag for clinic visit observation)
- Determination of family responsibility, and availability if medication administration support is needed

---

Medication Supports

Medication management is an important area. Seniors may need assistance with reminders. Devices for medication dispensing reminders can be as simple as a weekly/daily pill box or an electronic reminder device like "Google Assistant" or an Internet-connected device such as "Alexia." Medications in general have a stronger effect on the metabolism of older adults and take longer to eliminate from the body. Polypharmacy is a fact of life for many older adults related to multiple chronic conditions. Older adults are at risk for medication side effects and drug interactions because of the variety of meds they take and age-related changes in metabolism (Kim et al., 2018). Successful self-management requires consistent coordination and active participation of the patient, family, and other health professionals to achieve positive health outcomes. A list of all medications including over-the-counter supplements should be taken on appointments with primary care providers, so potentially dangerous interactions can be vetted and superfluous meds eliminated.

Box 19.4 covers key areas for medication assessment.

Advocacy Support

Nurses have an important role in explaining treatment to patients and families, helping them frame questions for physicians and hospitalists, and arranging for continuity of care with community agencies (see also Chapter 24). Role modeling is an indirect form of advocacy, which nurses provide in institutional settings. Treating older patients

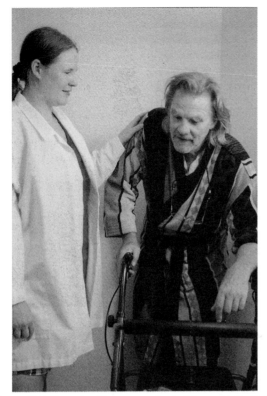

Figure 19.1 Home health nurse or physical therapist can assist ambulation. (Courtesy of K. Boggs.)

> ### BOX 19.5   Areas of Relevant Health Promotion Activities
>
> * Health protection: annual physical examinations; public health approaches promoting flu vaccines
> * Health prevention: environmental or home assessments to prevent falls
> * Health education: information about healthy eating; exercise; age-related sensory changes
> * Health preservation: seeking community social support activities at senior centers, churches, volunteer organizations, food banks, etc.; promoting optimal levels of functioning by increasing the control older adults have over their lives and health

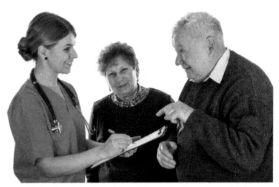

Figure 19.2 Cognitively intact older couples are an important source of information about their health issues. (Copyright © Ocskaymark/iStock/Thinkstock.)

with respect, not becoming impatient with primitive behaviors, and providing excellent care is noted by family and nonprofessionals. Holding nursing assistants accountable for maintaining quality care is a nursing responsibility.

Health Promotion for Older Adults

Health-damaging behaviors such as poor nutrition, inactivity, alcohol, and tobacco abuse contribute heavily to the onset of disability in the elderly. The Centers for Disease Control and Prevention (CDC) recommends an integrated health promotion approach to address common risk factors and comorbidities in older adults. Older adults benefit from health promotion activities tailored to their stage of life. Physical therapy and use of mobility devices such as walkers, wheelchairs, or electric scooters promote safer mobility (Fig. 19.1). It is never too late to practice good nutrition; engage in healthful exercise such as strength training, walking, and yoga; connect with social relationships on a regular basis; and improve safety factors. Most urban communities have groups specifically for older adults.

At the same time, healthy older adults have special needs. Health requirements change as a person ages; their nutrition, exercise, sleep, and other health needs are different. Health promotion strategies need to be modified to meet

the unique requirements of aging adult. Box 19.5 identifies areas of relevant health promotion activities for older adults.

Health Teaching

Health teaching for the elderly is critical if they are to master the tasks of old age and maintain their health. Healthy older adult learning capabilities remain intact for needing more time to think about how they want to handle a situation. Nurses explore what information is needed (Fig. 19.2). The sensitive nurse observes the patient before implementing teaching for the purpose of matching teaching strategies to the individual learning needs of each patient.

Suggestions for simple modifications to reduce age-related barriers to learning when teaching older adults include the following:

* Explain why the information is important to the patient.
* Use familiar words and examples in providing information.
* Draw on the patient's experiences and interests when creating an action plan.

SIMULATION EXERCISE 19.3 Health Promotion Teaching for Older Adults

Purpose
To provide a health teaching segment for an older adult.

Procedure
1. Develop a step-by-step mini–teaching plan related to fall prevention for a cognitively intact older adult.
   a. Consider what person-centered information you will need from the patient to effectively provide tailored content.
   b. Identify specific content you will need to include in your presentation.
   c. Describe teaching strategies you will use.
   d. What accommodations will you need to make?
   e. How will you evaluate the patient's understanding of the material?
2. Implement the teaching plan.
3. Share your experience with other students in small groups of three to six students.

Reflective Discussion Analysis
1. Were there any similarities/differences in themes, or patient responses to the teaching session?
2. Were you surprised at anything you found in preparing for the teaching session versus what occurred during the session?
3. If you had to provide patient education on another topic relevant to the older adult, what would you do differently, if anything?
4. What did you learn from doing this exercise that you could use in future practice with older adults?

- Make teaching sessions short enough to avoid tiring the patient and frequent enough for continuous learning support.
- Speak slowly, naturally, and clearly.

Communicating with elders who have sensory deficits is covered in Chapter 17.

Reflect on Simulation Exercise 19.3 for practice in health promotion teaching with older adults.

Communicating With Cognitively Impaired Older Adults

Dementia

Mild cognitive impairment (MCI) and dementia are neurological disorders characterized by a progressive decline in intellectual and behavioral functioning. **Dementia** is the greatest cause of years lost due to disability in developed countries and the second greatest worldwide. Approximately 6%–8% of the population older than 65 years and more than 30% of those who reach the age of 85 years will experience profound progressive cognitive changes associated with dementia. Dementia is characterized by working memory loss, particularly for recent events, significant personality changes, and a progressive deterioration in intellectual functioning.

When a person suffers with dementia, many people tend to focus on the cognitive and behavioral deficits and overlook the psychosocial, emotional, and spiritual personality components that make up the whole person.

Symptoms of cognitive impairment and communication difficulties in older adults can appear similar to those in patients suffering from depression, delirium, and dementia, so accurate diagnosis is important. Communicating with a patient suffering from dementia requires a different set of strategies than those for the patient with depression. Table 19.2 identifies important differences between the three disorders in older adults. Secondary clinical depression and/or delirium can be superimposed on dementia, making a difficult situation even more challenging.

Supporting Adaptation to Daily Life

Box 19.6 outlines early cognitive changes seen with dementia. Memory loss is a consistent finding. Structure and consistency in the environment are important themes to consider. In the early stages, nurses can help patients develop reminder strategies such as making notes to themselves and using colored labels, alarms, or calendars. Focusing on what the patient can do, rather than on deficits, taps into the functions still available to the patient and decreases feelings of hopelessness.

Apraxia, defined as the loss of the ability to take purposeful action even when the muscles, senses, and vocabulary seem intact, is a common feature of dementia. The person appears to register on a command but acts in ways that suggest he or she has little understanding of what transpired verbally. In the following case example, the caregiver observes the patient's difficulty. Notice how her response supports his ability to function.

Case Study: Ida Absolm Is Confused

The care staff member noticed Mrs Absolm's restlessness as she struggled to figure out which shoes to put on. Ida began looking around with darting eyes, quickly shifting her gaze from here to there. The care staff member said, "I am sorry. I have put two pairs of shoes here and it is confusing. Please put these on." Ida A. looked relieved, put on the shoes, and moved to a table where the care staff member placed a box that had many small articles brought from Mrs Absolm's company. The care staff member said, "Would you help us sort this?" She smiled and said, "Okay … I can see you need help here," as she began to organize the articles into piles.

TABLE 19.2   Sorting Out the Three D's: Delirium, Dementia, Depression

Disorder	Delirium	Dementia	Depression
Onset	Acute, over hours, days	Insidious, over months, years	Relatively rapid, over weeks to months
Acuity	Acute symptoms, medical emergency	Chronic symptoms, progresses slowly	Episodic symptoms, coincides with losses
Course	Short term; resolves with identification of cause, treatment	Gradual, progressive deterioration, memory loss	Self-limiting; recurrent symptoms; resolves with treatment
Duration	Lasts hours to weeks, resolves with treatment	Progressive and irreversible, ends in death	At least 2 weeks, may last months to years, responds to treatment
Alertness or consciousness	Fluctuates, intervals of lucidity and confusion, worse at night	Clear, stable during day, sundown syndrome	Clear, thinking may appear slowed; decreased alertness because of lack of motivation
Attention	Trouble focusing, short attention span, fluctuates	Usually unaffected	Minimal deficit, difficulty concentrating
Orientation	Disoriented to time and place, but not to person	Impaired as disease progresses; inability to recognize familiar people or objects, including self	Selective disorientation
Memory	Recent and immediate impaired	Impaired memory for immediate/recent events; unconcerned about memory deficits	Selective impairment, concerned about memory deficits
Thinking	Incoherent, global disorganization	Impoverished, inability to learn, trouble word finding	Intact, negative themes
Perception	Gross distortions; illusions, visual, tactile hallucinations	Prone to hallucinations as disease progresses	Intact, but colored by negative themes
Speech	Incoherent, disorganized, loud, belligerent	Impoverished, tangential, repetitive, superficial, confabulations	Quiet, decreased, can be irritable, language skills intact
Sleep/wake cycle	Disturbed; changes hourly	Disturbed; day/night reversal	Disturbed; early morning wakening, hypersomnia during day
Contributing factors	Underlying medical cause; toxicity, fever, tumor, infection, drugs	Degenerative disorder associated with age, cardiovascular deficits, substance dependence	Significant or cumulative loss; drug toxicity, diabetes, myocardial infarction

Adapted from Arnold, E. (2005). Sorting out the three D's: Delirium, depression, dementia. *Holist Nursing Practice, 19*(3), 99–104.

Supporting Communication

Difficulty with purposeful communication is a hallmark of dementia. The patient's loss is a gradual process initially, so many patients can maintain superficial conversation, with empathetic support. Dementia affects basic receptive (decoding and understanding) and expressive (conveying information) forms of communication. These deficits influence the person's capacity to think abstractly and solve

BOX 19.6 Signs of Early Cognitive Changes With Dementia

- Difficulty remembering appointments
- Difficulty recalling the names of friends, neighbors, family
- Forgetting words or using the wrong word when talking
- Jumbling words, using mixed up sentence
- Not following the conversation of others
- Not understanding an explanation or story
- Difficulty remembering when a task was completed (last hour verses last week)
- Difficulty keeping up with the steps to complete a task
- New difficulty filling out complex forms
- Different behavior/personality: restless, quick to get angry; quiet/withdrawn; craving sweets
- Loss of interest in meeting with friends or doing activities

BOX 19.7 Communication Do's and Don'ts With Dementia Patients

Communication Do's

- Simplify environmental stimuli before beginning to converse.
- Look directly at the patient when talking.
- Ask the patient what he or she would like to be called.
- Try to identify the emotions behind the patient's words or behavior.
- Identify and minimize anything in the environment that creates anxiety for the patient.
- Watch your body language; convey interest and acceptance.
- Repeat simple messages slowly, calmly, and patiently.
- Give clear, simple directions one at a time in a step-by-step manner.
- Direct conversation toward concrete, familiar objects.
- Communicate with touch, smiles, calmness, and gentle redirection.
- Structure the environment and routines, to allow freedom within limits.
- Use soft music or hymns when the patient seems agitated.

Communication Don'ts

- Don't argue or reason with the patient; instead, use distraction.
- Avoid confrontation.
- Don't use slang, jargon, or abstract terms.
- If attention lapses, don't persist. Let the patient rest a few minutes before trying to regain his or her attention.
- Don't focus on difficult behavior; look for the underlying anxiety and redirect.
- Avoid hand restraints if at all possible.
- Avoid small objects that could be a choking hazard.

problems. Although patients may speak in fragments, they are still capable of interacting with prompts, and especially when given your full attention. Caregiver issues are discussed in Chapter 12.

Difficulty with word retrieval can reflect short-term memory impairment. Patients may stop midsentence and look confused. They may ask for help with a word, or continue with phrases that have little to do with the intended conversation.

Providing *verbal cues* helps older adults with short-term memory impairment. Nurses can support patients by suggesting a missing word or providing a simple meaning. Check with the patient that your interpretation is accurate.

Sometimes you can grasp what the word might be from its context.

Case Study: Carol Buret

In a conversation with her nurse, Carol Buret could not retrieve the word "Halloween." Instead she said, "When people dress in costumes." The nurse said, "You mean like Halloween?" The patient said yes, and the conversation continued.

Short-term memory allows people to follow a conversation when the topic changes. Cognitively impaired patients lack short-term memory, so topic transitions can be difficult. Restate ideas using simple words and sequence and validate the meaning of a patient's response.

Using words directly applicable to daily routines, such as "before lunch," can anchor the patient's recognition of time frames better than saying a specific time such as 11:00 a.m.

Use plain language and simple questions that can be answered with a yes or no for patients. Be aware that the patient is acutely aware of your body language and may consider it as a measure of your acceptance. Your goal is to try and make each conversation a "person-centered" verbal connection. Box 19.7 summarizes communication guideline Dos and Don'ts for communicating with cognitively impaired patients.

Cognitively impaired patients often have trouble following instructions consisting of multiple steps. Breaking instructions into single steps helps these patients master tasks that otherwise are beyond their comprehension. Keep the conversation simple and focused only on one step at a time.

Do not explain why or what will happen if the directions are not followed. Scolding usually worsens confusion. Unlike children who can learn from a mistake, the patient with dementia cannot. If the patient does not do a task or follow directions incorrectly, keep the words simple. Proactively state a next step in pleasant calm tones, for example, "Let's see if we can …" (followed by a one-step directive). Table 19.3 lists suggested behavioral communication interventions for types of dementia symptoms.

Patients with dementia often retain many of their social skills, even when their cognitive memory significantly declines, especially in the early stages (Mace & Rabins, 2017). Asking mild to early moderate cognitively impaired older adults about their past life experiences is a way to connect verbally with those who might have difficulty telling you what they had for breakfast 2 h ago. Remote memory (recall of past events) is retained longer than memory for recent events. For the patient, the experience of connecting with another person is more important than having an in-depth conversation. Giving a compliment helps. Family members can be encouraged to reminisce with dementia patients. Even if the patient cannot respond verbally, sometimes behaviors will show through facial expression or garbled words an appreciation for the connection. Sometimes this occurs when least expected.

Touch

Touch is something patients with dementia can no longer ask for, create for themselves, or tell another of its meaning. Older adults generally experience gentle touch not only physically as sensation, but also affectively as emotion and behavior. Touch is a form of communication that immediately acknowledges a dementia patient's stress, calms an agitated patient, and provides a sense of security, particularly if accompanied by a smile, or a compliment, and a gentle approach. As dementia progresses, informal and professional caregivers can use gentle touch to gain a patient's attention, to guide a person toward an activity, or simply as an expression of caring. In general, patients with dementia appreciate the use of touch. But to some, it can be frightening, particularly if you move in too fast. Before using touch, make sure that the patient is open to it.

Sundowning

Sundowning is a term used to describe agitated behavioral symptoms, usually occurring later in the day with dementia patients. Common behaviors include fretfulness, anxiety, and demanding behaviors. Days and nights are reversed. This behavior can be very difficult for family members because their sleep is disturbed. Keeping the patient active during the day helps. Small doses of medication are used to alleviate symptoms.

Legal Issues

Patients with early dementia can still make simple decisions, if they are supported and are patiently respected.

Decisional capacity refers to the capability of a person to:
- Understand and process information about diagnosis, prognosis, and treatment options.
- Weigh the benefits, burdens, and risks of the proposed options.
- Apply a set of personal values to the analysis.
- Arrive at a decision that is consistent over time.
- Communicate the decision.

Mental competence represents a medicolegal determination, related to injury, disease, or intellectual disability of a person's ability to manage his or her personal legal affairs. By contrast with decisional capacity, **mental incompetence** occurs when a person lacks the capacity to negotiate legal tasks such as making a will, entering into a contract, or making certain legal decisions.

The time to execute legal documents to patient rights is before patients become unable to cognitively assign decision-making authority to someone they trust.

Once cognitive capacity is lost, a court procedure is necessary to establish a conservatorship or guardianship. This action is costly and emotionally painful for most families because it requires legally certifying the person as incompetent (Arnold, 2005).

Advocating for the Patient With Dementia

Nurses should refer patient family members to local Alzheimer's or Parkinson's or related dementia support groups. These support groups provide a place to talk about the challenges of caring for their family members. *The 36-Hour Day* (Mace & Rabins, 2017), developed from the insights of family members coping with dementia in a loved one, is a classic understandable resource for family members.

Caring for Patients With Advanced Dementia

Dementia is a progressive disease; patients gradually lose control over body functions and the capacity to handle even simple tasks. Meaningful verbal communication terminates. Attempts to communicate through behavior are primitive and not easily understood.

Treatment goals for patients with advanced dementia should emphasize dignity, quality of life, and supportive comfort strategies.

TABLE 19.3   Symptoms of Dementia With Suggested Behavioral Communication Interventions

Dementia Symptom Pattern	Suggested Intervention
Agitation/altered behavior, restless	• Identify and remove cause • Assess for physical problems • Reduce stimuli, suggest a walk • Use simple repetitive activities: folding towels, rolling socks • Use soothing music, Bible verses • Look for patterns that trigger agitation • Medication
Verbal or physical aggression: grabbing, hitting	• Avoid triggers • Recognize that the patient is frightened • Decrease stimuli, move patient to a quiet place • Do not take the patient's behavior personally • Respect and enlarge the patient's personal space • Identify and minimize cause • Make eye contact; speak in a calm voice • Acknowledge frustration; do not reprimand • Check medications
Withdrawal/loss of Interest: decreased socialization, apathy, social isolation	• Put GPS into shoe or other tracking device such as RDIF chip • Use simple activities, make tasks simple with one instruction at a time • Find simple socialization opportunities and support patient involvement
Refusal or resistance to suggestions	• Drop the topic or activity and reintroduce it later
Disturbed motor activity: wandering, pacing, raiding waste cans, shadowing caregiver	• Keep the environment safe • Remove trash • Use medical alert bracelets • Label drawers, room (photos help) • Use locks on doors at home
Sleep disturbances: day/night sleep reversal, calling out/moaning in sleep	• Medication • Keep active during the day • Toilet patient as needed during night without conversation • Control wandering at night; lead back to bed; avoid use of restraints • Use bed alarm, signals if senior does not return to bed after __ minutes
Altered cognition, memory problems Hallucinations, delusions, illusions	• Encourage talk of long ago memories • Use reminders: calendars, lists, computerized memory aids • Clock in every room • Respond to the emotion, not content • Reduce stimuli • Use good nonglare lighting • Use distraction (e.g., walk, simple activity) • Use touch, reassurance, postponement

Continued

TABLE 19.3 Symptoms of Dementia With Suggested Behavioral Communication Interventions—cont'd	
Dementia Symptom Pattern	**Suggested Intervention**
Disinhibition: inappropriate speech, touching, improper body exposure, entering other people's space	• Do not reprimand • Respond to the emotion • Redirect patient to other activities
Incontinence: urine, feces, eliminating in wrong places	• Check for bladder infection, fecal impaction • Note elimination pattern; establish corresponding toileting timetable • Schedule toileting at frequent intervals • Toilet before bedtime • Take patient to bathroom, verbally cue • Use washable clothing, Velcro closings
Swallowing difficulty: choking, stuffing mouth, not swallowing	• Cut food into small pieces, offer small quantities of liquid at one time • Check medications for size, modify as needed • Sit with patient while eating • Verbally cue to chew and swallow
Agnosia: difficulty recognizing faces, including one's own	• Remove or cover mirrors if patient is frightened by self-image • Verbally identify familiar people and their relationship to the patient

SUMMARY

This chapter described adaptations in communication strategies for use with older adults. Statistics reveal that older adults constitute the fastest growing population group in the United States. Aging is a universal life process with distinctive features. Typically there is a progressive decline in sensory and motor functions with appropriate supports; older adults can expect to live longer and enjoy a better quality of life than in previous generations.

Erikson's theory of psychosocial development identifies ego integrity versus despair as the central maturational crisis of old age. People who believe that their lives have purpose and meaning, and that they have few or no regrets about a well-lived life, demonstrate the ego strength of integrity.

Differential assessment of depression, delirium, and dementia is important, as symptoms can appear similar. Supportive communication and empowerment strategies to assist patients in maximizing their health and well-being were described as well as related communication strategies with patients and families. Health promotion activities that take into account the unique needs and cultural values of older adults are more likely to be successful. As a primary provider in long-term care and in the community, the nurse is in a unique role to support and meet the communication needs of older adult patients.

ETHICAL DILEMMA: What Would You Do?

Mrs Allan is an accomplished 82-year-old woman, living alone. She treasures her independence. While she realizes she is more frail, she does not want to leave her home or lose her independence. Her daughter is worried about her and wants her to move to assisted living. During your initial assessment for a recent fall, Mrs Allan confides that while she does have "some" memory lapses, she cannot bear the idea of what assisted living will mean for her independence and quality of life. She asks you to keep her confidence. You can understand Mrs Allan's concerns but you also know that keeping silent may not be in her best interest. How could you balance the ethical concept of beneficence with your patient's concerns? What would you do?

DISCUSSION QUESTIONS

1. What are some examples of ageism affecting older adults?
2. How is ageism perpetuated?
3. From an advocacy perspective, how could you as a nurse help create a more positive image of older adults?

REFERENCES

Arnold, E. (2005). Sorting out the 3 D's: Delirium, dementia, depression: Learn how to sift through overlapping signs and symptoms so you can help improve an older patient's quality of life. *Holistic Nursing Practice, 19*(3), 99–104.

Burnes, D., Acierno, R., & Hernandez-Tejada, M. (2019). Help-seeking among victims of elder abuse: Findings from the National elder Mistreatment study. *Journals of Gerontology Series B: Psychological Sciences and Social Sciences, 74*(5), 891–896.

Butler, M., Gaugler, J. E., Talley, K. M. C., et al. (2020). *Care interventions for people living with dementia and their caregivers. Comparable effectiveness review #231.* AHRQ Publication No. 20-EHC023 Rockville, MD: AHRQ. Retrieved from: https://effectivehealthcare.ahrq.gov/sites/default/files/pdf/cer-231-dementia-interventions-final_0.pdf. [Accessed 25 June 2021].

Erikson, E. (1980). *Identity and the life cycle.* New York: Norton.

Folstein, M. F., Folstein, S. E., & McHugh, P. R. (1975). "Mini-mental state." A practical method for grading the cognitive state of patients for the clinician. *Journal of Psychiatric Research, 12*(3), 189–198.

Kim, L. D., Koncilja, K., & Nielsen, C. (2018). Medication management in older adults. *Cleveland Clinic Journal of Medicine, 85*(2), 129–135.

Mace, N., & Rabins, P. (2017). *The 36-hour day: A family guide to caring for people with Alzheimer's disease, other dementias, and memory loss* (6th ed.). Baltimore, MD: Johns Hopkins University Press.

Macieira, T. G., Yao, Y., Smith, M. B., Bian, J., Wilkie, D. J., & Keenan, G. M. (2020). Nursing care for hospitalized older adults with and without cognitive impairment. *Nursing Research, 69*(2), 116–126.

Maslow, A. (1954). *Motivation and personality.* New York: Harper & Row.

Mayo Clinic. (n.d.). *Alzheimer's disease.* MayoClinic.org [website] Retrieved from: www.mayoclinic.org/diseases-conditions/alzheimers/. [Accessed 25 June 2021].

National Academies of Sciences, Engineering, and Medicine. (2020). *Social isolation and loneliness in older adults: Opportunities for the health care system.* Washington, DC: The National Academies Press.

Touhy, T., & Jett, K. (2015). *Ebersole and Hess' toward healthy aging: Human needs and nursing response* (9th ed.). St. Louis, MO: Elsevier.

U.S. Department of Health and Human Services (USDHHS). (2020). *Older adults. Healthy People 2030.* Retrieved from: https://health.gov/healthypeople/objectives-and-data/browse-objectives/older-adults. [Accessed 25 June 2021].

20

Communicating With Patients in Crisis

OBJECTIVES

At the end of the chapter, the reader will be able to:
1. Define crisis and related concepts.
2. Discuss theoretical frameworks related to crisis and crisis intervention.
3. Apply structured crisis intervention strategies in the care of patients experiencing a crisis state.
4. Apply crisis intervention strategies to emergency situations.

BASIC CONCEPTS

Definitions

Crisis

A **crisis** occurs when a stressful life event overwhelms an individual's ability to cope effectively in the face of a perceived challenge or threat. People in a crisis state experience an actual or perceived overwhelming threat to self-concept, an insurmountable obstacle or a loss that conventional coping measures cannot handle. Unabated, the resulting tension continues to increase, creating major personality disorganization and a crisis state.

Personal responses to crisis can be adaptive or maladaptive. Nurses can help patients with restorative coping strategies to lessen the damaging impact of crisis. Successfully working through a crisis has the potential to strengthen people's coping responses and encourage a sense of self-efficacy. Maladaptive responses can result in the development of acute or chronic psychiatric symptoms.

Crisis State. A **crisis state** as an acute but *normal* human response to severely abnormal circumstances. A crisis state is *not* a mental illness, although individuals with mental illness can experience a crisis state associated with their disorder. Crisis is a complex concept, which can defy easy cause/effect explanations. Because a crisis state represents a personal response, two people experiencing the same crisis event will respond differently to it. Understanding the patient's personal response to a crisis rather than an objective crisis stressor is critical to successful crisis intervention.

A crisis state creates a temporary disconnect from attachment to others, loss of meaning, and disruption of previous mastery skills. Individuals feel vulnerable. Crisis intervention strategies are designed to help support people experiencing crisis achieve psychological homeostasis. A favorable outcome depends on the person's combined interpretation of the crisis, perception of coping ability, resources, and level of social support. As you read this chapter, consider what you would do in the following case if you were dealing with Andy Rooney.

CASE STUDY: **Andy Rooney Threatens Suicide**

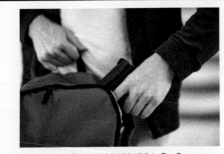

From iStock #687794504, FatCamera.

Andy is 15 years old, attending the school where you work as a school nurse. He approaches you and tells you he is going to kill himself, showing you a gun.
1. What can you do or say to deescalate this situation?
2. How do you protect other students nearby from this potential school shooting?

Types of Crisis. **Developmental Crisis.** A crisis is classified as developmental or situational. Erikson's (1982) stage model of psychosocial development forms the basis for exploring the nature of developmental crisis. Developmental crisis can occur as individuals negotiate developmental age-related milestones in their lives, for example, becoming a parent or retiring from long-term employment. Normative psychosocial crises are used as benchmarks for assessing signs and symptoms of developmental crisis. When a situational crisis is superimposed on a normative developmental crisis, the crisis experience can be more intense. For example, a woman losing a spouse at the same time she is going through menopause can experience a more intense impact.

Situational Crisis. A situational crisis refers to an unusually stressful life event, which exceeds a person's resources and coping skills. Examples include unexpected illness or injury, rape, a car accident, the loss of a home or spouse, or being laid off from a job. When the crisis impacts a large number of people simultaneously, for example, a disaster, it is referred to as an *adventitious crisis*. A situational crisis is *not* defined by the life event itself, but by the individual's personal response to it. How successfully a person responds to a crisis can depend on the following:

- Previous experience with crises, coping, and problem-solving
- Perception of the crisis event
- Level of help or obstruction from significant others
- Developmental level and ego maturity
- Concurrent stressors

Behavioral Emergencies. A **behavioral emergency** occurs when a crisis escalates to the point that the situation requires immediate intervention to avoid injury or death. Examples include any type of violent interpersonal behavior, psychotic crisis, suicide, or homicide. A behavioral emergency describes any type of thinking or behavior that places an individual in an immediate potentially injurious or lethal situation. A behavioral emergency is always an emotionally charged, unpredictable situation. In addition to assessing patient risk characteristics, it is important to evaluate the environmental features and other factors that can either increase or decrease suicidal risk. When this patient is discharged from the hospital, the family and patient should be provided suicide prevention information, for example, crisis hotline (The Joint Commission, 2019, 2021).

Crisis Intervention. **Crisis intervention** represents a systematic application of theory-based problem-solving strategies designed to help individuals and families resolve a crisis situation quickly and successfully. The desired clinical outcome is a return to an individual's precrisis functional level. Crisis intervention strategies should be adapted to fit each patient's preferences, beliefs, values, and individual circumstances. As a nurse, you cannot always change the nature of a crisis situation, but you can help defuse a patient's emotional reaction to it with compassionate professional support and guidance.

Crisis intervention is a *time-limited* treatment. Four to six weeks is considered the standard time frame for crisis resolution. Interventions should be present-focused and action-oriented. The emphasis is on *immediate problem-solving* and *strengthening the personal resources* of patients and their families. Full recovery can take a much longer period of time, particularly from a disaster crisis. Nurses function as advocates, resources, partners, and guides in helping patients resolve crisis situations, usually as part of a larger crisis intervention team.

Theoretical Frameworks

Lindemann (1944) and Caplan (1964) developed the most widely used models of crisis and crisis intervention. Lindemann's study of bereavement provides a frame of reference for understanding the stages involved in resolving emotional crisis and bereavement. His findings suggest that psychiatric management of grief reactions may prevent prolonged and serious alterations in the patient's social adjustment, as well as potential medical disease.

Caplan broadened Lindemann's model to include developmental crisis and personal crisis. Although the focus of crisis intervention is on secondary prevention because the crisis state is already in motion, Caplan's model of preventive psychiatry starts in the community. He introduced practical crisis intervention strategies, for example, crisis telephone lines, training for community workers, and early response strategies. He viewed nurses as key service providers in crisis intervention.

Caplan discusses a crisis response pattern. He identifies a person's initial response to a crisis state as *shock,* with varied emotions, ranging from anger, laughing, hysterics, crying, and acute anxiety to social withdrawal. An extended period of adjustment follows the state of shock with a period of *recoil,* which can last from 2 to 3 weeks. Behavior appears normal to outsiders, but patients describe nightmares, phobic reactions, and flashbacks of the crisis event.

Restoration or reconstruction describes the final phase of crisis intervention. This phase involves developing a plan and taking constructive actions to resolve the crisis situation. If successfully negotiated, the person returns to a precrisis functional level, which is the desired clinical outcome. Maladaptive coping strategies, such as drug or alcohol use, violence, or avoidance, prevents restoration and places the patient at risk for further problems. Simulation Exercise 20.1 is designed to help you to understand the nature of crisis.

Nursing Model

The nursing model developed by Aguilera (1998) approaches crisis intervention from a balancing perspective between a crisis situation and a patient's capacity to resolve it. The model proposes that a crisis state develops because of a distorted perception of a situation or because the patient lacks the resources to cope successfully with it. Balancing factors include a realistic perception of the event, the patient's internal resources (beliefs or attitudes), and the patient's external (environmental) supports. These factors can minimize or reduce the impact of the stressor, leading to resolution of the crisis.

Absence of adequate situational support, lack of coping skills, and a distorted perception of the crisis event can result in a crisis state, leaving individuals and families feeling overwhelmed and unable to cope. Interventions are designed to increase the balancing factors needed to restore a patient to precrisis functioning.

APPLICATIONS

Goal

The goal of crisis intervention is to return patients to their previous level of functioning. This goal is evidenced by
*   stabilization of distress symptoms,
*   reduction of distress symptoms,
*   restoration of functional capabilities to precrisis levels, and
*   referrals for follow-up support care, if indicated.

Structuring Crisis Intervention Strategies

Communication is the key to crisis deescalation (Dufresne, 2003). Roberts and Yeager (2009) provides a seven-stage sequential blueprint for clinical intervention, which can be used to structure the crisis intervention process in nurse–patient relationships. This model is compatible with the nursing process sequence of assessment, planning, implementation, and evaluation.

DEVELOPING AN EVIDENCE-BASED PRACTICE

One-third of global workplace violence occurs in healthcare settings with nurses being the most common recipients. Nearly all nurses report being the target of some type of violence sometime during their careers. Njaka's (2020) review examined 1650 articles and studies of relationships between workplace violence and outcomes for African nurses. Mento analyzed 27 publications also looking at these relationships (2020), while Price's 2015 metaanalysis of 38 studies looked at effects of deescalation training on staff handling violent behaviors.

Findings

Workplace violence in all studies was most commonly reported as verbal abuse, generally from patients and their families. Other violence included bullying, physical abuse such as slapping, and psychological abuse such as threats. Causes of violence by patients were attributed to frustration due to long waits for service, impolite communication by staff (Döndü & Yasemin, 2021), or patient intoxication. Outcomes for nurses included physical injury, psychological harm such as increased stress and anxiety, and job dissatisfaction or impairment. Evaluation of the impact of education training programs in deescalation skills showed some staff performance improvement when dealing with subsequent violent behavior.

Strength of evidence: High for demographic data: level of occurrence, causes, effects on staff; low for training/

education intervention effects perhaps due to wide variation in intensity and type of education.

Application to Your Clinical Practice

1. Request more education on assessment and intervention on deescalation techniques for the patient who is suicidal. During this education, it would be helpful for the nurse to evaluate and explore how their attitudes may influence assessment and identification of workplace violence.
2. Practice deescalation communication skills.
3. Be familiar with agency policy on workplace violence and how to report.
4. Treat every patient with respect (politeness).

References

Döndü, Ş., & Yasemin, B. (2021). Determination of the society's perceptions, experiences, and intentions to use violence against health professionals. *Safety and Health at Work*, *12*(2), 141–146.

Mento, C., Silvestri, M. C., Bruno, A., et al. (2020). Workplace violence against healthcare professionals: A systematic review. *Aggression and Violent Behavior*, *51*, 101381.

Njaka, S., Edeogu, O. C., Oko, C. C., Goni, M. D., & Nkadi, N. (2020). Work place violence (WPV) against healthcare workers in Africa: A systematic review. *Heliyon*, *6*(9), e04800.

Price, O., Baker, J., Bee, P., & Lovell, K. (2015). Learning and performance outcomes of mental health staff training in de-escalation techniques for the management of violence and aggression. *British Journal of Psychiatry*, *206*(6), 447–455.

SIMULATION EXERCISE 20.1 Understanding the Nature of Crisis

Purpose
To help students understand crisis in preparation for assessing and planning communication strategies in crisis situations in professional patient care situations.

Procedure
1. Describe a crisis you experienced in your life. There are no right or wrong definitions of a crisis, and it does not matter whether the crisis would be considered a crisis in someone else's life.
2. Identify how the crisis changed your roles, routines, relationships, and assumptions about yourself.
3. Apply a crisis model to the situation you are describing.
4. Identify the strategies you used to cope with the crisis.
5. Describe the ways in which your personal crisis strengthened or weakened your self-concept and increased your options and your understanding of life.

Reflective Discussion Analysis
1. What did you learn from doing this exercise that you can use in your clinical practice?

BOX 20.1 Field Expedient Tool to Assess Dangerousness to Self or Others

- **D**epression/suicidal
- **A**nger/agitation, aggressive
- **N**oncompliance with requests/taking medication
- **G**eneral appearance/inappropriate dress/poor hygiene
- **E**vidence of self-inflicted injury
- **R**esponding/reacting to delusions or hallucinations
- **O**wns/displays weapon(s)
- **U**norganized thoughts/appearance/behavior
- **S**peech pattern/substance/rate (too fast, too slow, jumps all over)
- **P**aranoid
- **E**rratic or fearful behavior
- **R**ecent loss of job/loved one/home
- **S**ubstance abuse
- **O**rientation to date/time/location/situation/insight into illness
- **N**umber and type of previous contacts with police, mental health, or crisis workers

From Officer Scott A. Davis, Crisis Intervention Tea (CIT) Coordinator. (2010) *Field expedient tool to assess dangerousness to self or others,* Rockville, MD, Montgomery County Police Department.

Step 1: Assessing Lethality and Mental Status
Initially, assessment should focus on determining the severity of current danger potential, both to self and to others as in the case of domestic violence. Box 20.1 presents a field expedient tool for initial assessment of a potential behavioral emergency. Crisis intervention teams (CIT) develop and use this tool to assess potential dangerous patient behaviors. CIT is collaboration between law enforcement officers and mental health providers that assists individuals in the community who are exhibiting a mental health crisis.

Step 2: Establishing Rapport and Engaging the Patient
Once the initial triage assessment of a patient in crisis is completed, the nurse performs a more comprehensive crisis appraisal. This assessment should be specific to the patient's current state and circumstances. Patients in crisis look to health professionals to structure interactions. Introduce yourself briefly, and quickly orient the patient to the purpose of the crisis questions and how the information will be used. Remember to abide by HIPAA confidentiality. If patients expect family members to give or receive information to health providers when the patient is not present, the patient needs to sign a consent form.

When engaging with patients, give them your full attention. People who are listened to feel validated. Patients experiencing a crisis state require a compassionate, flexible, but clearly directive calm approach from nurses. Place the patient in a quiet, lighted room with no shadows, away from the mainstream of activity. Avoid the use of touch, as the patient may be supersensitive to any form of unexpected response from a health professional. Be nonjudgmental. Use fewer rather than more words to explain. Utilize a clear, concrete communication style, with an emphasis on attending to the patient's needs.

Only a minimum number of people should be involved with the patient, until the patient is emotionally stabilized. If the patient is unable to cooperate, for safety reasons, more than one professional may be needed to stabilize the situation. Depending on the nature of the crisis and the patient's personal responses, a trusted family member may be included.

Interventions. **Communication.** Speak calmly and use close-ended questions to elicit the person's immediate intent. Use short, clear, direct phrases and questions. Use closed-ended questions in the *early* stages of crisis intervention related to safety issues, requesting specific information and eliciting a patient commitment to immediate action needed to stabilize the crisis situation. Careful, accurate listening skills are essential. It is important to discover the patient's perception of the crisis—how it developed, how it impacts the patient's life, etc. One suggested way is to ask "Is this the first time you have experienced a crisis like this? Have you had other crises? What were they like? How did you problem-solve these crises?"

Focus on Feelings. Assess the patient's perception of their emotional coping strength, asking questions such as, "How were you feeling about this before the crisis got so bad?" "Where do you see yourself headed with this problem?" Use reflective listening responses to identify feelings (e.g., "It sounds as if you are feeling very sad [angry, lonely] right now."). You can help patients focus on relevant points by repeating a phrase, asking for validation or clarification to focus the discussion. Allow silences. This person may need time to process their thoughts and think about your input. Simulation Exercise 20.2 offers an opportunity to understand reflection as a listening response in crisis situations.

SIMULATION EXERCISE 20.2   Using Reflective Responses in a Crisis Situation

Purpose
To provide students with a means of appreciating the multipurpose uses of reflection as a listening response in crisis situations.

Procedure
Have one student role-play a patient in an emergency department situation involving a common crisis situation (e.g., fire, heart attack, auto accident). After this person talks about the crisis situation for 3–4 min, have each student write down a reflective listening response that they would use with the patient in crisis. Have each student read their reflective response to the class. (This can also be done in small groups of students if the class is large.)

Reflective Discussion Analysis
1. Were you surprised at the variety of reflective themes found in the students' responses?
2. In what ways could differences in the wording or emphasis of a reflective response influence the flow of information?
3. In what ways do reflective responses validate the patient's experience?
4. How could you use what you learned from doing this exercise in your clinical practice?

Step 3: Identify Major Problems

Focus on the Here and Now. Questions should be short and relevant to the crisis.

Request more specific details (e.g., ask who was involved, what happened, and when it happened) if this information is needed. Ask about the feelings associated with the immediate crisis. Your responses should be brief, empathetic, and clearly related to the patient's story. Note changes in expression, body posture, and vocal inflections as they talk. Be alert for any escalation of agitation or verbal outbursts. If they show signs of agitation, ask what would be helpful right now? Identify central emotional themes in the patient's story (e.g., powerlessness, shame, stigma, hopelessness) to provide a focus for intervention.

- Proceed slowly with a calm tone and direct communication.
- Affirm patient efforts and offer encouragement.
- Summarize content often and ask for validation so that you are on the same page, with a comprehensive understanding of major issues. Have them summarize their thoughts.

Identifying Feelings. Patients can have difficulty putting crisis emotions into words because of high anxiety. Nurses can help patients clarify important feelings with observations about patient responses (e.g., "I wonder if because you think your son is using drugs [precipitating event], you feel helpless and confused [patient emotional response] and don't know what to do next [patient behavioral reaction]."). "Does that capture what is going on with you?" Checking in with a patient helps to ensure that your interpretations represent the patient's truth.

Patients in crisis tend to develop tunnel vision. Often, they feel there is no solution. Losing sight of personal assets and potential reserves, which could be used to defuse the crisis, some patients are frightened by the intensity of their emotional reactions. Patients appreciate hearing that most people experience powerful and conflicting feelings in crisis situations. The message you want to get across is "you are not alone, and together we can come up with a plan to deal with this difficult situation." Global reassurance is not helpful, but specific supportive comments that recognize patient efforts can help patients to deescalate a crisis event to workable proportions.

Affirm Personal Strengths. Evoking the person's social supports and calling attention to personal strengths can enhance coping skills. Reinforce personal strengths as you observe them or as the patient identifies them. Simulation Exercise 20.3 provides an opportunity to experience the value of personal support systems in crisis situations.

Providing Explicit Information. Being truthful about what is known and unknown and updating information as you learn about it helps build trust with patients

SIMULATION EXERCISE 20.3   Personal Support Systems

Purpose
To help students appreciate the breadth and importance of personal support systems in stressful situations.

Procedure
All of us have support systems we can use in times of stress (e.g., church, friends, family, coworkers, clubs, recreational groups).
1. Identify a support person or system you could or do use in a time of crisis.
2. Reflect on why you would choose this person or support system.
3. What does this personal support system or person do for you (e.g., listen without judgment; provide honest, objective feedback; challenge you to think; broaden your perspective; give unconditional support; share your perceptions)? List all relevant reasons.
4. What factors go into choosing your personal support system (e.g., availability, expertise, perception of support)? Which is the most important factor?

Reflective Discussion Analysis
1. What types of support systems were most commonly used by class or group members?
2. What were the most common reasons for selecting a support person or system?
3. After doing this exercise, what strategies would you advise for enlarging a personal support system?
4. What applications do you see in this exercise for your nursing practice?

in crisis. Even with unknowns, people cope better when uncertainty is briefly acknowledged, rather than not mentioned. Explain what is going to happen, step by step. Letting patients know as much as possible about progress, treatment, and the consequences of choosing different alternatives allows patients to make informed decisions and reduces the heightened anxiety associated with a crisis situation.

Step 4: Explore Alternative Options and Partial Solutions

Try broadening their perspective by looking at partial solutions. Breaking tasks down into small, achievable parts empowers people. Proposed strategies should accommodate both the immediate problems and patient resources. *It is important to encourage the patient to make autonomous choices, rather than giving advice.* You can assist patients in discussing the consequences, costs, and benefits of choosing one action versus another (e.g., "What would happen if you choose this course of action as compared with … ?" or "What is the worst that could happen if you decided to … ?"). Making choices helps patients reestablish control. Even a small decision encourages patients to become invested in the solution-finding process and hopeful about finding a resolution to a crisis situation.

Involving Immediate Support Systems and Community Resources. Accessing immediate social supports and available community resources provides a buffer and can act as a source of information and a sounding board for individuals in a crisis state. Support networks provide practical advice and a sense of security. They are a source of encouragement that can reaffirm a patient's worth and help defuse anxiety associated with the uncertainty of a crisis situation. In addition to inquiring about the number and variety of people in the patient's support network, find out, "who does the patient and/or family trust" and "who would the patient be most comfortable talking about their situation." It is helpful to learn when the patient and/or family last had contact with the identified person. In crisis situations, many patients and families temporarily withdraw from natural support systems and may need encouragement to reconnect.

Step 5: Develop a Mutual Realistic Action Plan

Crisis Intervention Is Action-Oriented and Situation Focused. Formulating a realistic action plan starts with prioritizing identified problems and related essential action steps. An effective crisis plan should have a practical, here-and-now, therapeutic, short-term focus and should reflect the patient's choices about best options. Stabilization of the patient through guidance, careful listening, and developing small viable plans helps to defuse the sense of helplessness in a crisis situation. When people begin to take even the smallest step, they gain a sense of control, and this stimulates hope for future mastery of the crisis situation. Thinking about crisis resolution as a whole is counterproductive.

Incorporate Previously Successful Coping Strategies. Looking at past coping strategies can sometimes reveal skills that could be used in resolving the current crisis situation. Ask, "What do you usually do when you have a problem?" or "To whom do you turn when you are in trouble?" Explore the nature of tension-reducing strategies that the patient has used in the past (e.g., aerobics, Bible study, calling a friend, participating in a hobby). With verbal encouragement, patients begin to identify successful coping mechanisms, which can be built on, for use in resolving the current crisis.

Establish Reasonable Goals. Becoming aware of choices, letting go of ideas that are toxic or self-defeating, and making the best choice are among viable options. Goal-directed activities should reflect the patient's strengths, values, capabilities, beliefs, and preferences. Tangible, achievable goals give patients and families hope that they can get to a different place with resolving their crisis.

Step 6: Implementing This Action Plan

Design Achievable Tasks. Help patients choose tasks that are within their capabilities, circumstances, and energy level. Achievable tasks can be as simple as getting more information or making time for self. You can suggest, "What do you think needs to happen first?" or "Let's look at what you might be able to do quickly." Engaging patients in simple problem-solving reduces crisis-related feelings of helplessness and hopelessness. Problem-solving tasks that strengthen the patient's realistic perception of the crisis event, incorporate a patient's beliefs and values, and integrate social and environmental supports offer the best chance for success. Helping patients tap into and use their personal resources to achieve goals facilitates crisis resolution and provides individuals with tools for further personal development.

Providing Structure and Encouragement. Patients need structure and encouragement as they perform the tasks that will move them forward. Setting time limits and monitoring task achievement is important. Resolving a crisis

state is not a straightforward movement. There will be setbacks. Patients need ongoing affirmation of their efforts. Supportive reinforcement includes validation of the struggles that patients are coping with, anticipatory guidance regarding what to expect, and discussion of ambivalent feelings, uncertainty, and fears surrounding the process. Comparing progressive functioning with baseline admission presentations helps nurses and their patients mutually evaluate progress, foresee areas of necessary focus, and monitor progress toward treatment goals.

Providing Support for Families. Crisis intervention strategies should include support for family members. A crisis affects family dynamics, such that each family member is coping with some sort of emotional fallout brought about by the patient's crisis. Additionally, there may be issues requiring family response to an unstable home environment created by the patient's absence or an inability to function in their previous roles. There may be legal or safety issues that family members also have to address.

Individual family members experience a crisis in diverse ways, so different levels of information and support will be required, giving families an opportunity to talk about the meaning of the crisis for each family member and offering practical guidance about resources. Communication strategies the nurse can use to help families in crisis are presented in Box 20.2.

BOX 20.2   Suggested Nursing Interventions for Initial Family Responses to Crisis

Anxiety, Shock, Fear
- Give information that is brief, concise, explicit, and concrete.
- Repeat information and frequently reinforce; encourage families to record important facts in writing.
- Determine comprehension by asking family to repeat back to you what information they have been given.
- Provide for and encourage or allow expression of feelings, even if they are extreme.
- Maintain a constant, nonanxious presence in the face of a highly anxious family.
- Inform family as to the potential range of behaviors and feelings that are within the "norm" for crisis.
- Maximize control within hospital environment, as possible.

Denial
- Identify what purpose denial is serving for family (e.g., Is it buying them "psychological time" for future coping and mobilization of resources?).
- Evaluate appropriateness of use of denial in terms of time; denial becomes inappropriate when it inhibits

the family from taking necessary actions or when it is impinging on the course of treatment.
- Do not actively support denial, but do not dash hopes for the future (You might say, "It must be very difficult for you to believe your son is nonresponsive and in a trauma unit.").
- If denial is prolonged and dysfunctional, more direct and specific factual representation may be essential.

Anger, Hostility, Distrust
- Allow for venting of angry feelings, clarifying what thoughts, fears, and beliefs are behind the anger; let the family know it is okay to be angry.
- Do not personalize family's expressions of these strong emotions.
- Institute family control within the hospital environment when possible (e.g., arrange for set times and set person to give them information in reference to the patient and answer their questions).
- Remain available to families during their venting of these emotions.

BOX 20.2   Suggested Nursing Interventions for Initial Family Responses to Crisis—(cont'd)

- Ask families how they can take the energy in their anger and put it to positive use for themselves, for the patient, and for the situation.

Remorse and Guilt
- Do not try to rationalize away guilt for families.
- Listen and support their expression of feeling and verbalizations (e.g., "I can understand how or why you might feel that way; however …").
- Follow the "howevers" with careful, reality-oriented statements or questions (e.g., "None of us can truly control another's behavior"; "Kids make their own choices despite what parents think and want"; "How successful were you when you tried to control _____'s behavior with that before?"; "So many things happen for which there are no absolute answers").

Grief and Depression
- Acknowledge the family's grief and depression.
- Encourage them to be precise about what it is they are grieving and depressed about; give grief and depression a context.

- Allow the family appropriate time for grief.
- Recognize that this is an essential step for future adaptation; do not try to rush the grief process.
- Remain sensitive to your own unfinished business, and hence comfort or discomfort with family's grieving and depression.

Hope
- Clarify with families their hopes, individually and with one another.
- Clarify with families their worst fears in reference to the situation. Are the hopes/fears congruent? Realistic? Unrealistic?
- Support realistic hope.
- Offer gentle factual information to reframe unrealistic hope (e.g., "With the information you have or the observations you have made, do you think that is still possible?").
- Assist families in reframing unrealistic hope in some other fashion (e.g., "What do you think others will have learned from _____ if he doesn't make it?" "How do you think _____ would like for you to remember him/her?").

Adapted from Kleeman, K.M. (1989). Families in crisis due to multiple trauma. *Critical Care Nursing Clinics of North America, 1*(1), 23–31.

Step 7: Evaluation: Termination and Follow-Up Protocol

Patients should receive verbal instructions, with *written* discharge or follow-up directives and phone numbers to call for added help or clarification. Although acute symptoms subside with standard crisis intervention strategies, many patients will need follow-up.

Mobilize Community Resources. There may be community agencies to provide essential supports. Having written referral information available regarding eligibility requirements, location, cost, and accessibility can make a difference in patient interest and adherence.

Debriefing. Dealing with crisis situations can be difficult emotionally for the healthcare team. Briefly meet to discuss and evaluate outcomes.

Mental Health Emergencies

Mental health emergencies present significant challenges for nurses. Whether encountered in the community or with patients admitted to an emergency department, these patients often present as a danger to themselves or others. They present with chaotic distress behaviors, which are not under the patient's control. The fact that they are not easily controllable makes them particularly distressing for.

Nurses should be aware that these patients may present at the emergency department sometimes seeking legitimate care for their symptoms or may present to obtain medications (narcotics, benzodiazepines) that they are either out of, or abuse regularly, which, in turn, can counter or repress their psychiatric symptoms.

Mental health emergencies require an *immediate* coordinated response designed to alleviate the potential for harm and restore basic stability. Examples of a mental health emergency include suicidal, homicidal, or threatening behavior; self-injury; severe drug or alcohol impairment; and highly erratic or unusual behavior associated with serious mental disorders. Unpredictability, acute emotions, and acting-out behaviors increase the intensity of mental health emergencies. Box 20.3 provides communication deescalation tips for use in community with mental health emergencies.

Model respect when communicating with mentally ill patients experiencing acute anxiety to avoid retraumatizing individuals already experiencing a chaotic, distressed state. Mentally ill patients respond best to respectful,

BOX 20.3   Communication Deescalation Tips for Mental Health Emergencies

Nonverbal

- Give the person your undivided attention.
- Respect personal space: stand 3 feet away; be sensitive to person's comfort zone.
- Use a nonthreatening, nonverbal stance: open, but not vulnerable. Ask them if you both can sit.
- Make eye contact: not constantly, but enough to show concern.
- Movement: avoid sudden movements, announce actions when possible, keep hands where they can be seen.
- Have a clear escape route: do *not* put the patient between yourself and the door.

Verbal

- Communication: focus on feelings.
- Be brief, slow, with simple vocabulary, moderate tone, only as loud as needed, repeat as needed.
- Attitude: remain calm, interested, firm, patient, reassuring, respectful, truthful.
- Be empathetic and nonjudgmental.
- Acknowledge legitimacy of feelings, delusions, hallucinations as being real to the patient "I understand you are seeing or feeling this, but I am not."
- Ignore challenging questions; redirect to the immediate issue.
- Remove distractions, upsetting influences.
- Keep the patient talking/focused on the here and now.
- Allow verbal venting within reason.
- Remove patient to a quiet space; remove others from immediate area (avoid the "group spectators").
- Give some choices or options, if possible.
- Set limits if necessary.
- Limit interaction to just one professional and let that person do the talking.
- Avoid rushing: slow things down.
- Allow silences to allow for reflection.

emergency patients usually require medication for stabilization of symptoms and close supervision.

Types of Mental Health Emergencies

Violence. **Violence** is a mental health emergency, which creates a critical challenge to the safety, well-being, and health of the patients and others in their environment. Nurses should always assume an organic component (drugs, alcohol, psychosis, or delirium) underlying the aggression in patients presenting with disorganized impulsive or violent behaviors, until proven otherwise.

Patient body language offers clues to escalating anxiety, particularly agitation, threatening gestures, or darting eye movements. Table 20.1 presents indicators of increasing tension as precursors to violence. A history of violence,

TABLE 20.1   Behavioral Indicators of Potential Violence

Behavioral Categories	Potential Indicators
Mental status	Confused
	Paranoid ideation
	Disorganized
	Angry
	Poor impulse control
Motor behaviour	Agitated, pacing
	Exaggerated gestures; fists clenched
	Rapid breathing
Body language	Eyes darting
	Prolonged (staring) eye contact or lack of eye contact
	Spitting
	Pale, or red (flushed) face
	Menacing posture, throwing things
Speech patterns	Rapid, pressured
	Incoherent, mumbling, repeatedly making the same statements
	Menacing tones, raised voice, use of profanity
	Verbal threats
Affect	Belligerent
	Labile
	Angry

calmly presented suggestions rather than commands. It is helpful to provide additional personal space for individuals who have experienced a crisis and who have a mental illness. Keep communication calm, short, compassionate, and well defined. Do not indicate that you feel threatened or argue the logic of a situation. Avoid intimidating the patient, but set reasonable limits. Proceed slowly with purpose. Avoid sudden movements. Whenever possible, offer simple choices with structured coaching. Psychiatric childhood abuse, substance abuse, neurodevelopmental disorders, problems with impulse control, and psychosis, particularly when accompanied by command hallucinations, are common contributing factors.

Treatment of violent patients consists of immediately providing a safe, nonstimulating environment for the patient. Often patients reduce the possibility of aggression if taken to an area with less sensory input. The patient should be checked thoroughly for potential weapons and physically disarmed, if necessary. Short-term medication is usually indicated to help defuse potentially harmful behaviors. The nurse should briefly identify why the medication is being given, and the patient should be carefully monitored for physical and behavioral responses. Collegial violence and bullying is discussed in Chapter 23.

Sexual Assault

Sexual assault and rape are serious forms of interpersonal victimization, which violate the core of self, in ways that are probably only second to murder. The patient's subjective stress is intense and long lasting. In the immediate aftermath of a sexual assault, everything should be done to help the patient feel safe and supported. The patient should be taken to a private room and should not be left alone. Evidence, if it is to be collected, requires that the patient not shower or douche prior to being examined. Larger emergency departments have a Sexual Assault Nurse Examiner (SANE) program, staffed by a specially trained nurse who provides first-response medical care and crisis intervention.

Adapting psychological first aid (PFA) to rape and sexual assault victims is a helpful comprehensive action-oriented intervention. PFA consists of eight core actions:
1. Contact and engagement
2. Safety and comfort
3. Stabilization
4. Information gathering
5. Practical assistance
6. Connection with social supports
7. Information on coping support
8. Linkage with collaborative services

In a sexual assault situation, there should be no blame or conjecture about the victim's role in the attack. Sexual assault is always an act of violence and control. It is not a voluntary sexual act, even if the perpetrator and victim are known to each other. Follow-up referral to a mental health professional can help the patient cope with stress symptoms, shame, and the intrusive thoughts that frequently develop in the days and weeks following the assault.

Psychosis

An acute psychotic break represents a serious mental health behavioral emergency. Psychotic and delirious patients have disorganized thinking, reduced insight, and limited personal judgment. Patients experiencing "command" hallucinations, defined as *hallucinations* that direct the person to carry out an act, are at a higher risk for suicide and aggression. Medication is almost always indicated to manage acute psychotic symptoms, and one-to-one supervision is required. Allow the patient sufficient space to feel safe, and never try to subdue a patient by yourself. Remain calm and positive. Use less, rather than more words. An open expression, eye contact, a calm voice, and simple concrete words invite trust. Do not use touch, as it can be misinterpreted.

Suicide

Definition. Suicide is defined as any self-injurious behavior that results in the death of an individual. This is classified as a behavioral emergency (Fig. 20.1).

Incidence. Suicide is the 10th leading cause of death in the United States, with 47,511 reported deaths (CDC, 2020). For every person who commits suicide, there are 25 other nonfatal suicide attempts. The World Health Organization (WHO) describes suicide as a public health priority with almost a million global cases annually, so access to weapons [guns] can make a difference in whether a person dies (WHO, 2021). Occurrences vary by race/ethnicity, age, and occupation. Males die by suicide at a rate almost four times higher than females. Veterans are in the highest risk group. Gay, bisexual, and lesbian people are at higher risk as are mine/extraction workers and nurses.

Behavior. The Joint Commission (2021) identifies suicide as a "**sentinel event**" and calls for appropriate screening in behavioral care units, medical surgical units, and the emergency department to avert a death. People turn to suicide as an option in times of acute distress, when under

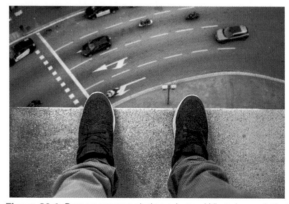

Figure 20.1 Person contemplating a jump: What deescalation strategies might you try? (From iStock #504859736, MarioGuti.)

the influence of drugs or when they believe there are no other alternatives. Impulsivity and hopelessness often go together with suicidal behaviors. Behavioral indicators of escalating suicidal ideation include a noteworthy change in behavior, often characterized by a burst of energy. The CDC offers suicide risk screening tips (CDC, 2020). Examples of changes in behavior of an individual who died by suicide include the following:

- A teen gave away all of electronics the week before his death.
- An 18-year-old young man went to friends at school apologizing for his "past" erratic behavior 3 days before he shot himself.

Screening and Assessment. Early identification and treatment for those at risk is a key prevention strategy. Be alert to cues (AFSP, 2021). Use a standardized screening tool such as SAFE-T (U.S. National Library of Medicine, 2020). Listen carefully to determine whether a person feels hopeless, trapped, and is a burden to others; is experiencing extreme mood swings; is increasingly using alcohol or drugs; has withdrawn from friends; or says they have no reason to live.

Pay attention to possible passive suicidal wishes and actions, such as not taking medications, not practicing safe sex, drinking too much, driving too fast, and not caring if you are in an accident, warrant exploration. Pay attention to statements such as "I don't think I can go on without …," "I sometimes wish I could just disappear," or "People would be better off without me," as they are examples of suicidal ideation. Such statements require further clarification (e.g., "You say you can't go on without … Can you tell me more about what you mean?"). Ask "Do you have any thoughts of hurting yourself?" (include frequency and intensity of thoughts). Do you have a plan? Individuals with a detailed plan and the means to carry it out are at greatest risk for suicide. If the patient answers yes, you should *assess the lethality of the plan* and inquire about the method and the patient's knowledge and skills about its use, along with the accessibility of the means to facilitate the suicide attempt. Refer to Box 20.4 for a list of risk factors.

Interventions. Stabilization of symptoms and patient safety are the most immediate concerns with patients experiencing a suicidal crisis. Possible weapons (e.g., mirrors, belts, knitting needles, scissors, razors, medications, clothes hangers) should be removed. In the general hospital, death by suicide occurs more frequently than one would suppose. Patients experiencing intense pain, a terminal prognosis, substance abuse, or a recent bereavement are at higher risk. Documentation of a suicidal risk assessment, interventions, and patient responses are essential. Included in the documentation should be quotes made by the patient,

---

BOX 20.4 Suicide Risk Factors

Risk Factors Include
- Previous attempts or family history of suicide
- Family history of child abuse
- History of alcohol and substance abuse
- Social isolation, lack of social support
- Recent major loss or history of trauma
- A sense of hopelessness
- Local epidemics of suicide
- Easy access to lethal means
- Within the first few weeks of discharge from a psychiatric hospital or emergency department

---

details of observed behavior, a review of identified risk factors, and patient responses to initial crisis intervention strategies. The names and times of anyone you notified and contacts with family should be documented.

Most psychiatric inpatient settings and emergency departments have written suicide precaution protocols that must be followed with patients presenting with suicidal ideation. Patients exhibiting high-risk behaviors require constant one-to-one staff observation; a potentially suicidal patient should never be left alone. Monitoring of suicidal patients ranges from constant 1:1 observation, to 15- or 30-minute observational checks. Less restrictive checks can include supervised bathroom visits, unit restriction or restriction to public areas, and supervised sharps. The frequency and type of observation is dependent on the suicidal assessment of the patient.

The American Nurses Credentialing Center Competencies. In 2015, the American Psychiatric Nurses Association wrote the Psychiatric-Mental Health Nurse Essential Competencies for Assessment and Management of Individuals at Risk for Suicide (APNA, 2015). This document is a guide for practice based on extensive literature review and peer review. The nine essential competencies are that the psychiatric nurse

1. understands the phenomenon of suicide;
2. manages personal reactions, attitudes, and beliefs;
3. develops and maintains a collaborative, therapeutic relationship with the patient;
4. collects accurate assessment information and communicates the risk to the treatment team and appropriate persons (i.e., nursing supervisor, on duty MD., etc.);
5. formulates a risk assessment;
6. develops an ongoing nursing plan of care based on continuous assessment;
7. performs an ongoing assessment of the environment in determining the level of safety and modifies the environment accordingly;

8. understands legal and ethical issues related to suicide; and

9. accurately and thoroughly documents suicide risk (APNA, 2015).

Develop a Safety Planning Intervention. This document is not a contract for safety, but rather, a collaborative plan that empowers the patient to determine ways to reduce the drive to die by suicide. The safety planning intervention helps the patient to identify the following:

- Warning signs of suicide
- Internal coping strategies: the patient identifies what he/she can do to interrupt thoughts about suicide
- People or social settings that can assist the patient to distract from the drive to commit suicide
- People in the patient's life that can be called to assist the patient to maintain safety
- Professionals or agencies that the patient can call during a crisis, including the National Suicide Prevention Line 800/272-TALK or by texting the CRISIS TEXT Line 741,741. Veterans can access specialists with 1-800-273-TALK (8255) #1. Online contact www.suicidepreventionlifeline.org/.

Crisis Intervention Teams

A team approach to managing at-risk patients is best. In the community, police with special training are important first responders in behavioral health emergencies. Police often bring such individuals to the emergency department. With the police reform movement, there may be increased access to mental health emergency sites (refer back to Box 20.1 to assess dangerousness to self or others in patients presenting as a mental health emergency).

Patients experiencing mental health emergencies may perceive necessary medical procedures as being intrusive and threatening. It is important to adhere to a nursing principle that before starting any procedure, you should tell the patient exactly what you are going to do and why the procedure is necessary, with a request to cooperate. If the patient refuses, do not insist, but explain the reason for doing the procedure in a calm, quiet voice. If you can help patients regain a sense of control, they are more likely to cooperate with you. Your movements should be calm, firm, and respectful.

Nurses: Death by Suicide. Long a hidden fact, nurses have a higher rate of suicide than the general population. Although the government collects data for registered nurse suicide rates, Davidson et al. (2020) suggest that data on nurse suicides are not fully reported, with limited data about causative factors. Nurses, both male and female, have significantly higher suicide rates than the general population (Davidson et al., 2019). Could this perhaps be due to stigma associated with mental health problems? Why

are professional nursing organizations silent about this problem? Furthermore, most agencies have not established protocols for how to handle staff after a colleague's suicide.

Prevention is a complex issue with a distinct lack of empirical evidence in the literature. Articles on stress management contain useful tips. Davidson et al. (2018) list risk factors for nurses as depression, access to means (meds and toxic substances), work related and personal stress, smoking, and substance abuse or use of Valium. Other factors include feelings of inadequacy, lack of role preparation, lateral violence (bullying), and transferring to a new work environment.

Prevention. It is clear that both healthcare organizations and individual nurses need to focus more on this issue. An evolving role in healthcare agencies is Chief Wellness Officer whose mission is to develop a structured wellness program for staff (Brower et al., 2021). Interventions include psychological first aid, peer support, and mental health services targeting prevention of posttraumatic stress disorder. Professional nurse organizations such as AACN, ANA, and American Organization of Nursing Executives have published workplace wellness standards. We need to create a culture in which "asking for help" is not stigmatized. Peer support is vital. Take a minute to offer a "job well done" affirmation to a colleague! Personal nurse interventions include increased awareness of suicide indicators, screening for depression, and establishment of personal routine daily for stress self-management. Each of us should set aside 15 min each day, every day, to destress. We need relaxation strategies to let go of the many demands and challenges of our day. Specific strategies are described in Chapter 27.

DISASTER MANAGEMENT

Disaster and Mass Trauma Situations

Definition. A **disaster** is defined as a calamitous event of slow or rapid onset that results in large-scale physical destruction of property, social infrastructure, and human life. Recent years have borne witness to more natural disasters, terrorism, and war than the world has seen in many decades. Mass shooting, natural disasters, and threats of domestic or foreign terrorist attacks have stimulated a fresh awareness of the need for community and national planned responses to disaster events. The components of mass trauma events are given in Table 20.2.

Planning for Disaster Management

In the United States, the Federal Emergency Management Agency (FEMA) is responsible for setting forth recommendations related to creating an effective disaster plan. FEMA recommendations provide guidelines for the creation

TABLE 20.2   Assessing Elements of Mass Trauma Events

Element	Example
Single versus recurring traumatic event	Type I (acute) trauma
	Type II (chronic or ongoing) trauma
Proximity to the traumatic event	Onsite
	On the periphery
	Through the media
Exposure to violence/injury/pain	Witnessed and/or experienced
Nature of losses/death/destruction	Personal, community, and/or symbolic loss
	Danger, loss, and/or responsibility traumas
	Loved one, missing or no physical evidence
	Death determined by retrieval of body or fragment
	Loss of status/employment/family income
	Loss of a predictable future
Attribution of causality	Random
	Act of God or deliberate
	Human-made

From Webb, N. (2004). The impact of traumatic stress and loss on children and families. In: Webb N (Ed.), *Mass trauma and violence: Helping families and children cope* (p. 6). New York: Guilford, reprinted with permission.

of local disaster planning team. The Sendai Framework was adapted by the United Nations to promote a prevention-based approach to international disasters. The emphasis in the Sendai Framework is on early warning when a disaster may take place; predicting the event and needs for prevention of causalities; recovery after the disaster; and rehabilitation once recovery of the disaster takes place. The Sendai Framework goals will be implemented and utilized between the years of 2015–30.

Disaster Management in Healthcare Settings

All hospitals are required to form disaster committees composed of key departments within the hospital, including nursing. Nurses interested in emergency volunteer activities should become aware of credentialing requirements to ensure their participation as part of a national emergency volunteer system for health professionals. Hospital and community disaster planning must be coordinated, so all phases of the disaster cycle are covered. Designated hospital personnel must receive training to carry out triage at the emergency department entrance. Protocols should contain the capability to relocate staff and patients to another facility if necessary, and a plan must be in place detailing mechanisms for equipment resupply. Policies regarding notification, maintenance of accurate records, and establishment of a facility control center are required (The Joint Commission, 2016).

Helping Children Cope With Trauma

Children do not have the same resources when coping with traumatic events as adults do. Preexisting exposure to traumatic events and lack of social support increases vulnerability. It is not unusual for children to demonstrate regressive behaviors as a reaction to crisis. While helping the child work through the emotional aspects of the trauma, utilize language appropriate to the child's level of development and cognitive ability. Assess how the child perceives the stressor, and determine the child's self-perception of how they are able to problem-solve.

Children will look for cues from key adults in their lives and tend to mirror their adult caregivers, so it is essential to communicate calmly and with confidence. More than anything else, children need reassurance that they and the people who are important to them are safe. Encourage the family to maintain regular routines. Parents need to provide children with opportunities both to talk about the crisis and to ask questions. Repetitive questions are to be expected. This often reflects the child's need for reassurance. Offering factual information helps dispel misperceptions.

Helping Older Adults Cope With Trauma

Reducing anxiety is especially important for the older adult disaster victim. Even the most capable older adult can appear confused and vulnerable in a disaster situation. Actions nurses can take include the following: assess for functional limitations associated with compromised physical mobility, diminished sensory awareness, and preexisting health conditions.

SUMMARY

Crisis is defined as an unexpected, sudden turn of events or set of circumstances requiring an immediate human response. People experience a crisis as overwhelming, traumatic, and personally intrusive. It is an unexpected life event challenging a person's sense of self and his or her place in the world. The most common types of crisis are situational and developmental crises. Most health crises are situational.

Theoretical frameworks guiding crisis intervention include Lindemann's model of grieving and Caplan's model, based on preventive psychiatry concepts. Aguilera's nursing model explores the role of balancing factors in defusing the impact of a crisis state. Erikson's model of psychosocial development provides a framework for exploring developmental crises.

The goal of crisis intervention is to return the patient to their precrisis level of functioning.

Crisis intervention is a time-limited treatment, which focuses on the immediate crisis and its resolution. Roberts's seven-stage model, used to guide nursing interventions, consists of assessing lethality, establishing rapport, dealing with feelings, defining the problem, exploring alternative options, formulating a plan, and follow-up measures. This chapter discussed some types of crises such as workplace violence or sexual abuse, but primarily discussed suicide as an exemplar of a mental health emergency crisis. The hidden issue of nurse suicide was discussed.

Guidelines for communication with patients experiencing mental health emergencies focus on safety and rapid stabilization of the patient's behavior. Assessment and deescalation communication strategies were listed. Collaboration between community law enforcement and mental health services designed to treat rather than punish individuals experiencing mental health emergencies is evolving.

Nurses need to understand the dimensions of disaster management and develop the skills to respond effectively in disaster situations. Disaster management is a special kind of crisis intervention applied to large groups of people.

ETHICAL DILEMMA: What Would You Do?

Sara Murdano is only 20 years old when she arrives at the mobile intensive care unit (MICU), but this is not her first hospital admission. She has been treated for depression previously. She states she is determined to kill herself because she has nothing to live for and that it is her right to do so because she is no longer a minor. As she describes her life to date, you cannot help but think that she really does not have a lot to live for. How would you respond to this patient from an ethical perspective?

DISCUSSION QUESTIONS

1. What are some explanations for patients who are in crisis?
2. What would you identify as the essential knowledge, skills, and attitudes required of a nurse confronted with a patient who is at high risk for a suicide attempt?

3. What questions would you ask to determine level of self-harm risk?
4. Why are nurses at higher risk for death by suicide?

ACKNOWLEDGMENT

The author would like to thank Pamela E. Marcus, who authored the previous edition of this chapter.

The purpose of this chapter is to describe communication strategies nurses can use with patients and families experiencing a crisis situation. This chapter describes the nature of crisis and identifies its theoretical foundations. The application section provides practical guidelines nurses can use with patients in crisis and during emergencies.

REFERENCES

Aguilera, D. (1998). *Crisis intervention: Theory and methodology* (7th ed.). St. Louis: Mosby.

American Foundation for Suicide Prevention (AFSP). (2021). *Suicide statistics*. Retrieved from: http://afsp.org/suicide-statistics/. [Accessed 25 June 2021].

American Psychiatric Nurses Association (APNA). (2015). *Psychiatric-mental health nurse essential competencies for assessment and management of individuals at risk for suicide.* Retrieved from: https://www.apna.org/files/public/Resources/Suicide%20Competencies%20for%20Psychiatric-Mental%20Health%20Nurses(1)(1).pdf. [Accessed 25 June 2021].

Brower, K. J., Brazeau, C. M. L. R., Kiely, S. C., et al. (2021). The evolving role of the Chief Wellness Officer in the management of crises by health care systems: Lessons from the COVID-19 pandemic. *New England Journal of Medicine, 2*(5).

Caplan, G. (1964). *Principles of preventive psychiatry.* New York: Basic Books.

Centers for Disease Control and Prevention (CDC). (2020). *Suicide and self-harm injury.* National Center for Health Statistics. Retrieved from: https://www.cdc.gov/nchs/fastats/suicide.htm. [Accessed 29 June 2021].

Davidson, J., Mendis, J., Stuck, A. R., DeMichele, G., & Zisook, S. (2018). *Nurse suicide: Breaking the silence.* National Academy of Medicine. Retrieved from: https://nam.edu/nurse-suicide-breaking-the-silence/. [Accessed 25 June 2021].

Davidson, J. E., Proudfoot, J., Lee, K., Terterian, G., & Zisook, S. (2020). A longitudinal analysis of nurse suicide in the United States (2005–2016) with recommendations for action. *Worldviews on Evidence-Based Nursing, 17*(1), 6–15.

Davidson, J. E., Proudfoot, J., Lee, K., & Zisook, S. (2019). Nurse suicide in the United States: Analysis of the centers for disease control 2014 national violent death reporting system dataset. *Archives of Psychiatric Nursing, 33*(5), 16–21.

Dufresne, J. (2003). *De-escalation tips.* Crisis Prevention Institute. Retrieved from: https://www.crisisprevention.com/Blog/De-escalation-Tips. [Accessed 25 June 2021].

Erikson, E. (1982). *The life cycle completed.* New York: Norton.

Lindemann, E. (1944). Symptomatology and management of acute grief. *American Journal of Psychiatry, 101,* 141–148.

Roberts, A. R., & Yeager, K. R. (2009). *Pocket guide to crisis intervention.* New York: Oxford University Press.

The Joint Commission. (2016). *Sentinel event alert 56: Detecting and treating suicide ideation in all settings Issue 56.*

The Joint Commission. (2019). *R3 report issue 18: National patient safety goal for suicide prevention.* Retrieved from: https://www.jointcommission.org/standards/r3-report/r3-report-issue-18-national-patient-safety-goal-for-suicide-prevention/. [Accessed 29 June 2021].

The Joint Commission. (2021). *Comprehensive accreditation manual for behavioral health care (CAMBHC).* Oak Brook, IL: TJC.

U.S. National Library of Medicine. (2020). *Suicide risk screening.* MedlinePLUS. Retrieved from: https://medlineplus.gov/lab-tests/suicide-risk-screening/. [Accessed 25 June 2021].

World Health Organization (WHO). (2021). *Suicide.* Retrieved from: https://www.who.int/en/news-room/fact-sheets/detail/suicide. [Accessed 25 June 2021].

21

Communication Approaches in Palliative Care

OBJECTIVES

At the end of the chapter, the reader will be able to:
1. Discuss the concept of loss and grief in own life.
2. Discuss the nurse's communication role in palliative care cases.

3. Apply evidence-based interventions to a simulated end-of-life situation.

This chapter introduces communication principles that can be used in dealing with families and patients in palliative critical care or end-of-life situations. Some say limited application of the end-of-life concepts is a crisis in our society (Belisomo, 2018). The National Cancer Institute recommends that all patients with advanced cancer receive palliative care. Selected theoretical frameworks useful for understanding stages of grief in dying patients are presented. The chapter highlights communication and care issues faced by nurses providing palliative care.

BASIC CONCEPTS

Nursing patients at their end-of-life can be stressful but very rewarding. Palliative care is an expanding field of specialization, but currently there are not enough nurses prepared to care for these patients (American Association of Colleges of Nursing, 2021). Reflect on the case with Ms Erb.

CASE STUDY: **Ms Evelyn Erb and Nurse Doug Dao, RN**

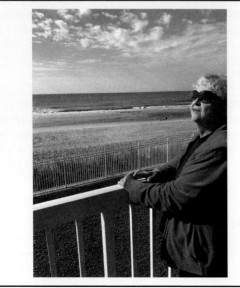

Evelyn Erb is 63 years old with a diagnosis of terminal lung cancer. She has chosen to remain at home with daily visits from her nurse on the palliative care team. Ms Erb is in moderate pain most of the time. As an alternative to narcotics, which she objects to as they make her so sleepy, she wants Doug to teach her some nonpharmacologic methods for pain management. Doug helps her use Guided Imagery for relaxation. With his help, Ms Erb pictures her favorite activity of sitting at the beach. Doug has her visualize the sparkling water and recall the familiar beach smell and the breeze blowing gently on her face.

Palliative Care

Definitions

Palliative care is a philosophy of care. The term refers to interdisciplinary care from a specialized team of personnel whose goal is to optimize quality of life and prevent or mitigate suffering among individuals with serious, complex terminal illnesses. The American Society of Clinical Oncology recommends that all patients with cancer use palliative care services. Services from the palliative team include treatment procedures and supportive services for patient and family who are dealing with grief and potential loss issues (ICN, 2012). Refer to Box 21.1 for the dimensions of palliative care. This care refers to care for critically ill individuals at any stage of life from the time of diagnosis. Everyone with a serious illness can benefit from palliative care (American Cancer Society, 2022). There is no time period specified.

    Hospice care usually refers to care that can be initiated after the patient has stopped all curative treatments and when they are nearing their end-of-life period. The differentiation is driven partially by regulations for Medicare reimbursement.

Incidence

By 2030, more than 72.8 million adults in America will be age 65 or older. Currently, nearly 18 million family members are caregivers for elders with diminished capacities (IOM, 2015). Kim et al. (2020) estimate that by 2060, 48 million people will die with serious suffering related to their illness. In addition to physical needs, many will have psychosocial and spiritual needs. There is a great need to expand palliative care providers to assist in providing resources to help these families. Connor et al. (2021) has estimated that over 7 million patients received palliative care in 2017 from approximately 25,000 providers. When the National Academies released their recommendations in their *"Dying in America"* report, they noted that nearly half of all physicians did not follow the patient's preferences and end-of-life desires.

Goal

Our goal is to maximize the quality of life of seriously ill or dying patients based on their desires and need for a pain-free situation while maximizing alertness (Blaževičienė et al., 2020; Huisman et al., 2020).

Healthcare Provider Role

The majority of physicians do not discuss psychosocial end-of-life problems with patients. Is it any wonder that half of families with end-of-life patients complain about

---

> **BOX 21.1   Dimensions of Palliative Care**
>
> - Provides relief from pain and other distressing symptoms
> - Affirms life and regards dying as a normal process
> - Intends neither to hasten nor postpone death
> - Integrates the psychological and spiritual aspects of patient care
> - Offers a support system to help patients live as actively as possible until death
> - Offers a support system to help the family cope during the patient's illness and in their own bereavement
> - Uses a team approach to address the needs of patients and their families, including bereavement counseling if indicated
> - Will enhance quality of life, and may also positively influence the course of illness
> - Is applicable early in the course of illness, in conjunction with other therapies that are intended to prolong life such as chemotherapy or radiation therapy, and includes those investigations needed to better understand and manage distressing clinical complications
>
> Data from World Health Organization (WHO). (2018). *Integrating palliative care and symptom relief into primary health care: A WHO guide for planners, implementers and managers.* Geneva, Switzerland: WHO.

---

inadequate communication? Nurses can play a pivotal role on the interdisciplinary team caring for these critically ill patients. We are a link between service providers and patients. While providing physical care and symptom management is important, studies show that providing culturally sensitive interventions, arranging for spiritual care, and providing emotional support are also important. The nurse mantra is "we save lives," but our toolbox also needs communication strategies to help dying patients. Specialized training is available for nurses who choose to work in palliative care or hospice care.

Communication in Palliative Care Situations

Patients value nurses who are competent, authentic, flexible, and supportive. Practice is helpful in increasing our comfort level when communicating with end-of-life patients. Use the simulation exercises provide, do some role playing, analyze case studies, or even view end-of-life discussions on YouTube, TED Talks, or other media platforms.

Professional Readiness

Most nursing graduates have little exposure to palliative and end-of-life care during their clinical rotations. Some feel uncomfortable with an expectation they will discuss related issues with families and patients in an effective, competent manner. Such communication is hard work for even experienced nurses (Blaževičienė et al., 2020).

Barriers to Communication

Contemporary society has almost placed a taboo on discussing dying. So, teach yourself what to say! We have been educated to focus on "cure." Some have assimilated the idea that death of a patient is a failure in healthcare. On occasions when a patient or family is angry or upset or reluctant to accept a poor prognosis, it is up to us to provide emotional support, difficult though that is. Limited time due to heavy workloads leaves less time for psychosocial support. Another communication problem surfaces when team members disagree about the treatment, especially when physician orders for medications do not meet patient needs (Huisman et al., 2020).

Communication Concerning Loss, Grief, and Bereavement

Important losses occur as part of daily living. Grief is part of a normal cycle of life. It is important that families complete this cycle. When any of us have invested our time and energy in a relationship with someone who is no longer with us, we experience a sense of lack of wholeness. Sometimes we even feel guilt. The intensity of the grief cycle varies with individuals but really only the person grieving knows their feelings. Sometimes loss is sudden, but often it is gradual such as with a family who has a member with Alzheimer's disease who has progressive loss of identity, role, and communication ability. Simulation Exercise 21.1 may help you understand the meaning of loss. In the case of multiple loss, a person can be overwhelmed. From a communication standpoint, it might help to focus on one thing at a time.

Death: The Final Loss

In the loss of a loved one, there is more than the physical absence. There are probably spiritual, social, cultural facets that color meaning. Nurses say patients report fear of dying alone, losing control, and being in pain are three major concerns. During the COVID-19 pandemic, nurses were stressed yet found creative ways to keep dying patients in touch with loved ones via Internet platforms.

Theoretical Frameworks

Kübler-Ross's Stages of Death and Dying

Kübler-Ross developed a five-stage model in 1969 that still serves as the premier framework for our understanding

---

SIMULATION EXERCISE 21.1   The Meaning of Loss

Purpose

To consider personal meaning of losses.

Procedure

Consider your answers to the following questions:
- What losses have I experienced in my life?
- How did I feel when I lost something or someone important to me?
- How was my behavior affected by my loss?
- What helped me the most in resolving my feelings of loss?
- How has my experience with loss prepared me to deal with further losses?
- How has my experience with loss prepared me to help others deal with loss?

Reflective Discussion Analysis

1. In the larger group, discuss what gives a loss its meaning.
2. What common themes emerged from the group discussion about successful strategies in coping with loss?
3. How does the impact of necessary losses differ from that of unexpected, unnecessary losses?
4. How can you use in your clinical work what you have learned from doing this exercise?

(Kübler-Ross, 1969). Not every person experiences each stage and some repeat a stage more than once. Others remain at a stage such as denial and never advance to complete all stages. Their right to do so should be respected. Her stages are as follows:

1. *Denial.* The initial thought is "not me" or denying what is happening. They may not have a realistic appraisal of their status, as apparent as it seems to others.
2. *Anger.* The second stage is characterized by the "Why me?" phase. Patients might verbalize about the unfairness of it all, or even express anger at Fate or God. Family members need your support to help them understand this is not a personal attack since angry feelings might get projected onto them. Reassure that this is a phase on the road to resolution.
3. *Bargaining.* This stage is characterized by a "yes me, but … I need a little more time." Bargaining is not a futile step. Sometimes the dying patient focuses on a goal, for example, living until a favorite grandchild graduates. This can add meaning to their struggle and enrich their

life. Nurses need to support their hope and avoid challenging them with a dose of reality.

4. *Depression.* The reality of the "Yes, me" stage is expressed through mood swings and sad feelings. You can help family members understand that this is an expected part of the grief process of anticipating loss. Mentally reviewing one's life and relationships can provide the patient with motivation to rework unfinished business. For the nurse, actively listening to the patient provides emotional support.

5. *Acceptance.* In Kübler-Ross's final stage of the grieving process, the patient acknowledges the inevitability of dying. Ideally, they come to a sense of peace and letting go. Again, it is helpful to all to view this as part of the process.

Lindemann's Grief Construct

Eric Lindemann (1944) pioneered the concept of grief work based on his interviews with bereaved people, finding both physical and emotional changes that occur. Grief responses can occur immediately following a death or they might be deferred until later. Three of Lindeman's concepts of interest for nursing communication interventions are as follows: use of open, empathetic communication; honesty in communication; and tolerance of emotions being expressed. If the grief work is exaggerated and persists over time, it is termed "complicated grief." Perhaps a psychological referral is needed.

Engle's Grief Constructs

George Engel's (1964) concepts build on Lindemann's work. He described three sequential phases of grief work: (1) shock and disbelief, (2) developing awareness, and (3) restitution.

Engle describes three sequences to grief: disbelief and shock; developing awareness; and resolution.

In the disbelief phase, the individual might feel detached from normal everyday life events, characterized by numbness rather than tears. Seeing or hearing the lost person or sensing his or her presence is a temporary altered sensory experience related to the loss, which should not be confused with psychotic hallucinations.

The second phase is developing awareness. This phase occurs slowly as the void created by the loss fully enters consciousness. Patients experience a loss of energy, not the kind that requires sleep, but rather recognizing that one lacks the functional energy to engage fully in normal everyday responsibilities.

Resolution is the last phase. During the resolution phase, the person becomes accustomed to life without the deceased and, while not forgetting, begins to rebuild a new life. The restitution phase is characterized by adaptation. There is a resurgence of hope and a renewed energy to fashion a new life. With successful grieving, the loss is not forgotten, but the pain diminishes and is replaced with memories that enrich and give energy to life.

Consider these theoretical concepts as you reflect on Sue Gen's case.

Case Study: Sue Gen Experience With Grief

Ms Gen: "Throughout the first year after my mother's death I was aware of a persistent feeling of heaviness. Not physical, but sort of an emotional and spiritual dark cloud. I tired very easily and seemed to have little energy to enjoy my life. My former sound sleeping routine turned into bouts of insomnia."

Trace Todd, RN: "Tell me more about this dark cloud" (allowing Ms Gen to vent, listening to her repeat herself and not interrupting or giving advice).

Patterns of Grieving

Acute Grief

In the acute phase, feelings are intense, and the emotional pain is almost beyond imagining. In some people, their feelings are somaticized being manifested in the form of physical symptoms such as fatigue, shortness of breath, or chest pain. Communication from the nurse consists of offering support, letting them vent feeling in a nonjudgmental manner, and reassuring them that such feelings are a normal part of grief process. Avoid offering platitudes such as "This will pass" or "You need to move on."

Anticipatory Grief

A loved one may begin to experience emotions associated with grief even before the patient dies. Ambivalent feelings are common, as described in the Marge Lubs case.

Case Study: Marge Lubs and Mr Lubs, Diagnosed With Alzheimer's Disease

Mrs Lubs husband of 30 years was diagnosed about 5 years ago. His condition has deteriorated until now he can no longer perform self-care. Mrs Lubs was unable to care for him at home any longer, and he was placed in a memory unit nearby where she visits daily. While she grieves over his impending loss, Mrs Lubs feels exhausted and tells the nurse on this unit that, at times, she wishes it was over. What would you respond?

Grief and Grieving

The concept of **grief** describes a holistic, adaptive process that a person goes through following a significant loss. Grief is an adaptive process, which is different for each person. There is an ebb and flow to the intense feelings that a death or significant loss stimulates in those who remain. Awareness of the loss creates recurring, wavelike feelings of memories and sadness. People describe it as "feeling unexpectedly punched in the gut." Intense feelings are particularly inclined to surface when the griever is alone, for example, while driving. Certain situations, holidays, and anniversaries, particularly during the first few years, make feelings of grief more poignant. Simulation Exercise 21.2 may help you explore grief from a personal viewpoint.

Grieving Concepts

Contemporary authors Neimeyer (2001) and Attig (2001) emphasize meaning construction as a central issue in grief work. The past is not forgotten. Instead, there is a continuous spiritual connection with the deceased, which illuminates different features of self, and possibilities for fuller engagement with life. Features of past experiences with the loved one are transformed and rewoven into the fabric of a person's life in a new form. The concept of a palliative approach to care represents an integrative model, which can guide the care of persons at any stage of chronic illness, dispelling the myth that palliative care is only for end-of-life.

Over time, grief feelings usually diminish in intensity, but there is no magic time frame. Grief over the loss of a child can be particularly pervasive, sometimes lasting a lifetime. Acceptance is characterized by living a life with feelings that acknowledge the blessings derived from have known the loved one.

Chronic Sorrow. **Chronic sorrow** is defined as a normal grief response associated with an ongoing living loss that is permanent, progressive, recurring, and cyclic in nature. Many parents of children with a physical, developmental, emotional, or chronic disorder experience chronic sorrow. Families need nurses to affirm their coping efforts and acknowledge the legitimacy of their sadness. Providing timely support for families when there is an exacerbation of symptoms can make the situation more manageable.

DEVELOPING AN EVIDENCE-BASED PRACTICE

Effective communication is vital in end-of-life nursing care situations. Recently, several researchers have analyzed studies examining racial disparities in care. Hart & Mathews (2021) analyzed 14 studies detailing end-of-life interventions for African-American patients, while Bonner (2021) focused on African-American caregivers. Collins et al. (2018) examined 24 articles discussing cultural aspects of end-of-life planning by African-Americans.

Results

An overwhelming conclusion is that racial disparities do exist both in use of advanced directives and in access to palliative care. This is support by prior studies such as Belisomo (2018) findings that African-American families have limited access to end-of-life services. Common themes that emerged were the greater number of comorbidities reported in this population; a higher distrust of the healthcare system; and a high level of family communal decision-making. Authors found patients reluctant to begin discussion and concluded providers need to initiate discussion of end-of-life issues. Nurses were repeatedly cited as "the ones who made things clear." Bonner (2021) used end-of-life education classes as a treatment, finding that the treatment group had a higher understanding about end-of-life care after attending than did the control group.

Strength of research evidence: Varied greatly. More research is needed.

Implications for Your Clinical Practice

1. Nurses need to initiate end-of-life issues discussions.
2. Communication should be culturally sensitive.
3. Recognize that end-of-life decisions may be more communally made by the families in the African-American population.

References

Belisomo, R. (2018). Reversing racial inequities at end-of-life: A call for health systems to create culturally competent advance care planning programs within African-American communities. *Journal of Racial and Ethnic Health Disparities, 5*(1), 213–220.

Bonner, G. J., Freels, S., Ferrans, C., et al. (2021). Advance care planning for African-American caregivers of relatives with dementias: Cluster randomized controlled trial. *American Journal of Hospice & Palliative Care, 38*(6), 547–556.

Collins, J. W., Zoucha, R., Lockhart, J. S., & Mixer, S. J. (2018). Cultural aspects of end-of-life care planning for African-Americans: An integrative review of the literature. *Journal of Transcultural Nursing, 29*(6), 578–590.

Hart, A. S., & Mathews, A. K. (2021). End-of-life interventions for African-Americans with serious illness: A scoping review. *Journal of Palliative Nursing, 23*(1), 9–19.

SIMULATION EXERCISE 21.2   A Personal Grief Inventory

Purpose
To provide a close examination of one's history with grief.

Procedure
Complete each sentence and reflect on your answers:
The first significant experience with grief that I can remember in my life was _____.
The circumstances were _____.
My age was _____.
The feelings I had at the time were _____.
The thing I remember most about that experience was

_____.
I coped with the loss by _____.
The primary sources of support during this period were

_____.
What helped most was _____.
The most difficult death for me to face would be

_____.

Adapted from Carson, V. B., & Arnold, E. N. (1996). *Mental health nursing: The nurse-patient journey* (p. 666). Philadelphia: W.B. Saunders.

APPLICATIONS

Communication in the Palliative Care Process

Effective communication is a competency listed by the American Association of Colleges of Nursing in preparing nurses for care of seriously ill patients. Their curricular guidelines "Peaceful Death: Recommended Guidelines for End-of-Life Nursing" specifically address communication competency.

Palliative care is patient-centered care, with an emphasis on care of patients with diagnosed, progressive, life-limiting health conditions (Sawatzky et al., 2016). Focus is on where the patient is at the grieving stages. Treatment goals move from disease control or cure toward maintaining quality of life and death with dignity. Palliative care considers care for the patient *and* the family as a single integrated care unit. As a patient's life-limiting condition progresses, palliative care supports patient comfort and symptom management, and a "good death." Unlike hospice, patients admitted to palliative care services can still receive active treatment for their disease. Aspects of palliative care nursing are listed in Box 21.2. The national End-of-Life Nursing Education Consortium (ELNEC) offers training courses providing nurses with skills to teach others how to manage end-of-life care.

The basic axiom for palliative care is to follow what patients want for themselves. After a patient's death,

BOX 21.2   Aspects of Palliative Nursing Care

- Structure and process of care
- Physical aspects of care
- Psychological and psychiatric aspects of care
- Social aspects of care
- Spiritual, religious, and existential aspects of care
- Cultural aspects of care

palliative care offers bereavement support for family members.

Location

Crowe (2017) writes of challenges faced by ICU nurses in their attempts to provide a peaceful death. ICUs are noisy, often highly illuminated, have restrictive visiting, and staffed by nurses with heavy workloads. Often treatment is in "cure" rather than "care" mode, with many invasive procedures. Yet it is still possible to attend to patient preferences, to be supportive, to refer ICU patients to a palliative care team.

Nursing Initiatives: Communication Strategies

Nurses have been at the forefront of developing guidelines for quality end-of-life care for many years. Finding in Canadian studies showed the quality of communication at end-of-life care was low (Heyland et al., 2017). They developed a conceptual model for decision-making, suggesting that advance care planning should be done early, prior to final hospitalization. So that patient preferences can be incorporated. Whittenberg-Lyles and colleagues (2013) proposed using the COMFORT communication model listed in Box 21.3.

Palliative Care Team Approaches

Palliative care is a team effort, designed to assess and manage patients' and families' care needs across physical, psychological, social, spiritual, and information domains. An **interdisciplinary palliative care team** usually consists of nurses, physicians, social workers, and clergy specially trained in palliative care. Patients are enrolled in palliative care, which operates as a 24-hour resource, providing comprehensive services to patients and families in hospitals, people's homes, nursing homes, and community settings.

Pain

Many conditions are accompanied by pain especially at the end-of-life. Morrow (2020) suggests keeping a pain log to identify trends, occurrences, and effectiveness of

BOX 21.3 The COMFORT Communication Model

C = Communicate with the family in ways they expect to elicit their main concerns and values, assessing what information they need and what their health literacy level is.

O = Orient yourself to family functioning being sensitive to their cultural beliefs about death.

M = Mindfully be there (presence) demonstrating empathy, using active listening and appropriate nonverbal communication.

F = Familiarize yourself with family dynamics, strengths, and vulnerabilities in their communication and coping, while helping them arrive at consensus about what end-of-life caring is acceptable.

O = Open yourself to recognize the pivotal moment when the patient's condition worsens so you can support family.

R = Relate to patient and family goals for a peaceful death.

T = Use team building communication skills to coordinate care among all providers.

interventions. It is recommended that we use a multimodal approach to pain management, combining some of the approaches listed here.

Pain Assessment. The therapeutic focus in palliative care is on patient comfort, pain control, management of physical symptoms, and easing the psychosocial and spiritual distress experienced by families and patients as they come to terms with coping with a life-limiting illness. Pain is what the patient says it is, occurring when and where they say (Morrow, 2020). Pain severity assessment tools have been developed and are widely used. One example is the Wong-Baker FACES pain rating scale depicted in Fig. 21.1. This tool can be used with children, aged 3 and older, for pain assessment only. Nurses perform screenings for pain, focused on the following:

- Onset and duration of pain
- Location of the pain
- Character of the pain (sharp, dull, burning, persistent, changes with movement, direct or referred pain)
- Intensity—using a 0 to 10 numerical rating scale, with 0 being no pain and 10 being unbearable pain
- History of substance dependence (needed to determine potential crossover tolerance)
- Aggravating factors such as difficulty breathing or turning
- Relief factors such as distraction with visitors, food or fluids, reassurance

Nonverbal Indicators of Pain. Children too young to meaningfully measure their pain level can be evaluated for behavioral indicators of pain such as abrupt changes in activity, inconsolable crying, inability to be consoled, listlessness or unwillingness to move, rubbing a body part, wincing, or facial grimacing (Morrow, 2020). Nonverbal behavior changes, particularly when associated with agitation, can indicate pain in cognitively impaired patients. Drawing up extremities and guarding the area of pain are also indicators.

Observation of behavioral distress indicators is particularly important with older adults. Estimates of older adults having significant pain range from upward of 40%. Some are able to evaluate their pain, using the suggestions above, but those with even mild cognitive changes may not be able to do so accurately when stressed.

Types of Pain/Degrees of Pain.

- *Acceptable.* Every patient is unique in terms of their tolerance of pain. Not all pain needs to be treated. It is important to find out what is an acceptable level of pain for your patient.
- *Acute pain.* Everyone has had some type of experience with acute pain. The range can be from minor such as a splinter, to severe such as might result from a severe car accident. Pain at end-of-life can also run this gamete. Severe pain associated with the patient's terminal condition can greatly impede quality of life and needs to be treated.
- *Chronic pain.* Many long-term conditions such as arthritis, cancer, diabetic neuropathy, osteoporosis, etc. involve pain of a chronic nature. These patients may not readily respond to pain medication. Guido (2010) maintains that pain in older patients can be under-treated because it is assumed that they cannot tolerate strong pain medications, or that their pain is due to chronic, persistent conditions which will not be as responsive. Misperceptions about addiction and medication strength can result in inadequate pain management, especially in these days of high opioid addiction in the general population.

Narcotic Medication for Pain Management. It is common for critically ill patients to fear pain. Patients needing palliative care often experience moderate to severe levels of pain, so part of the care plan is use of opioids. Some recommend that opioids be alternated with other nonnarcotic analgesics. Nurses need to educate patients and families about pain control, including the differences between pain associated with disease progression, and weigh adverse effects related to opioids, such as not being able to think clearly. Experts suggest using scheduled sustained release opioids for management of ongoing pain, with the option of an immediate acting medication for breakthrough pain.

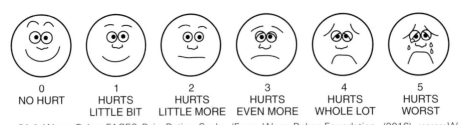

Figure 21.1 Wong–Baker FACES Pain Rating Scale. (From Wong-Baker Foundation. (2016). www.Wong-BakerFaces.org. Originally published in *Whaley & Wong's Nursing Care of Infants and Children*. Used with permission. Copyright, Elsevier.)

Noninvasive medication routes are preferred. When oral meds are no longer possible, some switch to transdermal patches. Rectal routes are also possible. Infusion routes are generally preferred to injections for ongoing pain management.

A use barrier is fear of addiction. Misperceptions about pain-relieving opioids are a major, unnecessary barrier in these critically ill patients All terminally ill patients are entitled to appropriate and adequate pain management of severe pain, without concern for addiction. The Joint Commission revised pain management recommendations in 2019.

Other barriers include a belief that suffering should be tolerated (stoicism) or is an unavoidable part of the dying process. Inability to swallow pain medication can be dealt with via alternative routes such as pain patches worn on the skin. Families sometimes attribute signs and symptoms of approaching death—such as increased lethargy, confusion, and declining appetite—to side effects of opioids. This is not usually true. With or without pain medication, actively dying patients become less responsive as death approaches.

Nonpharmacologic Pain Management Strategies. Our toolkit contains many alternatives to opioid administration for pain management such as meditation, relaxation exercises, guided imagery, or chiropractic or physical therapy. The Chinese have practiced cupping and acupuncture for thousands of years. There are TENS units that dispense electric shocks to disrupt the pain pathways. Massage such as myofascial release massage can help some people with their pain. Nutritionists recommend dietary supplements such as turmeric or omega supplements. There are many Apps available for download that can be easily used by people in self-managing their pain.

Key Issues and Approaches in End-of-Life Care
Nonpain Symptom Control
Management of disease- or treatment-related side effects such as nausea and vomiting disrupts the lives of our palliative care patients. These need to be alleviated to the extent possible. For many patients, especially those with cancer, physical symptoms also include shortness of breath, fatigue, and insomnia.

Self-Awareness
When caring for seriously or terminally ill patients, you must first recognize your own ethical, cultural, and spiritual attitudes and beliefs. Monitor your own responses continually during care. Liken it to taking your stress temperature. Caring for such patients on a continual basis can become distressing. How are you managing? Chapter 27 addresses such intrapersonal communication and suggests ways to self-manage your stress. Evaluate your work unit, perhaps using a tool such as AACN's "Healthy Work Environment Assessment."

As the body begins to shut down in preparation for imminent death, the gold standard for end-of-life care is to restrict nutritional support. However, a teaspoon of ice chips and mouth care can be a comfort measure. Patient preferences often change over time. Care directives often must be revisited, especially if there is a change in prognosis and the potential for quality of life diminishes significantly.

Supporting End-of-Life Decision-Making
Patients and families face difficult, irreversible decisions in the last phase of life. Preference decisions related to discontinuation of fluids, antibiotics, blood transfusions, and ventilator support require a clear understanding of a complex care situation. These are emotional issues with adaptive components for families. Families need support in meeting the adaptive challenges. End-of-life decisions present considerations, which cannot be resolved with technical intervention or clear-cut solutions. It is not uncommon for patients to avoid discussing their death preferences with family members, nor is it uncommon to find these family members in opposition to what the patient has chosen. Box 21.4 presents principles guiding end-of-life decision-making about care.

Decisions should be transparent, meaning that all parties involved in the decision should fully understand the implications of their decision. For example, to make an

BOX 21.4   Principles Guiding End-of-Life Care Decision-Making

- What if family requests that patient not be told: Our primary obligation is to the patient including the right to honest, open communication.
- Discuss of medical futility with patients and family will be more effective if they include concrete information about treatment, its likelihood of success, and the implications of the intervention and nonintervention decisions.
- Improve effective decision-making at the end of life influenced by use of advance directives and surrogate decision-makers, family spiritual practices.
- Ascertain the patient's perceptions about quality of life at the end of life; it is essential to ensuring optimal outcomes.

informed decision about use of life supports for terminal patients, patients and families need to know whether further treatments will enhance or diminish quality of life, their potential impact on life expectancy, financial cost, and whether the treatment is known to be effective or is an investigative treatment.

Ethical and Legal Issues

Nurses need to be aware of their states or provinces "right to die" laws. Families and patients must consider a number of legal issues as patients approach death.

Advance Directives. In 1990, the *Patient Self-Determination Act* became law. This law requires that all adult patients be given information about advance directives. Advance directives are written instructions detailing the process by which patient, together with their families and healthcare practitioners, specify preferences for future care. Advance directives specify a person's healthcare decisions should they become incapacitated. This includes "do not resuscitate (DNR) directives." Information should be documented and made available to caregivers directly involved in the patient's care. A copy of their advanced directive must accompany then to each place they go such as in the ambulance, in the emergency department, onto their hospital unit. Otherwise, it is not uncommon for EMTs or ED physicians to disregard them. An advance directive is not permanently binding; if the patient chooses to later revoke the document, the patient can do so.

The nurse's role is to provide the patient with full information about risks and benefits of prolonging life and to serve as patient advocate in support of the person's right to make decisions about treatment and care. When patients are decisionally competent, they should be key

decision-makers. If a patient is not competent, or is unable to articulate their wishes, a responsible family member or significant person can be designated to legally assume the responsibility of surrogate spokesperson.

Durable Power of Attorney for Healthcare. Competent adults can choose to appoint a surrogate decision-maker (durable power of attorney for healthcare) in the event that they cannot make important health decisions on their own behalf. This designation includes the surrogate's authority to accept or refuse treatment on the patient's behalf. Some patients have neither power of attorney for health nor advance directives. Box 21.5 provides guidelines for talking with families about care options when an advance directive or durable power of attorney is not in effect.

Assisted Suicide. It is worth mentioning again that nurses need to be aware of laws governing care. A number of European countries and several of the American states have passed laws that allow medically induced suicide. Yet in other areas, it remains a felony. What ethical considerations are involved in assisting a patient to kill themselves? What are your personal values?

Standards of Care. Nurses are required to routinely assess every patient for pain and document appropriate monitoring and pain management interventions.

Communication in End-of-Life Care

Family and Team Conferences

Family conferences are effective tools to alleviate family anxiety about the dying process, reduce unnecessary conflict between family members, and assist family members with important decision-making processes. This is especially important in decision-making related to withdrawing or withholding life support in end-of-life care, including withdrawing artificial feedings. Samara et al. (2021) has reported that telehealth Internet can be used in lieu of face-to-face family gatherings, so distant family can participate. Although a physician commonly leads the discussion, nurses often present data and answer questions. We should also assess for communication gaps among those present. Common concerns include conflicts among family members about care; tensions between the patient, family, and/or physician and family about treatment; where death should occur (home, hospital, hospice); and if/when hospice should be engaged. Anderson's (2019) research suggests one effective tool to promote discussion is use of a question prompt list. The Institute of Medicine (2015) has published a helpful book.

Family Education

Providing complete, understandable information, and psychological support are part of the nursing role. Like patients,

BOX 21.5   Talking With Families About Care Options

If neither durable power of attorney nor written directive is in effect, nurses can facilitate the process by helping to do the following:

- Determine who should be approached to make the decisions about care options.
- Determine whether any key members are absent. (Try to keep those who know the patient best in the center of decision-making.)
- Find a quiet place to meet where each family member can be seated comfortably.
- Sit down and establish rapport with each person present. Ask about the relationship each person has with the patient and how each person feels about the patient's current condition.
- Try to achieve a consensus about the patient's clinical situation, especially prognosis.
- Provide a professional observation about the patient's status and expected quality of life—survival versus quality of life. Ask what each person thinks the patient would want.
- Should the family choose comfort measures only, assure the family of the attention to patient comfort and dignity that will occur.
- Seek verbal confirmation of understanding and agreement.
- Attention to the family's emotional responses is appropriate and appreciated.

Modified from Lang, F., & Quill, T. (2004). Making decisions with families at the end of life. *American Family Physician, 70*(4), 719–723.

BOX 21.6   Imminent Death: Family Communication Needs

- Honest and complete answers to questions; repetition and further explanation if needed
- Updates about the patient's condition and changes as they occur
- Clear, understandable explanations delivered with empathy and respect
- Frequent opportunities to express concerns and feelings in a supportive, unhurried environment
- Information about what to expect—physical, emotional, spiritual—as death approaches
- Discussion of whom to call, legal issues, memorial or funeral planning
- Conversation about cultural and/or religious rituals at time of and after death
- Appreciation of the conflicts that families experience when the illness dictates that few options exist; for example, a frequent dilemma at end of life is whether life support measures are extending life or prolonging the dying phase
- Short private times to be present and/or minister to the patient
- Permission to leave the dying patient for short periods with the knowledge that the nurse will contact the family member if there is a change in status

families have different levels of readiness. Generally, if they ask a question, they are ready to hear the answer. Communication issues include the following: Which family member makes decisions? Who gives the care? How much do they know about the trajectory of the patient's illness? Are they able to access Internet portals to make appointments, be seen virtually, or request prescription refills? Education should also include information about what to expect in the dying process. Box 21.6 gives guidelines for talking with families when patient death is imminent.

Patients

Most patients know intuitively when their time is getting shorter, but the exact time frame may not be apparent until very close to death. It is not unusual for a patient to ask in the course of conversation, "Am I going to die?" or "How much longer do you think I have?" Before answering, find out more about the origin of the question. A useful listening response is, "What is your sense of it?" (National Cancer Institute, 2020).

Box 21.7 presents guidelines for communicating with patients when death is imminent.

Nursing Role in Palliative Care

Morgan (2001) identifies a protective coping and adjustment response that nurses can use with palliative care patients. This is a two-part intervention, which involves nursing conversations that protect, maintain, and support individual patient integrity, and explore the patient's preferences and values in end-of-life care. Nurses are key informants about patient status and changes in the patient's condition. Data sharing should be compassionate, accurate, and presented in language understandable to the family. Contradictory recommendations and incomplete information add to a family's confusion and cause unnecessary distress. A coordinated team approach prevents fragmentary and inconsistent care.

Addressing Cultural Needs
Incorporating Cultural Differences

Different cultures have distinctive communication and care standards for patients with life-threatening

BOX 21.7 Immanent Death: Guidelines for Communicating With Patients

- Avoid automatic responses and trite reassurances.
- Each death is a unique, deeply personal experience for the patient and should be treated as such.
- Avoid destroying hope. Reframe hope to what can happen in the here and now.
- Let the patient lead the discussion about the future. Be comfortable with focusing on the here and now. (This discussion is not a one-time event; openings for discussion should be encouraged as the patient's condition worsens.)
- Relate on a human level. Show humor as well as sorrow.
- Use your mind, eyes, and ears to hear what is said, as well as what is not said.
- Respect the individual's pattern of communication and ways of dealing with stress. Support the patient's desire for control of his or her life to whatever extent is possible.
- Maintain a sense of calm. Use eye contact, touch, and comfort measures to communicate.
- Do not force the patient to talk. Respect the patient's need for privacy, be sensitive to the patient's readiness to talk, and let him or her know that you will be available to listen.
- Humility and honesty are essential. Be willing to admit when you do not know the answer.
- Be willing to allow the patient to see some of your fears and vulnerabilities. It is much easier to open up to someone who is "human and vulnerable" than to someone who appears to have all the answers.

conditions. Cultural distinctions focus on (1) type of care that provides comfort to the dying person; (2) understanding of the causes of illness and death; (3) appropriate care of the body and burial rites; and (4) expression of grief responses. Asking patients/families directly about their cultural values and issues as a starting point helps ensure cultural safety for patients and families. For many cultures, spirituality is significantly embedded in a person's culture, and many cultures have special rituals. A simple question such as "Can you tell me about how your family/culture/spiritual beliefs views serious illness or treatment?" provides a framework for discussion. When cultural differences are considered, it is important to avoid stereotyping, as each person's interpretation of their culture is unique. Once cultural needs are identified, every effort should be taken to honor their meaning to patients and families by incorporating them in care. It is important to be aware of and sensitive to values in various cultures. For example, African-American families tend toward family decision-making about end-of-life care, as opposed to some other cultures where it is the patient who does the decision-making (Moss et al., 2018).

Attending to Spiritual Needs

Spirituality becomes a priority for many people at the end of their life. It is not unusual for patients who have previously declined spiritual interventions to desire them as they move into the final phase of life. Spiritual beliefs and religious rituals provide a tangible vehicle for individuals and families to express and experience meaning and purpose. Relevant religious practices and rituals can be important to patients even if the person no longer formally practices the religion. Facilitating these practices touches the patient's inner core and helps the person move toward a peaceful death. Nurses can ask the patient and/or family if they would like a visit from an appropriate clergy or hospital chaplain. Issues that may trouble patients relate to forgiveness, unresolved guilt issues, expressions of love, saying good-bye to important people, and existential questions about the meaning of life, the hereafter, and concern for their family and beliefs.

Childhood Death

It is not the natural order of things for a child to die. People are supposed to live into adulthood. When a child is diagnosed with a life-limiting condition, the effect on parents is devastating; it influences role functioning, friendships, and treatment of siblings. Children are such an integral part of their parents' identity that issues of parental protectiveness, guilt, responsible caregiving, balancing family demands, and helplessness parents feel should be part of the discussion. In addition to providing appropriate symptom management medications to make the child more comfortable, the following interventions are supportive to children with a life-limiting illness.

In hospital:
1. Open visitation for parents.
2. Ensure parents have respite (give permission).
3. Open communication: Involve and inform the child of everything that is going on, with developmentally appropriate language and content.
4. Encourage visits from family and friends, including using communication platforms such as Facebook.

In home:
5. Encourage the family to keep the child's life as normal as possible.
6. Suggest ways to enhance family functioning with attention paid to making special time for siblings.

7. Encourage families to maintain or adapt cultural, family, and religious traditions.
8. Encourage families to seek emotional support: support groups, extended family, friends.

Childhood Grief Issues

Children grieve within the context of the family, but they do not grieve in the same ways. Encourage parents to explain what is happening in a concrete, direct way using clear, concrete language suitable to the child's developmental level. Questions should be answered directly and honestly at the child's developmental level of comprehension, free of medical jargon. This type of discussion should *not* be a one-time event, and parents may need to be proactive in initiating the conversation.

Death of a significant person is difficult for children because they have neither the cognitive development nor the life experiences to fully process its meaning. A child younger than 5 years has no clear concept of what death means. Until children reach the formal operations stage of cognitive development, they can have fantasies about the circumstances surrounding the death and their part in it.

How a Child Grieves

Children do not express their grief in the same way adults do. Unpredictable acting-out behaviors, withdrawal, anger, fear, and crying are common responses. One minute the child may be playing, the next he is angry or withdrawn. Preschoolers may repeatedly ask when someone close to them will be coming home even if parents tell them that person has died. Developmentally, they do not understand the permanence of death. Elementary school children accept the permanence of death but view it in a concrete manner.

The National Cancer Institute (2013) identifies common concerns children may have about the death of someone important to them:

1. Did I cause the death to happen?
2. Is it going to happen to me?
3. Who is going to take care of me?

Parents can *create* opportunities for children to ask these questions. Asking the child about potential concerns can elicit a conversation that will not happen otherwise. Maintaining daily routines in the child's life after the death of a parent or primary caregiver is critical. Children need to know that they are safe and will be taken care of by the remaining adults in their life. If changes are needed, children should have the opportunity to discuss the reasons for them and time to absorb this information if at all possible.

Death

Death is a deeply personal experience. The Institute of Medicine (2015) defines a **good death** as one that is free from unavoidable distress and suffering for patients, families, and caregivers; in general accord with patients' and families' wishes; and reasonably consistent with clinical, cultural, and ethical standards. Mendoza (2020) suggests a good death is one in which the patient is reasonably free from avoidable distress, in the company of loved ones and trusted care providers, occurring in accord with cultural and religious practices. With some patients, the dying process is swift. With others, there is gradual downward spiral. Common symptoms include decreased need for food or liquids, long periods of sleeping or coma, decreased urinary output (dark urine), changes in vital signs, disorientation, restlessness and agitation, dyspnea (breathlessness), Cheyne stokes breathing, picking at bed clothes, plus skin temperature, and skin color changes. All of these changes are normal findings as a person prepares to leave this world. Dying patients experience profound weakness such that they cannot independently complete even basic hygiene.

A nurse's calming *presence* is perhaps the most important form of communication and emotional support for dying patients *and* families (Fig. 21.2). Most patients cannot carry on an in-depth conversation as death approaches. Flexibility in allowing family and/or significant others open access to the patient can reduce family anxiety and can be comforting for all concerned. At the same time, as patients approach death, it becomes an effort for the patient to respond to family and friends. Tell the family that it is their presence that matters.

In the following example, a nurse helps a terminally ill Mr Amos achieve a sense of spiritual completion.

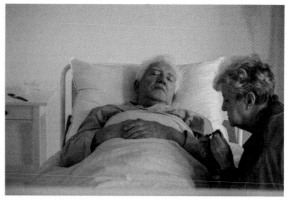

Figure 21.2 Nurses can facilitate meaningful family "presence" at life's ending, even when verbal communication is limited. (Copyright © KatarzynaBialasiewicz/iStock/Thinkstock.)

Case Study: George Amos Is Dying

Mr Amos was in the last stages of his end-of-life journey. He had repeatedly refused to have spiritual visits and had no desire for the sacrament of the living (a religious rite in the Catholic church). His nurse said the priest was on the floor at the hospital and asked him if he would like to receive communion. He answered, "Yes, but nothing else." The priest gave him communion, after which the patient asked him to hear his confession and requested the last rites. This would not have happened without the collaborative efforts of this nurse's advocacy. After the priest left, Mr Amos told his nurse, "You always seem to know what to do, and when to do it; thank you."

Simulation Exercise 21.3 provides you with the opportunity to personally think about what constitutes a good death.

Caring for the Patient After Death

Respect for the dignity of the patient continues after death. If the family is present at time of death, allowing uninterrupted private time with the patient before initiating postmortem care is important. If the family is not present, all excess equipment and trash should be removed from the room. You can offer presence and emotional support as you escort the family into the room. Some families will want privacy; others will appreciate having the presence of the nurse or chaplain. The nurse can obtain signatures to release the patient to the funeral home *after* the family has spent some time with the patient.

Stress Issues for Nurses in Palliative Care Settings

Nurses become invested in the care and comfort of patients and families facing immediate death; it is an emotional time for everyone involved. Nurses can experience **compassion fatigue**, a syndrome associated with serious spiritual, physical, and emotional depletion related to caring for end-of-life patients. Self-care and self-compassion are essential to avoid burnout and result in burnout and a nurse's decision to leave nursing.

SUMMARY

This chapter describes the stages of death and dying, and theory frameworks of Kubler-Ross, Lindeman, and Engel for understanding grief and grieving. Palliative care is discussed as a philosophy of care and an emerging discipline focused on making end-of-life care a quality life experience. A good death is defined as a peaceful death experienced with dignity and respect; one that wholly honors the patient's values and wishes at the end of life. Nurses can offer compassionate communication, presence, and anticipatory guidance to ease the grief of loss.

Nursing strategies are designed to help patients cope with the secondary psychological and spiritual aspects of having a terminal illness such that they achieve the best quality of life in the time left to them. Talking with patients about advance directives is a professional responsibility of the nurse, and it reduces unnecessary conflict among family members at this critical time in a person's life. Talking with children about terminal illness or death of a relative or in coping with a terminal diagnosis themselves should take into consideration the child's developmental level. Questions should be answered honestly and empathetically. As death approaches, nurses can help families understand the physiological changes signaling the body's natural shutdown of systems. Self-care is essential so nurses can avoid burnout.

SIMULATION EXERCISE 21.3 What Constitutes a Good Death?

Purpose

To help students focus on defining the characteristics of a good death.

Procedure

1. In pairs or small groups, think about, write down, and then share briefly examples of a "good" and a "not-so-good" death that you have witnessed in your personal life or clinical setting.
2. What were the elements that you thought contributed to its being a "good" or "not-so-good" death?

Reflective Discussion Analysis

Were there any common themes found in the stories as to what constitutes a "good" death? How could you use the findings of this exercise in helping patients achieve a "good" death?

ETHICAL DILEMMA: What Would You Do?

Francis Dillon has been on a ventilator for the past 3 weeks. He is not decisionally competent, and he is not able to communicate. Although he has virtually no chance of recovery, his family refuses to take him off the ventilator because "there is always the chance that he might wake up." What do you see as the ethical issues, and how would you, as the nurse, address this problem?

DISCUSSION QUESTIONS

1. What is meant by the statement, "There is potential for healing and meaning even in the face of impending death"?
2. What does the concept "quality of life" mean in end-of-life care?
3. How do you care for yourself when working with seriously ill patients and what would you recommend to avoid burnout?

REFERENCES

American Association of Colleges of Nursing (AACN). (2021). *End-of-Life Nursing Education Consortium (ELNEC) fact sheet.* Washington, D.C.: AACN. Retrieved from: https://www.aacnnursing.org/ELNEC/About. [Accessed 28 June 2021].

American Cancer Society (2022). Palliative care. www.cancer.org/treatment/treatments-and-side-effects/palliative-care.html.

Anderson, R. J., Bloch, S., Armstrong, M., Stone, P. C., & Low, J. (2019). Communication between healthcare professionals and relatives of patients approaching the end-of-life: A systematic review of qualitative evidence. *Palliative Medicine,* 33(8), 926–941.

Attig, T. (2001). Relearning the world: Making and finding meanings. In R. Neimeyer (Ed.), *Meaning reconstruction and the experience of loss* (pp. 33–53). Washington, D.C.: American Psychological Association.

Belisomo, R. (2018). Reversing racial inequities at end-of-life: A call for health systems to create culturally competent advance care planning programs within African-American communities. *Journal of Racial and Ethnic Health Disparities,* 5(1), 213–220.

Blaževičienė, A., Lars, L., & Newland, J. A. (2020). Attitudes of registered nurses about the end-of-life care in multi-profile hospitals: A cross sectional survey. *BMC Palliative Care,* 19(1), 131.

Connor, S. R., Centeno, C., Garralda, E., Clelland, D., & Clark, D. (2021). Estimating the number of patients receiving specialized palliative care globally in 2017. *Journal of Pain and Symptom Management,* 61(4), 812–816.

Crowe, S. (2017). End-of-life care in the ICU: Supporting nurses to provide high quality care. *Canadian Journal of Critical Care Nursing,* 28(1), 30–33.

Engel, G. L. (1964). Grief and grieving. *American Journal of Nursing,* 64(7), 93–98.

Guido, G. (2010). *Nursing care at the end of life.* Upper Saddle River, NJ: Pearson.

Heyland, D. K., Dodek, P., You, J. J., et al. (2017). Validation of quality indicators for end-of-life communication: Results of a multicentre survey. *Canadian Medical Association Journal,* 189(30), e980–e989.

Huisman, B. A. A., Geijteman, E. C. T., Dees, M. K., et al. (2020). Role of nurses in medication management at the end-of-life: A qualitative interview. *BMC Palliative Care,* 19(1), 68.

Institute of Medicine (IOM). (2015). *Dying in America: Improving quality and honoring individual preferences near the end of life.* Washington, D.C.: National Academies Press.

International Council of Nurses (ICN). (2012). *Nurses' role in providing care to dying patients and their families. Position statement.* Retrieved from: https://www.icn.ch/sites/default/files/inline-files/A12_Nurses_Role_Care_Dying_Patients.pdf. [Accessed 2 July 2021].

Kim, S., Lee, K., & Kim, S. (2020). Knowledge, attitude, confidence, and educational needs of palliative care in nurses caring for non-cancer patients: A cross-sectional, descriptive study. *BMC Palliative Care,* 19(1), 105.

Kübler-Ross, E. (1969). *On death and dying: What the dying have to teach doctors, nurses, clergy, and their own families.* New York: Scribner.

Lindemann, E. (1994). Symptomatology and management of acute grief. *The American Journal of Psychiatry,* 151(Suppl. 6), 155–160.

Mendoza, M. A. (2020). *What is a good death? How to die well. Psychology today.* Retrieved from: www.Psychologytoday.com/us/blog/understanding-grief/202003/what-is-good-death/. [Accessed 28 June 2021].

Morgan, A. (2001). A grounded theory of nurse-patient interaction in palliative care nursing. *Journal of Clinical Nursing,* 10(4), 583–584.

Morrow, A. (2020). *How to recognize and assess pain.* Verywell Health. Retrieved from: www.verywellhealth.com/pain-assessment-1131968#assessing-nonverbal-signs/. [Accessed 28 June 2021].

Moss, K. O., Deutsch, N. L., Hollen, P. J., Rovnyak, V. G., Williams, I. C., & Rose, K. M. (2018). Understanding end-of-life decision-making terminology among African-American older adults. *Journal of Gerontological Nursing,* 44(2), 33–40.

National Cancer Institute. (2013). *Grief, bereavement, and coping with loss (PDQ®)-patient version. Children and grief.* Retrieved from: http://www.cancer.gov/cancertopics/pdq/supportivecare/bereavement/Patient/page9. [Accessed 28 June 2021].

National Cancer Institute. (2020). *Grief, bereavement, and coping with loss (PDQ®)-health professional version.* Retrieved from: http://cancer.gov/cancertopics/pdq/supportivecare/bereavement/HealthProfessional. [Accessed 28 June 2021].

Neimeyer, R. A. (Ed.). (2001). *Meaning reconstruction and the experience of loss.* Washington, D.C: American Psychological Association.

Samara, J., Liu, W. M., Kroon, W., Harvie, B., Hingeley, R., & Johnston, N. (2021). Telehealth palliative care needs rounds during a pandemic. *Journal for Nurse Practitioners,* 17(3), 335–338.

Sawatzky, R., Porterfield, P., Lee, J., et al. (2016). Conceptual foundations of a palliative approach: A knowledge synthesis. *BMC Palliative Care,* 15, 5.

Wittenberg-Lyles, E., Goldsmith, J., Ferrell, B., & Ragan, S. (2013). *Communication in palliative nursing.* New York: Oxford University Press.

22

Role Relationship Communication Within Nursing

OBJECTIVES

At the end of the chapter, the reader will be able to:

1. Describe professional role relationships among nurses in healthcare.
2. Distinguish among the professional nursing role opportunities.
3. Discuss the components of professional role socialization in nursing.
4. Analyze evidence-based role research and apply to clinical practice situations.

Chapter 22 presents an overview of role relationships within professional nursing and their implications for professional communication, education, and practice. Being clear about your professional role is essential for meaningful functional relationships with others. Empirical evidence shows effective communication among members of the team reduces the potential for error and the consequences of error, aiding us in providing safe care. The communication skills and leadership style of nurse managers strongly predict the job satisfaction of direct care nurses (Jankelová & Joniaková, 2021). The applications section addresses the process of professional nursing socialization, role development, mentorship, and communication with supervisors, peers, and nursing assistant personnel. Leadership competencies are discussed. Chapter 23 will address communication in interdisciplinary teams.

BASIC CONCEPTS

Role

Role is a multidimensional psychosocial concept defined as characteristic behavior patterns and expression of self expected of an individual within a given society. People develop social, work, and professional roles throughout life. Some roles are conferred at birth (ascribed roles), and some are attained through circumstance during a lifetime (acquired roles). Personal ascribed role performance standards reflect social, cultural, gender, and family expectations. Nursing roles have flexibility. Consider the Ms Retha case.

Professionalism and Work Environment
Theoretical Constructs Related to the Nurse Role
Criteria that are characteristic of a profession were initially developed by Flexner more than a century ago (1915). Examine these criteria listed in Box 22.1 to determine whether nursing meets these criteria. A nurse's professional relationships and work environment play a big part in satisfaction. Job dissatisfaction contributes to high turnover rates at a time when there is a worldwide nursing shortage (World Health Organization [WHO], 2020). Even in developed countries, new graduates leave their jobs and even the profession in high numbers. Job attrition is cited as running between 15% and greater than 60% in various countries, as cited by numerous articles. Could creating

CASE STUDY: Ms Mary Retha and Adaptive Nursing Role

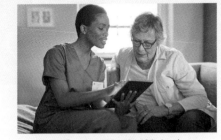

From iStock #1201491499, kupicoo.

As a community nurse, you make a home visit to Ms Retha, who has diabetes and multiple other health issues. She lives in a trailer park in a remote area with no public transportation. Her primary physician reports she does not follow the ADA diet he prescribed. Starting with an open-ended question, you ask her "Tell me about how you get your groceries?" During the discussion, you discover her only source of food is from the 24/7 gas/mart near her place. After an initial lack of success locating alternative food sources, you decide to adapt your teaching to Ms Retha's lifestyle resources and use the fast-food menu to help her select healthier, low-fat choices from what is available. Might you also explore the local foodbank as a resource?

Courtesy of Connie Bowler, DPN, RN, Lakeland Community College, 2017.

a supportive workplace with open communication and respect promote better retention?

Social Learning Theory. Bandura's work provides a useful framework for examining the role of a nurse. Bandura said that learning takes place in a social environment, in the nurses' case in the clinical setting. Learners aspire to be like, to identify with, those who hold positions to which they themselves aspire. Students are motivated to pay attention to a role model's behavior, to imitate it after cognitively processing observed behavior. They internalize their observations and then reproduce it. Bandura suggested this occurs in four stages: attention, retention, reproduction, and motivation. Reinforcement adds to motivation (Horsburgh & Ippolito, 2018).

Role Theory. Using concepts from sociology and social psychology, role theory encompasses socially defined norms, behaviors, and duties that are expected to be performed by an individual in a certain role within our social structure. Individuals who do not conform incur social disapproval. Everyone has multiple roles to fulfill as defined by society such as cultural roles, gender roles, work roles, social roles, etc. Problems occur when one role comes into conflict with another.

Professional Nursing Role Competencies

Competency is defined as a set of capabilities, skills, aptitude, and experience. In addition to development of technical nursing skills, technology, and communication skills, collaborative skills are needed to become a positive force in team-based healthcare. Nurse competencies have been defined by professional organizations, including QSEN, State Boards of Nursing licensure, and the government. Competencies include physical mastery of nursing skills and cognitive knowledge and attitudes needed to provide patient-centered care as illustrated in Fig. 22.1.

Professionalism in Nursing. Professional nurses comprise the largest professional group of healthcare providers. They spend more sustained professional time with patients and families than any other hospital care professional. Nursing roles have steadily evolved to include current expectations for nurses to assume leadership roles, to provide primary care, and to act as first-line providers in implementing healthcare reform initiatives.

Scope of Practice. The scope of practice for professional nurses continues to expand to include reimbursable health screening and promotion, risk reduction, and disease prevention strategies. Nurses increasingly provide care as part of interdisciplinary healthcare teams in hospitals and the community. All nurses are expected to advocate for healthcare transformation and to take a leadership role in addressing environmental, social, and economic determinants of health. Nurses are assuming public advocacy roles

BOX 22.1   Flexner's Criteria

- Members share a common identity, values, attitudes, and behaviors.
- A distinctive specialized substantial body of knowledge exists.
- Education is extensive, with both theory and practice components.
- Unique service contributions are made to society.
- Acceptance of personal responsibility in discharging services to the public.
- Governance and autonomy over policies that govern activities of profession members.
- A code of ethics that members acknowledge and incorporate in their actions.

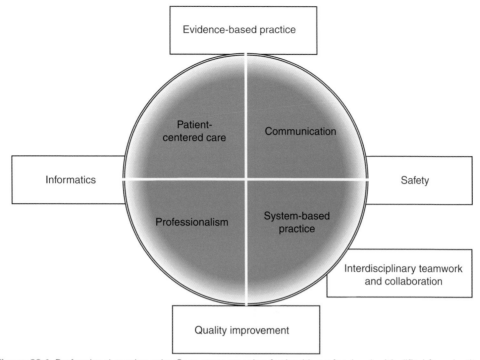

Figure 22.1 Professional nursing role: Core competencies for health professionals. Modified from Institute of Medicine (IOM). (2003). *Health professions education: A bridge to quality* (pp. 45–46). Washington, DC: National Academies Press.

to inform policy makers, educators, and other healthcare providers about health-related issues. Nurses also provide leadership and coordination in healthcare improvement through education and participation in research. Simulation Exercise 22.1 is designed to help you look at the different role responsibilities of practicing nurses.

Technology. Competency in use of technology is a QSEN goal. Technology permits swift transactions, universal access, and levels of portability unanticipated 20 years ago. Defining aspects of caring and patient communication are supported, not led, by technology. Nurses are more responsible than ever to devise communication strategies that preserve the caring aspects of nursing. Chapters 25 and 26 provide in-depth discussions of communication and technology use issues.

Leadership. Hesburgh's (1971) description of leadership, and its relationship to caring, still holds true: The mystique of leadership, be it educational, political, religious, commercial, or whatever, is next to impossible to describe, but wherever it exists, morale flourishes, people pull together toward common goals, spirits soar, order is maintained, not as an end in itself, but as a means to move forward together. Such leadership always has a moral as well as intellectual dimension; it requires courage as well as wisdom; it does not simply know, it cares.

Role Clarity. Professional role clarity is an essential quality for working with healthcare teams. If nurses are not clear about their professional roles, it is difficult for them to communicate their value as healthcare providers to other professionals. Yet, McKenna et al., 2017, study found new graduates still lack knowledge about their role. Role clarity about professional competencies is necessary to support patient safety initiatives that lead to improved client outcomes. Influencing change and making difficult decisions become easier when nurses have a clear vision of their professional role, because they are better able to stimulate confidence in others (Ward, 2020).

Nurse Practice Roles

An empowering aspect of the nurse role is the opportunity to evolve roles, change specialties of care, move into advanced roles, or take on new administrative roles. Nurses must put forth the value of nurses as skilled healthcare providers. Evolved scope of practice and professional standards serve as the foundation for practice accountability and decision authority in contemporary nursing practice.

Direct Patient Care Nurses. Direct patient care nurses are expected to exhibit competent care skills and also show competency in their communication skills. Contemporary professional nursing roles reflect the increasing complexities of healthcare, globalization, changing patient demographic characteristics and diversity, and the exponential growth of health information technology.

The bedside nurses' role consists of delivery and organization of care for multiple patients. This role includes quality control issues, problem-solving, patient education, and coordination of communication among the many health team members. There is a strengthened focus on health promotion/disease prevention, and self-management of chronic disorders also echoes new economic realities and provider availability. For more information, refer to AACN's Essentials of Baccalaureate Nursing (2021) document defining core professional **role competencies** required of contemporary nurses. To deliver high-quality, safe, patient-centered care, the focus is on collaboration, a hallmark of role competence. We need to know our own role so we can work together smoothly.

Nurse Managers. Most often a midlevel administrative position, these managers provide leadership for staff on hospital units. Administrative duties include work schedules, job goals, and evaluations. Their communication skills and transformative leadership styles have been shown to increase job satisfaction of staff nurses and decrease their stress (Jankelová & Joniaková, 2021). Effective managers provide support to team members and use their position to create better working conditions, thus increasing staff retention.

Advanced Practice Nurses. The IOM (2011) mandate to increase the number of professional nurses in advanced practice roles makes a strong statement in healthcare reform. An advanced practice nurse (APRN) is a licensed skilled practitioner holding a minimum of a master's degree in a clinical specialty, with the expert knowledge base, complex decision-making skills, and clinical competencies required for expanded specialty practice. Various countries have established many roles for APNs, including nurse practitioners, clinical nurse specialists, certified nurse midwives, nurse anesthetists, etc. Specialized training allows APRNs to diagnose and independently manage care, including prescriptive authority for some, as regulated by each state. In addition to clinical roles, APRNs function in research, educational, and administrative roles. A significant issue yet to be completely resolved is a lack of consistency that has lessened but still exists surrounding role responsibilities and scope of practice of APRNs.

The Clinical Nurse Leader. Leadership is the art of motivating people to act to achieve a common goal (Ward, 2020). In response to the IOM (2001) report, the American Association of Colleges of Nursing (AACN) developed the clinical nurse leader (CNL) model as a master's-prepared generalist role to provide leadership at the bedside. The CNL's focus is on quality of care, bridging the gaps between members of the health team. The CNL curriculum prepares students with a baccalaureate degree in another field to become an advanced generalist nurse (master's degree and eligibility for licensure as a registered nurse). Core competencies include clinical leadership skills, environmental management, and clinical outcome management. For CNLs to practice as an APRN in a specific *clinical specialty*, the CNL must complete further academic preparation.

The Doctor of Nursing Practice. The Doctor of Nursing Practice (DNP) is a *terminal practice* degree for professional nurses. It is a nonresearch clinical doctorate. The complexity of the nation's healthcare environment served as a major impetus for promoting transitions to practice doctorates, as did the need to position nursing professionally on a par with other major health professions, all of which offer practice-focused doctorates (AACN, 2020). The curriculum combines advanced nursing practice skill proficiency with a solid foundation in the clinical sciences, evidence-based practice methods, system leadership, information technology skills, health policy, and interdisciplinary collaboration. Think of the role as promoting implementation of research evidence developed by nurse researchers and many others.

Nurse Scientist. This position varies with the employing agencies. Often these are joint appointments between academia and healthcare agency. The nurse scientist is a knowledge broker who facilitates knowledge application in understandable terms to patient care. They use science to inform not just clinical practice but policy-making. This cuts down on the former average of 17 years it used to take for scientific evidence to make it into practice changes (Thompson & Barcott, 2019).

The PhD-Prepared Nurse Researcher. Doctoral research degree programs in nursing have grown substantially in developed countries. These nurses are prepared to conduct original research, to be primary investigators seeking substantial grants, working not only in university settings but also in many healthcare corporations.

Trends in Education That Develop Communication Skills

So much has changed due to the pandemic. Contact your State Board of Nursing for specific information. We will limit discussion to trends that impact communication.

Experiential Learning. Experiential learning is defined as active participation in learning scenarios, with self-reflection to analyze learning components. Contemporary healthcare education depends on experiential learning for developing both technical care skills and communication proficiency. Its competency-based goal is to provide students with the knowledge, skills, and attitudes needed to effectively collaborate and improve the quality of healthcare. Students use case study analyses, role play, exercise activities, computer simulations, standardized patient models, etc. The most vital part of the experiential learning process is the final activity of **reflection analysis** to recap what was learned and strategize about how to correct mistakes made.

Clinical Simulations. Problem-based learning scenarios provide innovative opportunities for students to analyze and find solutions in a safe, controlled environment. Clinical simulation is a preferred learning strategy because it allows interdisciplinary students to give close attention to all aspects of the clinical environment and to actively problem-solve solutions from a collaborative team perspective. Students construct and develop "live"

understanding of interdisciplinary health team functioning through shared reflection on their actions and interactions with each other in collectively meeting identified patient-centered goals.

Interdisciplinary Education. Interdisciplinary education is defined as educational occasions when two or more professions learn from and about each other to improve collaboration and the quality of care. Introducing interdisciplinary coursework early in the curriculum helps students to understand nursing roles and communication across other professionals. It gives some insight into the "mind set" of other professionals and encourages a pattern of collaboration. Cultivating interdependence between health professionals required for quality care in an era of cost containment is noted as being critical to success in meeting national health goals. Students gain firsthand understanding of the professional values held by other disciplines. In clinical scenarios, the decision-making process with team approaches is more complex than with single discipline methods, *acknowledging* and *respecting* the unique expected behaviors and skill sets of each health discipline fosters understanding. Frequent communication is essential to good results.

Examples of shared interdisciplinary electives include ethics, death and dying, culture, quality improvement (QI), genomics, emergency preparedness, gerontology, health policy, and legal issues. Clinical simulation courses open to students from multiple health disciplines provide unique opportunities for students in the healthcare professions to work together in the clinical management of complex disease health conditions.

Case Study: Interdisciplinary Project

A multidisciplinary learning opportunity was offered in collaboration with the University of Maryland and Montgomery County's Department of Health and Human Services involving nursing, pharmacy, and social work students. The students engaged in seeing patients and participating in collaborative discussions with faculty preceptorship related to their care at the Mercy Health Clinic. This outpatient clinic serves those without medical insurance and has a large culturally diverse clientele. The goals of the project were as follows:

1. To expose students to interdisciplinary collaborative practice in a community setting with diverse client values and needs.
2. To enhance the quality of care for clients with complex medical, cross-cultural, and social issues through interdisciplinary collaboration.

DEVELOPING AN EVIDENCE-BASED PRACTICE

Nurses can choose among so many roles both in acute care and within the community. Yet data show nurse retention to be a major problem. The literature identifies factors associated with job satisfaction, using a variety of measurement tools. Penconek and global colleagues (2021) reviewed 38 studies dealing with nurse manager satisfaction. These factors should be considered by those seeking the job.

Results

Correlates with job satisfaction were identified and classified into three categories:

Job characteristics: Autonomy to make decisions; a positive, supportive work climate; positive relations with staff.

Organizational characteristics: A shared model of organization and personal goals; assistance to accomplish goals including user-friendly technology, active participation in making changes.

Personal characteristics: Role meaningfulness; feelings of connectedness and positivity with others, including supervisors, physicians, staff.

As supported by multiple articles, job dissatisfaction was related to perceptions of heavy workload.

Strength of research evidence: Low. These were primarily correlational studies; it appears that study designs did not control for competing explanations.

Application to Your Clinical Practice

1. When seeking a job, look beyond the job description of the work to examine whether this is a positive working environment.
2. Ask about job retention statistics and factors such as workload.
3. Inquire about methods the organization uses to assist new nurses to adjust such as mentorships, preceptorships, organization-wide wellness programs, promotion opportunities reflected in such things as clinical ladders.

Reference

Penconek T., Tate K., Bernardes A., et al. (2021). Determinants of nurse manager job satisfaction: A systematic review. *The International Journal of Nursing Studies, 118,* 103906.

APPLICATIONS

Professional Role Socialization

Professional role socialization is a complex, continuous, interactive educational process through which student nurses acquire the knowledge, skills, attitudes, norms, values, and behaviors associated with the nursing profession. Novice nurses continue this process, as they acquire their professional identity. Role identity is thought to mitigate the negative effects of stress, helping you avoid "burnout." Transmission of the cultural value system inherent in the nursing profession is seen as the key element in role socialization. For example, beginners learn that nurses value their patients and their autonomy. Building on Leininger's (1991) ideas about the culture of nursing, we identify the process of mastering the knowledge, skills, and attitudes on our role. Although we still need greater understanding of the transition process, we know role modeling by academics and especially by expert clinicians is vital. Some say the clinical area is where we are really socialized.

Acquiring the Profession's Culture

This involves internalizing the values, standards, and role behaviors associated with professional nursing. As students begin to try out new professional behaviors, they receive feedback and support for their efforts from clinical staff, faculty, and clients. Positive feedback empowers students by acknowledging their clinical judgments and encourages them to perform successfully.

Academic Role Models as Socializing Agents

Initially, nursing students are absorbed in learning basic knowledge and skills. They depend on textbooks, instructors, and simulation labs to help them. As students become comfortable with foundational nursing knowledge, they interact with clinical staff. With increased experience, students begin to trust their reasoning in making clinical judgments.

Clinical Nurse Colleagues as Socializing Agents

Nursing faculty, clinical preceptors, and nursing mentors serve as important socializing agents, helping students learn the values, traditions, norms, and competencies of the nursing profession.

Clinical Preceptors

In a formalized, goal-directed clinical orientation relationship, the clinical preceptor is an experienced nurse, chosen for clinical competence and charged with supporting, guiding, and participating in the evaluation of student or new graduate clinical competence on a one-to-one basis. Perhaps designated by employers or by virtue of being on a career ladder, clinical preceptors' model professional behaviors give constructive feedback and promote clinical thinking in the novice nurse or nursing student.

Mentors

Mentoring describes a commitment to help another nurse become the best professional they can be. Mentors are seasoned, expert nurses who act as advisors for less experienced, novice nurses, generally over a long time period. The mentorship role is usually an informal arrangement. Mentors can be a sounding board for career option discussions and for providing guidance in looking at the whole picture, while considering what will fit in with our personal responsibilities. *Every nurse should seek out a career mentor, someone whose experience can help to guide your career.*

Organization/Agency Employment

Healthcare is rapidly evolving as it faces financial constraints, workforce shortages, and changing population needs (Sinclair, 2020). Healthcare in the 21st century will evolve into a different, more community-based model, rather than centering on hospitals whose original purpose was to provide acute care.

Steps in Role Socialization

Orientation of Direct Care Nurses

Accrediting agencies now recommend formal "residency" programs to orient and guide new graduate nurses, suggesting that to be effective, such programs need to be at least a year in length. Such programs combine some didactic instruction with clinical guidance by one or more clinical preceptors. Expectations about profession communication skills and agency goals, rules, and communication styles are imparted. The attitudes, actions, and directed support of the preceptor encourage students to adopt clinically appropriate professional behaviors. On the other hand, a clinician who does not follow good communication strategies, such as the tools provided by the TeamSTEPPS program, can negate all that the novice nurse has learned in the classroom (Amodo et al., 2017). In addition to clinical preceptors and peers, other informal socializing agents include patients, families, and peers. They promote understanding of the professional nursing role from a consumer perspective.

Employment Transition Socialization

Professional Skill Acquisition and Role Development. Transitioning to a new role is always stressful, even for experienced nurses. Personality traits that include resilience and inquisitiveness aid this transition. The Bauer and Erdogan's (2011) socialization model and organizational theories have been applied to understand what makes a

nurse effectively transition from student to novice nurse to competent practitioner.

Internationally, several authors developed models designed to describe the role transition process undergone by all new nurses during their first year of work (Benner, 1984, 2001). In her classic work discussing the theory–practice gap and subsequent "reality shock," Benner describes five developmental stages of formative role development in professional nursing. Based on the Dreyfus and Dreyfus model (1980) of skill acquisition, Benner specified each developmental stage in which a nurse demonstrates increasing proficiency in implementing the professional nursing role: novice, advanced beginner, competence, proficiency, and expert.

1. *Novice.* The first stage is referred to as the *novice stage.* Initially, students have limited or no nursing experience to perform required nursing tasks. Novice nurses need structure and exposure to the objective foundations upon which to base their nursing practice. They tend to compare clinical findings with the textbook picture because they lack the practice experience to do otherwise. Theoretical knowledge and confidence in the expertise of more practiced nurses and faculty serve as guides to practice. Schoessler and Waldo's model suggests that in the first 3 months of employment, the new graduate nurse struggles to develop organizational skills, master technical skills, and deal with coping with mistakes or the fear of making them.

2. *Advanced beginner.* In this stage, nurses understand the basic elements of practice and can organize and prioritize clinical tasks. Although clinical analysis of healthcare situations occurs at a higher level than strict association with the textbook picture, the advanced beginner is able to only partially grasp the unique complexity of each patient's situation. Preceptors can make a difference in helping new nurses cope with the uncertainty of new clinical situations and to hone their skills. They act as a guide by the side; in helping new nurses gain nursing proficiency. The new nurse's patients are also an important resource. For example, patients can help us to develop a greater appreciation for the complexity of social, psychological, and physical aspects of chronic disease as a result of their interactions. By paying close attention to their patients, and what seems to work best, advanced beginner nurses learn the art of nursing. In the Schoessler and Waldo model, this time is referred to as "neutral zone," the phase in which communication with others, including physicians or patients, is still problematic, while feeling more comfortable with organization and knowledge. After the first year and before 18 months, the new nurse enters a "new beginning" phase of feeling comfortable with nursing activities.

TABLE 22.1	Benner's Stages of Clinical Competence
Nurse Competency Level	**Description of Behaviors**
Advanced beginner	• Enters clinical situations with some apprehension • Sees task requirements as central to the clinical context, whereas other aspects of the situation are seen as background • Requires knowledge application to meet clinical realities • Perceives each clinical situation as a personal challenge • AIs typically dependent on standards of care, unit procedures
Competent	• Focuses more on clinical issues in contrast to tasks • Can handle familiar situations • Expects certain clinical trajectories on the basis of the experience with particular patients • Searches for broader explanations of clinical situations • Has enhanced organizational ability, technical skills • Focuses on managing patients' conditions
Proficient	• Responds to particulars of clinical situations in a broader way • Requires an experiential base with past patient populations • Understands patient transitions over time • Learns to gauge involvement with patients and families to promote appropriate caring
Expert	• Has increased intuition regarding what are important clinical factors and how to respond to these • Engages in practical reasoning • Anticipates and prepares for situations while remaining open to changes • Performs care in a "fluid, almost seamless" manner • Bonds emotionally with patients and families depending on their needs • Sees the big picture, including the unexpected • Works both with and through others

From Norman, V. (2008). Uncovering and recognizing nurse caring from clinical narratives. *Holistic Nursing Practice, 22*(6), 324–335, by permission. Data from Benner, P. A., Tanner, C. A., & Chesla, C. A. (1996). *Expertise in nursing practice: Caring, clinical judgment, and ethics.* New York: Springer.

3. *Competence.* This stage occurs 1–2 years into nursing practice. The competent nurse is able to easily manage the many contingencies of clinical nursing. Nurses begin to practice the "art" of nursing. They view the clinical picture from a broader perspective and are more confident about their roles in healthcare.

4. *Proficiency.* This stage occurs 3–5 years into practice. Nurses in this stage are self-confident about their clinical skills and perform them with competence, speed, and flexibility. The proficient nurse sees the clinical situation as a whole, has well-developed psychosocial skills, and knows from experience what needs to be modified in response to a given situation.

5. *Expert.* This last stage is marked with a high level of clinical skill and the capacity to respond authentically and creatively to patient needs and concerns. Expert nurses have confidence in their own ability and rarely panic in the face of a breakdown. They can recognize the unexpected and work creatively with complex clinical situations. Expert nurses demonstrate mastery of technology, sensitivity in interpersonal relationships, and specialized nursing skills in all aspects of their caregiving. Being an expert nurse is not an end point; nurses have the professional and ethical responsibility to continuously upgrade and refine their clinical skills through professional development and clinical skill training. Table 22.1 identifies behaviors associated with different levels of Benner's model.

Continuing Education

Professional development represents a lifelong commitment to excellence in nursing and requires regular upgrading of skills. As QSEN experts say "No patient wants a nurse who still practices only what she learned 10 years ago." Standard means of continued professional development include relevant continuing education presentations, staff development modules, conference attendance, academic education, specialized training, and research activities. Professional development also occurs through informal means such as consultation, professional reading, experiential learning, giving presentations, and self-directed learning activities such as Internet-based modules. The Profession and Governmental Licensure Bureaus encourage and, in some areas, require nurses to annually complete a certain level of continuing education activities to maintain licensure or certification. These offer unique opportunities to access new information and to network, share expertise, and learn different perspectives from others in the field.

Strategic Career Planning

Serious career plans should reflect careful appraisal of values, skills, interests, and different career possibilities. Mentors can be helpful in this area.

Role Relationships Within Nursing

It is inevitable that you will encounter some communication and collaboration problems with nurse colleagues. If managed appropriately, these difficulties can become opportunities for innovative solutions and improved relationships. A number of strategies discussed in Chapter 23 are useful in dealing with fellow nurses.

Communication With Peers. The nurse–patient relationship occurs within the larger context of your professional relationships with coworkers. Issues will arise. However, if we ignore relationship problems, others may unconsciously "act out" and undermine care. Historically, newly hired staff nurses encountered as much "hazing" as they received support. Bullying is discussed in Chapter 23. Occasionally, you may have to work with a peer with whom you develop a "personality conflict." Stop and consider what led up to the current situation. In general, it is due to the accumulation of small annoyances that occur over time. The best method is to verbalize occurrences rather than ignoring them until they become a major problem. Avoid "the blame game," and discuss in a private, calm moment what you both can do to make things better. Modeling positive interactions may assist in resolution. Holding an "intervention" or "crucial conversation" discussion is needed. The mnemonic CRIB can be used to guide the conversation:

C = Commit to seeking a mutual purpose (to move toward resolution of the conflict).

R = Recognize the purpose (can use a mentor to help)

I = Invent a mutual purpose (agree to a win-win purpose)

B = Brainstorm new strategies (agree to work together differently to move forward).

Whenever there is covert conflict among nurses, it is the patient who ultimately suffers the repercussions. The level of trust a patient has in the professional relationship is compromised until the staff conflict can be resolved. Getting accepted and building congenial working relationships take time and some energy.

Communication With Supervisors. Negotiating with persons in authority can be stressful, even threatening, because such people have control over your future as a staff nurse or student. Supervision implies shared responsibility in our overall goal of providing safe, high-quality care to patients. The wise supervisor is able to promote a nonthreatening environment in which all aspects of professionalism are allowed to emerge. In the supervisor–nurse relationship, conflict may arise when performance expectations are unclear or when the nurse is unable to perform at the desired level. Communication of expectations often occurs after the fact, within the context of employee performance evaluations. Effective management means these job expectations are known from the first day. Frequent feedback and performance reviews are used to let you know about areas needing improvement, as part of an ongoing, constructive relationship. When a supervisor gives constructive criticism, it should be in a caring, nonthreatening manner.

Supervision of Staff. Use of open communication techniques already discussed is effective in supervising others. If a problem occurs, use the same communication techniques described in Chapter 13: state your concern, state expectations, and mention outcomes that will occur if the problem behavior persists. There are two categories of personnel you as a staff nurse might be responsible for supervising: unlicensed and licensed personnel. The ANA Code speaks of delegation in Provision 4.4: Nurses are responsible for monitoring the activities and evaluation of the quality and outcome of others to whom they have delegated (patient care).

Communication in Delegating to Unlicensed Assistive Personnel. Our nursing workload demands have given rise to employment of several types of unlicensed personnel, such as nursing assistants and orderlies. Although we are ultimately responsible for the quality and safety of care given under our supervision, we delegate less complex tasks to assistants. Delegation is defined as the transfer of responsibility for the performance of an activity from one individual to another while retaining accountability. Whether delegating to a peer or unlicensed assistive personnel (UAP), the nurse is only transferring a task, not responsibility for care (ANA, n.d.). Delegation can free a nurse for attending to more complex care needs. In the current healthcare environment, some UAPs possess minimal knowledge or experience skills, whereas others have excellent abilities. Refer to your licensure organization for guidelines. Try Simulation Exercise 22.2 to apply principles of delegation.

SIMULATION EXERCISE 22.2   Applying Principles of Delegation

Purpose
To help students differentiate between delegating nursing tasks and evaluating outcomes.

Procedure
Divide class into two groups. Reflect on the following case study of a typical day for the charge nurse in an extended-care facility. Group A is to describe the nursing tasks they would delegate to UAP assistants and the instructions they would give. Group B is to describe the responsibilities of the professional nurse related to the delegated work.

   Reflective analysis and discussion: identify goals.

Case
Anne Marie Roach, RN, is the day shift charge nurse at Shadyside extended care facility. Today the unit census is 24, and her staff includes four nursing assistants (NAs) and two certified medicine aides (CMAs) who are allowed to administer oral medications. The NAs are qualified to give morning baths; assist with feeding; obtain and record vital signs, intake, and output; do fingersticks for blood glucose readings; and turn and reposition bed-bound patients and assist the others to ambulate. They also change decubitus dressings for the three needing this care. Of the residents, 12 are bed bound, requiring full baths and feeding assistance. The remaining 12 need some assistance with morning care and ambulation to the dining room. Nine residents need glucose levels; seven have weakness recovering from strokes. All residents are at risk for falls. Night shift reported all residents' conditions as stable. Time to make today's assignments.

Reflective Discussion Analysis
Discuss and evaluate groups' responses.

Communication in Delegating to Other Licensed Nurses. There are several categories of nurses who, while licensed, have a more limited scope of practice and may require your supervision. In some countries, these nurses are known as licensed practical nurses (LPNs) or licensed vocational nurses (LVNs). Role overlap, lack of clear distinctions in roles, power factors, and pay inequality still lead some to struggle with maintaining collegial relationships. Appropriate use of delegation can facilitate your ability to meet these challenges. More often than not, novice nurses are inadequately prepared for the demands of delegation. Reflect on the Monica Lewis case.

Case Study: Monica Lewis, RN
After receiving the report of her patient assignments, Ms Lewis assigns a newly hired nursing assistant Sally Smith (UAP) to provide routine care (morning bath, assistance with breakfast, vital signs, fingerstick for glucose level) to several patients, including Ms. Jones, who was admitted yesterday for exacerbation of her type 2 diabetes mellitus. While on rounds, Monica finds that Mrs Jones is unresponsive, cold, and clammy, with a heart rate of 110 beats/min. Her record shows that the 8 a.m. fingerstick reading of a glucose level was 60 mg/dL, as performed by Sally. Thinking that Mrs Jones is experiencing hypoglycemia, Monica requests Sally Smith obtain another glucose reading. While preparing to administer glucose intravenously, Monica observes Sally make several errors obtaining an accurate blood glucose test. Sally admits she was never taught the procedure but says she thought reading the instructions was sufficient. Monica had wrongly assumed all UAPs underwent training on principles of obtaining accurate fingersticks.

Inherent in effective delegation is an adequate understanding of the skills and knowledge of UAPs, as well as of legal parameters such as the Nurse Practice Act in the location in which you are nursing. Nurse Practice Acts clearly state what and what cannot be delegated and to what type of personnel these actions can be delegated. The employing agency and the nurse need to reinforce the UAP's knowledge base, assess current level of abilities, oversee tasks, and evaluate outcomes. This is a costly process both in time and in energy. Practice of Simulation Exercise 22.2 should help you to consider the principles of delegation.

Self-awareness
Self-awareness is defined as the capacity to accurately recognize emotional reactions as they happen and to understand your responses to different people and situations. Self-awareness helps nurses to work from their strengths and cope more effectively to minimize personal weaknesses in interactions with others. Developing self-awareness allows nurses to make higher-quality decisions because decisions are more likely to be based on facts than personal feelings.

It is not always easy to be completely honest about one's personal weaknesses, values, and beliefs. However, this level of self-awareness is a crucial component of effective professional leadership development. Self-awareness directly affects self-management and how we professionally respond to others. Professional self-awareness promotes recognition of the need for continuing education, the acceptance of accountability for one's own actions, the capacity to be assertive with professional colleagues, and the capability of serving as a patient advocate when the situation warrants it, even if it is uncomfortable to do so.

Nurses Have Rights

In addition to significant responsibilities, you as a nurse have rights in your professional relationships with colleagues and patients. See Box 22.2 for the Nurses Bill of Rights.

Think about your professional collegial relationships and your dual professional commitment to self and others. How can you balance your legitimate responsibilities to self and your responsibilities to patients and coworkers?

Transformational Leadership. Leadership plays a pivotal role in setting expectations regarding scope of practice, collaboration, optimal interdisciplinary teamwork, and empowered knowledge partnerships in professional nursing practice. Transformational leadership requires engaging the hearts, as well as the minds, of those in the workforce. The transformational leader is self-actualized, stays focused on group processes, influences others in a warm, trusting climate, inspires trust, challenges the status quo, and empowers

others. Simulation Exercise 22.3 provides an opportunity to examine nurse leadership behaviors.

Demonstration of transformational leadership is required for **magnet hospital** status designation. Transformational leadership qualities include a clear vision and commitment to excellence, with a willingness to take reasonable risks, consult with others, and persistent dedication to task completion. They understand leadership as a communication process, not an event or position. Transformational leaders are energetic, positive thinkers, who act as visible role models in helping other nurses to develop leadership skills.

Structural Empowerment. Structural empowerment is a concept that describes the organizational commitments and configurations that give informational and supportive power to healthcare workers to accomplish their work effectively in significant ways. Complex healthcare issues require different types and levels of expertise, working together to achieve an outcome greater than the sum of individual efforts. Communication among health professionals is open, and there is an appropriate mix of healthcare personnel to ensure quality care.

Communicating to Creating Safe, Supportive Work Environments

We are in a time of increasing nurse shortages but increasing acuity for hospitalized patients. Measures that attract nurses and improve clinical outcomes for patients need to be implemented. Improving work environments in healthcare shapes *both* nursing and patient outcomes. The literature suggests attention to the following.

Physical Space

Agency administrators have tried various strategies to promote healthy work environments, which support easier communication among staff. Space is integral for effective communication. For example, arranging in-patient beds and storing supplies in patient rooms to decrease the number of steps nurses walk. Communication devices such as smartphones or hands-free models such as VOCERA allow nurses to locate other personnel more easily. Computers or tablets at bedsides promote easier record keeping. Refer to Chapters 25 and 26.

Organizational Climate

Beyond the physical arrangements, the work environment is patient centered, not person centered. There is a supportive atmosphere with a commitment to seek solutions, value nurses, and provide quality patient-centered care. Likewise, nurses who are good communicators, competent, dependable, adaptable, and responsible are key variables in creating a satisfying, quality work environment.

SIMULATION EXERCISE 22.3   Characteristics of Exemplary Nurse Leaders

Purpose

To help students distinguish leadership characteristics in exemplary leaders and managers encountered in everyday nursing practice. Identifying leadership characteristics helps students become aware of professional behaviors associated with achieving the mission of professional nursing.

Procedure

This exercise is most effective when the reflections take place prior to class time and findings are discussed in small groups of four to six students.

1. Reflect on the professional characteristics and behaviors of a professional nurse you admire as a leader in your work or educational setting.
2. Write down what stood out for you about this person as a leader in your mind. What specific characteristics framed this person as a leader? How did this person relate to other health professionals including students?
3. Share and discuss your findings with your small group. Have one student act as a scribe. Identify commonalities and differences in student perceptions.
4. Share small group findings with your larger class group.

Reflective Discussion Analysis

1. Describe specific behaviors associated with effective leadership.
2. Distinguish ways nurses can demonstrate leadership in contemporary healthcare.
3. Evaluate ways nursing leadership is a dynamic, interactive process.
4. What are some of the ways nurses can demonstrate leadership in contemporary healthcare?

Open Communication

Collaborative relationships characterized by open communication are directly linked to optimal patient outcomes. Goals that focus on improvement rather than punitive measures are important to prevent future errors. Embracing use of technology also helps to reduce errors, such as bar coding for medicines or for lab specimens.

Team Collaboration

Components of collaboration include working with other nurses who are clinically competent, with a supportive manager, and with team members who respect each other's roles and respond to errors in a facilitative, nonpunitive manner.

Manageable Workloads

Safe work environments include safe staffing levels, provisions for adequate off-unit breaks, ongoing education, nurse autonomy and accountability, and adherence to standards of care with evidence-based interventions.

Magnet Hospitals

In an effort to develop and support quality work environments favorable to nurses, the ANA through its credentialing center developed the Magnet Recognition Program in 1993, to recognize nursing role excellence. Characteristics of a magnet culture include the following:

- Active support of education
- Clinically competent nurses
- Positive interdisciplinary professional relationships
- Control over and autonomy in nursing practice
- Patient-centered care for patients and families
- Adequate staffing and nurse manager support (ANCC, 2019a; 2019b)

Fig. 22.2 depicts magnet concepts.

Networking Roles

Networking is an essential component of professional role development and ultimately of advancing the status of professional nursing roles in healthcare delivery systems. Professional networking is defined as establishing and using contacts for information, support, and other assistance to achieve career goals. Nurses can use networking when they are in the market for a new job, need a referral, want to receive or share information about an area of interest, or need assistance with making a career choice. Networking is a two-way interactive process. As a form of communication, networking offers valuable professional opportunities for developing new ideas and receiving feedback that might not otherwise be available. Have your business cards with you. Follow up with contacts by sending a text, email, etc. Participating in activities of nursing organizations or continuing education events provides fertile opportunities. Networking with health professionals from other disciplines is also important.

Patient Advocacy Roles

The goal of patient advocacy support is to empower clients and to help them attain the services they need for self-management of health issues. Nurses are advocates for patients every time they protect, defend, and support a patient's rights and/or intervene on behalf of patients who cannot do so for themselves. The ANA (2015) affirms advocacy as an essential role in its Code of Ethics for Nurses. Patients who benefit from advocacy fall into two categories: those who need advocacy because of vulnerability caused by their illness and those who have trouble successfully navigating the healthcare system. Nursing patient advocacy includes facilitating access to essential healthcare services for patients and acting as a liaison between patients and the healthcare system to ensure quality care, improve health, and reduce health deviations. Skill sets and knowledge needed for patient advocacy are identified in Box 22.3. For more information on nurse involvement in community-based advocacy, see Chapter 24.

Advocacy should support autonomy. Patients need to be in control of their own destiny, even when the decision reached is not what you as the nurse would recommend. Referrals to community resources should be chosen, based on compatibility with the patient's expressed need, financial resources, accessibility (time as well as place), and ease of access.

Nurse–Patient Role Relationships

Nurse. Professional performance behaviors in the nurse–patient relationship include a sound knowledge base, technical competency, and interpersonal competency, as well as caring. On a daily basis, nurses must collect and process multiple, often indistinct, pieces of behavioral data. They problem-solve with patients and families to come up with workable, realistic solutions. Through words and behaviors in relationship with other healthcare providers and agencies, nurses provide quality care and act as advocates for patients and for the nursing profession.

Currently, nurses function in a high-tech, managed healthcare environment in which the human caring aspects of nursing are easier to overlook. Unique challenges to the nurse–patient relationship in clinical practice include shorter in-patient contacts, technology, and lower levels of trust in relation to these factors. The nurse–patient relationship will become increasingly important in helping patients feel cared for in a healthcare environment that sometimes neglects their psychosocial needs in favor of cost effectiveness.

Patient Role. In the current healthcare environment, patients are expected to take an active role in self-management of their condition to whatever extent is possible. The relational expectation is for an equal partnership, having shared power and authority as joint decision-makers in their healthcare. Is the patient-centered model of healthcare delivery actually true? Is every decision related to diagnosis and treatment based on combined input and joint responsibility for implementing the

---

BOX 22.3   Knowledge Base Needed for Patient Advocacy

- Patient values, beliefs, and preferences
- Alignment with treatment goals
- Informed consent procedures, patient's third-party insurance
- Nurse's personal, professional, and cultural biases
- Print materials and online resources relevant to patient needs
- Organizational system variables related to service delivery
- Current laws, service delivery policies, and regulations
- Community resources including referral processes, eligibility, and access requirements
- Effective communication strategies related to consultation and collaboration
- Understanding of required documentation, management, and interpretation of patient records

Reprinted from American Nurses Association. (2002). Know your rights. ANA's bill of rights arms nurses with critical information. *The American Nurse, 34*(6), 16, with permission.

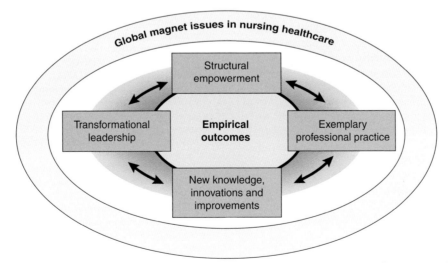

Figure 22.2 Magnet model components. (Used with permission from American Nurses Credentialing Center ©2008. All rights reserved.)

recommendations? Use of the patient's self-knowledge and inner resources allows nurses to more effectively respond to their needs.

SUMMARY

How nurses perceive their professional role and how they function as a nurse in that role has a sizable effect on the success of their interpersonal communication. The professional nursing role should be evidenced in every aspect of nursing care but nowhere more fully than in the nurse–patient relationship. A professional nurse's first role responsibility is to the patient. Because hospitals no longer are the primary settings for nursing practice, nurse practice roles take place in nontraditional and traditional community-based healthcare settings. Expanded nursing roles were described. Emphasis on health team roles and communicating with interdisciplinary team members will be further described in Chapter 23.

Socialization and role theoretical concepts were used to describe the transition to the professional role. Among other theorists, focus was given to Benner's five developmental stages of increasing proficiency to describe the nurse's progression from novice to expert. Professional development as a nurse is a lifelong commitment. Mentorship and continuing education assist nurses in maintaining their competency and professional role development.

NEXT-GENERATION NCLEX® EXAMINATION-STYLE CASE STUDY

Nursing Mentorship and Career Guidance

A nurse who completed a bachelor's degree in nursing 2 years ago has now been accepted into a master's degree program and successfully earned eight graduate level credits. The nurse with 8 years of medical–surgical experience as well as with 4 years of maternal–newborn experience is now interested in applying for a position in a new specialty area. When a position is posted for an emergency department (ED) nursing position, the nurse asks an experienced ED nurse to discuss the possible career move.

What topics should the discussion focus on initially? *Select all that apply.*

a. Transferral of existing skill sets
b. Professional challenges
c. Nursing responsibilities
d. Advancement potential
e. Required credentials
f. Needed experience
g. Personal rewards
h. Staffing policies

ETHICAL DILEMMA: What Would You Do?

As a new nurse on the unit, you witness diminished patient care quality due to poor communication and lack of provider continuity. If you raise the issue in a staff meeting with your supervisor and coworkers, you fear your opinion will not be taken seriously because the others have been working together for a much longer time. What should you do?

DISCUSSION QUESTIONS

1. Identify the critical indicators of professionalism in nursing.
2. Classify the skills you consider the most important in developing a collaborative team approach to clinical care.
3. Evaluate the statement "Every nurse should be a leader," and explain how this idea might be realized in contemporary healthcare.
4. What do you conjecture as the distinct and collaborative contributions of different professional roles to patient care and healthcare delivery?

REFERENCES

American Association of Colleges of Nursing (AACN). (2020). *AACN position statement on the practice doctorate in nursing.* Washington, DC: AACN. Retrieved from: https://www.aacnnursing.org/DNP/Position-Statement. [Accessed 15 June 2021].

American Association of Colleges of Nursing (AACN). (2021). *The essentials: Core competencies for professional nursing education.* Washington, DC: AACN. Retrieved from: https://www.aacnnursing.org/Portals/42/AcademicNursing/pdf/Essentials-2021.pdf. [Accessed 16 June 2021].

American Nurses Association (ANA). (2015). *Code of ethics for nurses.* Silver Spring, MD: ANA.

American Nurses Association (ANA). (n.d.). *Medication aides, assistants, technicians.* Retrieved from: https://www.nursingworld.org/practice-policy/medication-aides--assistants--technicians/. [Accessed 16 June 2021].

American Nurses Credentialing Center (ANCC). (2022). *2023 MAGNET® application manual.* Silver Spring, MD: American Nurses Association.
Retrieved from https://www.nursingworld.org/organizational-programs/magnet/magnet-model/. [Accessed 15 February 2022].

Amodo, A., Baker, D., Emery, D., & Hines, S. (2017). The TeamSTEPPS program. In *Presented at the 2017 TeamSTEPPS® national conference,* Cleveland, Ohio, June 5, 2017.

Bauer, T. N., & Erdogan, B. (2011). Organizational socialization: The effective onboarding of new employees. In S. Zedeck

(Ed.), *APA handbook of industrial and organizational psychology* (Vol. 3) (pp. 51–64). Washington, DC: American Psychological Association.

Benner, P. (1984, 2001). *From novice to expert: Excellence and power in clinical nursing practice.* Upper Saddle River, NJ: Prentice Hall Health.

Dreyfus, S. E., & Dreyfus, H. L. (1980). *A five-stage model of the mental activities involved in directed skill acquisition.* Berkeley: University of California at Berkeley.

Flexner, A. (1915). Is social work a profession? In *Paper presented at the 42nd annual session of the national conference on charities and correction, 1915.* Baltimore, MD: May 12–19, 1915 (p. 576).

Hesburgh, T. M. (1971). Presidential leadership. *Journal of Higher Education, 42*(9), 763–765.

Horsburgh, J., & Ippolito, K. (2018). A skill to be worked at: Using social learning theory to explore the process of learning from role models in clinical settings. *BCM Medical Education, 18*(1), 156.

Institute of Medicine (IOM). (2001). *The future of nursing: Leading change, advancing health.* Washington, DC: National Academies Press.

Institute of Medicine (IOM). (2011). *Health professions education: A bridge to quality.* Washington, DC: National Academies Press.

Jankelová, N., & Joniaková, Z. (2021). Communication skills and transformational leadership style of first-line nurse managers in relation to job satisfaction of nurses and moderators of this relationship. *Healthcare, 9*(3), 346.

Leininger, M. M. (1991). *Culture care diversity and universality: A theory of nursing.* New York: National League for Nursing.

McKenna, L., Brooks, I., & Vanderheide, R. (2017). Graduate entry nurses' initial perspectives on nursing: Content analysis of open-ended survey questions. *Nurse Education Today, 49,* 22–26.

Sinclair, S. K. (2020). *Getting nurses to stay: The retention challenge.* DailyNurse [website]. Retrieved from: https://dailynurse.com/?s=job+retention. [Accessed 16 June 2021].

Thompson, M. R., & Barcott, D. S. (2019). The role of the nurse scientist as a knowledge broker. *Journal of Nursing Scholarship, 51*(1), 26–39.

Ward, S. (2020). *What is leadership? Definition and examples of leadership.* The Balance Small Business [website]. Retrieved from: www.thebalancesmb.com/leadership-definition-2948275/. [Accessed 15 June 2021].

World Health Organization (WHO). (2020). *State of the world's nursing report - 2020.* Geneva, Switzerland: WHO. Retrieved from: https://www.who.int/publications/i/item/9789240003279. [Accessed 16 June 2021].

23

Interprofessional Communication

OBJECTIVES

At the end of the chapter, the reader will be able to:

1. Discuss application of teamwork communication concepts.
2. Discuss communication barriers in interprofessional relationships, including disruptive behaviors.
3. Discuss methods for communicating effectively and handling conflict with others in organizational settings.
4. Apply research to evidence-based clinical communication, including TeamSTEPPS Communication Tools to Enhance Performance and Patient Safety (TeamSTEPPS) approach.

To be effective as a nursing professional, it is not enough to be deeply committed to patient centered care. You need proficient communication skills to function as a member of an interprofessional team to effectively provide quality care safely (Munro & Hope, 2020). In this era of complex inpatient care, early discharge, and community care follow-up, follow-up interprofessional collaboration is essential. Criteria for effective interprofessional functioning include fostering open communication, demonstrating mutual respect, and sharing in decision-making (QSEN, n.d.).

An essential communication skill is the ability to adapt your own communication style to meet the needs of team members and to mindfully, continually scan changing situations. This chapter will focus on principles of communication with other professionals. Strategies will be suggested that you can use to function more effectively as an interprofessional team member and leader. Specific ways to communication with other health professionals are described to help you remove communication barriers.

BASIC CONCEPTS

Collaborative Practice

Definition

The Robert Wood Johnson Foundation says effective collaboration includes activities that promote active participation by each discipline involved in the patient's care. The healthcare team provides the mechanism for continual communication that enhances attainment of goals.

Communication

Effective communication is a bedrock principle of quality care. Such communication is frequent, timely, accurate, complete, unambiguous, and understood by the recipient. Communication breakdowns affect patient care. For example, the literature shows that the greatest determinant of intensive care unit death rates is how smoothly nurses and physicians work together in planning and providing care. Effective communication prevents errors. The Joint Commission (TJC) found team communication breakdowns were the root cause of preventable sentinel events in 70% of cases (TJC, 2011). Communication challenges are substantial when many different providers are involved. Deliberate, mindful, use of strategies to improve communication with colleagues is part of a nurse's job. Consider the F.R.O.G. case study.

Theoretical Model Concepts

The National Center for Interprofessional Practice and Education has provided leadership in developing models of collaboration. As yet though there is no comprehensive model, common components have been identified.

CASE STUDY: **Friction Rubs Out Germs** (F.R.O.G.)

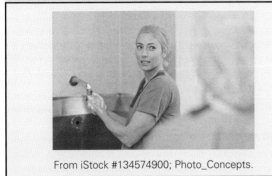

The quality analysis staff in a large hospital system introduced a "Friction Rubs Out Germs" (FROG) hand hygiene in-service for frontline staff, after evidence showed nurses only washed half the time before attending patients. Later, Liz Rice observes Mr Adam's nurse by-passing the sink, forgetting to wash. She whispers "rivet" into the nurse's ear as a fun reminder.

From iStock #134574900; Photo_Concepts.

Shared Common Goals

The goal of collaboration is to provide safe, high-quality care. As part of creating a culture of teamwork where staff is valued, a standard across organizations should be zero tolerance for disruptive or bullying behaviors. To accomplish this, each organization needs one well-defined code of behavior applied consistently to all staff. TJC mandates that each healthcare organization has a code of conduct defining acceptable and unacceptable behaviors, as well as an agency process for reporting and handling disruptive behaviors, discrimination, or disrespectful treatment (TJC, 2011).

Shared Mental Model

Team functioning especially in increasingly complex health situations requires effective teamwork to ensure patient safety (Polis et al., 2017). Every team member needs to "buy in" to the collaborative team concept. Collaboration is a dynamic process in which work groups from different professional backgrounds cooperate and share expertise to deliver quality healthcare. This involves an integration of knowledge, skills, and attitudinal values. Complex health issues are best addressed by an interdisciplinary team approach. Ideally, each team member understands the role of others and pools their own expertise with those of other team members.

Value of a Shared Mental Model

An interprofessional expert panel has specified core competencies for interprofessional practice including care that is patient-centered, community oriented, relationship focused, and process oriented and using common language, applicable across professions. The TeamSTEPPS program stresses the importance to develop a shared mental model (goal) for each patient's care.

Effective Open Communication

Open communication and trust are core elements for smooth effective teamwork. For example, you trust team colleagues to communicate honest feedback.

Collegiality

A culture of collegiality is essential for a work environment that is to provide high-quality patient care. The interprofessional team depends on recognition of and participation by representatives of each provider to deliver quality healthcare. **Collaboration** begins with communicating an awareness of each other's roles, knowledge, and skills. It fosters the development of shared values and respects the expertise of each team member. Such collaboration enhances the attainment of patient- and family-centered goals. This requires regular discussions based on patient needs. If team members do not **trust** and **respect** each other and communicate in an open and respectful manner, they are more likely to make mistakes. Standards of a healthy work environment are listed in Box 23.1. Consider the Ms Libby case for an attempt to work toward a better work climate. Collegiality is discussed as an aspect of healthy work environments. The American Association of Critical Care Nurses (AACN) (2019) has issued six *standards* characteristic of a healthy workplace (www.aacn.org):

1. Nurses must be as efficient in communication skills as they are in clinical skills.

BOX 23.1 **Standards of Healthy Work Environment Identified by Nursing Organizations**

- Collaborative culture of trust
- Respectful open communication and behavior
- Communication-rich culture that emphasizes trust and respect
- Clearly defined role expectations with accountability
- Adequate workforce
- Competent leadership
- Shared decision-making
- Employee development
- Recognition of workers' contributions

2. Nurses must be relentless in pursuing and fostering true collaboration.
3. Nurses must be valued and committed partners in making policy, directing and evaluating clinical care, and leading organizational operations.
4. Staffing must ensure the effective match between patient needs and nurse competencies.
5. Nurses must be recognized and recognize others for the value each brings to the work of the organization.
6. Nurse leaders must fully embrace the imperative of a healthy work environment, authentically live it, and engage others in its achievement.

Case Study: Ms Libby and Conflict on a Surgical Unit

Two nursing teams work the day shift on a busy surgical unit. As nurse manager, Ms Libby notices that both teams are arguing over computer use and have become unwilling to help cover the other team's patients. It is now taking longer to complete assigned work. To achieve a more harmonious work environment, she arranges a staff meeting to get the teams to communicate. Rather than just computer issues, multiple problems surface suggesting inadequate time management and overload. Ms Libby listens actively, responds with empathy, and provides positive regard and feedback for solutions proposed by the group. She asks the group to decide on two prioritized solutions. Recognizing that her staff feels unappreciated and knowing that compromise is a strategy that produces behavior change, she resolves to offer more frequent performance feedback, such as weekly evaluations via email, and providing specific data on overtime. She herself assumes responsibility for requesting an immediate computer upgrade purchase using the unit budget's emergency funding allocation. A team member who serves on the employee relations committee assumes responsibility for requesting that the human services department schedules an in-service training on time management and stress reduction within the next month. The group agrees to meet in 6 weeks to evaluate.

Teamwork and Communication

Interprofessional team functioning is both a role-focused process and task-based skills-focused process. Team members have unique personalities, egos, and skill sets, yet all must work together. We nurses are guided by our Code of Ethics and published workplace standards (AACN, 2016, 2019; ANA, 2015a). Playing to each team member's strengths enhances ability to deliver safe, quality care. Collaborating in planning care, in joint decision-making, and in care coordination requires knowing when to hold and when to let go of ideas and opinions. TeamSTEPPS training, offered by AHRQ, improves team communication. These concepts are listed in Table 23.1.

Communication is central to team functioning. Team communication requires trust, mutual support, and thoughtful, open communication. Information is shared for informed decision-making. AHRQ (2017) refers to several models, but suggests a new "holacracy model" in which every team members' opinion is valued, generating an attitude of "no one wins unless everyone wins." This open communication is based on patient needs and is undefined by status of team members. Overall treatment goals should be the guiding force in team conversation. For fun to dramatize team function, try the zoom situation in Simulation Exercise 23.1.

TABLE 23.1 TeamSTEPPS: Using a Team Training Program Improves Team Communication

Essentials of Communication	Sending Technique	Receiving Technique
Clear	Use common language/terminology; be specific.	Validate: use feedback or "talk back" to confirm understanding
Brief	Communicate only information essential for this situation	Clarify any nonverbal information
Timely	Verify message is received; respond quickly to requests for additional information; provide updates continuously	Verify receipt of information. Repeat to verify accuracy.
Complete	Give all relevant information; use standardized communication tools	Document: essential information validated, understood, and recorded

Data from Agency for Healthcare Research and Quality (AHRQ). (2006). *TeamSTEPPS multimedia resource kit.* Pub. No. 06-0020-2. Rockville, MD: AHRQ; and Agency for Healthcare Research and Quality (AHRQ). (2021). *Approach to improving patient safety: communication.* PSNet. Retrieved from https://psnet.ahrq.gov/perspective/approach-improving-patient-safety-communication/. Accessed 2 July 2021.

SIMULATION EXERCISE 23.1 Zoom

Procedure

Use one of the "Zoom" picture books (Banyai I. Zoom. NY: Viking: Penguin Books).

Duplicate enough sets of photos for use by groups of 10. Place each different photo into a manila folder. Mix up their order. Divide students into groups of 10 or so, and give each student group member a folder.

Activity Instructions

"Look at your photo but do not show to anyone else. Verbally describe your photo. Group task or goal is to interpret." Allow 5–7 minutes.

Reflective Discussion Analysis

After activity completion, ask each group to apply team principles to describe their roles. Who was group leader? Was there a clear goal? Did each team member feel free to speak up?

BOX 23.2 Interpersonal Sources of Conflict in the Workplace: Barriers to Collaboration and Communication

1. Different expectations
   - Role ambiguity
   - Being asked to do something you know would be irresponsible or unsafe
   - Having your feelings or opinions ridiculed or discounted
   - Getting pressure to give more time or attention than you are able to give
   - Being asked to give more information than you feel comfortable sharing
   - Differences in language
2. Threats to self
   - Maintaining a sense of self in the face of hostility or sexual harassment
   - Being asked to do something concerning a patient that is in conflict with your personal or professional moral values
3. Differences in role hierarchy
   - Differences in education or experience
   - Differences in responsibility and rewards (payment)
   - Lack of support from leadership/administration
4. Clinical situation constraints
   - Emphasis on rapid decision-making
   - Complexity of care interventions
   - Stressful workload

Barriers to Effective Team Communication

Ineffective communication has several root causes. Barriers include an obstructive attitude; role status that precludes sharing information among team members; a hierarchical structure inhibiting some members from speaking up; variations in communication styles or vocabulary (silos); complacency, defensiveness, and conflict (Sanchez et al., 2020). The "silo" system refers to professionals who are educated only within their own discipline and who are accustomed to operating independently.

Conflict

Antecedents. Ineffective communication often leads to disagreements, injured feelings, and unsafe care. It cannot be overemphasized that poor communication is the factor most frequently cited as an underlying cause of conflict. Refer to Box 23.2 for sources of conflict. Factors leading to conflict are changing away from the traditional doctor–nurse hierarchical structure and gender bias (Sanchez et al., 2020). Today's emphasis is on effective team functioning characteristics including effective formal and informal communication; mutual respect; team leadership and vision; role clarity; and accountability. Problems in any of these areas can be reflected as disruptive behavior and can compromise patient safety. For example, the vast majority of frontline staff report that care was not completed on the prior shift. Would open communication help resolve this?

Disruptive Behaviors

Conflict was defined in Chapter 13 as a hostile encounter. The nursing literature uses a variety of terms to refer to persistent lack of civil behaviors in the workplace: bullying; verbal abuse; horizontal violence; lateral violence; "eating your young"; in-fighting; mobbing, harassment, or scapegoating. The term we use in this book is *disruptive behavior*.

Definition. **Disruptive behavior** is defined as situations in which lack of civility or lack of respect occurs repeatedly in professional relationships that threatens the dignity of coworkers. It is dysfunctional. Disruptive behaviors may include *overt* behaviors: rudeness, verbal abuse, intimidation, put-downs; angry outbursts, yelling, blaming, or humiliating by criticizing team members in front of others; sexual harassment; or even threatening physical confrontations. Other disruptive behaviors are more *covert*: passive-aggressive communication withholding need-to-know information, withholding help, assigning excessively heavy workloads, refusing to perform an assigned task, being impatient or reluctance to answer questions, not returning telephone calls or pages, and speaking in a condescending tone. These behaviors threaten the well-being of nurses and the safety of patients. Are recipients of bullying less assertive?

Incidence of Incivility. The actual frequency of poor communication and incivility is unknown since most cases are unreported (Ebberts & Sollars, 2020).

Disruptive behavior is fairly common in large organizations, especially hospitals, but is largely unreported. When repeated over time, this behavior is termed "bullying." Ranging from half to three quarters of all nurses report being subjected to disruptive behavior at some time which they say compromised patient safety (Moore et al., 2017). Disruptive behavior can escalate to violence, putting staff at risk, The Joint Commission cites ineffective communication between team members as contributing to 60% of errors. Most studies have found that nurse-to-nurse disruptive behaviors occur more frequently than disruptive physician–nurse interactions and occur more often in high-stress areas such as surgical suites, psychiatric units, or emergency departments (AHRQ, 2019).

Process. All healthcare workers have the right to be treated with respect. As discussed earlier, avoidance is still the primary style used by nurses in conflict situations, even though this does not resolve the problem (Sherman, 2019). Acknowledge the issue. Know that if you are spoken to in a disrespectful manner, it is unacceptable. If upset, calm down. Plan your approach, requesting a discussion. "I am uncomfortable but we need to discuss …" State the problem behavior and how it made you feel. State your expectations.

Patient Outcomes. Disruptive behavior is a barrier to effective healthcare when it leads to miscommunication. Subsequently impaired communication compromises patient safety (AHRQ, 2019). Poor communication is associated with problems in patient safety (Anusiewicz et al., 2020). Good collaboration and communication has been shown to be associated with better patient outcomes, such as decreased infections.

Nurse Outcomes. As described earlier, failures in collaboration and communication affect nurses' physical and psychological health. Poor communication among health team members is among common factors cited for nurse frustration, job stress, poor morale, job abandonment, lost productivity, loss of confidence, absenteeism, and task avoidance. Do student nurses experience bullying or harassment?

Organization Outcomes. Failure to effectively deal with staff conflict creates a toxic work environment. Costs to agency center on financial issues related to absenteeism, increased staff turnover, losses in productivity, as well as increases in care errors and even legal action. Other outcomes include decreases in care quality, increases in care errors, and adverse patient outcomes. TJC states that healthcare organizations need policies facilitating collaboration. What does your organization's policy say?

Creating a Collaborative Culture of Regard to Eliminate Disruptive Behavior

To deliver safe, high-quality healthcare, corporate climate now emphasizes a collaborative **patient-centered care model** in which the hierarchical power model is replaced by a model in which all team members are valued. Organizational support is essential for success. **Collaboration** is broadly defined as working with all the members of the healthcare team to achieve maximum health outcomes for our mutual patient, and includes the following:

1. Common goal: Developing a **collaborative culture** in which all team members keep the delivery of safe, high-quality care foremost in mind requires that we trust and respect the decision-making of all team members. Different professionals were educated to hold differing beliefs and styles of communication. We need to develop an understanding of these various perspectives, not so we can change them, but so that we can utilize them.

2. Open, safe communication: Creating a communication-rich environment requires that all team members value open communication. We combine assertiveness (speaking up, giving and receiving feedback) with cooperation.

3. Mutual respect: Appreciation for each member's value. An important part of working together is developing mutual trust; you trust coworkers to "have your back."

4. Engaging in self-reflection to recognize own personal moments of incivility.

5. Shared decision-making: Leadership is required to avoid duplication of tasks and to ensure that all tasks are completed.

6. Role clarity: Members of a team that has been working together smoothly generally have developed complementary roles. We know our role and that of other team members and recognize when we need to call on their expertise.

7. Message clarity: Focus on salient facts, and avoid inconsequential comments.

Collaboration is a dynamic process benefiting from ongoing practice and evaluation. In the past, some organizations tolerated disruptive workplace behaviors. Pressures on nurses exist to increase productivity and cost-effectiveness. Accrediting organizations encourage agencies to practice zero tolerance of these behaviors. Individually, we need to become aware of how to discourage disruptive behaviors as we work to develop a healthy, collaborative workplace atmosphere to ensure high-quality patient care (TJC, 2008). Conflict resolution should be a part of every nurse's toolkit (Rux, 2020). A hallmark of a professional is acceptance of accountability for one's own behavior. Preventing conflicts is accomplished by avoiding public criticism, cultivating a willingness to help attitude, and doing one's fair share.

Respect

Feeling respected or not respected is an integral part of how nurses rate the quality of their work environment. Three key factors are as follows: a positive climate of professional practice; a supportive manager; and positive relationships with other staff. Nurses say they feel respected and appreciated if their opinions are listened to attentively and they receive feedback from authority figures as to the value of their work competence. Regard for another's knowledge and skills shown in collaborative actions promotes high level team functioning (Rux, 2020).

Factors That Affect Nurse Behavior Toward Other Team Members

Team training has been instituted to educate all team members to work in a collaborative manner. Inability to deal with conflict is a central characteristic of teams who do not work well together (Sherman, 2019). Other factors may adversely influence professional relationships including the following:

- *Gender.* Contemporary society continues to redefine gender role behavior, negating some of the traditional gender stereotypical behaviors.
- *Hierarchy.* Because healthcare authority traditionally was vested in a hierarchical structure, control rested with the physician. Changes in the physician–nurse communication process are occurring as nurses become more empowered, more assertive, and better educated. Most nurses occasionally encounter problems in the physician–nurse relationship. Differences in power, perspective, education, status, and pay may be barriers to workgroup communication and care.
- *Communication silos.* Traditionally, each healthcare profession was educated separately, evolving their own unique vocabulary. If you encounter a conflict situation at work, reflect on whether the problem is due to differences in communication style.
- *Generational diversity.* As mentioned, members of older and younger generations differ in their preferred communication styles. It is suggested that teams use a commonly understood communication style.

Constructive Criticism

Receiving. Distinguish between incivility and constructive feedback. Receiving appropriate criticism may not feel pleasant, but focus on the changes suggested. Interpret it as a learning moment rather than as a personal attack.

Giving. Discuss the issue privately. Use concrete examples, saying "I need to tell you somethings that make me uncomfortable. But the reason I am sharing is that I care for you, for our team, and our patients."

Outcomes of Successful Team Training in Communication

Evidence from many studies on effects of team training shows improved efficiency and increased patient safety for the team approach to healthcare. Refer to the TeamSTEPPS website for Team Strategies and Tools to Enhance Performance and Patient Safety strategies. Each nurse team member needs to participate and be accountable for facilitating team communication.

APPLICATIONS

As nurses, we can help to establish and sustain a healthy workplace. This requires continuous assessment of our own and others' current communication practices and implementation of "best practices" to prevent and deal with conflict. Reflect on Table 23.2 for suggestions to make communication more effective and improve care. Can you add to these? Communication and conflict resolution strategies can be learned but require continued reinforcement through ongoing communication training. Improving communication has been shown to improve patient safety. An essential component of communication in healthcare teams is leadership to set goals, provide feedback (care outcome data), and facilitate conflict resolution.

Conflict Resolution

As nurses, we have the responsibility to work effectively with others to provide care. Yet, whenever people work together, conflicts inevitably arise. Many of the same resolution concepts described in Chapter 13 can be applied to conflicts occurring among staff. Avoidance is still the primary style used by nurses although it is ineffective in the long run (Sherman, 2019). System conflicts arising from agency or system policies also need attention.

TeamSTEPPS: Team Strategies and Tools to Enhance Performance and Patient Safety

When AHRQ adapted the Department of Defense team training program to use in healthcare settings, they gave it the **TeamSTEPPS** acronym. A main component of this free program is training to use a toolbox of communication strategies (AHRQ.gov). How many times do we say good communication is essential to effective team function? Effective communication skills convey accurate information and provide awareness of your role responsibilities. As a team member, you communicate to keep all others informed and contribute to successful goal achievement.

DEVELOPING AN EVIDENCE-BASED PRACTICE

Researchers have investigated aspects of interdisciplinary collaboration especially as related to the quality of care outcomes. O'Leary's (2020) groups analyzed teamwork climate scores for 380 physicians, nurses, and nurse aides across four hospital settings. Reeves and colleagues (2017) reviewed 34 studies of interprofessional collaboration for the Cochrane Library Database. Whittington et al. (2020) used an interprofessional competency framework to have radiology students develop interprofessional communication strategies examining case studies.

Results

O'Leary found perceptions of team climate differ across hospital sites, and nurses reported lower quality of collaboration than did physicians though these differences were not statistically significant. Whittington and Walker found that case analysis is effective in teaching "best practice" interprofessional communication strategies. Reeves found evidence of some improvement in patient functional outcomes as well as better adherence to approved treatment practices with team collaboration.

Strength of evidence: Low. Authors recommend further research into the effects of team collaboration.

Applications to Your Clinical Practice

1. Goals: Keep your focus on the common goal of improving patient outcomes.
2. Role clarity: Work to understand each team member's role.
3. Communication skills: Practice your interdisciplinary communication skills perhaps through case study analyses.

References

O'Leary, K. J., Manojlovich, M., Johnson, J. K., et al. (2020). A multisite study of interprofessional teamwork and collaboration on general medical services. *The Joint Commission Journal of Quality and Patient Safety, 46*(12), 667–672.

Reeves, S., Pelone, F., Harrison, R., Goldman, J., & Zwarenstein, M. (2017). Interprofessional collaboration to improve professional practice and healthcare outcomes. *Cochrane Database of Systematic Reviews, 6*(6), CD000072.

Whittington, K. D., Walker, J., & Hirsch, B. (2020). Promoting interdisciplinary communication as a vital function of effective teamwork to positively impact patient outcomes, satisfaction, and employee engagement. *Journal of Medical Imaging and Radiation Sciences, 51*(4S), S107–S111.

Refer to Fig. 23.1 for a summary of patient-centered team collaboration.

Teamwork and collaboration are a major focus of both TeamSTEPPS and QSEN. Each team member shares a clear vision of expected outcomes for each patient. TeamSTEPPS (AHRQ, 2015) creates a transformed healthcare model. Tools and strategies are provided, which can be used to develop better system-wide communication knowledge, skills, and attitudes. Communication clarity is an important goal, as is the conciseness found on checklists. Experts recommend use of standardized communication tools such as SBAR (which stands for situation, background, assessment, recommendation), use of **C.U.S.** assertive statements ("I am **C**oncerned; I am **U**ncomfortable, this is a **S**afety issue"), followed by "the two-challenge rule" stating your concern twice, check-backs (to verify that your communication message is understood accurately), briefs, debriefs, and huddles. Consider the C.U. S. case study.

Case Study: Using CUS

Mr Michaels is scheduled for discharge today. During morning team rounds, you notice redness at the Intravenous site. Even though his temperature at 7 a.m. was recorded as 99.2°F, the Resident wants to sign off on the discharge. You use the "CUS" assertive statements technique:

C = "I am concerned about possible sepsis."
U = "I am uncomfortable discharging him today."
S = "This is a safety issue."

When your CUS is ignored, you use the "two-challenge rule" voicing your safety concern twice. The team leader acknowledges your concern, but if the discharge is still scheduled, you utilize your chain of command reporting this issue to your nurse supervisor.

TeamSTEPPS teaches team members, including nurses, how to increase their competencies in leadership, situation monitoring, and use of mutual support strategies (AHRQ, 2015). Examples of leadership competency are clarifying team goals and roles. Competencies for situation monitoring include use of decision-making skills in emergent situations and providing corrective feedback. Mutual support skills include assisting others and using communication tools. Other team behaviors are discussed at the AHRQ website.

Conflict Resolution Steps

Many of the same strategies for conflict resolution discussed for conflicts between patient and nurse can be applied to conflicts between the nurse and other health

TABLE 23.2 **Improve Interprofessional Communication**	
Ineffective Problem Communication	**Change to Effective; Proposed Solution**
Incomplete	Change to effective, complete, concise, clear communication
Silos (use of vocabulary jargon unique to the discipline)	Use common terms understood by all team members to focus on patient problems
Communication based on role status or hierarchy	Adopt open team-centered communication to share with all team members
Dominance	Develop role clarity with shared leadership
Disruptive communication or obstructive attitude	Periodically review mutual goals to emphasize common goals and values

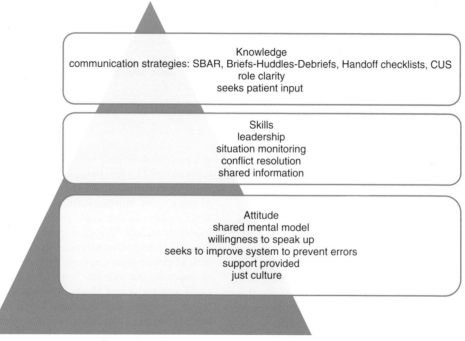

Figure 23.1 Patient-centered care team collaboration.

team members. (Review the principles of conflict management in Fig. 13.1 in Chapter 13.) As mentioned, conflict resolution can be a positive force for change. Instead of picturing a straight line of either you win or I win, envision the outcome of conflict resolution as a triangle with an outcome of mutual resolution as a peak, where you both have built something greater together.

Step 1. Identify Sources of Conflict
Conflict often stems from miscommunication. Recognize it early. Think through the possible causes of the conflict. Identify your own feelings about it and respond

appropriately, even if the response is a deliberate choice not to respond verbally. Interpersonal conflicts that are not dealt with leave residual feelings that will reemerge in future interactions.

Step 2. Set Goals
Be proactive, stay calm, and address just the issue of concern. Seek a solution.

Step 3. Implement Solutions
Your primary goal in dealing with workplace conflict is to find a high-quality, mutually acceptable solution: a win-win strategy.

Remembering that we all share the ultimate goal of delivering high-quality patient-centered care may help us work together even if we personally do not like each other. In many instances, a better collaborative relationship can be developed through the use of the following conflict management communication techniques adapted from Johansen (2012):

- *Reframe* a clinical situation as a cooperative process in which the health goals and not the status of the providers becomes the focus:
- *Assume responsibility* for one's own behaviors and for maintaining a "blame-free" work environment.
- *Identify your goal.* A clear idea of the outcome you wish to achieve is a necessary first step in the process. Remember the issue is the conflict, not your coworker.
- *Obtain factual data.* It is important to do your homework by obtaining all relevant information about the specific issues involved—and about the individual's behavioral responses to a healthcare issue—before engaging in negotiation.
- *Intervene early.* Be assertive. The best time to resolve problems is before they escalate to a conflict. Create a forum for two-way communication, preferably meeting periodically. Structured formats have been developed for you to use in conflict resolution, especially in team meetings. The format of *DESC* used by the TeamSTEPPS program is as follows:

D = describe the specific behavior (the problem) using concrete data

E = express your concerns, describing how this situation makes you feel

S = specify a course of action, suggesting alternatives, and state consequences to patient goals

C = obtain consensus

- *Avoid negative comments that can affect the self-esteem of the receiver.* Even when the critical statements are valid (e.g., "You do …" or "You make me feel …"), they should be replaced with "I" statements that define the sender's position. Otherwise, needless hostility is created, and the meaning of the communication is lost.
- *Consider the other's viewpoint.* Having some idea of what issues might be relevant from the other person's perspective provides important information about the best interpersonal approach to use. In addition to dealing with your own feelings, you need an ability to deal with the feelings of the others. Be cooperative, acknowledging the team's interdependence and mutual goals.

Communicate to Promote Effective Collaboration

Avoid Barriers to Resolution

How important is it to raise your awareness of and accountability in conflict situations? The authors suggest

---

BOX 23.3   Strategies to Turn Conflict Into Collaboration

1. Recognize and confront disruptive behaviors.
   - Use conflict resolution strategies.
   - Take the initiative to discuss problems.
   - Use active listening skills (refrain from simultaneous activities that interrupt communication).
   - Present documented data relevant to the issue.
   - Propose resolutions.
   - Use a brief summary to provide feedback.
   - Record all decisions in writing.
2. Create a climate in which participants view negotiation as a collaborative effort.
   - Develop agency behavior policies with stated zero tolerance for disruptive or bullying behaviors.
   - Model communicating with staff in a respectful, courteous manner.
   - Participate in organizational interdisciplinary groups.
   - Solicit and give feedback on a regular, periodic basis.
   - Clarify role expectations.

---

you participate actively to minimize staff member conflicts. Refer to Box 23.3 for strategies on how to turn conflict into collaboration. Individual behaviors such as avoiding the use of negative or inflammatory, anger-provoking words, or avoiding phrases that imply coercion have been described. Examples include "We must insist that …" or "You claim that …" Most individuals react to anger directed at them with a fight-or-flight response. Anyone can have a moment of rudeness, but monitor your own communications to avoid any pattern of abusive behaviors, including blaming or criticizing staff to others. When nurse supervisors become aware of how their behavior affects their nurses, they can increase the nurses' performance, increase their job involvement, and increase organizational identification. Participating in new hire mentoring or internship programs for novice nurses may help avert conflict.

Physician–Nurse Conflict Resolution

Remarkable increases in safety in airline and space programs were achieved by creating a climate in which junior team members were free to question decisions of more senior, powerful team members. Healthcare has adopted a similar philosophy. The American Medical Association (AMA, 2017) has specifically stated that codes of conduct define appropriate behavior as including a right to appropriately express a concern you have about patient care and safety. While this is being set forth as a medical code of conduct for physicians, should it also apply to nurses?

Nurses Influence Physician–Patient Communication. Nurses assess what physicians tell patients, encouraging them to seek clarification, and support our patient's right to ask questions. This is an important aspect of our belief that the patient is a valued member of our health team. Do you think it is ever appropriate for a nurse to criticize a physician's actions to a patient? A common underlying factor in at least 25% of all malpractice suits is an inadvertent or deliberate critical comment by another healthcare professional concerning a colleague's actions.

Make a Commitment to Open Dialogue. Listening should constitute at least half of a communication interaction. Foster a feeling of collegiality. Use strategies to defuse anger. During your negotiation, discussion should begin with a statement of either the commonalities of purpose or the points of agreement about the issue (e.g., "I thoroughly agree Mr Smith will do much better at home. However, we need to contact social services and make a home care referral before we actually discharge him; otherwise, he will be right back in the hospital again."). Points of disagreement should always follow rather than precede points of agreement. Empathy and a genuine desire to understand the issues from the other's perspective enhance communications. Solutions that take into consideration the needs and human dignity of all parties are more likely to be considered as viable alternatives. Backing another health professional into a psychological corner by using intimidation, coercion, or blame is simply counterproductive. More often than not, solutions developed through such tactics never get implemented. The final solution derived through fair negotiation is often better than the one arrived at alone.

Strategies to Remove Barriers to Communication With Other Professionals

Generally, conflict increases anxiety. When interaction with a certain peer or peer group stimulates anxious or angry feelings, the presence of conflict should be considered. Once it is determined that conflict is present, look for the basis of the conflict and label it as personal or professional. If it is personal in nature, it may not be appropriate to seek peer negotiation. It might be better to go back through the self-awareness exercises presented in previous chapters and locate the nature of the conflict through self-examination.

Sharing feelings about a conflict with others helps to reduce its intensity. It is confusing, for example, when nursing students first enter a nursing program or clinical rotation, but this confusion does not get discussed, and students commonly believe they should not feel confused or uncertain. As a nursing student, you face complex interpersonal situations. These situations may lead you to experience loneliness or self-doubt about your nursing skills compared with those of your peers. These feelings are universal at the beginning of any new experience. By sharing them with one or two peers, you usually find that others have had parallel experiences.

Individual Strategies to Deal With Workplace Conflicts

Consider using the behaviors that were listed in Table 23.3 when directly dealing with conflict in the workplace. Discussion of these behaviors may give you some ideas about how to implement them. Just as learning a new psychomotor nursing skill takes practice, conducting difficult conversations is a skill that takes practice, such as in Simulation Exercise 23.2.

Model Behaviors That Convey Respect

Prevent conflict by behaving with respect. Just as you treat patients with respect, you have an ethical responsibility to treat coworkers with respect. Nurses need to be appreciated, recognized, and respected as professionals for the work they do. Unsupportive and uncivil coworkers and workplace conflicts negatively influence retention of nursing staff. Unprofessional communication can range from rudeness or gossip to overt hostile comments. Communication can become distorted rather than open when you are concerned about offending a more powerful individual. Strategies for dealing with disrespectful or disruptive behaviors include establishing common communication expectations and skills, teaching conflict resolution skills, and creating a culture of mutual respect within the healthcare system. Ideally, the system has ongoing education, leadership and team collaboration support, and policies to evaluate behavior violations.

Mentor New Nurses

Can it really be true that 50% of newly hired nurses leave within the first 3 years? A number of these transfer to other places, but many actually abandon the nursing profession entirely. Orientation of novice nurses is expensive for the institution. QSEN and IOM encourage agencies to establish internships or mentoring programs for the first 1–2 years of each novice nurse's employment.

Clarify Communications

Poor communication is repeatedly cited as an influential factor leading to conflict. You can use the tools and skills taught throughout this textbook to improve both the clarity of message content and the emotional tone of interactions. Communication problems lead to a large percentage of disruptive behaviors, especially telephone communication.

TABLE 23.3   Examples of Reframing Unclear Communication

Situation	Cognitive Processes	Reframed to Improve Communication
Low self-disclosure	No one knows my real thoughts, feelings, and needs. *Consequently:* I think no one cares about me or recognizes my needs. Others see me as self-sufficient and are unaware that I have a problem. *Consequently:* Others are unable to respond to my needs.	Attitude: • Respect. • Value working with others. • Willingness to collaborate.Use skills: • Open communication—I verbalize aloud my needs clearly so others can have an opportunity to respond, to speak up. • Conflict resolution strategies.
Reluctance to delegate tasks	Other people think I do not believe that they can do the job as well as I can. *Consequently:* The others work at a minimum level. I do not expect or ask others to be involved. *Consequently:* Other people do not volunteer to help me. *Consequently:* I feel resentful, and others feel undervalued and dispensable.	Attitude: • Cooperate—I am part of a team. • Trust—I need to assign team members to do the tasks they can complete competently.Use skills: • Interdisciplinary communication.
Making unnecessary demands	I expect more from others than they think is reasonable. *Consequently:* I feel the others are lazy and uncommitted and I must push harder. Others see me as manipulative and dehumanizing. *Consequently:* Others assume a low profile and do not contribute their ideas. *Consequently:* Work production is mediocre. Morale is low. Everyone, including me, feels disempowered.	Attitude: • Shared mental team model—accept team model and shared decision-making • Willingness to listen. • Acknowledge shared accountability—relinquish some autonomy. Use skills: • Interdisciplinary communication strategies. • Role clarity—I need to clearly define my expectations and capabilities; I need to set clear work goals and deadlines. • Develop situational awareness—cross-check and offer assistance when needed. • Validation—I need to give feedback.
Using communication styles unfamiliar to other disciplines	*Consequently:* Communication is unclear to others.	Attitude: • Willingness to reflect on personal communication style. • Willingness to participate in conflict resolution.Use skills: • Adapt own style to the needs of others on the healthcare team. • Use standardized communication tools especially during emergent situations.

SIMULATION EXERCISE 23.2   Interprofessional Communication Case

Purpose
To help students understand the basic concepts of patient advocacy, communication barriers, and peer negotiation in simulated nursing situations.

Procedure
1. The following situation is an example of situations in which interprofessional communication barriers exist. Refamiliarize yourself with the concepts of professionalism, patient advocacy, communication barriers, and peer negotiation.
2. Formulate a response.
3. Compare your responses with those of your classmates, and discuss the implications of common and disparate answers. Sometimes dissimilar answers provide another important dimension of a problem situation.

Situation
Dr Tanlow interrupts Ms Serf, RN, as she is preparing pain medication for 68-year-old Mrs Gould. It is already 15 minutes late. Dr Tanlow says he needs Ms Serf immediately in Room 20C to assist with a drainage and dressing change. Knowing that Mrs Gould, a diabetic, will respond to prolonged pain with vomiting, Ms Serf replies that she will be available to help Dr Tanlow in 10 minutes (during which time she will have administered Mrs Gould's pain medication). Dr Tanlow, already on his way to Room 20C, whirls around, stating loudly, "When I say I need assistance, I mean now. I am a busy man, in case you hadn't noticed."

If you were Ms Serf, what would be an appropriate response?

Reflective Discussion Analysis
This situation could be discussed in class, assigned as a paper, or used as an essay exam.
1. Construct the best possible response.
2. Justify your response using the concepts of professionalism, patient advocacy, communication barriers, and peer negotiation.

If miscommunication occurs, seek clarity by owning your part in misunderstandings. Message clarity is enhanced when standardized formats such as SBAR are used: The nurse identifies self by name and position, the patient by name, diagnosis, the problem (include current problem, vital signs, new symptoms, etc.), and clearly states his or her request. In interprofessional communication, message clarity is crucial. Taking ownership of miscommunication allows recognition that no one is immune.

Clarify Roles
Since role ambiguity is a factor frequently contributing to conflict, seek role clarity.

More Conflict Resolution Strategies
Self-Reflection. Self-awareness is beneficial in assessing the meaning of a professional conflict. The strategies for communicating with angry patients, as described in Chapter 13, can be applied when disrespect or anger is directed toward you from colleagues. First take a moment to reflect on your own behaviors. Have you inadvertently triggered inappropriate behavior in others? Take responsibility for how you communicate both verbally and nonverbally. Understand your own role. Do you value the role of other team members? Do you treat each of them in a courteous manner?

Take Stress Reduction Measures
Because we know that you are at higher risk for conflict if you are highly stressed, take whatever steps are needed to reduce personal stress.

Commit to a Collaborative Resolution Process. Just as the agency should have a code of conduct defining respectful behavior, there should also be an established process for direct resolution of conflict issues, with support and even "coaches" who help staff resolve conflicts constructively. Steps to promote conflict resolution are listed in Box 23.4.

Process for Responding to Put-Downs. In addition, you need to develop a strategy to respond to unwarranted put-downs and destructive criticisms. Generally, the person delivering them has but one intention, to decrease your status and enhance the status of the person delivering the put-down. The put-down or criticism may be handed out because the speaker is feeling inadequate or threatened. Often it has little to do with the actual behavior of the nurse to whom it is delivered. Other times the criticism may be valid, but the time and place of delivery are grossly inappropriate (e.g., in the middle of the nurses' station or in the patient's presence). In either case, the automatic response of many nurses is to become defensive, embarrassed, or angry.

Recognizing a put-down or unwarranted criticism is the first step toward dealing effectively with it. If a comment from a coworker or authority figure generates defensiveness or embarrassment, it is likely that the

BOX 23.4 Steps to Promote Conflict Resolution Among Healthcare Team Members

1. Set the stage for collaborative communication.
   - Self-reflection: Assume responsibility for own behavior.
   - Privacy: Meet in an appropriate venue, bringing together all involved groups.
   - Acknowledge the conflict problem using clear communication.
   - Allow sufficient time for discussion and resolution process.
2. Attitude: Maintain a respectful, nonpunitive atmosphere.
   - Solicit the perspectives of each.
   - Define the problem issue and objectives clearly.
   - Stay focused while respecting the values and dignity of all parties.
   - Group members can be assertive but not manipulative.
   - Remember to criticize ideas, not people.
3. Be proactive: Initiate early discussion:
   - Use communication skills.
   - Identify the conflict's key points.
   - Have an objective or a goal clearly in mind.
   - Seek mutual solutions.
   - Have group members propose a solution: Identify the merits and drawbacks of each solution.
   - Be open to alternative solutions in which all parties can meet essential needs.
   - Depersonalize conflict situations.
4. Decide to implement the best solution.
   - Specify persons responsible for implementation (role clarity).
   - Establish timeline.
   - Decide on the evaluation method.
   - Emphasize common goal is our shared value of quality care.
   - Emphasize shared responsibility for team success.

Case Study: Student Nurse Heather Cox

Heather Cox, SN, examines a crying child's inner ears and note that the tympanic membranes (eardrums) are red, and reports this to her supervisor, Mr. Webb, saying that the child may have an ear infection.

Mr Webb: "When a child is crying, the drums often swell and redden. How about checking again when the child is calm?" *(Learning response)*

Or

Mr Webb: "Of course they are red when the child is crying. Didn't you learn that in nursing school? I haven't got time to answer such basic questions!" *(Put-down response)*

Which response would you prefer to receive? Why? Whereas the first response allows the nurse to learn useful information to incorporate into practice, the second response serves to antagonize, and it is doubtful much learning takes place. What will happen is that Heather may be more hesitant about approaching the supervisor again for clinical information. It is the patient who ultimately suffers.

Once a put-down is recognized as such, you need to respond verbally in an assertive manner as soon as possible after the incident has taken place. Waiting an appreciable length of time is likely to cause resentment and loss of self-respect. It may be more difficult later for the other person to remember the details of the incident. At the same time, if your anger, not the problem behavior, is likely to dominate the response, it is better to wait a few minutes for the anger to cool a little and then to present the message in a reasoned manner. Preparing your response is a form of "cognitive rehearsal." You can respond to put-downs in the following way:

- *Address the objectionable or disrespectful behaviors first.* Briefly state the behavior and its impact on you. *Emphasize the specifics of the put-down behavior.* Once the put-down has been dealt with, you can discuss any criticism of your behavior on its own merits. Refer only to the behaviors identified.
- *Prepare a few standard responses.* Because put-downs often catch one by surprise, it is useful to have a standard set of opening replies ready. Examples might include the following:
  - "I found your comments very disturbing and insulting."
  - "I feel what you said as an attack. That wasn't called for by my actions."

Use Open Communication

Use Standardized Communication Tools and Standardized Lists. These tools have been especially found effective during

comment represents more than just factual information about performance. If the comment made by the speaker contains legitimate information to help improve one's skill and is delivered in a private and constructive manner, it represents a learning response and cannot be considered a put-down. Learning to differentiate between the two types of communication helps the nurse to "separate the wheat from the chaff." Reflect on the Student Nurse Heather Cox case.

BOX 23.5 Constructive Criticism Example

Steps in Giving

1. Express sympathy. *Sample statement:* "I understand that things are difficult at home."
2. Describe the behavior. *Sample statement:* "But I see that you have been late coming to work three times during this pay period."
3. State expectations. *Sample statement:* "It is necessary for you to be here on time from now on."
4. List consequences. *Sample statement:* "If you get here on time, we'll all start off the shift better. If you are late again, I will have to report you to the personnel department."

Steps in Receiving

1. Listen and paraphrase. If unclear, ask for specific examples. *Sample reply:* "You are saying being late is not acceptable."
2. Acknowledge you are taking suggestions seriously. *Sample comment:* "I hear what you are saying."
3. Give your side by stating supportive facts, without being defensive. *Sample comment:* "My car would not start."
4. Develop a plan for the future. *Sample plan:* "With this paycheck I will repair my car. Until then I'll ask Mary for a ride."

SIMULATION EXERCISE 23.3 Communication to Promote a Healthy Work Environment

Suggestions include negotiating with nurse administrators to avoid being assigned to multiple shifts or allowing small breaks every few hours to recharge; texting or posting affirmation (positive) messages for all the staff to read; saying or texting a message of "good job" or "thank you" to a team member; using humor; putting a smile on your face.

Purpose

To brainstorm ideas about communicating with team members and administration to facilitate a healthier workplace.

Procedure

Gather in small groups to role-play ways to communicate which might help promote a pleasant, healthy work environment.

Reflective Discussion Analysis

Reflect on your communication, then compare ideas with your peers.

---

patient handovers. They are effective in improving interdisciplinary communication.

Criticize Constructively. Giving constructive criticism and receiving criticism is difficult for most people. Refer to Box 23.5 for examples of giving and receiving constructive criticism. When a supervisor gives constructive criticism, some type of response from the person receiving it is indicated. Initially, it is crucial that the conflict problem be clearly defined and acknowledged. To help handle constructive criticism, nurses can do the following:

- Schedule a time when you are calm.
- Request that supervisory meetings be in a place that allows privacy.
- Defuse personal anxiety.
- Listen carefully to the criticism and then paraphrase it.
- Acknowledge that you take suggestions for improvement seriously.
- Discuss the facts of the situation but avoid becoming defensive.
- Develop a plan for dealing with similar situations; become proactive rather than reactive.
- Maintain open dialog.

Document and Report Disruptive Behaviors

A crucial aspect of sustaining quality care is the ability to confront a team member whose behaviors violate accepted norms. Studies show that reporting a colleague to an authority figure without talking the objectionable behavior over with him or her is not effective in restoring harmony. Yet surveys show that the vast majority of physicians and nurses are reluctant to either confront or report. If your attempts to directly discuss behavior with the involved person fail to achieve behavior change, then you need to follow the agency's process and report the problem. In handling disruptive behavior occurrences, documentation is a key step. Hopefully, the agency has a no-blame process, but remember that when pushed, many people will retaliate. Be aware!

Some agencies may hold "communication training sessions" after the offenses have been documented. Simulations such as Simulation Exercise 23.3 offer you practice in developing strategies to promote a healthy workplace.

Develop a Support System

Collegial relationships are an important determinant of success for professionals. Since lack of support is associated with workplace conflicts, you need to make positive efforts to create a support system network. Don't just passively wait and hope it happens. Integrity, respect for others, dependability, a good sense of humor, and an openness to sharing with others are communication qualities people look for in developing a support system.

Positive Reinforcement

Everyone likes to be recognized for their efforts. Simple steps such as saying "thank you" or texting a "job well done" message to colleagues are appreciated. In organizations that have integrated team training and safety initiatives, participation in team activities is integrated into job evaluations. In some agencies, positive evaluations are tied to bonuses. Other organizations hold formal and informal affairs to recognize and celebrate efforts to improve communication and safety.

Organizational Strategies for Conflict Prevention and Resolution

Organizational Climate

The ANA Position Statement on "Incivility, Bullying & Workplace Violence" (ANA, 2015b) mandates that nurses and employers work to create a climate of respect using evidence-based strategies including building in accountability, negotiation, respect, and trust. The literature mentions specific strategies including the following:

- Zero tolerance policy for disrespect (Organizations Code of Conduct)
- Continuing education programs to raise awareness and teach conflict intervention skills
- Accountability follow-up
- Creating a corporate climate conveying respect for all workers

Promote Opportunities for Interdisciplinary Communication. Creating opportunities for interdisciplinary groups to get together is a highly effective strategy for enhancing collaboration and communication. Ideas include collaborative rounds, huddles, team briefings and debriefings, and committees to discuss problems. Some studies associate daily team rounds and joint decision-making with shorter hospital stay and lower hospital charges.

Promote Understanding of the Organizational System. Whenever you work in an organization, you automatically become a part of a system that has norms for acceptable behavior. Each organizational system defines its own chain of command and rules about social processes in professional communication. Even though your idea may be excellent, failure to understand the chain of command or

an unwillingness to form the positive alliances needed to accomplish your objective dilutes the impact.

Although sidestepping the identified chain of command and going to a higher or more tangential resource in the hierarchy may appear less threatening initially, the benefits of such action may not resolve the difficulty. Furthermore, the trust needed for serious discussion becomes limited. Some of the reasons for avoiding positive interactions stem from an internal circular process of faulty thinking. Because communication is viewed as part of a process, the sender and receiver act on the information received, which may or may not represent the reality of the situation.

Promote Clear Policies. As mentioned earlier, regulatory bodies are requiring that healthcare organizations have written codes of behavior and internal processes to handle disruptive behaviors.

Ongoing continuing education stressing awareness and safety training is advocated by OSHA (2016). Prevention strategies might include participation in assertiveness training in-services or the TeamSTEPPS program. Educational interventions that increase staff awareness are extremely effective, as are simulations similar to the exercises in this book. It is not enough to offer an educational intervention once. Team training is necessary. Literature recommends periodic reassessment of need and offering reviews of communication skills and conflict management strategies.

SUMMARY

In this chapter, the same principles of communication used with conflicts in the nurse–patient relationship are broadened to examine the nature of communication among health professionals on the healthcare team. Most nurses will experience conflicts with coworkers at some time during their careers. The same elements of thoughtful purpose, authenticity, empathy, active listening, and respect for the dignity of others that underscore successful nurse–patient relationships are needed in relations with other health professionals. Building effective communication with colleagues involves concepts of collaboration, coordination, and networking. Modification of barriers to professional communication includes negotiation and conflict resolution. Learning is a lifelong process, not only for nursing care skills but also for communication skills. These will develop as you continue to gain experience working as part of an interdisciplinary healthcare team.

ETHICAL DILEMMA: What Would You Do?

You are working a 12-hour shift on a labor and delivery unit. Today, Mrs Kalim is one of your assigned patients. She is fully dilated and effaced, but contractions are still 2 minutes apart after 10 hours of labor. Mrs Kalim, her obstetrician, Dr Mar, and you have agreed on her plan to have a fully natural delivery without medication. However, her obstetrician's partner is handling day shift today, and Dr Mar goes home. This new obstetrician orders you to administer several medications to Mrs Kalim to strengthen contractions and speed up delivery, because he has another patient across town to deliver. Your unit adheres to an empowering model of practice that believes in patient advocacy. How will you handle this potential physician conflict? Is this a true moral dilemma?

DISCUSSION QUESTIONS

1. Reflect on a time someone tried to intimidate or bully you. How did you feel? Assemble and support some productive strategies for responding in such situations.
2. Develop a list of strategies that seem to work best when communicating with team members from outside nursing to facilitate a collaborative environment.

REFERENCES

Agency for Healthcare Research and Quality. (2015). *TeamSTEPPS 2.0: Instructor manual: Table of contents.* Retrieved from: https://www.ahrq.gov/teamstepps/instructor/contents.html. [Accessed 29 June 2021].

Agency for Healthcare Research and Quality (AHRQ). (2017). *TeamSTEPPS webinar: Models for functional collaboration.* Retrieved from: https://www.ahrq.gov/teamstepps/events/webinars/feb-2017.html. [Accessed 29 June 2021].

Agency for Healthcare Research and Quality (AHRQ). (2019). *PSNet: Patient safety network. Patient safety primer: Disruptive and unprofessional behavior.* Retrieved from: https://psnet.ahrq.gov/primer/disruptive-and-unprofessional-behavior. [Accessed 29 June 2021].

American Association of Critical Care Nurses (AACN). (2016). *AACN standards for establishing and sustaining healthy work environments.* Aliso Viejo, CA: AACN. Retrieved from: https://www.aacn.org/WD/HWE/Docs/HWEStandards.pdf. [Accessed 2 July 2021].

American Association of Critical Care Nurses (AACN). (2019). *AACN Position Statement: Zero tolerance for bullying, incivility, and verbal abuse.* Retrieved from: https://www.aacn.org/policy-and-advocacy/~/link.aspx?_id=D766B121F3CE4BD8933DBA72B66A80CF&_z=z. [Accessed 30 June 2021].

American Medical Association (AMA). (2017). *Code of medical ethics opinion 9.4.4. Physicians with disruptive behavior.* Retrieved from: www.ama-assn.org/delivering-care/ethics/physicians-disruptive-behavior. [Accessed 30 June 2021].

American Nurses Association (ANA). (2015a). *Code of ethics for nurses with interpretative statements.* Washington, D.C.: ANA.

American Nurses Association (ANA). (2015b). *ANA position statement: Incivility, bullying, and workplace violence.* Retrieved from: https://www.nursingworld.org/practice-policy/nursing-excellence/official-position-statements/id/incivility-bullying-and-workplace-violence/. [Accessed 29 June 2021].

Anusiewicz, C. V., Ivankova, N. V., Swiger, P. A., Gillespie, G. L., Li, P., & Patrician, P. A. (2020). How does workplace bullying influence nurses' abilities to provide patient care? A nurse perspective. *Journal of Clinical Nursing, 29*(21–22), 4148–4160.

Ebberts, M., & Sollars, K. (2020). Educating nurses about incivility. *Nursing 2020, 50*(10), 64–68.

Johansen, M. L. (2012). Keeping the peace: Conflict management strategies for nurse managers. *Nursing Management, 43*(2), 50–54.

The Joint Commission (TJC). (2008). *Behaviors that undermine a culture of safety. Sentinel event alert No. 40, July 9, 2008.* Retrieved from: http://www.jointcommission.org/assets/1/18/SEA_40.pdf. [Accessed 29 June 2021].

The Joint Commission (TJC). (2011). *Patient-centered communication standards for hospitals R3 Report: Requirement, Rationale, Reference, 1, 1–4.* Retrieved from: https://www.jointcommission.org/~/media/tjc/documents/standards/r3-reports/r3-report-issue-1-20111.pdf. [Accessed 30 June 2021].

Moore, L. W., Sublett, C., & Leahy, C. (2017). Nurse managers speak out about disruptive nurse-to-nurse relationships. *The Journal of Nursing Administration, 47*(1), 24–29.

Munro, C. L., & Hope, A. A. (2020). Healthy work environment: Resolutions for 2020. *American Journal of Critical Care, 29*(1), 4–6.

Polis, S., Higgs, M., Manning, V., Netto, G., & Fernandez, R. (2017). Factors contributing to nursing team work in an acute care tertiary hospital. *Collegian, 24*(1), 19–25.

QSEN Institute. (n.d.). *Pre-licensure KSAS.* Retrieved from: https://qsen.org/competencies/pre-licensure-ksas/. [Accessed 29 June 2021].

Rux, S. (2020). Utilizing improvisation as a strategy to promote interprofessional collaboration within healthcare teams. *Clinical Nurse Specialist, 34*(5), 234–236.

Sanchez, E. S., Tran-Reina, M., Ackerman-Barger, K., Phung, K., Molla, M., & Ton, H. (2020). *Implicit biases, interprofessional communication, and power dynamics.* Agency for Healthcare Research and Quality. PSNet. Retrieved from: https://psnet.ahrq.gov/web-mm/implicit-biases-interprofessional-communication-and-power-dynamics. [Accessed 29 June 2021].

Sherman, R. O. (2019). *Dealing with conflict on your team.* Emerging RN Leader. Retrieved from: https://www.emergingr nleader.com/dealing-with-conflict-on-your-team/. [Accessed 29 June 2021].

U.S. Department of Labor, Occupational Safety and Health Administration (OSHA). (2016). *Guidelines for preventing workplace violence for healthcare & social service workers.* OSHA Publication 3148-06R, Retrieved from: https://www.osha.gov/sites/default/files/publications/osha3148.pdf. [Accessed 29 June 2021].

24

Communicating for Continuity of Care

OBJECTIVES

At the end of the chapter, the reader will be able to:
1. Apply continuity of care concepts to transitional care handover across agencies or at hospital discharge.
2. Apply evidence-based practices to case situation involving patient transfers.
3. Analyze current goals and problems in providing continuity of care across healthcare systems.

There has been a remarkable shift to a community-based healthcare model (National Academies, 2021). Change factors include early hospital discharge; aging population; increases in behavioral/mental problems; and inequitable healthcare services. Hospitals originated as institutions for acute care, but currently the majority of patients have chronic condition diagnoses. Medical advances and reimbursement policies are decreasing acute care postpandemic. The Future of Nursing 2020–30 report says nurses will have new roles in new work settings. Future healthcare models will need to address community care for increased chronic conditions. Transitions between hospital, rehabilitation facilities, long-term care institutions, and home care require increased attention to promoting care continuity. Smooth transitions require clear, accurate communication to provide safe care.

BASIC CONCEPTS

Definitions

Continuity of care is defined as a multidimensional, longitudinal coordination of care by different providers across clinical settings in an integrated manner over time. By definition, it is care over time. Clear communication is the basis of transitions in care whether responsibility for care is being transferred to the next shift, to a different unit, to a different healthcare facility, or to the patient's own home. Open communication sharing patient information is important in providing continuity of care (Mendes et al., 2017).

Incidence

Lack of continuity is often equated in the literature with hospital readmissions within 30 days. Up to 40% of the time readmission is due to miscommunication about medications (Family Caregiver Alliance, 2009).

On the other hand, better continuity is associated with less morbidity and mortality, and substantial reductions in cost to hospitals. Significant declines in readmissions have occurred since the Centers for Medicare and Medicaid Service (CMS) instituted their nonpayment policy, withholding payment for preventable complications for readmissions within 30 days.

Goal. Our goal is to develop and use a successful continuity model to ensure a smooth transition of care and to improve patient outcomes (Spehar et al., 2005). Reflect on the Jay West case.

CASE STUDY: Jay West Needs Help With Continuity

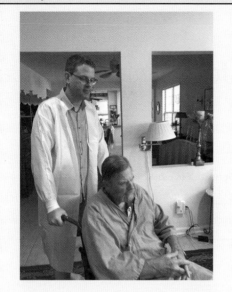

Mr West, 50 years old, was diagnosed with ALS 2 years ago. He experienced a progressive loss of muscle control. Now he has advanced to swallowing difficulties. Jay complains "I am not able to handle this." His neurology team arranges for a J-tube to be inserted through his abdomen (gastrostomy). This will allow liquid feedings, eliminating risks of tracheal aspiration. Three days after discharge, his case manager nurse calls to follow up, discussing his progress. After listening to Jay's complaints, he displays empathy by commenting "You sound frustrated that you are not yet gaining weight and still feel so weak. Would you be willing to have some therapy at home to work on these issues?" He arranges for a nurse, physical therapist, and speech therapist to make home visits.

Continuity Characteristics

Fig. 24.1 depicts aspects of patient-centered continuity of care. This chapter uses the transition model specifying three components: relational, informational, and management continuity. Continuity decreases the potential for duplication of services, conflicting assessments, or gaps in service. Discharge discontinuity contributes to rehospitalizations, patient confusion, and poor quality of care postdischarge.

Chronic Disease

Chronic disease has become the major cause of death and disability nationally and globally. According to the Agency for Healthcare Research and Quality (AHRQ), over 66% of older adults suffer from chronic disease, often with other comorbid conditions (AHRQ, 2020). Chronic disorders often have periods of exacerbation and remission. They require ongoing healthcare interventions by multiple providers best provided using a continuity of care model.

Theory-Based Conceptual Frameworks

According to Olson and Juengst (2019) who were studying discharge of stroke patients, there is no clear best practice yet for transitioning at the time of hospital discharge. Several frameworks have been applied to this transition process.

Transition Care Model: Care Over Time Concept

Transition Care Model was designed to promote a smooth transition. It provides a healthcare system with discharge-related time-limited interventions, including predischarge and postdischarge elements. This is an interdisciplinary model with one person designated as the case manager or care coordinator (Ridwan et al., 2019). The patient has an enduring trusting relationship with their team of healthcare providers who cooperate in providing safe, cost effective healthcare for the duration of illness.

Relational Continuity. This concept includes care that spans more than one episode of care and leads, in the practitioner, to a sense of clinical responsibility and accumulated knowledge of the patient's personal and medical circumstances. Relational continuity also describes an active ongoing alliance among professionals from various disciplines and different agencies who work together to provide integrated health services.

Informational Continuity. Clear, understandable communication among health team members working on discharge care and among family members is needed. Data about treatment and care should be tailored to meet patient needs. Ascertaining the ability of patient and caretaker to manage care and medications, tubes, dressings, ambulation, and other care is an essential part of the process. Technology is used to promote real-time communication among all providers and between providers and patients as needed. Patients and their families are engaged early in the hospitalization in planning for meeting needs postdischarge. AHRQ has developed a "Guide to Patient and Family Engagement" that is available on their website under the TeamSTEPPS program (AHRQ, n.d.).

Management Continuity. Utilization of a consistent, coherent approach to patient care management is essential. Continuity-of-care concepts link acute care with primary care, creating a "smooth seamless flow" of care across facilities and caregivers. Patients should be able to rely on a coordinated transition from one healthcare setting to another, with personalized care designed to meet their specific needs.

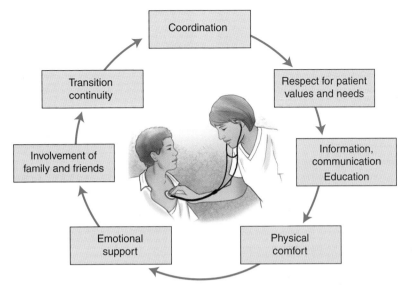

Figure 24.1 Dimensions of patient-centered care in continuity of care.

The Chronic Care Model

Sources give credit to Dr Edward Wagner for developing this model designed to provide better management and continuity in the care of patients with chronic diseases. In Dr Wagner's experience, patients did not change behaviors as a result of hearing a physician's didactic lecture about what to do, but did respond to a more collaborative effort. The model has been refined over the years and made broad use of health system and community resources. Concepts from the Chronic Care model including using a team to coordinate care with all providers and to support patient self-management and decision-making. Electronic record formats keep all providers up to date on the patient's status. Outcomes include better informed patient, better health, fewer exacerbations, and cost savings.

The Johns Hopkins Mobile Integrated Healthcare Model

Known as the "Guided Care" model, the focus is on the care of patients with multiple chronic conditions, especially older patients. A nurse is designated to coordinate care closely among different physicians and works closely with patients to optimize resources in the community to provide care. Outcomes have been measured in over 35 studies showing patients decrease use of the emergency department by up to 17%, decrease hospital admissions, resulting in decreased costs. Clarke et al. (2017) cite those who project this could save Medicare up to half a billion dollars.

Case Management

More a role than a model, case management seeks to assist the flow of patients throughout the healthcare system.

A nurse or a social worker is the case manager or case coordinator assigned to a patient, evaluating the patient's need for services and collaborating with various providers in the community to obtain these services. See Box 24.1 for a list of case manager activities regarding discharges for some patients. There are over 30 definitions of "case manager" and every employing agency or physician practice has a unique version of what the job entails. The goal is to provide quality care to promote better patient outcomes. Finances is a limiting factor. Who pays for the case manager position? Who pays for services?

Discharge and Transition Guidelines to Promote Continuity

Quality discharge planning is correlated with lower rates of readmission within a 30-day time frame (Henke et al., 2017). The 30-day readmission rate is an arbitrary measure which CMS uses to penalize hospitals through nonpayment of services, when the cause is poor discharge planning. The Joint Commission (2021) has developed guidelines for the discharge process. Improving the level of collaboration among healthcare professionals is identified as a primary strategy for improving the level of continuity. Carefully read Table 24.1 to identify key elements in planning care transitions, especially ones which decrease readmission rates.

Barriers to Continuity

Kable et al. (2019) showed that lack of resources for post-discharge services is the main barrier to continuity. Other concerns include the following.

BOX 24.1　Nursing Actions in Comprehensive Discharges

Case manager nurses promote smooth discharge transitions by activities such as follows:

- Using a language translator program or assistant, if needed
- Making follow-up appointments if needed
- Reviewing written, easily understandable discharge plan with patient and family
- Expediting transmission of discharge plan to primary provider and/or next case manager
- Involving the family in planning early enough to arrange for needed home equipment and community services professional help
- Assessing the ability of patient or family/caretaker to manage care and medication regimen; having them explain it back in own words
- Emphasizing medication information, dose, time for administration, side effects, adverse effects, and where to obtain prescribed medications, verifying patient's plan to obtain
- Making plan for follow-up laboratory tests and interpretation, if necessary
- Providing a written list of case manager and community support contacts with telephone numbers or portal URLs, including options for home healthcare. Teaching how to initiate services
- Reviewing what to do if a problem arises, and reinforcing who and when to call for follow-up appointments with outpatient departments or primary provider; as well as ensuring transportation
- Verifying patient understanding by having them restate the plan
- Doing a follow-up contact within 2 weeks, by telephone or virtually

Data from PSNet. https://psnet.ahrq.gov/primer/discharge-planning-and-transitions-care and Tahan, H. M., & Treiger, T. M. (2017). *CMSA core curriculum foe case management* (3rd ed.). Philadelphia: Wolter Kluwer.

TABLE 24.1　Key Elements in Planning for Care Transitions

Assess needs	1. Assess the ability of patient and family/caretaker to manage care at home 2. Assess understanding of medication purpose, time, amount 3. Assess total person needs and nature of support systems
Assist family to select best care setting	1. Extended care facility 2. Rehabilitation facility 3. Assisted living facility 4. Own home with supportive services
Make referrals	1. Involve family early on in discharge planning for care, equipment 2. Verify financial resources: private insurance coverage or government eligible services
Review discharge clinical summary	1. Review written copy with patient and family 2. Expedite transmission to primary provider and all community clinical assistive agencies involved
Medication teaching	1. Emphasize relevant medication information using "teach-back" method. Include purpose, dose, time for administration, side effects, adverse effects, where to obtain med immediately, who to report problems to 2. Reconciliation: what meds were stopped and why.
Follow-up care	1. Who will be contacting family 2. Who family should contact: provide list of telephone numbers, patient portals 3. Ensure transportation to follow-up appointments
Education	1. Assess understanding of disease trajectory and treatment plan 2. Assess ability to use Internet resources 3. Assess knowledge for virtual visits

Miscommunication

Unclear discharge instruction has been cited as one of the biggest risk factors associated with transitions in healthcare. Poor care coordination or inadequate communication leads to failures in transmitting essential patient information, increases in medication adverse effects, causes delays in service, increases costs, and diminishes health outcomes (Clarke et al., 2017). Communication is the glue that holds the complex health system together (Spehar et al., 2005).

Organization Problems

Communication Deficits

Primary care and secondary care institutions do not always communicate easily. Outdated reimbursement protocols restrict billing flexibility. One example is the use of EMS ambulances to transport patients with minor, nonacute conditions to emergency departments for care, which Clarke et al. (2017) estimate costs CMS (Medicare/Medicaid) over half a billion dollars annually.

Role Funding

The role of case manager has evolved to fill the need for discharge coordination. The ability of family caregivers to assume care at home is assessed, family is involved in the discharge planning process, and appropriate referrals for home health services are arranged. But this role filled by a nurse or social worker is not always recognized as a budget line item. The Case Management Society of America developed standards of practice, which describe the role of case manager as extending across the continuum of multiple settings. As mentioned, financial considerations limit scope of practice.

System Problems

Limited time may lead to inconsistent discharge teaching. Other problems include lack of involvement of the patient's primary care provider; lack of resources, fragmentation of healthcare systems, as well as lack of follow-up. All these lead to gaps in care.

Relational or Personal Characteristics

On the individual's level, demographic variables such as language barriers, lack of knowledge (low health literacy), and cultural barriers have been implicated in discontinuity of care. Sometimes, patients are simply not ready to learn (AHRQ, 2020).

Promoters of Continuity

Assets of implementing a care transition model are as follows:

- *Timely follow-up.* Handover to primary provider. According to AHRQ (2020), up to half of patients and families told to make a follow-up appointment fail to do so. Verification of patient condition is ascertained via telephone calls or virtual internet visits within 72 h after discharge.
- *Discharge checklist.* Gao and associates (2018) explored use of a discharge timeout checklist. In their study of 429 discharges, 27.8% of patients were shown to need additional education about their condition. The use of this checklist tool allowed staff to identify knowledge deficits and remediate. Some community pharmacies will deliver patient medication to the bedside prior to discharge. Since medication misinformation is a major problem, this allows one more point for verification of understanding.
- *Meds to the bed programs.* Many pharmacies are willing to deliver postdischarge medications to the patients' bedside the day of discharge, so there is no interruption in medication.
- *Deprescribing.* Many senior citizens receive multiple medications from a variety of providers (polypharmacia). AHRQ (2020) reviewed 27 studies finding many medications to be unnecessary for managing the patient's current condition. They developed the STOPP screening tool (Screening Tool of Older Person's Inappropriate Prescriptions) to verify whether a certain med is needed and whether its dosage is appropriate.

DEVELOPING AN EVIDENCE-BASED PRACTICE

Many studies have assessed hospital readmission rates. Some deal with specific diagnoses or age groups; others analyze general readmissions. For example, Burr and associates (2020) analyzed readmissions for patients with chronic obstructive pulmonary disease (COPD) following implementation in Los Angeles of a Hospital Readmissions Reduction Program. Facchinetti et al. (2020) looked at older adult readmissions, while Wasfy and associates (2017) analyzed large cohort hospital readmissions after the Centers for Medicaid and Medicare Services (CMS) instituted their nonpayment policy for preventable readmissions.

Results

All studies found statistically significant reductions in readmissions after institution of continuity of care interventions (driven by the CMC financial consideration).

Strength of evidence: Research is high and has strong evidence for application.

Application to Your Clinical Practice

Consult the AHRQ websites for broad information. Specifically, you as a direct care nurse or case manager should do the following:

1. Review the written discharge plan with patient and family and identify any gaps in needed services.
2. Educate your patients to understand their postdischarge plan by having them explain it back to you and provide them with written instructions, as well as forwarding it to their primary provider and next case manager.
3. Advocate for better discharge planning and follow-up procedures.

References

Buhr, R. G., Jackson, N. J., Kominski, G. F., Dubinett, S. M., Mangione, C. M., & Ong, M. K. (2020). Readmission rates for chronic obstructive pulmonary disease under the hospital readmissions reduction program: An interrupted time series analysis. *Journal of General Internal Medicine, 35*(12), 3581–3590.

Facchinetti, G., D'Angelo, D., Piredda, M., et al. (2020). Continuity of care interventions for preventing hospital readmission of older people with chronic diseases: A meta-analysis. *International Journal of Nursing Studies, 101*, 103396.

Wasfy, J. H., Zigler, C. M., Choirat, C., Wang, Y., Dominici, F., & Yeh, R. W. (2017). Readmission rates after passage of the Hospital Readmissions Reduction program: A pre-post analysis. *Annals of Internal Medicine, 166*(5), 324–331.

APPLICATIONS

Continuity of care offers a care pathway to safeguard care stability and to provide a secure safety net for individuals and families that they can rely on for support and information. Ideally, we communicate effectively to work together to establish a direction and implement coordinated interventions throughout the health system. We will discuss each of the three dimensions of continuity: relational, informational, and managerial.

Relational Continuity

Characteristics of Collaboration and Continuity

Patient and family should be active decision-makers in care collaboration. The decision-making process starts with providing sufficient information on which to make informed decisions. Information must be presented in an understandable format, relevant to this particular patient's diagnosis and treatment plan. Be alert to the differences in what level of information the patient desires at this time. Collaboration among team members who then present one uniform postdischarge plan increases patient satisfaction and efficacy of care, producing better health outcomes. See Fig. 24.2 for characteristics of collaboration.

Communication as a Promoter of Continuity

Care transitions are cited as a prime risk time for miscommunication by The Joint Commission (2017). This accreditation group has made accurate communication during "hand-off" care transition, a National Patient Safety Goal. They define "hand-off as a transfer and acceptance of care responsibility achieved through effective communication. A real time process of passing patient specific information … for the purpose of ensuring the continuity and safety of the patient's care."

The Medical Home. This implies that the patient is consistently seen by the same group of primary care providers. They are a patient in that practice. These providers assume responsibility for providing regular, accessible, comprehensive primary care services for designated patients in a familiar medical setting. This practice is the first point of contact when the patient needs healthcare. They take responsibilities for external referrals for specialty services and community agencies.

Coordination

Effective coordination depends on the development of dynamic relationships among involved professionals. Relationships are as important to success as content. Shared goals and basic knowledge regarding each provider's work contributing to the whole of patient care facilitates positive outcomes.

Shared Goals. Shared goals are an essential product of effective patient-centered collaboration. Problem-solving communication should be respectful, accurate, timely, and frequent. Aim for developing shared meanings rather than simple information exchanges. Mutual trust and respect for differences offer powerful reinforcement for open dialog. Once agreement is reached, the entire team, including the patient, needs to take full responsibility for implementing clearly described action plans.

Role Clarity

An essential for working on an interdisciplinary team is role clarity. Effective collaborative participation requires clarity about own level of skill and scope of practice role and respect and knowledge of roles of others on the team. Roles are discussed in Chapter 22. Simulation Exercise 24.1 gives an opportunity to examine roles of other health professionals.

Mutual Trust

In time working together, team members develop trust and rely on each other's competence. This is fostered by team meetings with collaborative dialog, where conflicts can be resolved. Patients can sense when team members have conflict, and this leads to confusion and less positive health outcomes. Consistent consultation with fellow team members improves process and commitment to delivery of

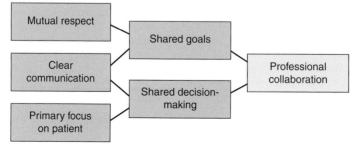

Figure 24.2 Characteristics of collaboration.

SIMULATION EXERCISE 24.1 Learning About Roles of Other Health Professionals

Purpose

To recognize similarities and differences in roles.

Procedure

1. Break into groups of four, giving each student a different professional role to explore, including educational requirements and skill sets.
2. Write or present to the larger group a concise description of each role.

Reflective Discussion Analysis

In what ways do the different skill sets compliment the roles of the others on the healthcare team? What can you do to create better communication among these professionals?

SIMULATION EXERCISE 24.2 Collaborative Decision-Making

Purpose

To help learners explore strategies for working together to achieve consensus in an uncertain situation.

Procedure

Break up into groups of three, with one assuming responsibility to record interactions. One presents an experience with a patient undergoing a complex clinical situation, with others asking clarifying questions.

Reflective Discussion Analysis

Discuss the dynamics of the interaction, rather than the solution arrived upon!

quality care. Simulation Exercise 24.2 provides an opportunity for you to understand collaborative communication.

Informational Continuity

Informational continuity refers to data exchanges among providers and provider systems and between providers and patient. Our goal is to continuously give coordinated care with an uninterrupted flow of information among participants and between primary and secondary agencies. Data need to be easily accessible. For example, information about current medications, start and stop dates, and patient responses helps provide safe care. Lack of information especially at times of transference of care can result in treatment delays, which unnecessarily increases family anxiety. The ability of family to communicate easily with various providers and treatment centers helps prevent family caregivers from becoming overwhelmed with the number of procedures, appointments, and directions.

Transition and Discharge Planning

Patients with multiple comorbidities or complex needs typically experience multiple care transitions. As mentioned, these transitions are a time of increased risk for miscommunication, leading to adverse events of "near misses and avoidable errors." Box 24.2 presents core functions for transition sending and receiving teams. It also diagrams collaborative nursing actions associated with complex discharges. In the community, informational continuity can empower patients through appointment reminders, call-back checks, and careful verification of care instructions and options. Knowing what to expect, with contingency plans in place, increases patient security. Notifying family about changes in patient condition or treatment is an essential part of ensuring continuity.

Management Continuity

Strong system-based management continuity facilitates self-care management. Management continuity uses a consistent, coherent approach to patient care that is responsive to changing needs. Part of management continuity is aligning patient needs with community resources through care coordination and case management.

Patient System Navigation

The goals of the care coordinator are to assist the patient in navigating the complexities of the healthcare system and to coordinate services. This works to decrease fragmentation to improve the flow of needed services.

The process begins with self-knowledge about possible bias and then develops a nonjudgmental collaborative relationship with patients to identify their needs, goals, and any barriers, which might impede success. It is easy to become overinvolved, so be sure to maintain professional boundaries. Coordination activities include the following:

- Establishing relationships based on trust
- Using communication skills to engage patients, providers, and community resources
- Providing needed health education
- Assessing strengths and needs
- Implementing a proactive plan of care
- Monitoring progress and assist with follow-up
- Supporting patients to self-manage
- Facilitating informed decision-making
- Facilitating care transitions
- Locating community resources to patient needs
- Measuring and evaluating the process and patient outcomes

- Using open communication to encourage flow of information
- Working within treatment recommendations

Case Management Communication

Not all patients need a case manager, but for those who are unable to safely maintain self-management of their complex chronic conditions, a case manager can improve quality of the healthcare experience.

Goal. The goal of coordinating care from multiple sources is to help patients function at their highest level in the least restrictive environment. Open, direct, honest communication among patient, family, case manager, the payer, and other team health professionals is the guiding principle of case management practice (Tahan & Treiger, 2017).

National Guidelines. AHRQ established the Re-Engineered Discharge Toolkit (RED) (AHRQ, 2013). Information includes discharge sample forms. Actively participate in the Ray Bolton case.

Case Study: Ray Bolton Needs a Case Manager

Mr Bolton is a 48-year-old with severe Crohn's disease. He has a permanent ileostomy, is on multiple medications, and has periodic flare-ups causing him severe pain. His only income is through the Social Security Disability Insurance program. His neurologic issues affect his gait and balance. He has negligible support systems, so he is referred to a nurse case manager after his recent hospitalization. Simulation Exercise 24.3 provides you with an opportunity to use a case management approaches in planning care and discharge.

Case Management Strategies

Case management strategies are designed to coordinate and manage care across a wide continuum of health services. Strategies rely on continuity concepts such as effective

SIMULATION EXERCISE 24.3   Planning Care and Discharge for Ray Bolton

Purpose
Provides practice with planning care and discharges.

Procedure
Break up into groups of three. Read and discuss the Ray Bolton Case. Identify the relevant data. What are the best ways to address each of Mr Bolton's complex needs? What kinds of resources will he need to effectively self-manage his care after discharge? If you are the nurse case manager, what steps would be included in your discharge plan? Make a list.

Reflective Discussion Analysis
In the larger classroom, compare the lists from other groups. What things did your group not think of?

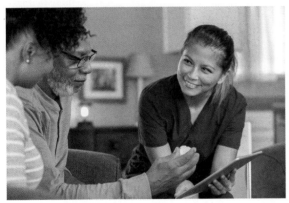

Figure 24.3 Home health nurse using tablet to access patient's EHR to verify his medications. (From iStock #1189837637, Courtney Hale.)

communication skills, openness, team building, and use of electronic health records as depicted in Fig. 24.3.

Case Finding. A proactive strategy is to seek out individuals at high risk for potential health problems post-discharge. Your intake assessment should include all the contact information for health providers, social service providers, school and work contacts, and insurance information. Available supportive community groups such as church contacts can be helpful. Important data such as "do not resuscitate" orders and advance directives should already be on the electronic health record (EHR).

Management of Chronic Conditions. Helping patients customize goals and preferences for management requires meeting with patients and families on a longitudinal basis. It is important to empower patient and family to control

their condition management. Can you envision a revamped health system in which a nurse case manager is assigned to specific families to follow them throughout their life, as is done to some extent in Europe? Management most likely involves interacting with multiple community care agencies especially when needed for home healthcare. At times, such interactions require dealing with agencies not directly concerned with the patient's diagnoses such as Fair Housing Bureaus, Social Security Disability benefit representatives, addiction support groups, etc.

Advocacy. A large part of a case manager's role is acting as an advocate for the patient. Case managers educate community workers. Advocacy focuses on options that are in the patient's best interest.

Outcome Evaluation. A case manager evaluates clinical condition changes and institutes necessary changes in the plan of care. Case managers document all information from a variety of involved agencies. In addition, the case manager evaluates patient satisfaction. Having a case manager saves patients much frustration, facilitates getting needed services to enhance quality of life, and as mentioned saves readmissions. While it is crucial to evaluate the cost of services, there is need for comparison to a larger picture. What would have the outcomes been had no case services been provided?

Large Data Sets/Big Data

As you can discern from the EBP example, many evaluation measures involve analyses of very large data sets. Individual case managers may have little to do with these analyses, but their results have massive impacts on services and personal job viability. For example, the CMS analyses already discussed involved savings in the billions of dollars. Could awareness of such information persuade agencies to employ more case managers?

Continuity for Family Caregivers

Living with chronic disease is often a home care responsibility, with unpaid family caregivers providing the majority of care. It is estimated that 1:4 Americans act as caregiver to an ill family member and that 74% of these care providers give care 7 days per week (American Geriatrics Society Health in Aging Foundation, 2021). This certainly gives continuity but can lead to exhaustion! Caregiver burden is discussed in Chapters 19 and 21. Assess for signs of caregiver stress such as fatigue, changes in sleep or eating patterns, increased irritability, or feelings of isolation and depression (U.S. National Library of Medicine, 2021). There are both positive and negative aspects to the caregiver role. Being cared for in one's own home can be a continuity asset since the patient receives care in familiar surrounds from loved ones. Caregiver's functional capacity has wide variations. A supportive case manager can arrange for others to fill the gaps. To do so requires the manager carefully assess the situation and level of needed knowledge, as well as problems being encountered. It is important also to validate feelings about this caregiver role such as frustrations fulfilling demands on their time. Providing a list of contact numbers, reviewing medication changes, and giving information about worsening symptoms and when to call for expert help are useful strategies. Case managers can provide financial considerations when selecting a home health agency or directly hiring a home helper, with general information about what services Medicare will reimburse for.

SUMMARY

Providing continuity of care is a dynamic process, consisting of relational, informational, and managerial functions. Though ideally the multidisciplinary team contributes, usually there is one identified coordinator or case manager with ability to arrange for services across agencies or request multiple services in the patient's home.

Relational continuity embraces interdisciplinary collaboration. Informational continuity allows for uninterrupted flow of data between all involved professionals and agencies, to families and patients, and to supportive services within the community. Management continuity provides coherent, updated care by supportive personnel across the complex healthcare community, helping the patient obtain needed services.

Although there are many names for the role of coordinator, the one used here is "case manager." Case management is the process for ensuring continuity of care, as patients transition across services.

ETHICAL DILEMMA: What Would You Do?

Mr Paul is nearing discharge after hospitalization for chronic pulmonary obstructive disease (COPD). It is clear to all that he cannot manage independently, especially since he has a hard time managing his diet and insulin injections to treat his diabetes. He is not an easy person to live with, but is sure his daughter will welcome into her home since he is "family." His daughter reluctantly agrees but is busy with her own family and job. She does not have a positive relationship with Mr Paul and resents that he just assumes she will take care of him. It is clear to staff that he cannot live independently in the community.

1. What would you do as case manager in this situation?
2. What are the implications of this situation as an ethical dilemma?

DISCUSSION QUESTIONS

1. What are barriers and facilitators of continuity in your clinical setting?
2. How is the healthcare system changing to provide greater continuity of care?

REFERENCES

Agency for Healthcare Research and Quality (AHRQ). (2013). *Re-engineered discharge toolkit: Samples and forms.* Retrieved from: www.ahrq.gov/sites/default/files/publications/files/redtoolkitforms.pdf. [Accessed 1 July 2021].

Agency for Healthcare Research and Quality (AHRQ). (2020). *Making healthcare safer III: A critical analysis of existing and emerging patient safety practices.* Publication no. 20-0029-EF. Retrieved from: https://www.ahrq.gov/research/findings/making-healthcare-safer/mhs3/index.html. [Accessed 30 June 2021].

Agency for Healthcare Research and Quality (AHRQ). (n.d.). *TeamSTEPPS program.* www.ahrq.gov/teamstepps/. [Accessed 30 June 2021].

American Geriatrics Society Health in Aging Foundation. (2021). *Caregiver health.* [website]. Retrieved from: HealthinAging.org. [Accessed 1 July 2021]. https://www.healthinaging.org/a-z-topic/caregiver-health.

Clarke, J. L., Bourn, S., Skoufalos, A., Beck, E. H., & Castillo, D. J. (2017). An innovative approach to health care delivery for patients with chronic conditions. *Population Health Management, 20*(1), 23–30.

Family Caregiver Alliance. (2009). *Hospital discharge planning: A guide for families and caregivers.* Retrieved from: www.caregiver.org/hospital-discharge-planning-guide-families-and-caregivers/. [Accessed 30 June 2021].

Gao, M. C., Martin, P. B., Mortal, J., et al. (2018). A multidisciplinary discharge timeout checklist improves patient education and captures discharge process errors. *Quality Management in Health Care, 27*(2), 63–68.

Henke, R. M., Karaca, Z., Jackson, P., Marder, W. D., & Wong, H. S. (2017). Discharge planning and hospital readmissions. *Medical Care Research and Review, 74*(3), 345–368.

Kable, A., Baker, A., Pond, D., Southgate, E., Turner, A., & Levi, C. (2019). Health professionals' perspectives on the discharge process and continuity of care for stroke survivors discharged home in regional Australia: A qualitative, descriptive study. *Nursing and Health Sciences, 21*(2), 253–261.

Mendes, F. R. P., Gemito, M. L. G. P., Caldeira, E., Serra, I., & Casas-Novas, M. V. (2017). Continuity of care from the perspective of users. *Ciência & Saúde Coletiva, 22*(3), 841–852.

National Academies of Sciences, Engineering, and Medicine. (2021). *The future of nursing 2020-2030: Charting a path to achieve health equity.* Washington, D.C.: The National Academies Press.

Olson, D. M., & Juengst, S. B. (2019). The hospital to home transition following acute stroke. *Nursing Clinics of North America*, 54(3), 385–397.

Ridwan, E. S., Hadi, H., Wu, Y. L., & Tsai, P. S. (2019). Effects of transitional care on hospital readmission and mortality rate in subjects with COPD: A systematic review and meta-analysis. *Respiratory Care*, 64(9), 1146–1156.

Spehar, A. M., Campbell, R. R., Cherrie, C., et al. (2005). Seamless care: Safe patient transitions from hospital to home. In K. Henriksen, J. B. Battles, E. S. Marks, & D. I. Lewin (Eds.), *Advances in patient safety: From Research to implementation, vol 1: Research findings*. Rockville, MD: Agency for Healthcare Research and Quality.

Tahan, H. M., & Treiger, T. M. (2017). *CMSA® core Curriculum foe case management* (3rd ed.). Philadelphia: Wolter Kluwer.

The Joint Commission (TJC). (2017). *Sentinel alert #58: Inadequate hand-off communication*. Retrieved from: https://www.jointcommission.org/resources/pati ent-safety-topics/sentinel-event/sentinel-event-alert-newsletters/sentinel-event-alert-58-inadequate-hand-off-communication/. [Accessed 30 June 2021].

The Joint Commission (TJC). (2021). *National patient safety goals*. Retrieved from: https://www.jointcommission.org/s tandards/national-patient-safety-goals/. [Accessed 30 June 2021].

U.S. National Library of Medicine. (2021). *Caregiver health*. MedlinePLUS [website]. Retrieved from: https://medlineplus.gov/caregiverhealth.html. [Accessed 30 June 2021].

25

e-Documentation in Health Information Technology Systems

OBJECTIVES

At the end of the chapter, the reader will be able to:

1. Identify purposes for documentation, describing legal, business, and research use for health information technology (HIT).
2. Discuss electronic health records (EHRs), computerized provider order entry (CPOE), and clinical

decision support systems (CDSS) as part of larger electronic HIT systems, evaluating whether "meaningful use" requirements have improved care quality.
3. Apply concepts about use of electronic longitudinal plans of care (LPC), decision support, CPOE, and other aspects of HIT systems to patient cases.

Technology has changed how nurses manage patient care (Ihlebaek, 2020). Two key elements of collaborative work are communication and documentation. The process of obtaining, organizing, and conveying patient health information to others in print or electronic format is referred to as *documentation.* Fig. 25.1 illustrates why we document, especially in terms of improved communication and evidence gathered from aggregated **electronic health records (EHRs)** to establish "best practice" interventions for quality improvement, a Quality and Safety Education for Nurses (QSEN) competency (QSEN, n.d.). Nursing will increasingly move into community settings, including home health (National Academies, 2021). We will become more dependent on technology for nursing communication.

The process of interdisciplinary communication has been increasingly integrated into EHRs as the method nurses use to document outcomes of care given. However, EHRs are only a component of the larger **health information technology** (HIT) system. Use of **computerized provider order entry** (CPOE) systems are also described in this chapter. Your use of EHR technology to communicate and manage patient information is a skill specifically cited as part of QSEN's informatics competency. Regulatory and ethical implications of documentation will also be described in this chapter, concluding with a brief discussion of coding and nursing taxonomies. New technology

and devices for medical communication at the point of care, CDSSs, remote monitoring, secure messaging, and telehealth are discussed in Chapter 26.

BASIC CONCEPTS

Computerized Health Information Technology Systems

Computers make information more accessible to all involved healthcare providers, including your patient. Globally, governments and professional organizations believe computerized systems not only improve the quality of healthcare but will also eventually reduce its cost. At the organization level, as part of agency accreditation processes, The Joint Commission (TJC) requires that hospitals and long-term care facilities demonstrate measurable quality results. At the individual nurse level, EHRs allow instant availability of patient information in real time, as well as to other providers simultaneously.

Goal

The goal is to use HIT to improve population health outcomes and healthcare quality (U.S. Department of Health and Human Services, n.d.). EHRs not only store information, but they can also improve care outcomes by improving clinical decisions, facilitating communication, fostering

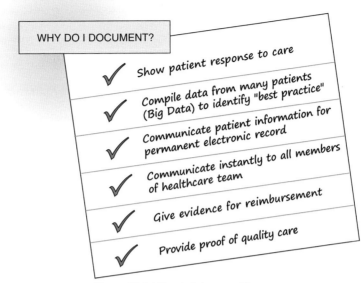

Figure 25.1 Why do I document?

collaboration with health team members, and increasing productivity by automating some care tasks (Rudin et al., 2020). Part of the larger HIT system can make care safer by engaging patients as partners in their healthcare, promoting better communication, and increasing use of preventive practices and evidence-based "best practices." How does this affect you? Use of HIT skills is an expectation at the beginning staff nurse job level. Studies show EHR use skills can be successfully integrated into simulations labs teaching these skills. Your ability to use information technology is among items tested on licensure exams. Consider the case of Sue Smith, RN.

CASE STUDY: Sue Smith, RN, and Computerized Care Documentation for Mr Robert

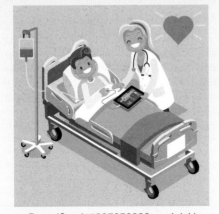

From iStock #827252328, aurielaki.

Sue Smith, RN, has worked on this medical unit for 3 years since graduation. She is notified that 34-year-old Mr Rob Robert is newly admitted via the Endocrine Outpatient Clinic to her floor. She carries her tablet with his electronic medical record to his assigned room as he is wheeled off the elevator. His A1c blood test results are already posted, along with orders to add 10 units of regular insulin to his IV drip per clinic nurse practitioner order. This order was simultaneously transmitted to the pharmacy, who dispatched a robot to the unit with this insulin. Mr Robert's medical history in his EHR has been forwarded to the intensivist assigned to this unit, who received an alert about this admission. She texts Sue that she will be in to see Mr Robert in 1 hour. As soon as Mr Robert is settled in his assigned bed and his family is reassured, Sue completes her intake assessment, documenting it via her tablet. Mr Robert's primary physician will receive an alert as soon as the intake exam is completed.

1 Do you feel that HIT has expedited care so far?

Meaningful Use

Adoption of HIT creates an interactive computerized information and communication system. Far more complex than just putting existing paper documentation on a computer, HIT systems are designed to support the multiple information needs required by today's complex patient care; provide you and others on the health team with *clinical decision support*; and achieve safer care for your patient.

In the United States, the Centers for Medicare and Medicaid Services (CMS) has specified EHR components required for use by providers and agencies who serve their patients. Mandatory crucial "meaningful use" information is listed in Table 25.1. In addition to using EHRs, providers

TABLE 25.1 Components of an Electronic Health Information Technology System in Our Journey to Consumer-Driven Healthcare

Mandatory (Required by CMS Under Its "Meaningful Use" Criteria)	Desirable (Some of Which Must be Chosen to Be Used)
An integrated, accessible electronic repository of patient data with easy access by a variety of healthcare providers for exchange of information. Contains and records changes in: Updated problem list Hx; Dx; VS; PE data Medication list Allergy list (cross-checks for drug–drug–allergy problems and sends alerts to providers) Imaging files with real-time access at the point of care	EHR system needs ease of access, perhaps by use of templates that the provider checks or customizes/modifies, e.g., a box is checked when an ECG was done and results are checked "normal" or "abnormal." Information is accessed before and after each task, with nurse documenting not only care given but progress toward goals. EHR can be remotely accessed by providers who can work from anywhere at any time. HIT system has financial tools, as well as clinical tools, e.g., it is able to generate newest ICD codes, do billing information, schedule appointments, etc. Incorporates accommodations to improve work flow and thus increase productivity. Ease of access allows provider to access many screen files with one login.
Has clinical decision support capabilities. Incorporates standard "evidence-based best practice" protocols that monitor your care and send you prompts if care is not recorded.	Sends alerts to providers
Uses CPOE	
Reports quality outcome measures to the government (CMS); public health agencies; state or local governmental agencies while safeguarding privacy/HIPAA requirements	Each year the percentage of total patients for whom your agency must submit reportable information increases.
Required use of EHRs also mandates capability to generate written prescriptions to avoid handwriting errors	May electronically send prescriptions to preferred pharmacy.
On request can provide patient with clinical summaries: copies of records, laboratory findings, discharge instructions, educational resources, forms for advanced directives, etc.	Patient may not have access to all levels of information. Has online portals to access their information. Sends electronic reminders or alerts to patients.
Provides summary of care at each point of transition, and for referrals	
Aggregates data	

CMS, Centers for Medicare and Medicaid Services; *CPOE,* Computerized physician/provider order entry; *Dx,* Diagnosis; *ECG,* Electrocardiogram; *EHR,* Electronic health record; *HIPAA,* Health Insurance Portability and Accountability Act; *HIT,* Health information technology; *Hx,* History; *ICD,* International Statistical Classification of Diseases and Related Health Problems; *PE,* Physical examination; *VS,* Vital signs.
Data from multiple sources, including HealthIT.gov, accessed June 30, 2021.

must submit electronic patient data to government agencies, as well as share data across agencies, to demonstrate quality outcomes and to facilitate care coordination. "Meaningful use" requires that patients can view their records. This is an example of how new regulations directly impact the way you document.

Definition of Terms

The authors use the term *EHR* in this book, although electronic records are also known as electronic patient records, person-centered health records, or electronic medical records. Fig. 25.2 depicts a page on the EHR screen. Most of these terms initially applied to computerized records within a provider's office or agency. Although this chapter focuses on the communication aspect of HIT systems, it should also be mentioned that there are business, financial, and legal aspects. For example, HIT provides the agency with the data necessary for billing without extra effort to providers, as well as establishing legal records.

Three Keys to Electronic Record Use

The three keys to electronic records are *interoperability*, *portability*, and *ease of use*.

Interoperability (Interagency Accessibility)

Currently, there are many different versions of electronic systems in use, lacking interoperability (cross-compatibility); exchanging health information among agencies is critical to smoothly delivering comprehensive patient-centered care. Interoperability means disparate systems can "talk to each other" to share patient information. This can reduce costs by eliminating redundancy. For example, when your patient's laboratory results or imaging files are available to multiple providers, unnecessary repetition of tests or procedures can be eliminated and costs reduced. However, incompatibility of software or privacy regulations can interfere with the communication of information. According to Shah and Prabhutendolkar (2020), rapid progress is being made to facilitate interoperability

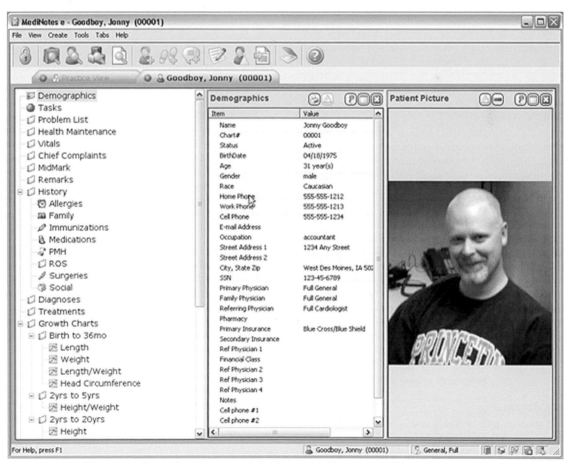

Figure 25.2 Example of an electronic health record. (Courtesy MediNotes Corporation.)

across agencies. Governments, the healthcare industry, and the insurance industry are working to enable different systems to exchange information—to "talk" to each other. In the US Office of the National Coordinator for HIT, a certification process was created to harmonize EHR products for better interoperability. The CMS lists interoperability as a minimum requirement (Stearns, 2020).

EHR data are integrated in multiple departments such as pharmacy, radiology, physical therapy, and nursing, and also across agencies. Consider the Levine case example.

Case Study: Mrs Levine's Electronic Health Records

Mrs Levine's laboratory results can be directly entered into her primary provider's EHR by an outside laboratory and then accessed by you, the nurse working in a specialty outpatient clinic. With interoperability, information flows to providers as needed, allowing seamless transitions. With interoperability, we can have anytime, anywhere access of healthcare records using remote devices. Using her home computer, Mrs Levine can access her provider's portal to read case notes and look at her lab test results, scheduling another appointment if needed.

Portability

Ideally, EHRs have portability and can follow your patient to other providers or specialists, or other hospitals, nursing homes, and so forth. Technology exists for secure storage on supercomputers in "the cloud," which would allow anytime, anywhere remote access by multiple providers (with patient permission). Electronic records are more durable than paper charting and are portable. They are easily transferable. For example, the Veterans Administration record system is fully integrated with the Department of Defense. Therefore, if a soldier is wounded abroad, diagnosed and treated, shipped home, and eventually discharged, records are seamlessly available to Veterans Administration doctors. Consider another example: you celebrate graduation by traveling across the country on vacation. If you are in a car accident and are admitted to an emergency department (ED), your records stored "in the cloud" are potentially available to the ED physician via the Internet. At the very least, you can carry them with you on a flash drive or CD.

Ease of Access

Ease of access ideally means access at the point of care or remotely using various digital devices. While maintaining record security, patients can give permission for access by multiple caregivers for anytime, anywhere communication.

However, several studies show this multiple access generates large records which may not easily allow access to specific data of immediate interest to the nurse. This 24/7 access from remote devices has markedly changed the way healthcare is practiced. Through use of Internet **portals,** patients can also access some of their health information.

HIT system barriers currently include cost, incompatible hardware and software, government privacy regulations, and most importantly, the great difficulty in keeping stored data secure. Individual related barriers include a tendency to delay entry of salient information until the end of day, which impedes the intended improved communication channel of shared view of a patient's condition across many providers (Chao, 2016).

Better Communication With Health Information Technology Use

Advantage: Improved Information Flow

A comprehensive computer information system changes the way information flows through the healthcare delivery system. Communication is streamlined rapidly. HIT can simultaneously communicate to doctors, nurses, patient, and families, and across agency departments. Continue to follow the Levine case:

Case Study: Continuation of the Levine Case Study

Mrs Levine develops trouble breathing. She is admitted via the ED to a medical unit at General Hospital at 11 a.m. with a diagnosis of congestive heart failure. Her ED physician had accessed her prior EHR, updated information, and documented his notes and her electrocardiogram (ECG) results. The ED nurse documented medications and treatments given. The HIT system flags her own physician, who comes in to examine her and enters diagnostic and treatment orders using a CPOE system. He does not need to repeat the ECG, because the system already contains these data. These orders are simultaneously and instantly transmitted to the pharmacy, the laboratory, and radiology, as well as to you, the nurse assigned on her unit.

Partnering With Patients in Documenting

In accord with making patients active partners in their healthcare, new "meaningful use" regulations require that they have access to some areas of their EHRs, allowing them to look at information or even possibly add additional data as needed. Studies repeatedly show that when patients are actively involved in decision-making about their health, they manage their illnesses better, complying with treatment protocols especially with chronic conditions. For example, Kaiser Permanente's nearly 9 million members can access their immunization records at any time from anywhere. Or through use of portals, patients can read their latest laboratory test results. We have the technology by which the patient can communicate home health–monitored data such as blood pressure, glucose level, weight, and so forth, to the primary provider's office electronically. In fact, some systems automatically input these data. Thus, the provider is immediately aware of significant changes. Use of biosensors to transmit patient generated data via Internet portals will be further described in Chapter 26.

Patient Access to Their Electronic Health Records Data

CMS rules require increasing patient access to their own records. Studies suggest access to health record information improves patient compliance (Bowen, 2021). For example, Neves et al. (2020) found access to lab results correlated with better A1c results. It has been shown that access to records improves patient engagement in the treatment process and improves their decision-making (AHRQ, 2020). Concerns expressed by nurses include increases in time/workload when patients ask about information they do not understand. Another concern is legal liability if there are inaccuracies or content upsetting to the patient.

Essentials of Nursing Documentation

Our documentation is guided by accreditation standards, third-party payers, and the legal system. Every healthcare agency has its own version of what constitutes complete clinical documentation. Medicare has published guidelines for primary providers saying documentation should include a patient history (a database that often includes a summary list of health problems and needs); physical examination findings; a description of the presenting problem; and rationales for decision-making, counseling, and coordination of care in a patient-centered care plan. Nursing documentation contains a daily record of patient progress and evaluation of outcomes. Daily records may include flow sheets, nursing notes, intake and output forms, and medication records. Some data, such as vital signs, are automatically recorded into the EHR.

Clarity

Information should flow in an efficient manner so all members of the team have access to current data, so they are able to do ongoing evaluations of treatment outcomes. Such improvements in communication lead to improved outcomes for patients. Try thinking of it this way: every task sequence you perform requires you to access data before and after completion to maintain continuity. As you chart continually, entering information into the system, communication among the health team is improved. For example, nurses making home visits can access current laboratory test results at the point of care, allowing them to discuss changes. Consider whether instant access to laboratory results on blood clotting time would allow you to contact the physician for a change in anticoagulation medication levels while you are still at your patient's home.

Clear documentation means using standardized terms that are understood by every member of the health team. Documentation of care must be accurate. For example, you are expected to document the presence on admission of catheters and intravenous lines, as well as facts about the status of any decubitus (bed sore).

Efficiency

Access time to records should be enhanced using HIT systems. For example, when using paper files, it took a lengthy time to do audits for agency quality assurance (QA) or by insurance companies verifying reimbursement.

Some literature suggests that nurses feel caught between the demands for meeting all their patient care needs and the agency requirements for complete documentation. However, the majority of evidence shows that EHRs actually save time, allowing direct care nurses more time at the bedside, especially when devices for charting are at the bedside. Concerns about documentation time may be alleviated as eventually "natural language" computers are able to use voice entry rather than typed data entry. Computerization improves the efficiency and quality of charting, by prompting for information needed, while eliminating duplication. For example, instead of requestioning patients about health history, this information is already available on their EHR. Efficiency is increased because providers all across the agency have immediate access to information. The literature lists HIT benefits that improve nursing efficiency in other "downstream" ways beyond what is apparent in documentation activities, such as medication record resolution, automatic medication calculations, automatic downloading of bedside monitoring records, automated nursing discharge summaries, and so forth. Capability to document your care from your patient's bedside or home is known as "*point of care.*"

Safety

As discussed in Chapter 2, HIT systems have made care safer. HIT systems force standardization of nursing terminology, eliminate use of inappropriate abbreviations, and avoid problems of illegibility. Errors are prevented because assistance is given with drug calculations, as well as assistance with decision support such as checking drug incompatibility, allergies, and so on. Studies of the medication process show significant reductions in errors.

Outcome Advantage: Improved Completeness of Nursing Documentation

Evidence shows EHR use results in more complete records (AHRQ, 2017). This may be due to e-prompts to nurses about including certain data; the features that download data such as vital signs automatically; the format that includes check-off boxes; the drop-down menu boxes; and the electronically generated standard interventions for each diagnosis. The Joint Commission (TJC) cautions us to be aware of patient safety risks evolving from use of technology (TJC, 2015). We need to communicate care our patient received. Timely and accurate documentation of care given is crucial to providing team members with the information they need to make informed decisions. The primary purpose of documentation is to maintain an exchange of information about the patient among all care providers *including staff nurses*. Documentation in EHRs supports the continuity, quality, and safety of your care. Quality documentation not only improves communication about the admitting diagnosis but also may increase recognition of comorbid conditions that can then also be treated.

Is it possible to fully document all nursing care given? Lack of visibility seems to be a recurring theme. Nurses report that the individualized care they give to their patients is not visible in the format demanded by the computer, especially when a checklist format is used for care. Consequently, some nurses are said to rely on "informal" communication passed along during change of shift, as well as the information on the patient's EHR. Records that are inaccurate, incomplete, or not reinforced verbally compromise clinical decisions and quality of care reporting. So we need to communicate current condition information and response to treatment both in the record and verbally.

Enhanced Quality of Care

There are many secondary uses of data contained in patient records. There has been a significant shift from rewarding quantity of care toward evaluating and rewarding quality care. For example, providers are no longer reimbursed for the number of lab tests they order, rather for interventions that improved health outcome. When masses of data are analyzed, information is generated to add to our knowledge of what care measures lead to improved and effective nursing "best practice" care.

Documentation to Demonstrate Quality Assurance

Healthcare has shifted to emphasize measurement of quality outcome indicators. Financial incentives reward evidence of clinical quality rather than volume. The United States has adopted a National Quality Strategy outlining three aims: better health care, healthier people, and more affordable care.

Reviews are done to determine the extent to which evidence-based care standards are being met. Ongoing reviews of care are done by internal agency review committees, as well as external audits by entities such as insurance companies or government regulatory bodies, such as those associated with the CMS. Assessments as to quality of care are based on what was documented and coded. Data are examined to see whether the care listed is in compliance with quality and safety guidelines and established standards of care. Clear documentation also provides evidence of effective care and outcomes during accreditation reviews. Evidence is slowly accumulating that shows HIT systems can make healthcare more patient-centered, promote better coordination of care, and make communication more effective.

Health Outcome Determinations Through Analyses of Large Datasets (Big Data)

Aggregation to Find "Best Practices"

Computerized systems offer ease of access to aggregate information from many patients for reports and disease surveillance and to research "best practice" nursing care. **Aggregated data** from a number of records can be analyzed to determine patient health outcomes. For example, information about the number of postoperative infections that have occurred on your unit can be obtained. Or you may want to find out how many diabetic patients in your primary care practice failed to return for follow-up teaching and then generate a list for call-backs for more education. HIT systems can be used to obtain reports about predictors of patient outcomes in home health care. For example, you can easily get information identifying the most effective specific nursing interventions to establish "best practice" and identify other interventions that need to be changed. By combining data, nurses identify better treatment methods and evaluate the outcomes of their interventions on groups of patients.

Timely feedback from data compilation organizations can help you to improve your practice. As an example, participation in centralized disease registries can give real-time feedback to providers, such as the users of the National Cancer Data System who can receive electronic "alerts" if best practice care is not started within a certain time frame.

Epidemiological Data

Analyses of large amounts of data show health trends, treatment outcome patterns, and disease outbreaks. For example, Furrow (2020) points out that a hospital-wide system can use an algorithm to search for hospital acquired conditions such as MRSA (medication-resistant staph infection), or an agency such as the CDC can identify disease "hot spots" such as occurred during the COVID-19 spread.

Quality Analyses

Accrediting agencies, government agencies, and private insurers use data to establish compliance with standards.

Better Outcomes. Combining data from many electronic records can identify better healthcare. Analyses of aggregated data add to our knowledge of which care measures are "best practices" leading to better patient outcomes.

Adverse Outcomes. Combining data from multiple records can also show patterns of adverse health outcomes. A classic example is when Kaiser Permanente was able to analyze information from 1.3 million patients receiving Vioxx to identify potential harm from this medication, which led to its removal from the market.

Epidemiological Trends

Combining large data sets can help public health agencies analyze information to identify disease trends to generate epidemiological information. One example would be when a government agency such as the Centers for Disease Control and Prevention analyzes the spread of influenza or COVID-19 infections across the world.

Financial Considerations

Third-party payers use electronic data to determine eligibility for reimbursement payments (Schmaltz & Barrett, 2019). Government insurance programs use Big Data to discern outcomes of care policies and practices.

Use of Computerized Provider Entry System

CPOE refers to that part of HIT in which providers such as physicians, physician assistants, nurse practitioners, or sometimes staff nurses directly enter their orders for diagnosis or treatment, which then transmits the order directly to the recipient responsible for carrying out that order, such as the pharmacy, the laboratory, or radiology. CPOE may reduce communication errors (Furrow, 2020), such as giving an alert when two incompatible medications are ordered. At a minimum, this aspect of the system ensures that orders are complete, use standard terms, and are available in a legible format. This system not only processes an order, but it also cross-compares it with data in the patient's EHR such as whether the patient is allergic to this newly ordered medication or has a potential for a drug–drug adverse interaction or whether the dose or route ordered exceeds standard guidelines for safety. CPOE may also check for errors of omission. For example, it would give a prompt about a need to also order a laboratory test to verify acceptable blood level of the new medication. CPOE systems are usually paired with computer-assisted **clinical decision support systems** (CDSSs), which are discussed in Chapter 26.

Outcomes for Use of Computerized Provider Entry. Evidence is beginning to suggest that use of these systems improves the appropriateness of orders, affects positively our communication, and improves patient outcomes, particularly by reducing adverse drug events and even increasing compliance (AHRQ, PSNet). CPOE is one of 30 "safe practices for better health care" recommended by AHRQ and the National Quality Forum. However, there is still some potential for error, such as entering data on the wrong patient. We still need to use critical thinking skills to evaluate for safe practice, especially in the area of medication administration.

Other Formats for Documenting Nursing Care

Use of structured documentation has been found to be associated with more complete nursing records, better continuity of care, more meaningful nursing data, and perhaps better patient outcomes. In charting electronically, the nurse can call up a template to record today's data.

Flow Sheets or Checklists. Electronic charting can use **flow sheets** with predefined progress parameters based on written standards with preprinted categories of information. They contain daily assessments of normal findings. For example, in assessing lung sounds, the nurse needs to merely indicate "clear" if that information is normal. Deviations from norm must be completely documented. By marking a flow sheet or checklist, you are saying all care was performed according to existing agency protocols.

Longitudinal Plan of Care

Nursing care plans are still valued by nursing instructors as a tool for student learning. However, in the age of electronic records in hospitals, clinics, and long-term care facilities, the traditional nursing care plans for each patient are being replaced by electronic **longitudinal plans of care** (LPCs). Clinical pathways stating daily patient goals have mostly either been incorporated into the EHR or been replaced by electronic prompts.

Electronic Longitudinal Plans of Care

In an effort to reduce regulations for hospitals in the United States, CMS recommends that nurses coordinate care through use of interdisciplinary care plans (replacing nursing care plans). The US Department of Health and Human Services, the national HIT office, and CMS issued a single plan of care format to assist in communication, coordination, and continuity. The plan of care needs to be accessible to all providers across all settings. Data from every discipline on the healthcare team are used to develop a single individualized interdisciplinary plan of care that sets mutual goals for each patient's progress and is documented by the nurse and other team members daily. The LPC must harmonize data requirements for home care, long-term care, and acute and postacute care; this is the patient-centered LPC.

Health Information Technology Standards: Ethical, Regulatory, and Professional

Standards of documentation must meet the requirements of government, health care agency, professional standards of practice, the use of electronic medical records, and storage of personal health information in computer databases has refocused attention on the issues of ethics, security, privacy, and confidentiality that are described earlier in this book. For example, a nurse in one unit of a hospital who accesses the electronic medical record of a patient who is in another unit and for whom the nurse has no responsibilities for care is violating confidentiality. Ethical professional practice requires that you do not allow others to use your access log on. Other ethical issues with electronically generated care plans and standard orders center on how to determine who is responsible for the computer-generated care decisions.

Confidentiality and Privacy

As discussed in earlier chapters, EHRs are subject to HIPAA confidentiality standards. **Confidentiality** is the act of limiting disclosure of private matters appropriately, maintaining the trust that an individual has placed in an agent entrusted with private matters. Electronic storage and transmission of medical records have sparked intense scrutiny over privacy protection. Many breaches have been reported in popular media. More than 70% of consumers have expressed concerns that their personal health records stored in an EHR with Internet connections will not remain private, and 89% say they withhold health information (Gordon, 2017). Indeed, experts say a breach of your health records is not a matter of whether but is a matter of when. With written permission, a patient's records can be shared with other providers via hard copy, USB thumb drives, etc.

Ethical and legal parameters limit when you can share patient information. When computers are located at the bedside, the screen displays information to anyone who

stops by the bedside. You need to be alert to this potential privacy violation. Violations of confidentiality because of unauthorized access or distribution of sensitive health information can have severe consequences for patients. It may lead to discrimination at the workplace, loss of job opportunities, or disqualification for health insurance. Personal information in health records such as Social Security numbers, home address, etc., can be used in identity theft. Issues of privacy will dominate how nurses and other healthcare providers address clinical documentation in the years ahead. Currently, a *personal medical identification number* is used on patient records, often one's Social Security number. Hardware safeguards such as workstation security, keyed lock hard drives, and automatic log-offs are used in addition to user identification and passwords to prevent unauthorized access. Some advocate that individuals be able to choose how much of their information is shared and be notified when their information is accessed. In the United States, federal law now requires patients be notified in the event of a breach of their EHR. Authorization is not needed in situations concerning the public's health, criminal, or legal matters.

Legal Aspects of Charting

Management literature emphasizes the need for quicker documentation that still reflects the nursing process. At the same time, documentation must be legally sound. The legal assumption is that the care was not given unless it is documented in the record, which is a legal document, even though it is digital (Merriweather et al., 2017). Malpractice settlements have approached the multimillion-dollar mark for individuals whose charts failed to document safe, effective care.

"If it was not charted, it was not done." This statement stems from a legal case (*Kolesar v. Jeffries*) heard before Canada's Supreme Court, in which a nurse failed to document the care of a patient on a Stryker frame before he died. Because the purpose of the medical record is to list care given and outcomes, any information that is clinically significant must be included. Aside from issues of legal liability, third-party reimbursement depends on accurate recording of care given. Major insurance companies audit records and contest any charges that are not documented. Every nurse should anticipate having their patients' records subpoenaed at some time during their nursing career.

Any method of documentation that provides comprehensive, factual information is legally acceptable. This includes graphs and checklists. By signing a protocol, check sheet, pathway, and so forth, you are documenting that every step was performed. If a protocol exists in a healthcare agency, you are legally responsible for carrying it out.

DEVELOPING AN EVIDENCE-BASED PRACTICE

Digital communication between providers and patients in increasing. This includes use of patient portals and even bedside computers in the hospital. Patient access to their own records is advocated by government. Neves (2020) did a metaanalysis of 20 studies to measure outcome, while Zanaboni (2020) examined effects on 1037 users of Norway's national health portal. A Cochrane Library Database analysis of 10 studies also examined effects of patient access to their health records (Ammenwerth, 2021).

Results

Among other finding, Neves showed that sharing EHR information with diabetic patients resulted in better controlled A1c levels. They concluded that patient access can improve safety and effectiveness in healthcare. Patients in Zanaboni's study reported increased satisfaction and perceived that they had better control over their health and easier communication with their provider. Patients in Ammenwerth's studies demonstrated slightly better compliance with risk factor monitoring. No effect, however, was demonstrated for medication adherence nor satisfaction levels. More evidence of impact on healthcare practices and on nursing is needed. Researchers do describe incidents when patients or their families are upset about nurse documentation of patient psychological state.

Strength of research evidence: Unable to establish due to conflicts in findings.

Implications for Your Clinical Practice

These studies do not specifically address nursing practice, but studies do suggest EHRs are affecting the way nurses document. Remember EHRs are legal documents. When patients have access to nursing entries, they may often have questions about items they do not understand.

1. Document facts, not opinions. Use objective assessment tools especially for mental status so you can document scores.
2. If future research continues to show patient access correlates with better treatment compliance, then encourage patients to become computer literate and to monitor their records.

References

Ammenwerth, E., Neyer, S., Hörbst, A., Mueller, G., Siebert, U., & Schnell-Inderst, P. (2021). Adult patient access to electronic health records. *Cochrane Database of Systematic Reviews, 2,* CD012707.

Neves, A. L., Freise, L., Laranjo, L., Carter, A. W., Darzi, A., & Mayer, E. (2020). Impact of providing patients access to electronic health records on quality and safety of care: A systematic review and meta-analysis. *BMJ Quality and Safety, 29*(12), 1019–1032.

Zanaboni, P., Kummervold, P. E., Sørensen, T., & Johansen, M. A. (2020). Patient use and experience with online access to electronic health records in Norway: Results of an online survey. *Journal of Medical Internet Research, 22*(2), e16144.

APPLICATIONS

Computer Literacy

One of the QSEN competencies expected of the new graduate is ability to use **informatics.** To practice nursing in coming years, you will need to continually upgrade your technology skills. As students, you learn skills such as data entry, data transmission, word processing, Internet accessing, spreadsheet entry, and use of standard language and codes describing practice. Will voice recognition software for clinical documentation make documentation easier for nurses?

Data Processing Problems

Though HIT has widespread adoption in healthcare, not all the "bugs" have been worked out. On one hand, errors occur due to overspecificity of choices, yet other problems arise from failure of IT developers to take into account the complexity required to describe nursing care and communication (Virginio & Ricarte, 2015). The complexity of nursing interventions cannot always be captured in the EHR (Ihlebaek, 2020).

Communicating Medical Orders

Written Orders

Nurses are required to question orders that they do not understand or those that seem to them to be unsafe. Failure to do so puts the nurse at *legal risk.* "Just following orders" is not an acceptable excuse. Conversely, nurses can be held liable if they arbitrarily decide not to follow a legitimate order, such as choosing to withhold ordered pain medication. Reasons for such a decision would have to be explicitly documented. With computerization, it is possible to have standing orders, such as for administering vaccines. The computer is programmed to recognize the absence of a vaccination and then to automatically write an order for a nurse to administer. What might the legal implications be?

Persons who are licensed or certified by appropriate government agencies to conduct medical treatment acts include physicians, advance practice nurses, and physician assistants.

In the United States, these providers have their own state prescribing numbers and must abide by government rules and restrictions. To prescribe controlled substances, they must also have a Drug Enforcement Agency (DEA) number. Nurse practitioners may choose not to apply for a DEA number. Consult your agency policy regarding who is allowed to write orders for the nurse to carry out.

Although electronic anytime, anywhere digital access should have replaced older communication, you may need to consider some other routes.

Faxed Orders

Occasionally, a provider may choose to send a faxed order. Because this is a form of written order, it has been shown to decrease the number of errors that occur when transcribing verbal or telephone orders. However, there is the risk for violating confidentiality when faxing health-related information.

Verbal Orders

Often, a change in condition requires the nurse to text or telephone the primary physician or hospital internist or resident to obtain new orders. Most primary providers work in group practices, so it is necessary to determine who is "on call" or who is covering your patient when the primary provider is unavailable. It may be necessary to call for new orders if there is a significant change in the physical or mental condition as noted by vital signs, laboratory value reports, treatment or medication reactions, or response failure. Before calling for orders, access the EHR and familiarize yourself with current vital signs, medications, infusions, and other relevant data. Read Chapter 2 on using the SBAR (situation, background, assessment, recommendation) format to communicate with doctors. Use of verbal orders is discouraged in an era of easy remote Internet access.

Nursing Action Problems Involving Electronic Documentation

Charting for Others

It is not acceptable to chart for others. Reflect on what you would do in the following case if you were called by Juanita Diaz, RN.

Case Study: Juanita Diaz, RN, Forgets to Chart Procedure

Juanita Diaz worked the day shift. At 6 p.m., she calls you and says she forgot to chart Mr Reft's preoperative enema. She asks you to chart the procedure and his response to it. Can you just add it to your notes? In court, this would be portrayed as an inaccuracy. The correct solution is to add an addendum to your EHR notes, "1800: Nurse Juanita Diaz called and reported …"

Workload and Work-Arounds

Nurses are trained as problem-solvers. They are constantly tinkering to improve. In their review of multiple studies. Nurses carry heavy workloads and do not like technology that disrupts or adds to their work flow. For example, "alarm fatigue" was described in Chapter 2. If nurses perceive HIT adds to their workload, they may create shortcuts to bypass aspects of the computerized system, known as "work-arounds." This raises safety concerns and may alter a system that is designed to improve safety and make it less safe (Finkel & Galvin, 2017). If we report system problems, we may work together to seek ways to improve the system.

Documenting on a Patient's Health Record

Documenting electronically requires learning the specific system at your agency. There is a learning curve; that is, initially it may take longer, but as you become familiar with each agency system, EHRs should increase your nursing efficiency. Electronic charting for nurses usually combines dropdown boxes with forced choice pick lists with free text boxes for narrative information. Keep in mind the need to use standardized terminology and, where possible, to use checklists. These allow for combining information into large data sets.

You are encouraged to document completely. Tips for documentation are listed in Table 25.2. Use the narrative box section to describe changes in your patient's outcomes. Remember that free text boxes may have word count limits. In addition, narrative comments may provide needed detail, but they may also perpetuate the electronic invisibility of nursing unless information can be captured into categories. Tips for efficient documentation include not repeating checklist information, use of autocorrect/proofreading narrative comments, checking all numbers to detect transpositions, and avoiding abbreviations.

Data Entry Errors

Sometimes there is a mismatch between technology and nursing workflow. Nurses are cautioned to avoid temptations to use input shortcuts, such as "cut and paste," which can lead to errors. Care too needs to be taken to log on and off properly, to avoid charting on the wrong patient record, or to use nonstandard terminology.

Keeping the Interpersonal While Doing Computerized Charting

Nurses have also reported reservations about unintended effects on their communication with patients. Although some individuals complain, most have adapted to providers

TABLE 25.2 Tips for Electronic Health Record Use Which Promotes a Culture of Patient Safety

Do	Do Not
Change your electronic health record (EHR) password frequently.	Avoid sharing your EHR password. Do not rush: ask for administrative time for data entry.
	Do not rush when typing data. Avoid short cuts such as "copy and paste."
Enter notes in "real time" as much as possible (chart promptly).	Avoid saving all charting until end of shift. Do not make "untimely" entries (after another shift has charted).
Maintain confidentiality (e.g., enter data in way that visitors cannot see).	For security, do not just rely on the "sleep" screen.
Verbalize a summary of what you enter at the bedside, so patient can validate.	Avoid the "cut and paste" that is a common data entry work-around.
Explain to patient the e-documentation process, letting them know they can ask questions as you enter data.	Do not speak about entries the patient could interpret negatively.
Review or mentally read back crucial data you have entered. Do document any ordered care which was omitted and state the rationale.	Verify unclear outcomes by speaking to the patient.
Make eye contact periodically.	Try not to depersonalize, by ignoring patient as you type.
Document progress: all changes in patient condition, any bizarre behavior.	Do not fail to record any ordered care which is omitted and who was notified.
Verbally reinforce crucial info with staff, even though you entered it into patient's record.	Do not let confusing information in the record stand unremarked.
Participate in all offered e-training updates.	
Correct errors per agency protocol, usually by adding addendum to your notes, listing correct info with explanation.	Avoid using "soft" or "hard" delete.

who spend time not making eye contact or pausing the dialog because they are busy typing data into the EHR. According to HealthIT (ONC, 2019), 74% of patients report that EHRs have enhanced their care. How would you manage communication rapport during an interview, when the HIT system keeps prompting you to obtain data?

Make documenting at the bedside warmer in a human relation sense. If your patient seems to be bothered by the lack of interpersonal contact while you are busy typing on the bedside computer, what steps could you take? One suggestion is to face the computer terminal toward the patient, so you do not turn your back while typing information. Some nurses comment aloud about the general information they are inputting, stopping every minute or so to make eye contact with their patient. Asking for information and then typing it in may make them realize they are actively contributing to

their EHR information. In addition, explaining about how these entries are keeping the team aware of updated information about the patient's condition may help them to value this process.

Classification Systems

Coding

Coding allows nursing information to be easily communicated and extracted from EHRs for the purpose of compiling information to make cross-comparisons: evaluations, audits, research, or develop standards of care. A prerequisite for this was to move nursing terminology to a standard taxonomy. It is crucial to nursing that nursing terminologies become embedded into EHRs, both to improve communication between nurses, such as at change of shift, and to allow data to be extracted to describe nursing care. Fig. 25.3 depicts reasons for coding.

Coding Nursing Practice Provides Information:

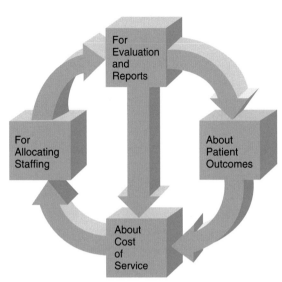

Figure 25.3 Coding in nursing practice.

Use of Standardized Terminologies and Taxonomies

The nursing profession was very active in developing standardized terminology, an essential element of EHRs. The International Council of Nurses (ICN) developed a unified nursing language system, the International Classification for Nursing Practice (ICNP). As nurses, our goal is to classify the care provided and document outcomes of care, to effectively communicate. Global adoption requires adequate translation into local languages, a difficult task.

In the past, nursing has been unable to describe the units of care and its effect on patient outcome or to establish a cost for its contributions to patient care. Nowhere on one's hospital bill does the cost of our nursing care appear. It traditionally has been part of the "room charge." Our goal in developing standardized terminology and classification codes is not only to improve communication but also to make nursing practice visible within computerized health information systems and to assist in establishing evidence-based nursing practice. Currently, little of nursing classification has been incorporated into HIT.

Taxonomies: Standardized Language Terminology in Nursing

Taxonomy is defined as a hierarchical method of classifying a vocabulary of items according to certain rules. For example, the Bloom taxonomy was used to develop chapter learning objectives. The ANA recognizes a number of different taxonomies for describing nursing care, based on specific criteria. Because no one system meets the needs of nurses in all areas of practice, technological applications are needed to communicate across classification systems. The North American Nursing Diagnosis Association International (NANDA-I) is the best researched and most widely implemented nursing classification internationally. The N3 terminologies (NANDA-I, Nursing Interventions Classification [NIC], and Nursing Outcomes Classification [NOC]), used together to plan and document nursing care, are sometimes referred to as **NNN.** Other nursing coding systems include the Omaha System designed for use in the community. Simulation Exercise 25.1 gives practice in using nursing data.

Other Coding Systems in Healthcare

Medical Classification Systems

The National Library of Medicine maintains a metathesaurus for a unified medical language. Reflecting the complexity of healthcare, multiple medical classification systems have emerged. Often providers use several in combination.

SIMULATION EXERCISE 25.1   Application of Nursing Data

Purpose
Practice making use of aggregated data.

Procedure
Reflect on these sample data compiled from EHRs on one medical unit, and then answer the questions.

On day 2 of hospitalization, nurses averaged four intravenous therapy interventions for patients with a diagnosis of hip fracture but averaged only two interventions for (oral) fluid management.

1. How could you use this information to justify the need for skilled nursing care?
2. Suppose data showed that by day 4, skilled care activities had been cut in half. How might the nurse manager readjust the patient assignment for her UPAs (nurse aides)?

On day 3, patients with hip fractures received three times as many nursing interventions encouraging proper coughing as were made for patients with colitis.

1. If the hospital units with more nursing interventions to encourage coughing were shown to have greatly decreased rates of patients with pneumonia complications. Could this information be used to justify a better nurse-to-patient ratio?
2. Reflect on how nationally aggregated data could identify outcomes leading to better nursing practice.

Examples of common medical classification and coding systems include 10th revision of the *International Statistical Classification of Diseases and Related Health Problems (ICD-10)* codes for medical diagnoses by body system; ICD-10-PCS codes for medical procedures; SNOMED CT (a disease management terminology similar to ICD), and the fifth edition of the *Diagnostic and Statistical Manual of Mental Disorders* (DSM-5) diagnoses for psychiatric conditions. Health Care Financing Administration's (HCFA) Outcome and Assessment Information Set (OASIS) assessment for the purpose of describing home care patients, developing outcome benchmarks, and providing feedback regarding quality of care to home health agencies. The OASIS assessment is required for home health agencies to receive reimbursement for the care provided to Medicare recipients. To learn more, visit HCFA's Medicare website (www.medicare.gov/).

SUMMARY

This chapter focuses on electronic documentation of care in the nurse–patient relationship as a major aspect of communication. Documentation refers to the process of obtaining, organizing, and conveying information to others in the patient record. The broad aspects of health information systems, as well as the nurse's role in using EHRs, were discussed. Emphasis on EHR's role in reducing redundancy, improving efficiency, reducing cost, decreasing errors, and improving compliance with standards of practice was stressed. The many secondary uses of compilations of electronic records for generation of knowledge were described, especially those which identify nursing care "best practice" outcomes. Classification systems were briefly described. Chapter 26 discusses eMobile technology that can facilitate communication among healthcare workers, increase patient education, increase engagement, and assist the providers of healthcare with decision-making.

ETHICAL DILEMMA: What Would You Do?

A coworker mentions that a staff nurse you both know, Alice Jarvis, RN, has been admitted to the medical floor for some strange symptoms and that her laboratory results have just been posted in her EHR, showing she is positive for hepatitis C, among other things.

1. Identify at least two alternative ways to deal with this ethical dilemma. (What response would you make to your coworker who retrieved information from the computerized system? What else might you do?)

From Sonya R. Hardin, RN, PhD, CCRN.

DISCUSSION QUESTIONS

1. Explain why "use of technologies to assist in effective communication in a variety of health care settings" is listed as an expected nurse competency by QSEN and other nursing organizations.
2. Documentation is an important aspect in your nursing. Of the reasons to document, determine the one of greatest concern to the novice nurse. Defend your selection.

REFERENCES

Agency for Healthcare Quality and Research (AHRQ). (2017). *Teams, TeamSTEPPs and team structures: Models for functional collaboration*. [Webinar]. Retrieved from https://www.ahrq.gov/teamstepps/webinars/index.html#2017. [Accessed 30 June 2021].

Agency for Healthcare Research and Quality (AHRQ). (2020). *Digital healthcare research: 2019 year in review*. Retrieved from https://digital.ahrq.gov/sites/default/files/docs/page/2019-year-in-review.pdf/. [Accessed 30 June 2021].

Bowen, R. (2021). *Patient access: Road to compliance*. [Webinar]. MRO. Retrieved from https://mrocorp.com/blog/webinar-recap-patient-access-and-the-road-to-compliance/. [Accessed 30 June 2021].

Chao, C. A. (2016). The impact of electronic health records on collaborative work routines: A narrative network analysis. *International Journal of Medical Informatics*, *94*, 100–111.

Finkel, N., & Galvin, H. (2017). Electronic Health Records: Medication decision support for inpatient medicine. *Hospital Medicine Clinics*, *6*(2), 204–215.

Furrow, B. R. (2020). The limits of current A.I. in health care: Patient safety policing in hospitals. *Northeastern University Law Review*, *12*(1), 1–55.

Gordon, L. T. (2017). Connecting consumers to their health information. *Journal of AHIMA*, *88*(3), 13.

Ihlebaek, H. M. (2020). Lost in translation – silent reporting and electronic patient records in nursing handovers: An ethnographic study. *International Journal of Nursing Studies*, *109*, 103636.

Merriweather, K., Slater, L., & Bohley, M. (2017). CDI in the outpatient setting: Finding the "hidden gems" of opportunity for improvement. *Journal of AHIMA*, *88*(7), 48–51.

National Academies of Science, Engineering, and Medicine. (2021). *The future of nursing 2020–2030: Charting a path to achieve health equity*. Washington, D.C.: The National Academies Press.

Neves, A. L., Freise, L., Laranjo, L., Carter, A. W., Darzi, A., & Mayer, E. (2020). Impact of providing patients access to electronic health records on quality and safety of care: A systematic review and meta-analysis. *BMJ Quality and Safety*, *29*(12), 1019–1032.

Office of the National Coordinator for Health Information Technology (ONC). (2019). *What information does an electronic health record (EHR) contain?* HealthIT.gov. Retrieved from https://www.healthit.gov/faq/what-information-does-electronic-health-record-ehr-contain. [Accessed 2 July 2021].

QSEN Institute. (n.d.). *Quality and safety education for nurses.* Retrieved from www.QSEN.org/.

Rudin, R. S., Friedberg, M. W., Shekelle, P., Shah, N., & Bates, D. W. (2020). Getting value from electronic health records: Research needed to improve practice. *Annals of Internal Medicine, 172*(11 Suppl. l), S130–S136.

Schmaltz, S., & Barrett, S. (2019). *Electronic health record data still limited in publicly reported risk factors.* The Joint Commission. Retrieved from https://www.jointcommission .org/resources/news-and-multimedia/blogs/improvement-insights/2019/06/electronic-health-record-data-still-limited-in-publicly-reported-risk-factors/. [Accessed 30 June 2021].

Shah, D., & Prabhutendolkar, S. (2020). Forging ahead with interoperability amid a pandemic. *Journal of AHIMA.* Retrieved from https://journal.ahima.org/forging-ahead-with-interoperability-amid-a-pandemic/. [Accessed 30 June 2021].

Stearns, M. (2020). Quality payment program 2020: Changes and requirements. Part III: MIPS promoting interoperability performance category in 2020. *Journal of AHIMA,* 22–29.

The Joint Commission (TJC). (2015). *Sentinel event alert 54: Safe use of health information.* Retrieved from https://www.jointcommission.org/-/media/tjc/documents /resources/patient-safety-topics/sentinel-event/sea_54_hi-t_4_26_16.pdf. [Accessed 30 June 2021].

U.S. Department of Health and Human Services. (n.d.). *Health IT. Healthy people 2030.* Retrieved from https://health.gov/he althypeople/objectives-and-data/browse-objectives/health-it. [Accessed 2 July 2021].

Virginio, L. A., Jr., & Ricarte, I. L. M. (2015). Identification of patient safety risks associated with electronic health records: A software quality perspective. *Studies in Health Technology and Informatics, 216,* 55–59.

26

Mobile-Health and Communication Technology

OBJECTIVES

At the end of the chapter, the reader will be able to:

1. Discuss the advantages and disadvantages of various technologies for continual communication at point of care, as well as anytime, anywhere access.
2. Apply clinical guidelines and clinical decision support systems to a case, demonstrating increased efficiency in delivery of safe, quality healthcare.
3. Analyze strengths and weaknesses of various health technologies in improving nurse–patient communications and facilitating patient self-management.

Advances in technology continue to revolutionize healthcare through digital communication. In most countries, mobile devices are essential healthcare tools (Mauzey, 2020). Everywhere, including in developing countries, Mobile-Health (m-Health) has changed how healthcare workers deliver care. This chapter will focus on use of mobile Internet access devices ("smart" devices) as an essential nursing competency. Smartphone applications with biomedical sensors are becoming widely used by patients to communicate with health providers. Nurses are playing a part in changing the focus from illness care to healthcare. We employ the latest in technology to communicate with other providers and with patients. "Smart" devices are used at the point of care, be it hospital bedside or in our patient's home. Tablets and smartphones are becoming indispensable for engaging our patients in their own healthcare for health promotion and self-management. Mobile devices and voice-activated systems allow continual real-time interactive communication of information, customized clinical decision-making, and *decentralized, remote access* to information at the point of care. Technology that has easy access enhances our work flow through expanded use of devices, which input data automatically, provide "alerts," improve feedback, and enable us to give remote care via telehealth (Odendaal et al., 2020). Since our focus is nurse communication, we describe pertinent e-Mobile technology concepts. Changes are happening so rapidly, new specific applications are constantly emerging.

BASIC CONCEPTS

Definition

The term *mobile health care* (*m-Health*) can mean the use of any wireless device and its downloaded health-related applications (Apps). These use the Internet and are independent of location.

Incidence. Globally, the majority of the world's 7 billion people have access to Internet devices, with over 200 billion "smart" devices in use. Seventy-seven percent of American adults use smartphones, including more than 75% of teenagers (Bianco et al., 2021).

Communication Facilitation

Evidence shows that technologies facilitate our communication and teamwork to provide more effective, safe care. Ideally, we work to establish fully integrated computerized systems that share information across the entire healthcare system. Globally, care focus is shifting toward engaging persons in their own care. Technology helps us shift from providing just "sick" care to a "preventative" mode.

Handheld Internet devices are small enough to be easily carried. Their Internet access is termed "wireless." Decentralized access to information and ability to document your care at your patient's location are referred to as **"point-of-care"** capability. You can use your smartphone or tablet to access nursing information databases to obtain evidence-based clinical care interventions. You document at the "point of care" either at your patients' bedsides or in their homes, as in the Sulif case.

CASE STUDY: Mrs Sulif Is Admitted to the Hospital

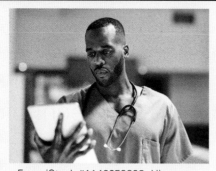

From iStock #1146652828, Hiraman.

Sam Esteves, RN, is employed by Medical Center on a medical unit. This hospital is part of a large healthcare system of primary care offices, clinics, laboratories, nursing homes, and three hospitals, all of which use the fully integrated computer system affectionately termed "Simon." Sam is notified at 0800 that his new patient, Mrs Sulif, is in admissions getting her bar-coded name bracelet with her photo image affixed to it. In admissions, she is entering her own history information into a "Simon"-affiliated tablet, which has also scanned and uploaded her history from her own smart card into her EHR. Dietary is flagged because she has nut allergies. Preadmission laboratory results are already in her EHR, having been uploaded by a lab tech, who notes the system has flagged her low hematocrit results and sent an "alert" to Sam and her admitting physician's office. Sam is also advised as to her need for handicapped-accessible equipment. On the unit by 0845, a robot has delivered equipment to the room, while Sam has summoned a patient care technician by text to help lift Mrs Sulif into bed wearing linen stored right in her room (refer to Transforming Care at the Bedside [TCAB]). Sam reviews the reason for admission, discusses her history with Mrs Sulif, and enters additional information at the bedside using his tablet, correcting some minor misinformation. Dr Chi, the intensivist physician, arrives to examine her. Dr Chi enters his orders into the computerized provider order entry (CPOE) system, which simultaneously notifies the lab and pharmacy. Sam then prints out bar-coded labels with Mrs Sulif's identity number, sending off urine for analysis. He then checks for robot delivery of her STAT meds, which he administers after scanning her name band and double verifying her name orally. Sam uses his tablet to find the latest clinical guidelines associated with Mrs Sulif's diagnosis.

1. How is the care described so far both safe and efficient?
2. What additional steps could make care safer or more efficient?
3. When it is time for her discharge and follow-up by a home health nurse, what other communication should occur?

Technology, especially eMobile devices with Apps, has revolutionized the way we communicate healthcare information (Wilson et al., 2021). eMobile devices promote greater patient control of their own care, potentially improving health outcomes. Patients are using more technology for education, self-monitoring, and support. Use of smart devices and Apps has revolutionized the way we use healthcare information (Wilson et al., 2021).

Apps

There are thousands of health Apps (application programs) for mobile devices. Apps can track patient physical states and health-related behaviors. Caution is needed since the vast majority of these are not medically approved. Providers use technology to communicate with patients and encourage patients to engage in self-care. As nurses, what interventions can we adopt to increase patient engagement?

Decentralized Access: Technology for Communicating at the Point of Care

Wireless technology extends into the patient's home, helping achieve a *Healthy People 2030* goal to increase the proportion of people who communicate with their healthcare providers over the Internet (U.S. Department of Health and Human Services, n.d.).

Nurses believe that technology should be designed to reduce the burden associated with work flows in documentation, medication administration, communication, implementing orders, and obtaining equipment and supplies. Nurses also say it is essential to have smart, portable, point-of-care devices to document and transmit information. But this technology must be user friendly, function well, and not add to existing workload or nurses will be dissatisfied. For technology to be effective and congruent with nursing expectations, nurses need to seek input into software design. If use is cumbersome, nurses will devise workarounds so they can

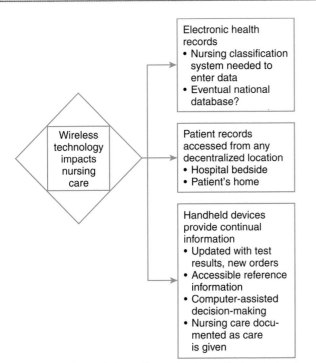

Figure 26.1 Health information technology: wireless technology impacts nursing care.

complete their assigned care in a timely manner. Some work-arounds are potentially unsafe, as described in Chapter 2.

"Smart" devices allow nurses decentralized access to patient records, incorporating point-of-care information and documentation. Mobile wireless devices allow continual use of updated information and reference material at any patient location. Communication in a timely manner is a standard of effective communication. Communication in "real time" is the hallmark of bedside nursing in the age of technology. Refer to Fig. 26.1 for a graphic diagram of HIT. With fiscal cutbacks, fewer nurses per patient, and increased acuity of conditions, use of technology can enhance our critical thinking, clinical decision-making, and delivery of safe, efficient care.

Information Collection

Information can be stored and sent to your agency computer or directly to a printer. You can update your patient's records including history, your assessment, the problem list, or other data and nursing notes. Your wireless device can also be used to track information such as a patient's medications and dosages or laboratory test results in a flow sheet format. For example, a nurse practitioner using a handheld device can call up previous prescriptions, renew them at a touch, record this new information in the agency server, correctly calculate the dosage of a new medication, write the order, and send this prescription to the patient's pharmacy instantly—all without writing anything on paper.

m-Health Devices

Smartphones

Smartphones represent the convergence of cellular phones and complex computers.

Resources. In addition to making calls, they enable you to download and access information resources; use healthcare Apps; provide Internet access to patient information (new laboratory results or physician orders); and do texting/instant messaging (IM). Some downloaded apps provide alerts by beeping when there are new orders or newly available test results.

Decision Support. Smartphones may have computer-assisted decision support systems. For example, downloadable Apps for drug programs not only provide drug information but, when you type in patient information such as age, weight, and diagnosis, they provide you with guidelines for correct dosage, contraindications, and side effects. New information alerts are sent to your device in a timely manner. Guidelines for best practice can also be downloaded to smartphones.

Tablets and Laptop Computers

Laptop computers are more powerful than tablets, yet both are still small and portable enough to be taken into the patient's hospital room or home. Uses of tablets to chart and to transmit and receive data are described throughout this book. Try Simulation Exercise 26.1 for practice in using SBAR format on your mobile device.

Mobile Health Monitoring Systems

Apps for Healthcare Providers

Apps useful to nursing care are available in IOS and Android operating systems. Downloadable protocols are available from the government and from most professional nurse organizations, as well as private for-profit companies. Using free, downloadable apps and guides for care, you can search by age, sex, and risk factors Most hospitals and larger agencies have resident experts, such as medical librarians or clinical nurse specialists, to help nurses access information about evidence-based care guidelines.

Apps for Individuals in the Community

As mentioned, there are an incredible number of Apps available. Search your favorite App store. Most of these are of interest to individuals rather than vectors to enhance patient–nurse communication.

Mobile Health Apps for Patients. Digital devices are perfect for anytime, anywhere learning. Because tablets and smartphones have mobility, available health Apps have become common. They provide effective communication at minimal cost. Try downloading one App for monitoring your diet. Do you use a wearable wrist device to monitor your exercise?

Disease-Specific Apps. One example of such an App is mySugr, designed for providers caring for patients with

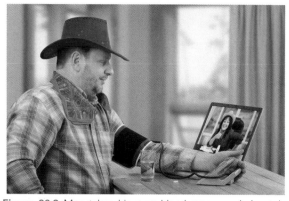

Figure 26.2 Man takes his own blood pressure during tele-health appointment. (Copyright © verbaska_studio/iStock/Thinkstock.)

diabetes mellitus. Check your App Store for disease related programs.

The trend is to skip Internet access issues and charges to go to use of high-technology phones.

Apps for Communication With Nurse or Physician

A number of monitoring devices have Apps that monitor vital signs such as blood pressure as demonstrated by the man in the cowboy hat in Fig. 26.2. There are sensor pads that, when touched, use algorithms to monitor your blood pressure. Apps can also monitor glucose levels, electroencephalograms, oxygen levels, etc. Some devices have attachments which enhance the remote provider's ability to examine the patient, such as stethoscopes. Other sensors can obtain and transmit ultrasounds, image organs, or obtain electrocardiograms.

Biomedical Sensors

Wearable Biomedical Sensors. These sensors can detect and treat some diseases as well as monitoring patient's health status (Surantha et al., 2021) and detect and measure patient activities. Wearable sensors monitor for patient lack of movement to detect falls or recognize epileptic seizures. They monitor for increased tremors in diseases such as Parkinson's (Ozanne et al., 2018). Other sensors can be embedded into pills to monitor whether a patient has taken his prescribed medication (Journal of AHIMA Staff, 2017).

Data Analysis. Algorithms receive then analyze copious input data, notifying a healthcare professional when there is an anomaly. What roles do you see evolving for nurse–patient communication as all these data accumulate?

In-Hospital Technology to Enhance Work Flow

Remote Site Monitoring, Diagnosis, Treatment, and Communication

Technological innovations can help make our care more efficient. Formerly, staff nurses in hospitals spent less than 40% of their day in actual patient care and spent at least 25% of their time walking to answer phones, obtain charts, gather supplies, locate other staff, and so on. Nurses can now use new technology systems to improve their work flow and allow them more time at the bedside!

Hands-Free Communication: Voice-Activated Systems

Voice-activated communication systems use wearable, hands-free devices that use the existing wireless network to support instant voice communication and messaging among staff within an agency. The nurse wears a small, lightweight badge that permits one-button voice access to other users of the system. It also will connect to the telephone system. One example is Vocera. It is said to reduce the time for key communications, such as looking for the medication keys, looking for others (a 45% reduction), paging doctors, or walking to the nursing station telephone (a 25% reduction). Nurses report that voice-activated communication results in fewer interruptions, promotes better continuity of care, and improves their work flow.

In-Hospital Biomedical Monitoring

When the point of care is at the hospital bedside, several of the technologies already mentioned, such as noninvasive automatic recording of vital signs, wireless telemetry, or the use of "smart" beds with sensors, automatically transmit and upload data into the patient's EHR. In another example, telemetry sensors might monitor information such as whether nurses wash hands. Or you might receive a signal if a patient falls and does not get up.

Radio Frequency Identity Smart Technology

Information can also be communicated to providers via data transmitted by **radio frequency identity (RFID) chips** or sensors inside our identification cards that we wear or have implanted. If we need to locate a member of our team, such sensors assist in tracking that doctor or other team member. Staff nurses walk hundreds of miles a year trying to locate and gather equipment and supplies they need to carry out their bedside care. RFID technology could instantly locate equipment, such as a needed infusion pump stored in the supply room. Perhaps robots will then deliver needed supplies to you! In a large review of this topic, Ajami and Rajabzadeh (2013) concluded that RFID technology needs to be integrated into an agency's health information technology system (HIT) to best reduce clinical and medication errors.

Computer-Mediated Communication in the Community

Radio Frequency Identification Chips

Lots of us have chips implanted into our pets so they can be located if lost. Is it ethical to implant similar devices into Alzheimer's patients who wander or others who are unable to function without supervision? Families are using sensors (tiles or chips) at home to monitor for potential problems (such as a serious fall) or a health crisis (such as an epileptic seizure).

Telehealth

Definition. **Telehealth**, also called eHealth in England, is changing the way healthcare is delivered. Telehealth is a general term for any real-time interactive use of Internet technology and information for delivery of healthcare across a distance (HRSA, 2021). In our definition, telehealth involves a prescheduled appointment with your regular healthcare provider, across a distance into your location.

Incidence. According to Schwenk (2021), virtual healthcare contacts are replacing many in-person visits and are becoming the new norm. There are approximately 3 billion smartphones globally. Technology has so improved that smartphones or tablets with Internet access are all that is needed for diagnosing and treating illnesses (ATA, 2021). Telehealth technology allows multiple providers in one visit, use of virtual translators, and ease of access, eliminating patient travel to seek care. Advanced practice nurses can monitor diagnostic and lab tests and assess for physiological changes remotely even for patients requiring intensive care. For the nurse using telehealth, clinical skill expertise and communication skills are indispensable. Security can be a concern if the provider is using social media platforms rather than secure sites. Fig. 26.3 shows a cartoon depicting a telehealth appointment.

Outcomes. Studies show positive outcomes including reductions in hospital admissions and in the number of home visits, increased patient and provider satisfaction, and

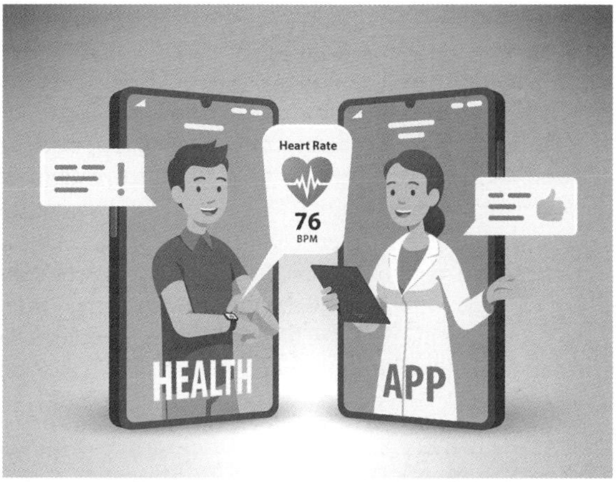

Figure 26.3 Patient talking to nurse practitioner during a video call with his smartphone App recording and sending his heart rate data. (From iStock #1224142396, IconicBestiary.)

similar health outcomes as compared with face-to-face visits. Studies tend to show telehealth decision-making, and diagnosing improves health outcomes with no difference between face-to-face encounters and remote intervention (Gonçalves-Bradley et al., 2020). Telepsychiatric encounters show better outcomes than occur with in-person visits. Telehealth originated at health facilities, but now telehealth often originates from the patient's home using cameras in smartphones.

E-Visits in Healthcare

Definition. In our definition, an e-visit is a one-time contact with a provider to deal with an acute health concern. A patient logs on, fills out a history questionnaire about their symptoms, and receives a return contact from a provider.

Incidence. E-visits are gaining in popularity. Often, a contact URL is offered by one's insurance company as it is more economical than an emergency department visit. Many sites such as "Doctor on Demand" exist.

E-visits offer opportunities for diagnosis, treatment, and monitoring of patient status via Internet portals. This makes care more affordable and convenient. Information is exchanged across geographic distances and is often used for specialist consultations. Technology may allow the distant consultant to manipulate an ophthalmoscope attachment to assess retinas or to use a stethoscope attachment to auscultate breath sounds. Use of this communication technology is commonplace, greatly accelerating during the recent pandemic.

Outcomes. Although study results are mixed, the majority show use of this technology reduces hospitalizations, increases quality of care and patient satisfaction, decreases emergency department visits, and decreases healthcare costs. Virtual contacts eliminate travel costs, childcare costs, and time off work costs for patients. According to the American Telemedicine Association (2021), more than 80% of patients report satisfaction with the virtual care they received. Use barriers are legal, such as privacy concerns, and financial costs. Especially since the onset of the pandemic, third-party payers such as Medicaid and Medicare Services have provided reimbursement even for annual well visits (Reeves et al., 2021).

Most studies do not differentiate type of virtual encounter. Generally, e-visits have been shown to resolve problems 86% of the time, with an average time of a visit being 3 min. While some patients prefer to be in contact with their own provider, some like the convenience of e-visits. Reflect on the case of Mr Dakota.

Case Study: Mr Dakota Uses Telehealth Technology

Jim Dakota, age 69 years, runs Eagleview, a bed and breakfast business in rural South Dakota. He recently was discharged after bowel surgery in a hospital 3 hours away. Instead of closing his business and traveling 3 hours to the medical center, he is able to self-manage his wound healing by taking "selfie" photos of his wound to send to his nurse, allowing the nurse to provide guidance and monitor for complications remotely.

Computerized Clinical Decision Support Systems

Decision Support System Information to Assist Critical Thinking and Decision-Making

An important asset of HIT adoption is the provision of computerized **clinical decision support systems (CDSS)**. CDSSs are cloud-based information programs designed to assist your decision-making. You input your patient information and the database provides you with patient-specific care guidelines. This is intended to enhance the quality and safety of your care. CDSS is often integrated with order entry systems in the hospital, but versions can be available to nurses working in the community. Key CDSS issues are speed and ease of access. CDSSs are useful but, of course, do not take the place of your own clinical critical thinking. The following case about Mrs Sanchez is an example of how this technology is designed to assist us to deliver better and safer nursing care more efficiently.

Case Study: Mrs Sanchez and Gail Myer, RN

Gail Myer, RN, is assigned to Mrs Sanchez as one of her eight patients on an obstetrical unit. Mrs Sanchez is in preterm labor. Gail's CDSS automatically lists desired patient outcomes based on her work assignment, lists "best practice" interventions, and then gives real-time feedback about outcomes. Her tablet receives electronic prompts to assist in clinical decision-making. For example, the hospital's CDSS program calculates expected delivery date for Mrs Sanchez and supplies the correct dose of the prescribed medication based on her weight. It alerts Gail if the prescribed dose she intends to administer exceeds maximum standard safety margins, and also cross-checks this new drug for potential drug interactions with the drugs Mrs Sanchez is already taking. It pops up a screening tool for Gail to use to assess Mrs Sanchez's current status and then alerts Gail if she should forget to document today's results.

1. What parts of this CDSS would you find most helpful?

The more-sophisticated CDSS systems give interactive advice after comparing entries of your data with a computerized knowledge base. The information offered to you is personalized to your patient's condition (filtered) and is offered at appropriate times in your workday.

Since the National Academies of Science, Engineering and Medicine (formerly IOM) and the Canadian Institutes of Health Research began advocating CDSS programs or supporting research into CDSS effect on patient care, the suggested types of data in the CDSS system have come to include the following:

- Diagnosis and care information displays with care management priorities listed
- A method for communication, that is, for order entry and for entering data (system offers prompts so you enter complete data; offers smart or model forms)
- Automatic checks for drug–drug, drug–allergy, and drug–formulary interactions
- Ability to send reminders to patients according to their stated preference
- Medication reconciliations and summary of care at transitions of patient care
- Ability to send electronic alerts or prompts if problems occur or you have not acknowledged receipt of information, such as the patient's laboratory test results

The hardware can be computer terminals on your hospital unit or wireless handheld devices anywhere. A software database can be information residing in the agency server or a central repository such as a disease registry or government database.

For the nurse, some CDSS software can generate specific information for your particular patient, including assessment guidelines and forms, analyses of their laboratory test results, and use of best practice protocols to make specific recommendations for safe care. Ideally, this is integrated into the EHR system your agency is using. Ease of use is crucial. Studies continue to show that the majority of time, staff nurses still prefer to rely on colleagues to validate their decisions.

Based on input about your patient's current condition, the CDSS is programmed to provide you with appropriate reminders or prompts. For example, after you complete care for your first assigned patient, specific information is presented to you if you have not yet documented a needed intervention. This assists you in preventing treatment errors or omissions, helps improve your documentation, and may speed up the time to intervention. More timely interventions should lead to fewer patient complications. Our central focus remains patient-centered care, so we include our patient's preferences in our clinical decisions.

Outcomes of Computerized Clinical Decision Support Systems. CDSS technology is slowly being adopted. Early systems were stand-alone, but technology is rapidly advancing, leading to more user-friendly systems integrated into HIT to provide timely, relevant content. Because the system stores your information about your activity, you can, for example, obtain reports about your overall compliance with standards of care or provide data for research.

Safer Care. In Chapter 2, we noted that IOM attributed over 70% of healthcare errors to poor communication. Constant improvements to our electronic healthcare technologies are geared to improving the flow of communication, increasing safety, and improving the quality of our care. Reviewers who analyzed more than 15,000 articles concluded that the evidence is *strong* that CDSS use effectively improves health outcomes on a range of measures for patients in diverse settings.

Alerts. The literature shows mixed results when reminders or alerts are sent. Nurses have been found to be more likely to chart when an electronic reminder is received. Patients respond positively to reminders such as texts and to CDSS coaching about their self-care.

Clinical Practice Guidelines: Access to Online Information

By standardizing interventions based on outcome evidence, practice guidelines promote quality and safety. Nurses have the opportunity to search databases when they need information, using computers or smartphones. Clinical practice guidelines need to be easily accessible, usable in your daily practice, with content from trusted, credible sources. Clinical guideline databases should allow input from you about your patient, and then provide customized clinical decision guidance. Clinical databases have been systematically developed to provide appropriate care recommendations for your patient's specific diagnoses based on available research evidence.

Patient Engagement With m-Health Opportunities
Mobile Nurse–Patient Healthcare Communication

Mobile technology has not only changed the way we document, it now provides communication resources which we can use for patient education. This information can be specifically tailored for each individual patient.

To review technologies involved in nurse–patient communication, we mention the following.

Email. Email can be a convenient, rapid, inexpensive method of communicating between providers and patients. Yet, while most patients express a desire to communicate with their healthcare providers via email, not all providers choose to do so, citing concerns about confidentiality, malpractice, and time factors. Instead, professionals and agencies use secure patient **portals**. Some practices require signed patient permission to use their portal. Read the case about Ms Trooper.

Case Study: Elsie Trooper, RN

Ms Trooper RN, an office nurse, uses the patient's individual's portal for posting test results, providing prescription refills or sending health reminders. She also texts appointment reminders. For example, she tracks the response of patients who are on new medication, instead of waiting until their next office appointment.

Texting: Secure Instant Messaging. Text IM is commonly used in daily life. Secure IMs can be used to improve communications between members of the health team or between patients and providers. For example, you want to request an additional pain medication from the resident on call. (You recognize, however, that you are not supposed to accept texted orders back.) IM can be used by patients to communicate self-monitored information to their care provider. In the aforementioned case, Ms Trooper could text reminders to monitor blood glucose today to her patient.

Technology for Patient Health Self-Management
Patient Disease Management: Gaining Information

The government is encouraging patients to access their electronic health records, using portals and even smartphone Apps to improve engagement in their healthcare (U.S. Department of Health and Human Services, 2020).

Online learning has been found to be as effective as traditional learning. Most people have searched the Internet for health information, using one of the many consumer health information sites. There is strong potential for improved health learning associated with interactive computer teaching programs.

Patient Disease Management: Recording Data

Active participation is said to increase the likelihood of producing positive health outcomes. Surveys show consumers hold positive attitudes toward use of technology including m-Health Apps. Patients can use Apps to record glucose levels, dietary intake, sleep deprivation, etc. The Agency for Healthcare Research and Quality's analysis of 146 studies on the impact of computer health modules on outcomes found that these programs succeeded in engaging patient attention, but more significantly they improved health. Just as studies have documented positive health outcomes after telephone support from nurses, contact with providers using interactive computer programs for health education or to provide answers to illness-related questions leads to positive health outcomes.

Lifestyle Management

Can you cite an example of use of devices and websites to increase patient knowledge about health promotion? Information about health conditions has been shown to positively impact outcomes. What is the role of nurses in recommending reliable Internet sites to patents?

Other Technology for Assisting Patients in Self-Management

Portal Technology to Assist Patients to Communicate and to Self-Manage

Portals are HIPAA-secure software gateways interfacing with a patient's EHR information, giving providers and patients a shared view of that patient's health. Portals can be "view only" or they can be "interactive." Patients have continuous *access to their health information,* such as immunizations or lab results.

More-sophisticated interactive portals allow the patient to pay bills, to record and share results of their home monitoring, to access the status of their insurance claims, and to schedule appointments. They also provide a mechanism for secure texting between patient and providers, and for downloading personalized health information or requesting prescription refills. Studies report highest patient use occurs in viewing lab tests, making appointments, and viewing visit summaries. Providers use portals to send reminders about appointments. They are important for care coordination and allow us to give self-management support to patients. Insurance and pharmaceutical companies have portals that provide consumer and healthcare provider access to drug information. Some agencies ask patients to preregister for a health/illness visit, asking a series of questions about their condition. Potentially their care provider could make a diagnosis, order treatment, write a progress note in the EHR, and reply to the patient, as in the Mr Williams case. This not only decreases use of staff time to answer phone calls and so

on, but it also records that this patient accessed and received certain information.

Case Study: Mr Williams: Portals and e-Visits

Mr Williams is traveling on an important business trip. Having ignored a random area of numbness and itching across his chest and back for several days, he now notices a linear blistering rash forming across the right side of his trunk. Recalling the Herpes Zoster vaccination TV commercials, he suspects shingles. He accesses his primary provider's interactive patient portal, and because he has completed a check-up within the last 12 months, the e-visit feature is unlocked and available for certain complaints, including rashes. Selecting the option to initiate an e-visit related to the topic of rashes, the software prompts him to provide the necessary relevant information, including a digital "selfie" photo that he uploads from his smartphone. Mr Williams is able to add free text comments to request his prescription be sent to an alternative pharmacy at his current travel location. Mr Williams receives an email confirming the suspicion of shingles, followed by a text notifying him that his prescription is ready for pick up at the preferred destination.

Contributed by Laura Holbrook, MSN, RN.

Personal Health Records

The literature speaks of portals and personal health records (PHRs) somewhat similarly. PHRs are records of one's health history which the patient maintains, entering data to provide a lifelong medical history compellation, able to be accessed by all providers. This system allows patients to control their own data and is said to assist them in self-management. PHRs are seen as a tool to overcome the fragmentation of information that occurs when a patient is seen by multiple providers and agencies. They were intended to be a centralized source for self-management, to provide communication tools similar to portals for making appointments, receiving reminders for prescription refill, and decision support tools. To be effective and to appeal to users, they need to be a seamless component of the patient's EHR, perhaps in the form of a compatible App.

Outcomes of Use of m-Health Technology for Nurses

For nurses, technology is said to improve work flow, provide safer care, provide automatic monitoring and documentation of some patient data, allow more nurse independence, and improve communications among team members. Acute care providers quickly adopted wireless devices at the bedside for communication. Evidence is mixed about the effects of technology. There is an expectation that it will decrease long-term costs. Generally, it seems to improve the flow of communications. Yet some view having to use technology as adding to workload. This may decrease as "natural language" computers that recognize vocal data entry become more widely used. Do you think new technology assists or impedes work flow?

Outcomes for Patient–Nurse Communication

Few studies are available showing effects of technology on nurse–patient communication. Generally, care may be less labor intensive and easier if delivered remotely via smartphones to patients. Technology is said to facilitate self-monitoring, improve self-management, improve cognitive functioning, reduce time spent in physician offices, provide needed information, provide support, decrease rehospitalization, increase markers of quality of life, and improve timely communication with health providers. Smartphone Apps are effective methods for teaching preventive care. It may be the preferred modality for some.

DEVELOPING AN EVIDENCE-BASED PRACTICE

Use of telehealth technology has significantly increased until some say it is the new preferred norm. The technology has improved to the point that smartphones can be used not just for consultation but also to transmit imaging, tests, and so on. Cochrane Database published Gonçalves-Bradley et al. (2020) analysis of 19 studies dealing with use of this technology for provider-to-provider communication. ARHQ did a similar but larger analysis of 233 articles (Totten et al., 2019).

Results

Both analyses reported positive health outcomes for real-time consultations including decreased mortality, decreased wait times for patients, and decreased number of clinic visits. Cost analyses brought mixed results, with some of the included studies finding no cost differences. In terms of convenience, patients reported increased satisfaction. This outcome is supported by other studies such as Tian and associate's 2021 review. Provider opinion showed variations in willingness to use telehealth and some cited concerns about security.

These results are consistent with prior studies showing positive health improvements or no difference in outcome.

Strength of the evidence: Moderate. Gonçalves-Bradley says strength of evidence is probably hampered by reporting bias.

Application to Your Clinical Practice

1. Telehealth provides opportunities for expert consultation in real-time for nurse practitioners, especially those practicing in rural areas.
2. Try using an opportunity for a telehealth visit, evaluating the pros and cons.

References

Gonçalves-Bradley, D. C, Maria, A. R. J., Ricci-Cabello, I., et al. (2020). Mobile technologies to support healthcare provider to healthcare provider communication and management of care. *Cochrane Database of Systematic Reviews, 8*(8), CD012927.

Tian, E. J., Venugopalan, S., Kumar, S., & Beard, M. (2021). The impacts of and outcomes for telehealth delivered in prisons: A systematic review. *PLoS One, 16*(5), e0251840.

Totten, A. M., Hansen, R. N., Wagner, J., et al. (2019). *Telehealth for acute and chronic care consultations.* Comparative effectiveness review no. 216. AHRQ Publication No. 19-EHC012-EF. Rockville, MD: AHRQ.

APPLICATIONS

Nursing Competencies in Technology Use

Every year there are new innovations in m-Health, highlighting the need for lifelong learning for every nurse. Technology cannot replace your accumulated knowledge and expertise in making a decision, but it can provide supplementary tools to help make these decisions. Competency in HIT use has broadly been cited by national nursing organizations, accrediting agencies, government agencies, and policy organizations as an essential of basic nursing practice. Use of informatics is an expected competency for new nurse graduates. Under this competency, *knowledge* objectives include ability to identify information available in a common database to support care. *Skills* include ability to respond appropriately to clinical decision-making supports and alerts. We are expected to demonstrate an *attitude*, which values use of technology for making decisions, preventing errors, and coordinating care. In addition to employers, regulatory agencies, professional agencies, and academic agencies, we, as professional nurses, are each responsible for maintaining this competency (American Nurses Association [ANA], 2014).

Electronic Nursing Competencies

Competencies required of nurses communicating virtually include clinical knowledge and skills; ethical knowledge; communication skills; coaching skills; supportive attitudes such as empathy; and ability to see things from the patient's point of view (Lu & Zhang, 2021; van Houwelingen et al., 2016).

Standards of Care

The same standards applicable to direct bedside care are required of nursing using digital devices. Specific standards can be accessed at various nursing organizations.

Point of Care

Wireless entry of data at the point of care can increase your access to and use of evidence-based resources in your practice. If smartphones are used for personal business, as well as in work situations, secure separate email and/or messaging accounts would be needed. Handheld devices at point of care provide timely access to patient information, are convenient, and are cost-effective in the long run. Their prompts should help you provide safer, more comprehensive care.

Device Use Guidelines

Infection Control

Prevention of device contamination is an issue of concern. When we give hands-on care or set our device down in the patient's space, we need to avoid contamination. Some suggest enclosing your device in a plastic bag, but the easiest method is to use ultraviolet light. Hand hygiene is crucial. Some reports say nurses fail to wash half the time. Hand hygiene sensors are available which does increase compliance.

Electronic Mail and FAX Use Guidelines

Faxing of orders is strongly discouraged (Young, 2021). The Federal Health IT Strategic Plan for 2020–25 states that healthcare should be connected with Health Data (records). We are discouraged from using any technology that does not become part of the patient's EHR, so data can be retrieved by others.

Smartphone Use Guidelines

Although just about every nursing student has seen or used a wireless device, not everyone has used them as an aid to giving patient care. Apps are available giving nurses access to databases to improve clinical decision-making. Some database suggestions for practice guidelines are listed in Table 26.1. There are still hospitals that prohibit nurses from using cell phones, even though studies show these devices can save time, decrease errors, and simplify information retrieval at the point of care. Ethically, you do not use electronic devices in your workplace for personal, nonprofessional use. All information needs to be Health Insurance Portability and Accountability Act (HIPAA) secure.

Texting/Instant Messaging Guidelines

In the work environment, electronic provider–patient IM can be used to communicate simple data. Both telephone and IM have been shown to be as effective as in-person

TABLE 26.1   Selected Resources for Accessing Clinical Guidelines

Organization Source	URL
AHRQ	www.ahrq.gov/
American Association of Critical Care Nurses	www.aacn.org/
British Medical Journal Clinical Evidence	www.bestpractice.bmj.com/evidence
Cochrane Database for Systematic Reviews	www.cochrane.org/cochrane/cc-broch.htm#cc/
Guide to Clinical Preventive Services	www.ahrq.gov/clinic/pocketgd.htm/
DANS EASY	https://easy.dans.knaw.nl/
Nursing Research	http://www.nursingresearchonline.com/
PubMed	www.ncbi.nlm.gov/pubmed/
PsychINFO	www.apa.org/pshchinfo/
RN Association of Ontario	http://mao.ca/
US Preventive Services Task Force	www.epss.ahrq.gov/

Internet URLs change rapidly. Some suggested sources for developing clinical care protocols are listed. Often you need to type in a search for the specific disease. Continue to search online for the best resources, CINAHL, MEDLINE/PubMed, Goggle Scholar, Science Direct, PsychINFO. When on these sites, use Medical Subject controlled terms (MeSH) such as "asthma."

education for patients with chronic conditions. Texts can increase time-efficient communication with patients. Texting reminders for immunizations have proven effective in significantly increasing compliance (Stockwell, 2020). Texts remind patients of appointments, services, or to take a medication or perform self-monitoring care. This may promote better quality care and improved patient utilization. The Joint Commission continues to say it is *not* acceptable for the physician or licensed independent practitioner to text orders for patients (TJC, 2021).

Multiple articles in the literature describe the efficacy of using personalized IM for helping patients manage their conditions, as illustrated in the Ryan case.

Case Study: Ann Ryan, RN

Mr Simpson, 47 years old, is newly diagnosed with hypertension. He is taking a new medication and texts his self-monitored blood pressure readings daily to Ms Ryan, RN, his nurse. She could text message a reminder to take his evening dose. Next, she texts a reminder to Ms Sweet, an elderly diabetic patient who has forgotten to submit her blood glucose level this morning, However, there are concerns about violations of patient privacy. See Social Media Guidelines listed in Chapter 3. Other concerns involve threats to safety. When an incoming message distracts a nurse during a crucial procedure, this distraction could potentially contribute to making an error (Shaw & Abbott, 2017).

Use of Wearable Biosensors

The potential for managing care using biosensors is exponential. Already smart watches and smart eyeglasses can detect health anomalies, such as irregular heart beat or blood pressure. Lack of motion detection can alert us to a potential patient fall. Sensors in back braces are beginning to be used to treat scoliosis (Surantha et al., 2021). Patients value using wearable sensors if they are user friendly and provide data useful in treating their disease (Ozanne et al., 2018).

Use of Social Media

Guidelines for nurse use of social media were discussed in Chapter 3. According to the National Council of State Boards of Nursing (NCSBN) and HIPAA, nurses breach patient privacy and HIPAA rules when they post photos or videos or comment about patients. We differentiate between the general open-to-all social sites, such as Twitter, from secure sites with restricted access, such as those created by hospitals as internal professional staff social networks.

Clinical Decision Support System Use

While use of CDSSs never eliminates the need for us to think critically, such systems are another tool to help us manage our nursing care. Use of CDSSs allows you to align your clinical decisions for your specific patient with best practice guidelines, as in the case of Ms Esteves.

Case Study: Ms Ella Esteves's CDSS Alert

As the staff nurse in the CCU unit, you sign on to the Esteves electronic record. The CDSS offers you a reminder (alert) about a medication order. You are given information about possible harmful interactions with other medications she is already taking. This CDSS "reminder" then gives you a suggestion to obtain a lab INR result prior to considering giving this med. Thus, the CDSS is integrated with your work flow, giving you suggestions about interventions based on researched best practice. Perhaps the CDSS next reminds you that later meds be held since Ms Esteves has an NPO (nothing by mouth) order beginning at midnight. It might offer you a suggested alternative if you fail to document this intervention.

In another example, nurses working with pediatric cancer patients have long used calculators to determine correct fractional dosage based on the child's weight. Now instead, they can use this automated support system because it automatically predetermines the correct doses.

Clinical Decision Support System Concerns

Alarm Fatigue. A common problem is that the CDSS might send you so many alerts that you ignore them. **Alarm fatigue** is a commonly reported problem. This is particularly true for drug–drug interactions. Studies suggest that as many as 90% of alarm alerts are overridden. Customizing alerts to your patient assignment or gradating the warning into low-priority (warning but no alarm) and high-priority (audible alarm) might overcome this. More studies are needed to examine effects of CDSS on communication, but data suggest a positive effect. In Canada, nurses use mobile devices to access the Registered Nurses' Association of Ontario best practice guidelines to receive timely information specific to their assigned patients. Try Simulation Exercise 26.2 to critique a nursing resource database and explore usability.

Cost and Ease of Use. Cost and ease of use are the main concerns in adopting this technology.

Application of Clinical Guidelines to Practice Integration into your workflow and relevance to your care are two serious concerns. Access at the point of care

SIMULATION EXERCISE 26.2   Critique of an Internet Nursing Resource Database

Purpose

To encourage students to gain familiarity with Internet resources.

Procedure

As an out-of-class assignment, access any nursing resource database, preferably using a smartphone or tablet. Many sites are listed in the online references.

Reflective Discussion Analysis

1. Discuss results, listing sites you think useful.
2. Evaluate each website's credibility for professional use.

BOX 26.1   Use of m-Health Devices (Wireless, Wi-Fi-Enabled, Handheld Devices)

Advantages

- Improve the flow of communication, as well as workflow
- Easily portable; can be used at the point of care (patient's bedside, in the home, etc.)
- Quick charting when nurse enters information by tapping menu selections
- Can contain reference resources about treatment, for medication dosage, and so forth, if uploaded
- Assists with customized decision-making, reminders about standards of care, sends alerts
- Instant communication (e.g., nurse is signaled by beep regarding receipt of new information)
- Provide quick access to patient records
- Provide patients with self-management tools
- Build support networks
- Provide a method of connecting with hard-to-reach patients

Disadvantages

- Possible threats to patient's legal privacy rights
- Nurse does not have a printed copy of information (until downloaded to agency printer)
- Small screen does not allow view of entire page of information
- Technical problem may result in dysfunction and/or downtime

---

to databases containing evidence-based guidelines for care means you have resources specifically tailored to suggest interventions for a specific patient.

Criteria for Downloadable Clinical Practice Guidelines

- They are evidence-based.
- They are easily accessible on your wireless device.
- They allow you to enter patient data to customize the interventions (data from EHR).
- They contain hotlinks to allow you to obtain and print more information.

m-Health: Technology for Patient Engagement

Use of Health and Lifestyle Monitoring Apps

This chapter describes possible App uses, but, of course, use of Apps is not quite as easy as it sounds, requiring devices, science-based programs, and use skills. Would you recommend consumers owning smartphones download some of the many Apps that assist them in tracking their self-assessment? For example, should a diabetic patient try using Glucose Buddy (an iPhone App) that allows them to enter glucose testing results and record carbohydrate consumption and other parameters? Or maybe uChek, which is a digital log of urinalysis testing results with data entered using the smartphone camera to record urine dipstick results? What factors would you consider before making this recommendation? Some advantages and concerns are listed in Box 26.1.

Outcomes of m-Health

Cyber Health Education for Health Promotion. There is considerable evidence about the efficacy of providing healthcare education and information online. See Chapter 15 for discussion of health promotion concepts.

Postdischarge Patient Education. New technology increases our options for providing needed information. One hospital example would be unit-owned tablets containing disease management information in skill-based learning modules which are lent to patients. Similar modules could be provided after discharge. Use of national website-based modules would eliminate the need for each agency to develop their own programs.

Disease Management and Follow-Up. Health information about controlling their chronic disease conditions can be provided to patients effectively, quickly, and inexpensively via the Internet. Nurse-provided information, often to their mobile device, allows patients to make better self-management decisions, such as reminding a diabetic patient to submit A1c results this week. Actively engaging and giving decision support is another way to provide patient-centered care, shifting the focus to self-care in their own home. One problem for patients accessing Internet health information is that not all online information is accurate or easy for the user to verify in measurable *outcomes*. Internet-based education programs have been shown to lead to better understanding and to greater disease control.

In the United States, documentation of each patient education session must contain the following:
- The topic discussed
- The time spent
- Your mutual behavioral goal
- Your assessment of patient's readiness to learn
- Your observations about the patient's level of understanding of their disease
Reflect on the Anna Smith case describing use of alerts.

Case Study: Anna Smith: Management of a Teen With Asthma

Anna, age 14, has asthma. Her treatment regimen significantly improved as technology became available to facilitate communication in several ways. Anna uses smart devices with mobile Apps for both her preventive maintenance and rescue medications as well as her peak flow meter. Bluetooth technology allows her inhalers to be paired with her smartphone for administration tracking. She can receive an alert if she forgets a routine dose. The frequency of use of rescue doses is also tracked. Her App automatically sends compiled information to her care provider and parents regarding treatments used and peak flow meter readings, and provides urgent alerts when an increase in rescue inhaler use or marked decrease in forced exhale volume is detected. When paired with a wearable smart device, this App can also integrate biometric data such as heart rate and episodes of waking in the night. By trending data, this individualized App can facilitate communication, improve treatment effectiveness, and prevent hospitalizations related to unrecognized asthma exacerbations.

Contributed by Laura Holbrook, MSN, RN.

Internet Support Groups

Chat Rooms. Computers are used to mediate support groups for families and patients with various health problems. These formal Internet groups not only provide information, but they also importantly have been shown to provide improved social support for those who are ill. Studies show group participants report decreased stress, less depression, increased quality of life, and improved ability to manage their disease condition. The chat rooms are usually synchronous, in real time, providing immediate feedback. Usually, discussion forums are asynchronous with time delays between postings and responses, allowing for more reflection before posting. More studies are needed

before we can specify the needed frequency, duration, or quality of content for optimal support.

Caregivers. Caregivers of people with chronic conditions can use Internet support groups, chat rooms, email, or direct communication with care providers to gain support. Nurses can gain insight and better understand the "lived experiences" of their patients by participating in these Internet opportunities. Internet or telephone support has been shown to be a cost-effective method for improving functioning and quality of life for patients with chronic conditions, and similar beneficial effects in nurse–caregiver relationship support are occurring. Do you believe chat rooms can improve nurse–patient communication?

Issues. The main concerns with technology are interoperability and security. Other things to consider are as follows.

Access. Barriers to use of new technologies include user resistance, lack of broadband, and literacy issues. The transition to use of eHealth technology in nursing implies constant adaptation to new ways of providing care. In all cases, our communication needs to be tailored to the needs and literacy level of our patient.

Competency. For nurses, rapid advances in technology mean we need to continuously transform the way we communicate. For patients, new technology offers tools to become more engaged in self-management of their own health. Information needs to be in a context which they understand.

Guidelines for professional relationships apply to use of electronic media. Caution is advised in communicating with patients outside the professional relationship. Online contact with former patients blurs the relationship boundary.

Costs. Major costs are involved in developing and obtaining software and hardware. A big consideration for providers is cost recovery. How will patients be billed for the time physicians, nurses, dieticians, therapists, etc., devote to interacting with patients using Internet modalities?

Liability Issues. Use of the Internet presents many questions about how to maximize its communication potential with an increasingly diverse population. Liability and regulatory statutes are outdated. For example, if transmission (and treatment) crosses state lines, in which region does the provider need to be licensed? If malpractice occurs, in which region or state would legal action occur?

Privacy and Security Issues. Separate organizations providing care to the same patient need to share information securely. Any information you learn during the course of treatment must be safeguarded. With any computer use, we are concerned about maintaining *security*. Many surveys of consumer concerns cite breach of privacy as their biggest concern. As HIT systems become more sophisticated and accessibility is a top priority, mechanisms and regulations to ensure privacy become more complex. As m-Health devices, wearable devices, and implanted devices interconnect on the internet, there is potential for harm from unintended or malicious actors. Major breaches of healthcare databases have occurred and attempts are likely to increase since these data sets are worth millions to thieves. Security experts recommend data encryption and always using a required login password, which is changed frequently.

SUMMARY

Mobile health has transformed the way nurses communicate with patients and with other professional heathcare providers. Technology provides nurses with powerful tools for communication and for new ways of care delivery, such as point-of-care documentation. Handheld devices, wearable devices, and use of patient portals all serve to provide the patient consumer with easier access to communication and care. HIT will continue to impact our practice. Technology gives us new tools to partner with patients, helping them manage their own care.

ETHICAL DILEMMA: What Would You Do?

One of the staff nurses you work with "friends" you on Facebook, allowing you to read postings sent to her by a student nurse assigned to her unit. The student has posted information about a 17-year-old former patient who threatens to commit suicide. You do not personally know either the student nurse or the patient.

1. Since this information is openly available on the Internet, what ethical responsibility do you have to intervene?
2. Did the student nurse violate the patient's legal right to privacy?
3. If you were the student, what steps would you take as soon as you receive this information?

DISCUSSION QUESTIONS

1. Social media sites have become a prominent component of our society. Identify any future professional uses for social media that you can envision.
2. AHRQ sites described in this chapter could provide you with useful information. Argue for or against use, including ease of access and whether they should implement periodic emails or tweets.
3. Construct a set of criteria for determining if websites are providing reliable information for your clinical practice.

REFERENCES

Ajami, S., & Rajabzadeh, A. (2013). Radio frequency identification (RFID) technology and patient safety. *Journal of Research in Medical Sciences, 18*(9), 809–813.

American Nurses Association (ANA). (2014). *ANA position statement: Professional role competence.* Retrieved from: https://www.nursingworld.org/practice-policy/nursing-excellence/official-position-statements/id/professional-role--competence/. [Accessed 1 July 2021].

American Telemedicine Association (ATA). (2021). *Patient satisfaction with virtual care.* Retrieved from: https://www.americantelemed.org/wp-content/uploads/2021/05/Patient-satisfaction-1.pdf. [Accessed 1 July 2021].

Bianco, C. L., Myers, A. L., Smagula, S., & Fortuna, K. L. (2021). Can smartphone Apps assist people with serious mental illness in taking medications as prescribed? *Sleep Medicine Clinics, 16*(1), 213–222.

Gonçalves-Bradley, D. C., Maria, A. R. J., Ricci-Cabello, I., et al. (2020). Mobile technologies to support healthcare provider to healthcare provider communication and management of care. *Cochrane Database of Systematic Reviews, 8*(8), CD012927.

Health Resources & Services Administration (HRSA). (2021). *What is telehealth?* Retrieved from: https://telehealth.hhs.gov/patients/understanding-telehealth/. [Accessed 1 July 2021].

Journal of AHIMA Staff. (2017). Reporting live from your stomach. *Journal of AHIMA, 88*(8), 56.

Lu, X., & Zhang, R. (2021). Impact of information behaviours in online health communities on patient compliance and the mediating role of patients' perceived empathy. *Patient Education and Counseling, 104*(1), 186–193.

Mauzey, S. (2020). *UV-C: A tool for disinfecting mobile devices.* American Nurse. Retrieved from: https://www.myamericannnurse.com/uv-c-a-tool-for-disinfecting-mobile-devices/. [Accessed 1 July 2021].

Odendaal, W. A., Anstey Watkins, J., Leon, N., et al. (2020). Health workers' perceptions and experiences of using mHealth technologies to deliver primary healthcare services: A qualitative evidence synthesis. *Cochrane Database of Systematic Reviews, 3*(3), CD011942.

Ozanne, A., Johansson, D., Hällgren Graneheim, U., Malmgren, K., Bergquist, F., & Alt Murphy, M. (2018). Wearables in epilepsy and Parkinson's disease-a focus group study. *Acta Neurologica Scandinavica, 137*(2), 188–194.

Reeves, J. J., Ayers, J. W., & Longhurst, C. A. (2021). Telehealth in the COVID-19 era: A balancing act to avoid harm. *Journal of Medical Internet Research, 23*(2), e24785.

Schwenk, T. L. (2021). Characteristics of clinical care provided through e-visits. *NEJM Journal Watch.* www.jwatch.org/.

Shaw, P. A., & Abbott, M. R. B. (2017). Distracted nursing: Strategies to teach nursing students about mobile devices. *Nurse Educator, 42*(4), 203.

Stockwell, M. S. (2020). Texting reminders to low-income, minority patients improves vaccine rates. In Agency for healthcare research and quality. *AHRQ digital healthcare research 2019 Year in review.* AHRQ publication No. 20-0047 (p. 17). Rockville, MD: AHRQ.

Surantha, N., Atmaja, P., & Wicaksono, M. (2021). A review of wearable Internet of Things device for healthcare. *Procedia Computer Science, 179*, 936–943.

The Joint Commission (TJC). (2021). *Standards FAQ: Texting – use of secure text messaging for patient orders*. Retrieved from: https://www.jointcommission.org/standards/standard-faqs/laboratory/leadership-ld/000002173/. [Accessed 2 July 2021].

U.S. Department of Health and Human Services. (2020). *Draft Federal Health IT strategic plan supports patient access to their own health information*. Retrieved from: www.hhs.gov/abo ut/news/2020/01/15/draft-federal-health-it-strategic-plan-supports-patient-access-health-information.html. [Accessed 2 July 2021].

U.S. Department of Health and Human Services. (n.d.). Healthy people 2030. Retrieved from: www.health.gov/healthypeople.

van Houwelingen, C. T. M., Moerman, A. H., Ettema, R. G. A., Kort, H. S. M., & Ten Cate, O. (2016). Competencies required for nursing telehealth activities: A delphi-study. *Nursing Education Today, 39*, 50–62.

Wilson, M. A., Fouts, B. L., & Brown, K. N. (2021). Development of a mobile application for acute pain management in U.S. military healthcare. *Applied Nursing Research, 58*, 151393.

Young, L. (2021). Death to faxes: COVID-19 highlights the need for interoperability. *Journal of AHIMA*, e1–e3.

27

Intrapersonal Communication to Self-Manage Stress and Promote Nurse Wellness

OBJECTIVES

Upon completion of this chapter the reader will be able to:

1. Differentiate between "good stress" and chronic deleterious stress.

2. Identify triggers and symptoms of own stressors.
3. Discuss techniques to apply to own stress prevention and treatment to focus on wellness.

Nurses regularly save lives, each caring for hundreds of patients every year (McSpedon, 2021). Many areas of nursing practice have been identified as especially stressful such as palliative care or intensive care. The recent pandemic stretched many nurses beyond their ability to cope with work-related **stress**. But who says to us that we need to take care of ourselves too? This chapter will discuss our inner or intrapersonal communication to help us recognize, prevent, or treat our stress to help us promote nurse wellness by emphasizing intrapersonal communication.

BASIC CONCEPTS

Definitions

Stress

Stress responses can be triggered by either physical or psychological threat, which induces specific physical change to prepare your body to ward off the threat. In the occasional short-term, the cascade of physical response is good. It prepared you for "fight or flight." However, in the long-term, chronic stress responses endanger your mental and physical health. The National Institute for Occupational Safety and Health (NIOSH) defines job stress as a harmful physical and emotional response that occurs when the requirements of the job do not match the capabilities, resources, or needs of the worker.

Resilience

Though there is no agreed-upon definition, **resilience** is defined as an ability to "bounce back." It refers to the individual's ability to positively adjust to adversity. It is a dynamic, variable response determined by our personality and the situation, which helps us adapt positively following adversity (Hartwig et al., 2020; Hollywood & Phillips, 2020). Attributes to maintaining resilience include willingness to work at maintenance, social support, and self-efficacy, as well as use of humor, optimism, and the ability to set realistic goals (Cooper et al., 2020). Some nurses are able to cope better than others with a given situation, but this varies over time. Resilience is considered to be a protective factor, helping prevent "burnout" in nurses. This syndrome occurs over a period of time. Burnout is a commonly used term to refer to folks who have become exhausted by their job. Nurses working in highly acute areas are particularly susceptible to adverse effects of stress and need to proactively take measures to manage stress, as illustrated in the case of Nancy.

Incidence of Stress

Not much scientific data are available about how widespread stress is among nurses. Certainly, we all experience job-related stressors. Generally, up to 40% of all workers report they feel significant stress at times in their job.

CASE STUDY: Nancy Cox, RN, Deals With Stress

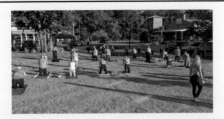

Nancy, age 21, is an intensive care nurse whose unit was repurposed to care for COVID-19 patients during the pandemic. She had never expected to care for patients dying by the dozens every week.

She developed severe headaches and stomach upsets and felt exhausted. Her nurse manager initiated debriefing sessions during which a therapist taught all the nurses stress-relieving strategies such as meditation and progressive relaxation. The nurse manager encouraged nurses to support each other and share feelings to help each realize they shared common feelings. Nancy and two colleagues were talking about needing to unwind, so they agreed to start holding 20-minute yoga sessions on the hospital lawn after the end of shift. Soon a dozen or so folks had joined their group sessions!

Intrapersonal Communication: Self-Talk

As nurses our brains are constantly processing incoming data, decoding verbal and nonverbal messages, interpreting environmental factors such as changes in our patient's condition. When we are stressed, we lose our objectivity. To counter feeling stressed out, we engage in intrapersonal "self-talk" as we prepare to give care.

Goals

- Reframe negativity. The goal is to become aware of negative thoughts and replace them instantly with positive ones. It is surprising how hard it can be to rid ourselves of negativity. Track down the event that led to the negative thought. Reframe this situation to focus on a positive thought.
- Cultivate positivity with self-talk. Develop a mantra which you repeat to yourself when a negative thought enters your consciousness, such as "I can do this."

Theory

Various theories about stress were discussed in Chapter 16, the classic being general adaptive syndrome.

Hans Selye

Selye described the human response to stress as the same neurological–endocrine cascade to either a physical or a psychological stressor. This prepares our body for "fight or flight" to ensure survival. But when the stressors are chronic, these responses damage our cardiovascular system, our gastrointestinal system, etc. Chronic stress can also damage mental health. We can work to prevent or modify our stress responses. For example, to control our response, we can increase our physical exercise, which releases endorphins and endocannabinoids that can improve sleep, block pain, etc. (Smith, 2020).

Orem's Self-Care Deficit Nursing Theory of Nursing

Dorothea Orem began developing her theory in the late 1950s. It describes why and how people care for themselves, how nurses can help, and the use of a nursing system of relationships so that nursing can occur. One of three main components is "self-care agency." Self-care is an active regulatory function, initiated by individuals, deliberately performed, to maintain their life, health, and well-being (Orem, 1995). Self-care must be learned and continuously performed in relation to the person's stage of development and environment. Orem adherents use these conceptualizations to guide care for individual patients, but in our case, we are using it to apply to the nurses' care of themselves, on their own behalf.

Burnout

Definition

Burnout is a syndrome characterized by emotional exhaustion. Think of it as a continual draining off of our emotional coping over time. It is a growing problem with no easy remedies. The International Classification of Diseases (ICD-11) categorizes burnout as an occupational phenomena rather than a medical diagnosis.

Incidence of Burnout in Nurses

Over time, chronic stress leads to burnout, which has been reported in more than half of nurses, with physicians also reporting intense burnout during the COVID-19 pandemic. This was increasingly apparent as nurses had high workloads and serious concerns about becoming infected and transmitting the virus to their families (Roberts et al., 2021). Burnout has been acknowledged as a problem for years, exacerbated by organizational policies. Fundamental rights for nurses are undermined when they are asked to work long hours, pass up breaks, and carry heavier workloads (Halsted & Hart, 2021). What do you see in the face and posture of the nurse in Fig. 27.1?

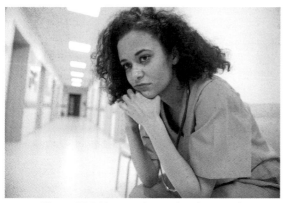

Figure 27.1 Nurse: exhausted and stressed.

In 2018 prior to the pandemic, Molina-Praena and colleagues analyzed 38 studies, finding 31% of nurses reported emotional exhaustion. Melnyk's 2021 studies of critical care nurses found up to 47% experiencing burnout with 30% reporting depression. In 2020, Bozdağ and Ergün found that 50% of nurses surveyed reported depression. Nurse responses to debilitating stress vary from thoughts of quitting, to actually leaving the field of nursing. Reports cite absenteeism, lateness coming on duty, detachment, increased use of sick days, and job turnover. Some reports cite suicide as a response by a few, although there are no concrete statistics (Halsted & Hart, 2021).

Signs and Symptoms

Stress affects everyone. Short-term stress can even be good for us, activating us for "fight or flight." But chronic stress can affect our mental and physical health, causing somatic symptoms such as achy muscles, changes in appetite, poor sleep, irritable gastrointestinal upsets, headaches, hypertension, as well as psychological symptoms such as feelings of exhaustion, detachment, depression, or irritableness and anger (Sampaio et al., 2021). Typically, the literature characterizes the nurse with burnout as emotionally detached, exhausted, and operating at decrease efficiency levels, making more errors and feeling irritable or hopeless (Institute for Healthcare Improvement [IHI], 2021; WHO, 2019).

Sequalae

Physically, burnout weakens our immune system (Leichtman, 2021) and is a significant predictor of later physical conditions such as high cholesterol, type 2 diabetes, and coronary disease. Psychologically, burnout leads to somatic symptoms such as headaches, stomach aches, insomnia, or feelings of hopelessness and depression.

Suicide

The National Institute of Mental Health (n.d.) has a suicide risk screening tool available. For anyone so distressed as to be contemplating suicide, the need for professional help is urgent. Contact any of the help lines listed on the Internet. The exact degree of the problem is difficult to obtain, since statistics are generally not available about nurse suicide. Data on nurses are shrouded in silence (Davidson et al., 2018). This is a critical matter needing attention, especially after the extraordinary demands placed on nurses caring for patients with COVID. Prior to the pandemic, the CDC reported significantly higher rates of suicide for female nurses compared with the general female population, and significantly higher rates for male nurses compared with the general male population (Davidson et al., 2019). The National Institute of Mental Health has a screening tool you can use (NIMH, n.d.). When the need for help is URGENT: call the National Suicide Hot Line 1-800-273-8255.

Treatment

As with so much in the healthcare field, prevention, early recognition, support and treatment are needed. General categories of intervention include stress reduction and use of interventions to build nurse resilience.

Implications for Nurses

Self-Talk

Analysis. We need to do a self-examination to evaluate our stress level each day. If reflection are difficult, try journaling your stress, recording exactly what circumstance acted as a trigger to initiate your stress response.

Action. Resolve to take preemptive action. Incorporate at least one of the stress preventive measures described in this chapter. With nurses, job-related stress occurs when work demands exceed our capacity to provide quality care, especially when needed resources are limited. This was even more apparent during the recent pandemic, but burnout has been acknowledged as a problem for years, exacerbated by organizational policies (Roberts et al., 2021). Burnout is a syndrome characterized by emotional exhaustion. It is a growing problem with no easy remedies. This leads us to feel a loss of control. All of us experience stress at times. Many interventions are available which allow us to control this stress.

Social Support

Social support buffers the deleterious effects of chronic stress. It is defined as the emotional comfort, advice, and instrumental assistance that a person receives from others. Families can be a major source of support, but can fade over time. In this digital age, there are many online support groups. Convince yourself to actively seek support. Remember if you are venting online, defaming an agency online can get you into legal trouble, so do not name names! The ANA has a "Mental Health Help for Nurses" webpage (ANA, n.d.) with advice and resources. Talk yourself into making extra efforts to sharing a meal, go to a gym, and seek company as a means of relieving stress. How can you convince yourself to actively cultivate more social support networks?

DEVELOPING AN EVIDENCE-BASED PRACTICE

Multiple studies of burnout in healthcare providers have demonstrated high levels of burnout exist in clinicians giving direct care, especially for nurses who have been employed for a year but not for over 10 years. Kelly and associates (2021) found more than half of 1688 nurses surveyed reported burnout. This was especially true for nurses working with critically ill patients whose chances of recovery were minimal. Sampaio's (2021) survey of 829 Italian nurses caring for patients with COVID-19 reported high levels of stress symptomology, both physical and mental. Individual resilience was an ameliorating factor helping nurses reduce the adverse impact of stress.

Results
Research supports nursing is stressful. High workload and long hours are contributing factors. Nurses and physicians in Sampaio's study worked over 100 h per week. In Chen's metaanalysis of 10 studies, strategies using mindfulness interventions significantly lowered anxiety and depression.
   Strength of research: low to moderate, since studies ranged from surveys to controlled trials.

Application to Your Clinical Practice
1. Resilience can be learned. Orientation programs should include stress-coping strategies, as should preceptorship programs.
2. Individual nurses need to practice resilience building using any of the strategies described in this chapter.
3. The National Academy of Medicine has established a consortium to explore strategies to reverse burnout and increase clinician well-being. Monitoring their website will increase your knowledge.

References
Chen, X., Zhang, B., Jin, S. X., Quan, Y. X., Zhang, X. W., & Cui, X. S. (2021). The effects of mindfulness-based interventions on nursing students: A meta-analysis. *Nursing Education Today, 98,* 104718.

Kelly, L. A., Gee, P. M., & Butler, R. J. (2021). Impact of nurse burnout on organizational and position turnover. *Nursing Outlook, 69*(1), 96–102.

Sampaio, F., Sequeira, C., & Teixeira, L. (2021). Impact of COVID-19 outbreak on nurses' mental health: A prospective cohort study. *Environmental Research, 194,* 110620.

APPLICATIONS

Promoting well-being is defined by Orem and others as behaviors practiced by individuals to maximize their health and wellness. This chapter is focusing on intrapersonal communication strategies to reduce stress and increasing coping. There are hundreds of websites that provide recommendations. Nurses and other healthcare providers are often said to put self-care low on their priority list (Chipu & Downing, 2020). As nurses, we need to commit ourselves to "practice what we preach." We need to practice wellness activities and to recognize and manage our stress.

Recognition
Take your emotional temperature daily to monitor your level of stress. Or use a stress inventory instrument. When you become aware of increased stress, this early recognition can let you begin to work on destressing activities. Identify triggers that increase your stress level. Table 27.1 has a quick self-stress assessment checklist.

Prevention: Building Resilience Promotes Wellness

Prioritize Self-Care
Recognize that if you are going to care for others, you need to proactively promote your own well-being. Various

TABLE 27.1 Quick Self–Stress Assessment		
	QD	q/week
How often do you experience demands you cannot meet?		
How often do you feel stressed?		
How often do you experience signs of stress such as sleep problems?		
How often do you feel powerless?		
How often do you feel like your work in meaningless?		
How often are you reluctant to go to work?		

surveys reveal that up to 70% of nurses do not make self-care their priority! Healthcare providers including nurses are encouraged to build in "wellness moments" during their workday (Fessell & Cherniss, 2020). Fig. 27.2 illustrates healthy habits.

Maintain a Balance
Leave work at work! Balance your work and home life so you are not putting all your energy into one or the other.

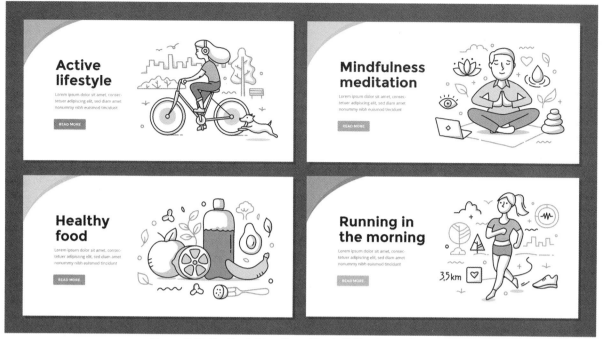

Figure 27.2 Healthy habits. (From iStock #1031904944, Rassco.)

Exercise

Follow a daily 30-minute exercise routine. Experts recommend exercising outdoors, when possible, even if it is only a walk during your lunch time. Others stress the helpfulness of exercising in the sunshine. Try talking the stairs instead of elevator, parking farther away from the entrance to your agency.

Center Mind and Body

While sanitizing your hands, waiting for the computer to boot, taking a bathroom break, or doing some other mindless task, do focus on your breathing. The secret to each stress prevention activity is consistent repetition. Box 27.1 lists strategies you can use. Pick a few of these suggestions and try to incorporate them into your daily schedule.

- *Practice prevention.* Rather than waiting until you develop symptoms of maladaptation to stress, make it a daily habit to practice prevention. If some exercises are ingrained, it makes it easier to reactivate them at the point when you encounter a major stressor.
- *Stress reduction.* Many websites have stress reduction suggestions, especially regarding dietary intake. Example: "eat protein for breakfast" to increase

serotonin levels, which decreases anxiety. Other sites offer dietary supplements, medications, and suggestions for staying connected with friends or for dialog with others such as therapists. Since this chapter is focusing on self-management, stress reduction can be managed by using one of dozens of free Apps for download. Perhaps downloading a relaxation App to your smartphone could make it accessible at work. Try downloading some meditation music.

- *Set boundaries.* At work, protect your time. Take all assigned breaks. Do not overcommit. Prioritize what has to be done. Set realistic goals. Do not bring work home. Accept that all of us are less than perfect.
- *Positivity.* Practice positive "self-talk," substituting positive thoughts each time a negative thought occurs. Balance job and personal life. Try not to take your work home with you. Set aside a time for yourself daily for an activity you enjoy such as crafting.

Interventions: Types of Intrapersonal Communication Strategies to Manage Your Stress

Mindfulness

Practice **mindfulness** as a stress-reducing exercise. Mindfulness is merely purposeful awareness of your immediate

BOX 27.1   Strategies for Preventing and Self-Managing Stress

Wellness Maintenance
- Prioritize self-care.
- Set boundaries.
- Protect your time.
- Balance work life and personal life.
- Practice positive self-talk.
- Exercise daily.
- Practice mindfulness.
- Meditate.
- Power down before sleep.
- Follow a sleep relaxation program.

Reduce Stress at Work
- Use relaxation techniques:
  - Use deep breathing exercises.
  - Take all breaks.
  - Do stretching exercises: head rolls; shoulder shrugs.
- Increase your exercise:
  - Take a walk outside on breaks.
  - Try minimeditation and relaxation exercises.
- Do periodic self-check-ups to identify your feelings.
- Psychological relief:
  - Use humor.
  - Learn to guard your time (say "no").
  - Prioritize your tasks.
  - Listen to meditation music briefly on your smartphone.
  - Use reflection, or journaling.
  - Actively seek support.
  - Reframe irritants to keep the "Big Picture" in mind.

SIMULATION EXERCISE 27.1
Developing Mindfulness

Procedure

Amy Sullivan of the Cleveland Clinic suggests a mindfulness exercise taking an orange (Levine, 2020). Hold it. Observe its shape and skin. Touch it, turning it in your hand. Smell its flavor. Peel it and eat a slice, tasting it. By focusing only on the orange you are slowing respirations and engaging your parasympathetic nervous system for relaxation.

Reflective Discussion Analysis
1. Compare your experience with classmates.
2. Discuss how you could use mindfulness in the clinical area.

internal experience. Studies show meditating for 10 min increases alpha waves associated with relaxation (Meditation, n.d.). To meditate, choose a quiet spot and assume a comfortable position, usually lying down. Focus on your breathing, turning your mind inward. Focus on a thought (mantra), or even on some body part. If distracting thoughts flit through your mind just dismiss them, exhaling and blowing them away. Repetition is important, so practice daily. Reflect on Mary's case for a variation on meditative practice.

Case Study: Mary Rachel, RN

Mary tells her coworkers on her coronary care unit that she gets up 15 min early daily to pray to Jesus in a private corner of her house. Sue, her young agnostic coworker, snickers. Others remind Sue that this is the same as practicing meditation and actually promotes good mental health as they learned in a recent in-service. Put in this light, Mary has an "aha" moment of understanding.

Eastern Mind–Body Programs

Try yoga or Tai Chi for relaxation. These exercises usually occur in a class but could be adapted at home. Yoga and other programs stress meditation along with stretching exercises.

Sleep

Get the best, most adequate sleep possible.
- Power down before bed. Establish a relaxing routine. Avoid exercising just prior to bed. Try to have a consistent sleep time. Establish a de-stress prebedtime routine.

internal and external environment without judgment to develop mind-body awareness. Mindfulness keeps you grounded in the current moment, not worrying about past or future events. Numerous studies show the effectiveness of practicing mindfulness to decrease stress and change the brain to improve mental health (Snow, 2020). Mindfulness exercises have been shown to decrease anxiety and depression in nursing students (Chen et al., 2021). To practice mindfulness, you focus only on the moment, noticing what is present. Consider practicing a mindfulness exercise as in Simulation Exercise 27.1.

Meditation

Practicing meditation is a formal commitment of time which you schedule to still your body to focus your mind on an

Have a 1-hour moratorium prior to retiring when you turn off all electronic communication, television, social media platforms, etc. Take a hot bath. Experts also suggest it is more conducive to sleep if our bedroom is dark and cool.

- Facilitate deep sleep. When retiring, you could play a relaxation program. Some recommend that if you read to relax, avoid blue light. Consider downloading a relaxation App which take you through a muscle tightening, deep breathing, and muscle relaxation program. Use *guided imagery or guided visualization.* This is a technique that uses your imagination to simulate mental images of "happy places" to stimulate healing and promote relief of stress. The process asks you to imagine a scene, previously experienced as safe, relaxing, and peaceful. Supportive prompts can help engage all your senses. Use self-talk to paint yourself as a strong, competent person. Or choose a downloadable guided imagery program that focuses on a relaxing scene such as rocking with ocean waves or soaring in a glider. This is a great intervention strategy for our patients as well. Try Simulation Exercise 27.2 to experience guided imagery yourself.

Resilience Training

Resilience is defined as the ability to adapt well to and adjust to adversity (Mayo Clinic, n.d.). Some agencies are developing "wellness office" positions to help staff. Some agencies offer resilience training programs to help staff adapt to stressful clinical situations. The goal is to teach you to view life's challenges as opportunities for personal growth.

Agencies may offer counseling services or cognitive behavioral therapy, which has shown some success in teaching people to reframe their stress. Nurses can also seek counseling services on their own. Our goal is to build resilience. This can be taught. A formal program of resilience training focuses on these areas:

- *Emotional attitude.* Accept that everything is always changing, and we need lifelong learning. Learn to view adversity as an opportunity for learning. Use reflection to increase your emotional insight. Some people journal and reflect on their comments. If humor is your thing, watch a comedy show. A good belly laugh is a great stress reducer!
- *Cognitive.* Remind yourself of your sense of purpose: why you became a nurse, and what the good things about your job are. Reflect on what is satisfying (Bozdağ & Ergün, 2020). Prioritize what must be done.

SIMULATION EXERCISE 27.2   Using Guided Visualization

Procedure
1. Sit in a chair, feet on ground.
2. Relax muscles.
3. Take three deep breaths, in through the nose, hold, blow out slowly through the mouth.
4. Close your eyes and imagine walking through forest, hear the birds.
5. Repeat.
6. Walk out from forest onto beach to the ocean edge.
7. Feel the sun on your face.
8. Wade through the water, listening to the waves.
9. Repeat deep breaths.
10. Open your eyes. Congrats on a job well done!

Reflective Discussion Analysis
Did this sooth you? By repeating this exercise for several days, it becomes ingrained and gets more effective at reducing stress.

From Lewis, K. (2021). Guided visualization: Dealing with stress [video]. National Institute of Mental Health. Retrieved from: https://www.nimh.nih.gov/news/media/2021/guided-visualization-dealing-with-stress. Accessed July 6, 2021.

- *Social.* Actively work to build collegiality with a scenario of "I've got your back."
- *Physical.* Incorporate some physical activity you enjoy in your self-care routine, such as biking, dancing, etc.
- *Spiritual.* Practices such as prayer can be comforting.
  At Work: Intrapersonal Communication Tips to Maintain Wellness.

Deep Breathing

Before responding to an irritating demand at work, inhale deeply through your nose; hold the breath for a 6-second count; then purse your lips; and exhale slowly taking as long as possible. This activates your parasympathetic nervous system's "rest and digest" function.

Humor

Use humor or jokes. Some of us have a naturally ebullient personality, others not so much. But we can cultivate a good joke daily. Why even "Alexia" can tell us a joke! Or maybe we can watch a comedy show on television and get a good laugh.

Mini-Meditation

Take an opportunity for a 3-minute sitting meditation at work as in Simulation Exercise 27.3.

Relaxation Routines

In addition to the aforementioned relaxing suggestions above, you can improvise short exercises for use at work, especially if you notice you are moving into a "fight or flight" response. You can say "give me a minute" and then do tummy breathing: take a deep breathe then counting mentally to 10, before responding, as in Simulation Exercise 27.4.

Reflection and Analysis

When you feel yourself getting upset, stop and identify your feeling. This shifts brain activity from the amygdala (emotional center) to the prefrontal cortex (thinking area) and helps calm you (Fessell & Cherniss, 2020).

Take a Break, Take a Walk

On your coffee break choose instead to do a purposeful walk, outside if possible, such as the one described in Simulation Exercise 27.5. Or try a download from AprilSnowConsulting.com/stress-workbook.

SIMULATION EXERCISE 27.3   Sitting Meditation

Procedure

Set a 3min timer perhaps on your smart watch. Take your pulse. Sit comfortably, body relaxed and in good alignment. Focus on breathing slowly and deeply. Use a "mantra" word you have practiced to activate parasympathetic brain activity. Retake your pulse.

Reflective Discussion Analysis

Was this effective? Did your pulse rate decrease?

SIMULATION EXERCISE 27.4   Tummy Breathing

Procedure

Breathe in slowly through your nose, expanding your abdomen, hold the breath for 6s, and then purse your lips to exhale slowly as if blowing out candles on a birthday cake. Repeat this 8–10 times.

Reflective Discussion Analysis

Could this be used automatically to reduce stress before entering a difficult situation?

SIMULATION EXERCISE 27.5   Simple Purposeful Walking Meditation

Snow (2020) describes a walking exercise that incorporates some meditation with exercise.

Start by planting both feet firmly on the ground, hands at rest. Take a deep breath through your nose. As you exhale, be aware of your left foot. As you breathe in again, become aware of your right foot. Place both feet side by side on the ground. After taking a deep nasal breath, exhale, lifting left foot, and placing your heel on the ground in front, allowing your weight to rock forward. Repeat with right foot and return both feet to the ground as you focus on sensations and environment.

Reflective Discussion Analysis

What response did you have? Would you do this again?

SUMMARY

The focus of this chapter was intrapersonal communication "*self-talk*" measures to help manage your stress levels. Self-care is an essential aspect of nursing, if we are to maintain our abilities to care for others. A review of Selye's general adaptive stress principles and Orem's Self-care agency need review. Practices for chronic stress prevention, recognition of our increasing stress level, self-care measures to control or decrease stress were discussed. Suggestions of specific exercises and practices were listed to help you in self-management of stress.

ETHICAL DILEMMA: What Would You Do?

Mary Denium, RN, has worked on a large medical unit for 15years. Lately she has mood swings alternating between irritableness and looking mellow. She focuses poorly on completing her patient care assignments. As an observant nurse on her team, you suspect she is skimming her patient's opioids. She never wants a day off (this would limit her access to drugs). The situation stresses you out since you really have no evidence. What do you do?

DISCUSSION QUESTIONS

1. What symptoms of stress have you recognized in yourself?
2. How do you manage your stress? Analyze whether each of these is maladaptive, such as comfort eating, or if they do help maintain health.

REFERENCES

American Nurses Association (ANA). (n.d.). *Mental health help for nurses.* Healthy nurse; healthy nation. Retrieved from: www.nursingworld.org/practice-policy/hnhn/2017-year-of-the-healthy-nurse/mental-health-wellness/. [Accessed 6 July 2021].

Bozdağ, F., & Ergün, N. (2020). Psychological resilience of healthcare professionals during COVID-19 pandemic. *Psychological Reports*, 124(6), 2567–2586. 33294120965477.

Chen, X., Zhang, B., Jin, S. X., Quan, Y. X., Zhang, X. W., & Cui, X. S. (2021). The effects of mindfulness-based interventions on nursing students: A meta-analysis. *Nursing Education Today*, 98, 104718.

Chipu, M., & Downing, C. (2020). Professional nurses' facilitation of self-care in intensive care units: A concept analysis. *International Journal of Nursing Science*, 7(4), 446–452.

Cooper, A. L., Brown, J. A., Rees, C. S., & Leslie, G. D. (2020). Nurse resilience: A concept analysis. *International Journal of Mental Health Nursing*, 29(4), 553–575.

Davidson, J., Mendis, J., Stuck, A. R., DeMichele, G., & Zisook, S. (2018). *Nurse suicide: Breaking the silence. NAM perspectives.* Discussion Paper Washington, D.C: National Academy of Medicine. Retrieved from: https://nam.edu/nurse-suicide-breaking-the-silence/. [Accessed 6 July 2021].

Davidson, J. E., Proudfoot, J., Lee, K., & Zisook, S. (2019). Nurse suicide in the United States: Analysis of the center for disease control 2014 national violent death reporting system dataset. *Archives of Psychiatric Nursing*, 33(5), 16–21.

Fessell, D., & Cherniss, C. (2020). Coronavirus disease 2019 (COVID-19) and beyond: Micropractices for burnout prevention and emotional wellness. *Journal of the American College of Radiology*, 17(6), 746–748.

Halsted, C., & Hart, V. T. (2021). Mental health in nursing: A student's perspective. *Nursing*, 51(1), 52–55.

Hartwig, A., Clarke, S., Johnson, S., & Willis, S. (2020). Workplace team resilience: A systematic review and conceptual development. *Organizational Psychology Review*, 10(3–4), 169–200.

Hollywood, L., & Phillips, K. E. (2020). Nurses' resilience levels and the effects of workplace violence on patient care. *Applied Nursing Research*, 54, 151321.

Institute for Healthcare Improvement (IHI). (2021). *Joy in Work. A global results-oriented learning network to combat burnout.* Retrieved from: http://www.ihi.org/Topics/Joy-In-Work/Pages/default.aspx. [Accessed 6 July 2021].

Leichtman, K. (2021). *How to fight burnout.* Edutopia. [website]. Retrieved from: https://www.edutopia.org/article/how-fight-burnout. [Accessed 6 July 2021].

Levine, H. (2020). *Natural stress remedies for right now.* AARP. [website]. Retrieved from: https://www.aarp.org/health/healthy-living/info-2020/natural-stress-reducers.html?CMP=KNC-DSO-Adobe-Google-Health-Conditions-Stress/. [Accessed 6 July 2021].

Mayo Clinic Staff. (n.d.). *Resilience training.* Retrieved from: www.mayoclinic.org/tests-procedures/resilience-training/about/pac-20394943/. [Accessed 6 July 2021].

McSpedon, C. (2021). A conversation with Annette Kennedy. *American Journal of Nursing*, 121(5), 66–68.

Meditation (n.d.). *Psychology today.* Retrieved from: https://www.psychologytoday.com/us/basics/meditation. [Accessed 6 July 2021].

Melnyk, B. M., Tan, A., Hsieh, A. P., et al. (2021). Critical care nurses' physical and mental health, worksite wellness support, and medical errors. *American Journal of Critical Care*, 30(3), 176–184.

National Institute of Mental Health (NIMH). (n.d.). *Ask suicide-screening questions (ASQ) toolkit.* Retrieved from: https://www.nimh.nih.gov/research/research-conducted-at-nimh/asq-toolkit-materials/. [Accessed 6 July 2021].

Orem, D. E. (1995). *Nursing: Concepts of practice.* St. Louis: Mosby.

Roberts, N. J., McAloney-Kocaman, K., Lippiett, K., Ray, E., Welch, L., & Kelly, C. (2021). Levels of resilience, anxiety and depression in nurses working in respiratory clinical areas during the COVID pandemic. *Respiratory Medicine*, 176, 106219.

Sampaio, F., Sequeira, C., & Teixeira, L. (2021). Impact of COVID-19 outbreak on nurses' mental health: A prospective cohort study. *Environmental Research*, 194, 110620.

Smith, M. W. (2020). *Ways to manage stress.* WebMD. [website]. Retrieved from: www.webmd.com/balance/stress-management/stress-management#1. [Accessed 6 July 2021].

Snow, A. (2020). *Mindfulness workbook for stress relief.* Emeryville, CA: Rockridge Press.

World Health Organization (WHO). (2019). *Burn-out an "occupational phenomenon": International classification of diseases.* Retrieved from: www.who.int/mental_health/evidence/burn-out/en/. [Accessed 6 July 2021].

FURTHER READING

Lewis, K. (2021). *Guided visualization: Dealing with stress [video].* National Institute of Mental Health. Retrieved from: www.nimh.nih.gov/news/media/2021/guided-visualization-dealing-with-stress. [Accessed 6 July 2021].

Molina-Praena, J., Ramirez-Baena, L., Gómez-Urquiza, J. L., Cañadas, G. R., De la Fuente, E., & Cañadas-De la Fuente, G. (2018). Levels of burnout and risk factors in medical area nurses: A meta-analytic study. *International Journal of Environmental Research and Public Health*, 15(12), 2800.

Next-Generation NCLEX® Examination-Style Case Study Answers

CHAPTER 2, CLARITY AND SAFETY IN COMMUNICATION

Addressing Communication Errors During In-hospital Patient Transfers

A community hospital has provided surgical treatment for 10 patients involved in multiple car accidents on the interstate. The surgical department's nursing staff has been required to work mandatory overtime to meet the needs of the patients recovering from anesthesia. A nurse preparing to move three patients to the postsurgical unit is asked to delay the transfer process to help admit two new patients from the surgical suite. One of the patients ready for transfer has a chest tube in place to reinflate a collapsed lung. Another patient while now presenting with stable vital signs has a history of congestive heart failure. The third patient with a history of substance abuse is awake and alert with stable vital signs. Due to the current situation, the nurse gives the transfer reports over the telephone to the nurses who will be accepting the patients on the various postsurgical units.

Which issues present risks for incomplete communication between staff during the transfer of these patients from one care site to another? *Select all that apply.*

a. Staff fatigue
b. Frequent interruptions
c. Ineffective staff training
d. Inconsistent report format
e. Omission of key information
f. Lack of relevant safety protocols
g. Poor adherence to established practice guidelines

Rationale: Miscommunication errors most often occur during a handoff procedure, when one staff member transfers responsibility for care to another staff member. More than half of all incidences of reported serious miscommunications occurred during patient handoff and transfer, when those assuming responsibility for the patient (coming on duty) are given a verbal, face-to-face synopsis of the patient's current condition by those who had been caring for the patient and are now going off duty. Patient care responsibility is transitioned or handed off when the patient is transferred to another unit. Transition times are high risk for incomplete communication and consequently result in more errors. This has been attributed to frequent interruptions, inconsistent report format, and omission of key information. General barriers to effective communication have been identified and include staff fatigue, lack of effective staff training, and poor adherence to established, relevant guidelines. In this scenario, the nursing staff is likely experiencing fatigue related to the mandatory overtime and intense patient load. The chaos is created by influx of new admissions to the postanesthesia unit while the need to transfer patients to the postsurgical units contributes to frequent interruptions. In this situation, the staff are not adhering to established practice guidelines but are rather giving the transfer report by telephone rather than the standard face-to-face format. There is no indication that the nursing staff in either of the patient care areas are ineffectively trained or that there has been an omission of key patient information. Hospitals are required to have patient safety protocols in place so it is highly unlikely this hospital would not have relevant protocols in place.

CHAPTER 4, CLINICAL JUDGMENT: CRITICAL THINKING AND ETHICAL DECISION-MAKING

Ethical Support of a Patient's Right of Autonomy

After learning of their cancer diagnosis, a patient has a long conversation about proposed treatment options with the oncologist. The next morning the patient shares with the nurse that they are very likely going to choose the option that includes a new chemotherapy treatment. **The nurse responds with personal stories regarding the outcome of several patients with a similar diagnosis, adding that new therapies tend to be very expensive.** The nurse stresses that while the decision is the patient's to make, **it is worth considering that the traditional therapies have proven to be very effective.**

In the aforementioned scenario, highlight the assessment findings that require immediate follow-up.

Rationale: Autonomy is the patient's right to self-determination. In the medical context, respect for autonomy is a fundamental ethical principle. It is the basis for the concept of informed consent, which means your patient makes a rational, informed decision without coercion. External factors, such as coercion by a care provider, may interfere with this process. In this situation, the nurse is interjecting personal biases, thus interfering with the patient's ability to make their own decision concerning treatment.

CHAPTER 7, INTERCULTURAL COMMUNICATION AND PATIENT DIVERSITY

Addressing Communication Barriers

A 19-year-old Latino migrant worker presents at the local hospital's emergency department (ED) after sustaining a 3-inch laceration to the right forearm. The patient neither speaks nor understand English sufficiently to give a medical history or details concerning the accident leading to the wound. The patient appears nervous and teary eyed. After the wound is cleansed and bleeding is controlled, it is determined that stitches and an antibiotic will be required. Postdischarge care will include wound care and follow-up appointment for stitch removal in 2 weeks.

Complete the following sentences by choosing from the list of options.

At this time, to best address the patient's needs, the nurse would first _____(1)_____ to _____(2)_____.

Options for 1	Options for 2
Arrange for a medical translator to be present	Provide emotional support and as well as supplement missing medical history information
Request that a friend or family member be called to the ED to translate	**Assure the patient is able to effectively participate in care planning**
Contact the hospital's social services department	Assist with postdischarge recovery care needs

Rationale: The patient has the right to participate in the planning of medical care. In this situation, informed consent is required for needed treatment. For care needs to be appropriately addressed, the patient will need to clearly understand the information being given. The language issues are a severe barrier to achieving those goals. A competent translator is necessary to best ensure the patient and staff are communicating effectively. The patient appears, understandably, to be emotional distressed. Being unable to fully understand what is happening contributes to an already stressful situation. While having friends or family present would likely help the patient manage this stress, being able to communicate effectively would serve to minimize some of the factors contributing to the stress. Social services can provide needed assistance, but the lack of effective communication with the patient could negatively affect this process as well.

CHAPTER 15, COMMUNICATION IN HEALTH TEACHING

Patient Instructional Needs

Sara, a 17-year-old emancipated minor, has presented at a community-based free clinic requesting medical treatment of a foot wound. Sara's physical confirmed the presence of a 2-inch laceration on her left foot that is reddened, edematous, and producing purulent drainage. The primary care provider determines the wound is infected and will require medical interventions including laceration cleansing, dressing, and antibiotic therapy.

During her history interview, Sara stated she left her home 2 years ago after years of being physically and emotionally abused by her parents, who were both seriously abusing drugs. She moved in with extended family and went to school while working to support herself financially. When she was eventually awarded legal emancipation by the court 7 months ago, she moved to the city and joined a group of teenagers who reside in a local park. Sara volunteered that she is a diagnosed asthmatic but ran out of medication 3 weeks ago and does not know where to get more. When asked, Sara expressed in interest in being vaccinated but stated, "I'm just not sure about getting the COVID shot."

Complete the following sentences by choosing from the list of options.

The nurse would first provide verbal and written information to _____(1)_____ to ____(2)_____.

Options for 1	Options for 2
Discuss the benefits and safety of the COVID-19 vaccine options	Manage existing health needs
Explain the options for immediate treatment of laceration	Provide for environmental safety
Review options for securing prescribed medication	**Secure informed consent to treat**
Present community housing resource options	Minimize risk of contracting a communicable disease

Rationale: The nurse has an obligation to provide appropriate information/education to address patient needs in a timely manner. When presented with several different health risks, addressing acute needs such as treatment for Sara's infected foot laceration will take primary since it presents an immediate risk to her health. To provide the necessary care, Sara must provide informed consent for the treatments. This consent requires that she understands both the condition and the needed treatment options being considered. Since she is an emancipated minor (legally able to independently provide such consent), the nurse needs to provide the information and evaluate her ability to apply the knowledge to the decision-making process. It is then that treatment can be initiated. While all the other option 1's present risks to the patient, none are acute in nature and should be addressed after the immediate infection management has been initiated. The need for medication prescribed for a chronic illness then has priority since lack of appropriate management of her asthma is associated with potential risk to her health. Discussions related to housing and vaccination needs should be initiated after existing health risks are addressed.

CHAPTER 22, ROLE RELATIONSHIP COMMUNICATION WITHIN NURSING

Nursing Mentorship and Career Guidance

A nurse who completed a bachelor's degree in nursing 2 years ago has now been accepted into a master's degree program and successfully earned eight graduate level credits. The nurse with 8 years of medical-surgical experience as well as for with 4 years of maternal-newborn experience is now interested in applying for a position in a new specialty area. When a position is posted for an ED nursing position, the nurse asks an experienced ED nurse to discuss the possible career move.

What topics should the discussion focus on initially? *Select all that apply.*

a. Transferal of existing skill sets
b. Professional challenges
c. Nursing responsibilities
d. Advancement potential
e. Required credentials
f. Needed experience
g. Personal rewards
h. Staffing policies

Rationale: The nurse is embarking on a career change that will require assuming a novice role in this new specialty area. The initial focus should be on hiring criteria, understanding of position responsibilities, and the aspects of the position that are personally and professionally challenging and gratifying. The issues of staffing, advancement possibilities, and the transferal of skill sets can be explored once the fundamental issues of interests, qualifications, and motivation to make such a change have been determined.

GLOSSARY

A

Accommodation: A desire to smooth over a conflict through cooperative but nonassertive responses.

Acting-out behavior: Displaying emotions physically, often in a disruptive or violent manner.

Active listening: A communication skill embodying listening with full attention on the patient for the purpose of developing and understanding collaboratively constructed meanings.

Aging: A universal life process of advancing through the life cycle.

Aggregated data: Compilation of multiple bits of factual information into large groupings allowing analysis.

Aggressive behavior: A response in which the individual acts to defend self, deflecting the emotional impact of personal attack, with an extreme reaction.

Alarm fatigue: Habituating the sound of a machine alert so as to not pay attention to it.

Allostasis: A theory of stress response that describes how the human organism maintains physiological homeostasis through changing circumstances.

Anticipatory guidance: A proactive provider strategy of sharing information to help patients cope effectively with stressful situations, thereby reducing unnecessary stress.

Anxiety: A vague, persistent feeling of impending doom.

Aphasia: A neurological linguistic deficit that is most commonly associated with neurological trauma to the brain.

Assertive behavior: Setting goals, acting on those goals in a clear, consistent manner, and taking responsibility for the consequences of those actions.

Assimilation: When an individual from a different culture fully adopts the behaviors, customs, and values of the mainstream culture as part of his or her social identity.

Attending behaviors: Behaviors designed to facilitate empathy that include an attentive, open posture; responding to verbal and nonverbal cues through appropriate gestures and facial expressions; using eye contact; and allowing patient self-expression.

Authoritarian group leadership: A leadership style in which leaders take full responsibility for group direction and control group interaction.

Avoidance: A coping mechanism in which a person changes their behavior to avoid thinking about, feeling, or doing difficult things. Nurses using avoidance distance themselves from their patients or provide less support.

B

Behavioral emergency: Refers to crisis escalation to the point that the situation requires immediate intervention to avoid injury or death.

Behavioral objectives: Guides to action that begin with the phrase "the patient will" followed by step-by-step achievable, measurable patient behaviors toward treatment goals.

Best practice: Nursing interventions derived from research evidence demonstrating successful outcome for patient.

Biases: Prejudices or beliefs associating negative characteristics to those perceived as different from oneself, often occurring unconsciously.

Body image: The physical dimension of self-concept.

Body language (also kinesics): Involving the conscious or unconscious body positioning or actions of the communicator.

Boundaries: Represent invisible structures imposed by legal, ethical, and professional standards of nursing that respect nurse and patient rights and protect the functional integrity of their relationship.

Briefing: Oral statement of roles and responsibilities prior to activity.

Burnout: A state of fatigue or frustration brought about by devotion to a cause, way of life, or relationship that failed to produce an expected reward.

C

Callouts: The team reviews the situation aloud.

Caring: An intentional human action characterized by commitment and a sufficient level of knowledge and skill to allow the nurse to support the basic integrity of the patient.

Care transition: The traditional patient report from one nurse handing over care to another nurse. The report should be accurate, specific, and clear, and allow time for questions to foster a culture of patient safety.

Chronic sorrow: A normal grief response associated with an ongoing living loss that is permanent, progressive, recurring, and cyclic in nature.

Clarification: A therapeutic active listening strategy designed to aid in understanding communication by asking for more information or for elaboration on a point.

Clinical decision making: Problem-solving by processing patient data and own knowledge to arrive at an appropriate intervention or diagnosis.

Clinical decision support system (CDSS): Software programs that input specific information about a patient, analyze it, and make recommendations for care based on best practice outcomes as established by research.

Clinical judgment: A combination of research, clinical expertise, and patient preferences. It requires both the ability to think critically and the knowledge as to how to apply ethical principles.

Closed-ended questions: Question format which requires a yes or no or single-phase response; they are used in emergency situations to quickly gather information.

Cognition: Refers to the thinking processes people use to make sense of their perceptions.

Cognitive dissonance: The holding of two or more conflicting values at the same time.

Cognitive restructuring: Changing beliefs to make them more positive.

Cohesion (group): An essential curative factor in therapeutic groups defined as the value a group holds for its members and underscores the level of member commitment to the group.

Collaboration: 1) Working with all the members of the healthcare team to achieve maximum health outcomes for our mutual patient. 2) A solution-oriented response to conflict in which we work together cooperatively to solve problems.

Collaborative culture: A care culture in which all team members keep the delivery of safe, high-quality care foremost in mind; requires that we trust and respect the decision-making of all team members.

Communication: A combination of verbal and nonverbal behaviors integrated for the purpose of sharing information that is timely, accurate, complete, unambiguous, and is understood by the receiver.

Communication deficit: An impairment in the ability to receive, send, process, and comprehend concepts or verbal, nonverbal, and graphic symbol systems. Deficits include compromised hearing, vision, speech, or language or problems with cognitive processing.

Community: Any group of citizens that have either a geographic, population-based, or self-defined relationship and whose health may be improved by a health promotion approach.

Compassion fatigue: A syndrome associated with serious spiritual, physical, and emotional depletion related to caring for those who are seriously ill.

Competency: A set of knowledge, skills, and attitudes.

Competition: A response style to conflict characterized by domination, exercising power to gain your own goals at the expense of the other person.

Compromise: A response style to conflict in which each party gives a little and gains a little; it is effective only when both parties hold equal power.

Computerized provider order entry (CPOE): Part of the health information system which allows providers to order tests and treatments.

Confidentiality: The respect for another's privacy that involves holding and not divulging information given in confidence except in case of suspected abuse, commission of a crime, or threat of harm to self or others.

Conflict: Disagreement arising from differences in attitudes, values, or needs in which the actions of one party frustrate the ability of the other to achieve his or her expected goals.

Connotation: A more personalized meaning of the word or phrase.

Continuity of care: Describes a multidimensional longitudinal construct in healthcare, which emphasizes seamless provision and coordination of patient-centered quality care across clinical settings.

Crisis: A crisis describes a stressful life event, which overwhelms an individual's ability to cope effectively in the face of a perceived challenge or threat.

Crisis intervention: The systematic application of problem-solving techniques, based on crisis theory, designed to help the individual move through the crisis process as swiftly and painlessly as possible with a return to their precrisis functional level.

Crisis state: An acute normal human response to severely abnormal circumstances; it is not a mental illness.

Critical thinking: An analytical process in which you purposefully use specific thinking skills to make complex clinical decisions.

Cultural competence: A set of cultural behaviors and attitudes integrated into the practice methods of a system, agency, or its professionals, which enables them to work effectively in cross-cultural situations.

Cultural diversity: Variations among cultural groups.

Cultural humility: A process of openness, self-awareness, being egoless, and incorporating self-reflection and critique after willingly interacting with diverse individuals.

Cultural identity: Awareness of beliefs and practices associated with one's ethnic, religious, or family background.

Cultural patterns: The social customs, expected behaviors, cultural beliefs, values, and language passed down from generation to generation by a group of people.

Cultural relativism: The belief that each culture is unique and should be judged only based on its own values and standards.

Cultural sensitivity: The ability to be appropriately responsive to the attitudes, feelings, or circumstances of groups of people that share a common and distinctive racial, national, religious, linguistic, or cultural heritage.

Culturally competent communication: A willingness to try to understand and respond to your patient's cultural beliefs.

D

Debriefing: A short meeting after an event to review the incident.

De-escalate: A tension-reducing action that strives to defuse and resolve a crisis.

Dementia: A general term for a neurological disorder characterized by a progressive decline in intellectual and behavioral functioning.

Democratic group leadership: A group leadership style in which the leader involves members in active open discussion and shared decision-making.

Denotation: The generalized meaning assigned to a word.

Deontological model (duty-based model): A duty-based model for making ethical decisions.

Disaster: A calamitous event of slow or rapid onset that results in large-scale physical destruction of property, social infrastructure, and human life.

Disruptive behavior: Conduct that interferes with safe care by negatively affecting the ability of the team to work together, such as bullying, harassment, blaming, etc.

Distress: A negative stress causes a higher level of anxiety and is perceived as exceeding the person's coping abilities.

Documentation: The process of obtaining, organizing, and conveying health information to others in print or electronic format.

E

Effective communication: A two-way exchange of information among patients and health providers ensuring that the expectations and responsibilities of all are clearly understood. It is an active process for all involved.

Ego defense mechanisms: Conscious and unconscious coping methods used by people to protect themselves by changing the meaning of a situation in their minds.

Ego integrity: Relates to the capacity to look back on your life with satisfaction and few regrets.

Electronic health record (EHR): Various types of computerized health records.

Empathy: The ability to be sensitive to and communicate understanding of the patient's feelings.

Empowerment: Helping a person become a self-advocate; an interpersonal process of providing the appropriate tools, resources, and environment to build, develop, and increase the ability of others to set and reach goals.

Environment: The internal and external context of an individual, as affected by their healthcare situation.

Ethical dilemma (also moral dilemma): The conflict of two or more moral issues; a situation in which there are two or more conflicting ways of looking at a situation.

Ethnicity: Personal awareness of a shared cultural heritage with others based on common racial, geographic, ancestral, religious, or historical bonds.

Ethnocentrism: The belief that one's own culture should be the norm and has the right to impose its standards of "correct" behavior and values on another because it is better or more enlightened than others.

Eustress: A short-term mild level of stress.

Evidence-based nursing practice: Implementing nursing interventions which are based on sound clinical research and professional judgment in real-time situations.

Expressive aphasia: A type of aphasia in which an individual can understand what is being said but cannot express thoughts or feelings in words.

F

Family: A self-identified group of two more or individuals whose association is characterized by special terms, who may or may not be related by bloodlines or law, but who function in such a way that they consider themselves to be a family.

Feedback: A message given by the nurse to the patient in response to a message or observed behavior.

Flow sheets: Charting patient's status information in preprinted categories of information.

Focused questions: Inquiries that require more than a yes/no one-word response to a specific discussion topic.

Functional status: A broad range of purposeful abilities related to physical health maintenance, role performance, cognitive or intellectual abilities, social activities, and level of emotional functioning.

G

Gender roles: Socially constructed roles and behaviors that occur in a historical and cultural context, and that vary across societies and over time.

Global aphasia: A type of aphasia in which an individual has difficulty with both expressive language and reception of messages.

Good death: A death that is free from unavoidable distress and suffering for patients, families, and caregivers; in general accord with patients and families' wishes; and reasonably consistent with clinical, cultural, and ethical standards.

Grief: Represents a holistic, adaptive process that a person goes through following a significant loss.

Group dynamics: Communication processes and behaviors occurring during the life of the group.

Group norms: Refer to the unwritten behavioral rules of conduct expected of group members. Norms can be universal (present in all groups) and group specific referring to those constructed by group members.

Group-specific norms: Rules constructed by group members representing the shared beliefs, values, and unspoken operational rules governing group functions. They help define member interactions and are often implicit.

H

Handoff (also handover): Transfer process taking place when patients are reassigned to another team of healthcare providers.

Hardiness: A protective factor that can minimize the effects of stress that consists of three basic elements: challenge, commitment, and taking control.

Health: A multidimensional concept having physical, psychological, sociocultural, developmental, and spiritual characteristics that is used to describe an individual's state of well-being and level of functioning.

Health disparity: A particular type of health difference that is closely linked with social, economic, and/or environmental disadvantage.

Health information technology (HIT): An electronic interactive system designed to support the multiple information needs required by today's complex healthcare.

Health literacy: The degree to which people have the capacity to obtain, process, and understand basic health information and services needed to make appropriate health decisions.

Health promotion: An educational support process that enables people to take control over their health.

Homeostasis (also dynamic equilibrium): A person's sense of personal security and balance.

Hospice care: Care that can be initiated after the patient has stopped all curative treatments and when they are nearing their end-of-life period.

Huddle: Brief, informal health team gathering to review a course of action.

Human rights–based ethical decision model: Based on the belief that each person has basic rights.

I

Identity: An internal construct about one's abilities, self-image, characteristics.

Informatics: The science of how to use data, information, and knowledge to improve human health and the delivery of healthcare services.

Informed consent: A focused communication process in which a clinician discloses all relevant information related to a procedure or treatment, with full opportunity for dialogue, questions, and expressions of concern, prior to asking for the patient's signed permission.

Input: Component of the transactional communication model where the patient/family receives information from the environment.

Intercultural communication: Conversations between people from different cultures that embrace differences in perceptions, language, and nonverbal behaviors, and recognition of different interpretative contexts.

Interdisciplinary palliative care team: A health care team usually consisting of nurses, physicians, social workers, and clergy specially trained in palliative care.

Interpersonal competence: The ability to interpret the content of a message from the point of view of each of the participants and the ability to use language and nonverbal behaviors to achieve the goals of the interaction.

Intrapersonal communication: Takes place within the self in the form of inner thoughts; beliefs are colored by feelings and influence behavior.

J

Just culture: A work environment in which staff are empowered to safely speak about their safety concerns.

L

Laissez-faire group leadership: A disengaged form of leadership style in which the leader avoids decision-making and is minimally available to group members.

Linear communication model: Consists of sender, message, receiver, channel, and context.

Longitudinal plan of care (LPC): Electronic multidisciplinary care plan used across sites to improve continuity of care.

M

Magnet hospital: A hospital that has been identified by a unique national program that recognizes quality patient care and nursing excellence in health care institutions and agencies as a work environment that act as a "magnet" for professional nurses desiring to work there because of their excellence.

Malpractice: Negligence or incompetence on the part of a professional.

Meaning: Interpretation of a message. Meaning is influenced by past experience and current circumstances of the message to the receiver, and is affected by nonverbal cues the sender conveys.

Medical home: A medical home is a place that serves as a central first contact point in primary care and provides regular, accessible, comprehensive primary care services for designated patients and families within a single familiar setting.

Medical jargon: Medical terms unfamiliar to a patient.

Mental incompetence: Occurs when a person lacks the capacity to negotiate legal tasks such as making a will, entering into a contract, or making certain legal decisions.

Message: Consists of the transmitted verbal or nonverbal expression of thoughts and feelings.

Message competency: The ability to use language and nonverbal behaviors strategically in the intervention phase of the nursing process to achieve the goals of the interaction.

Metacommunication: A broad term which describes all the verbal and nonverbal factors used to enhance or negate the meaning of words.

Metaparadigm: The four core nursing concepts: person, environment, health, nursing.

Microaggressions: Communicating subtle and often unintentional discrimination pertaining to self-concepts of race, ethnicity, gender, or any other demographic.

Microassaults: Explicit negative verbal or nonverbal communication that offends an individual through criticism, slighting, or purposeful prejudicial actions.

Microinsults: Subtle unintended rebuffs, but the insinuation would clearly offend the recipient.

Microinvalidations: Communications that discount or invalidate a person's values, feelings, or lifestyle.

Mindfulness: Refers to awareness within the present moment, especially regarding safety issues.

Miscommunication problem: Failure in communication in one or more categories: the system, the transmission, or in the reception.

Motivational interviewing: Techniques used to identify a patient's beliefs about current health behaviors with the goal of fostering change or improving self-care behaviors.

Mutuality: An agreement on problems and the means for resolving them; a commitment by both parties to enhance well-being.

N

Negative attributions: A person's less-than-optimal characteristics.

NNN: Abbreviation designating the combination of North American Nursing Diagnosis Association (NANDA), Nursing Interventions Classification (NIC), and Nursing Outcomes Classification (NOC).

Nonverbal communication: Refers to physical expressions and behaviors not expressed in words, which help clinicians understand the emotional meanings of messages.

Nursing process: Embodies five phases in healthcare delivery: assessment, problem identification/diagnosis, planning, implementation, and outcome evaluation.

O

Open-ended questions: A question format designed to help individuals express health problems and needs in their own words. Open-ended questions are open to interpretation and cannot be answered by yes, no, or another one-word response.

Output: Component of the transactional communication model where information has been received and interpreted/processed by the receiver.

P

Pain assessment scales: Tools used to rate the severity of a person's discomfort; these tools can come in different forms such as a numerical list (1 to 10) or a pictograph (Wong-Baker FACES Pain Rating Scale).

Palliative care: A philosophy of care aimed at primarily relieving symptoms associated with terminal illness and providing support for seriously ill patients and their families.

Paralanguage: The oral delivery of a verbal message expressed through tone of voice and inflection, sighing, or crying.

Paraphrasing: Transforming the patient's words into the nurse's words while keeping the meaning intact.

Patient-centered care (PCC) model: Clinical collaborative team partnership with patients, according to their preferences, needs, and values.

Patient-centered care relationship: A subset of the professional therapeutic relationship, in which nurses and other health professionals engage with their patients to understand the patient's experience of an illness, help them learn to self-manage chronic health problems, develop healthy lifestyle behaviors to prevent or minimize the development of chronic disorders, and increase their satisfaction with clinical outcomes and well-being.

Patient education: A set of planned educational activities, resulting in changes in health-related behaviors and attitudes as well as knowledge.

Patient safety: The prevention of errors and adverse effects to patients associated with healthcare.

Point of care: Whatever location the nurse is in to provide care to the patient, whether at the bedside in the hospital room, in an outpatient clinic, or even in the patient's own home. Health information can be updated via wireless Internet devices.

Portals: See Web portal.

Possible selves: Used to explain the future-oriented component of self-concept.

Presbycusis: Decrease in hearing associated with aging.

Presbyopia: Decrease in visual adjustments associated with aging.

Primary group: A group membership with an informal structure and close personal relationships.

Primary disease prevention: Actions taken to preclude illness or to prevent the natural course of illness from occurring; strategies target modifiable risk factors with health education to promote a healthy lifestyle.

Professional role socialization: A complex, continuous, interactive educational process through which student nurses acquire the knowledge, skills, attitudes, norms, values and behaviors associated with the nursing profession.

Proxemics: The study of an individual's use of space.

Q

Quality of life: A personal experience of subjective well-being and general satisfaction with life that includes, but is not limited to, physical health.

R

Radio frequency identity (RFID) chips: Small embedded computerized chips that can be located remotely.

Receptive aphasia: A type of aphasia in which an individual has difficulty receiving and processing written and oral messages.

Reflection: A listening response focused on the emotional implications of a message used to help patients clarify important feelings related to message content.

Reminiscence: An empowerment strategy that reminds older adults of personal strengths and meaningful goals already achieved.

Resilience: Strength and stability during change and stressful life events with rapid recovery from adversity; the ability to "bounce back."

Respect: A positive feeling or action shown towards someone to convey a due regard for the feelings, wishes, rights, or traditions of others.

Restatement: An active listening strategy used to broaden a patient's perspective or when the nurse needs to provide a sharper focus on a specific part of the message.

Role: A multidimensional psychosocial concept defined as a traditional pattern of behavior and self-expression, performed by or expected of an individual within a given society.

Role competencies: A set of skills, abilities, and related knowledge needed to perform a specific task or an activity within a specific function or role.

S

SBAR (situation, background, assessment, recommendation): A standardized communication tool.

Scientific method: Used in research, this is a logical, linear method of systematically gaining new information, often by setting up an experiment to test an idea.

Secondary group: A group membership that is time-limited with a prescribed formal structure, a designated leader, and specific goals and functions.

Secondary disease prevention: Interventions designed to promote early diagnosis of symptoms through health screening or timely treatment after the onset of the disease, thus minimizing their effects on a person's life.

Self-awareness: An intrapersonal process in which a nurse reflects on how their own feelings and beliefs influence professional behaviors.

Self-clarity: The extent to which sense of self is stable and well-defined; a feature of self-concept.

Self-concept: A term describing peoples' complex understanding of their cultural heritage, their environment, their upbringing and education, their basic personality traits, and cumulative life experiences.

Self-efficacy: A term which refers to a person's perceptual belief about their capability to perform tasks and execute courses of action successfully.

Self-esteem: The emotional degree to which people approve of themselves in relation to others and the environment.

Self-management: A patient's ability to manage the symptoms and consequences of living with a chronic condition, including treatment, physical, social, and lifestyle changes.

Sentinel event: A life-changing health care occurrence; The Joint Commission specifically uses this term to refer to serious errors in healthcare, which harm patients.

Shared decision-making: Process in which healthcare professionals work together with patients to use evidence-based data to access treatment options, risks involved, and possible outcomes to make the best health choices for individuals.

Silence: A powerful listening response delivered as a brief pause.

Simulations: Experiential exercises, such as applications to clinical cases or scenarios in simulation labs. Simulations are used after graduation in continuing education, team training, and systems testing.

Social cognitive competency: The ability to interpret message content within interactions from the point of view of each of the participants.

Standardized communication tools: Uniformly used formats for communication of patient information among all care providers, such as the SBAR tool.

Stereotyping: The process of attributing characteristics to a group of people as though all persons in the identified group possessed them.

Stress: A natural physiological, psychological, and spiritual response to the presence of a stressor.

Stressor: A demand, situation, internal stimulus, or circumstance that threatens a person's personal security or self-integrity.

Stress responses: A response to stress triggered either by a physical or psychological threat which induces specific physical change to prepare your body to ward off the threat.

Summarization: An active listening skill used to pull several ideas and feelings together, either from one interaction or a series of interactions, into a few succinct sentences.

Surrogate: A legal guardian or personal health care agent who provides consent for the medical treatment of adults who lack the capacity to consent on their own behalf.

T

Taxonomy: A hierarchical method of classifying vocabulary of items according to certain rules.

TCAB: An acronym for the program Transforming Care At the Bedside, which empowers nurses to make changes that improve patient safety.

Teach-back method: A teaching strategy used in patient education to evaluate and verify their understanding of health teaching; their ability to repeat a demonstration of requisite knowledge and skills.

TeamSTEPPS: A program (Team Strategies and Tools to Enhance Performance and Patient Safety) which emphasizes improving outcomes by improving communication.

Telehealth: Any use of Internet-transmitted visualization for healthcare diagnosis or treatment. Also known as telemedicine, telenursing, eHealth.

Tertiary disease prevention: Rehabilitation strategies designed to minimize the handicapping effects of a disease or injury once it occurs.

Therapeutic communication: A goal-directed form of communication used in healthcare to achieve objectives that promote patient health and well-being.

Therapeutic relationship: A professional alliance in which the nurse and patient join for a defined period to achieve health-related treatment goals.

Throughput: Component of the transactional communication model where the patient/family internally processes and interprets the meaning of the information received.

Timeout: A communication tool used by teams to stop and review a situation.

Transactional communication models: Communication models that employ systems concepts to describe communication context, feedback loops, and validation; each person influences the other and is both a sender and receiver simultaneously within the interaction.

Trust: A dynamic relational process, involving perceptions of reliance reflecting the deepest needs and vulnerabilities of individuals.

U

Universal norms: Explicit behavioral standards, which must be present in all groups to achieve effective outcomes.

Utilitarian or goal-based model: A framework for making ethical decisions in which the rights of the patient and the duties of the nurse are determined by what will achieve maximum welfare or overall good.

V

Validation: A focused form of feedback involving verbal and nonverbal confirmation that both participants have the same basic understanding of a message. Feedback loops validate information or allow the human system to correct its original information.

Veracity: Truthfulness.

Violence: A health emergency, which can create a critical challenge to the safety, well-being, and health of patients, staff, or others in their immediate environment.

Vocalics: Aspects of the voice, such as tone, volume, pitch, and rhythm.

W

Web portal: An agency website that provides opportunities for consumers to use hyperlinks to access a variety of information, receive cyber support, make appointments, pay bills, etc.

Well-being: A person's subjective experience of satisfaction about his or her life related to six personal dimensions: intellectual, physical, emotional, social, occupational, and spiritual.

Wisdom: The virtue associated with Erikson's final stage of ego development represents an integrated system of "knowing" about the meaning and conduct of life.

Work-arounds: Use of nonapproved shortcuts in giving healthcare.

INDEX

Note: Page numbers followed by "f" indicate figures, "t" indicate tables, "b" indicate boxes.

A

AACN. *See* American Association of Colleges of Nursing
Absent stimulation, communication deficit, 240
Academic role models, 318
Acceptable pain, 305
Acceptance, loss stage, 302
Accommodation, 176
   allostatic, 221
Acculturation, 89
Acting-out behaviors, 262–263
Active listening, 67–68
   child communication, 264
   responses, 68
   simulation exercise, 68b
Activities of daily living (ADLs), 272
Activity groups, 111
Actual self, 118
Acute grief, 302
Acute pain, 305
Acute stress, 220
Adjourning phase
   group, 107
   therapeutic groups, 113
Adolescents (child communication), 260–261
Advanced beginner, 319
Advance directives, 307
Advanced practice nurse (APRN), 316
Adverse medication event, 17b
Advocacy, support (aging), 275–276
Age-appropriate communication, 254–255
Age cohort diversity, 81–82
Ageism, 269
Agency for Healthcare Research and Quality (AHRQ), 30, 267
Aggregated data, 362
Aggressive behavior, 178–179
Aging
   advocacy support, 275–276
   applications, 271–280
   apraxia, 277
   case study of, 268b, 277b
   concepts of, 267–271
   connectedness, 274
   daily life, supporting adaptation, 277
      case example of, 277b, 279b

Aging *(Continued)*
   definition, 267
   delirium, dementia, depression, 278t
   education, 274
   elder abuse, 270
   Erikson's ego development model, 269–270
   functional status, assessment, 272–273
   fundamental rights, 268b, 271
   health
      promotion activities, 276b
      teaching, 276–277
   healthcare communication and, 268
   illness incidence, 267
   legal issues, 280
   life review, 274
   Maslow' s hierarchy of needs theory, 270
   medication self-management, teaching, 275b
   medication supports, 275
   mental health issues, 270–271, 271b
   quality of life functionality framework, 270
   reminiscence groups, 274
   safety supports, 275
   social and spiritual supports, 274–275
   socialization, amount of, 274
   story, exercise, 272b
   successful
      definition of, 267
      goal, 267–268
   sundowning, 280
   supporting communication in, 278–280
   theoretical models, care and, 269–270
   touch, relationship, 280
   transition healthcare model, 269
   treatment, barriers, 268–269
   wisdom, 270
Alarm fatigue, 381
Alcoholism, approaches/statements, 194t
Alexia, Google Assistant, 275
Allostasis, 221
   model of stress, 221f
Allostatic accommodation, 221
Allostatic load, 221
Alternative communication, of child communication, 264

Altruism, 111t
Ambulatory clinic, physically ill children (communication), 257
American Association for Critical Care Nurses, 30
American Association of Colleges of Nursing (AACN), 30
American Nurses Association (ANA), 30
   Bill of Rights for Registered Nurses, 323, 323b
   Code of Ethics for Nurses, 31–33, 33b, 52
   standards for communication, 61b
American Nurses Credentialing Center Competencies, 294–295
American Speech-Language-Hearing Association (ASHA), 235–236
ANA. *See* American Nurses Association
Anger, 228–229
   anxiety, relationships, 227b
   clinical encounters, 189
   creation, nurse behaviors, 173b
   expression, 189
   loss stage, 301
   nonverbal clues, 185
   signs, recognition, 185–188
   stage, 175
Anticipatory grief, 302, 302b
Anticipatory guidance, 231
   in community, relationship, 265
   provision, 264
Anxiety
   anger, relationships, 227b
   care problem and, 262
   decrease, nursing interventions to, 230t
   impact, 152–153
   levels, 153t
   nonverbal behaviors, association/iden-tification, 153b
   reduction, nursing strategies, 154b
   stranger, 257
   verbal behaviors, association/identifi-cation, 153b
Aphasia, 238, 244
   expressive, 238, 244
   global, 238, 244
   receptive, 238
Applications (apps), 377

Apraxia, 277
APRN. *See* Advanced practice nurse
Artistic groups, 111
Art of nursing, 7
ASHA. *See* American Speech-Language-Hearing Association
Assertive behavior, 178
  communication, 188
  components, 178–179
  development, characteristics, 179b
  nature, 178–179
Assertive message, pitching, 178b
Assertive responses, 180b
Assessment, 96–97
  interviews, communication guidelines, 272–274, 272b
Assessment and Management of Individuals at Risk for Suicide, 294
Assimilation, 89–90
Assisted suicide, 307
Assumptions, identification, 53
Attending behaviors, usage, 156
Attitudes, 18–19, 49, 99
  communicating with children and, 249–250
  technology and, 379
Audiovisual aids/hobbies, usages, 260
  case example of, 260b
Auditory learners, 209–210
Augmentative and alternative communication (AAC) methods, 244
Authenticity, of child communication, 264
Authoritarian group leader, 109
Autism spectrum disorder, 263
Autonomy
  case example, 46b
  concept, application, 46
  exercise, 50b
  medical paternalism *versus*, 46
Avoidance, 176

B
Bad news, 168
Bandura's social cognitive model, 207–208
Bandura's social learning theory, 194–195, 195b
Barcoded name bands, 24, 24f
Bargaining, loss stage, 301–302
Bedside, transforming care at, 25
Behavioral emergencies, 285
Behavioral objectives, 208
  classifying, 208, 209f
Behavioral reaction, 288
Behavior change, 184
Behaviors, disruptive, 331–332

Beliefs, 91–92
Beneficence, 46–47
  case example, 47b
  challenge, 46–47
  exercise, 51b
Bereavement
  concepts, 301
  study, 285
Best practices, 17, 362
  fostering safety, 15
  interprofessional communication, 333
Bias, impact, 151–152
Big data, 353
Bill of Rights, for Registered Nurses, 323, 323b
Bioethical principles, 46
Biomedical sensors, 374
Bloom taxonomy, 208
Body image, 115
  nursing strategies and, 123
Body image disturbance, 122–123
  assessment, 123
  case example, 123b
  nursing strategies, 123
  patient-centered assessment, 123
Boundaries, 61
Bowen's systems theory, 162
Brainstorming, group, 107
Breakthrough pain, 305–306
Breathing, 393b
Briefing, 22
Burnout, 175, 232, 387–389
  definition, 387
  implications for nurses, 388
  incidence of, 387–388, 388f
  prevention, 232t
  sequalae, 388
  signs and symptoms, 388
  social support, 388–389
  suicide, 388
  treatment, 388

C
Calgary family assessment and family interaction models, 162
  development, 162
  instrumental and expressive functions, 162
  structure, 162
Callouts, 23–24
Cancer, 231b
Care
  continuity
    advocacy, 86–87
    communicating for, 345–355, 354b
  coordination, 350
  options, discussion, 308b

Care *(Continued)*
  palliative care, 304–306
  point of care, 372–373
  standardized communication as an initiative for, 17–18
  transitions, planning for, 348t
Career guidance, 3
Caregiver, support, 169
Caretaker burden, 168
Care transition model, 349
Care transitions, 23
Caring, 148
  absence, 148
  application, 149b
  leadership and, 315
  process, steps, 156
  relationship, provision, 148
  technology and, 315
Carl Rogers' client-centered model, 136
Case finding, 353
Case management, 347
  advocacy, 353
  chronic conditions, management of, 353
  communication, 352, 352b
  national guidelines, 352
  strategies, 352–353
Case studies, usage, 57
Catharsis, 111t
Cellular telephones, 373
Center mind and body, 390, 391b
Centers for Medicare and Medicaid Services (CMS), reporting required by, 14
Change, stages (Prochaska), 194t
Charting
  computerized, 366–367
  legal aspects of, 364–365
Chat rooms, 383
Checklists
  in documenting nursing care, 363
  patient safety outcomes, 19
  usage, 19
Child communication, 249–266, 266b
  active listening, 264
  adaptation, 254b
  adolescents, 260–261
  age-appropriate communication, 254–255
  age-appropriate medical terminology, 260b
  agency environment, evaluation, 258, 258f
  alternative communication strategies, 264
  anticipatory guidance, provision, 264
  anxiety, 262

Child communication *(Continued)*
applications, 253–266, 253f
authenticity, 264
care problems, 261–263
cognitive development, 250
community
anticipatory guidance in, 265
nurse advocacy, 265–266
support groups, 265
decision-making, mutuality, 260
incidence, 249
limit-setting plan, development
guidelines, 263b
location, 249
mutual storytelling technique, usage,
259b
parents
communication guidelines, 265b
healthcare partnership formation,
264–265
pediatric nursing procedures, 262b
play, communication strategy, 258–259
points in, 255b–257b
in preschoolers, 258–259
regression, 254
respect, convey, 264
school age, 259–260
speech development, 250
storytelling, communication strategy,
259
strategies for, 263–264
toddlers, 257–258
veracity, 264
Childhood, definition, 249
Children
acting-out behaviors, 262–263
assessment, 260
attitude, 249–250
cognitive processing, impairment, 239
community, nurse advocacy, 265–266
coping strategies, 252
death, 309–310
developmental level, nursing strategies,
253f
end-of-life care for, 264
in grief, 264
grieving, 310
hearing loss, 237
illness
assessment, 253–255, 254b
information, understanding
(overestimating), 257
needs (nurse-child communication
strategies), 251f, 254b
outpatient procedures, location, 249
psychological behavioral problems,
communication, 255–257

Children *(Continued)*
with special healthcare needs, 251, 263
autism spectrum disorder, 263
hyperactive disorders, 263
mental health problems, 263
parental communication, 265–266
stress issues, 229
vision loss, 238
Choice talk, 144
Chronic Care Model, 347
Chronic conditions, management of, 353
Chronic disease, 346
Chronic disorders, self-management, 200
Chronic pain, 305
Chronic sorrow, 303
Chronic stress, 220
CINAHL. *See* Cumulative Index to
Nursing and Allied Health
Circular questions, 69
Civil laws, 34–35
Clarification, 69
communication, 337–339
documentation, 361
exercise, 69b
roles, 339
Client
anger
anxiety, reduction (nursing strategies), 154b
clinical encounters, 189
expression, 189
nursing behaviors, 186t–187t
dementia, advocacy, 280
difficulty, clinical encounters, 189
feelings, meaning (understanding),
150
problems, analysis, 188
rights/responsibilities, 138–139,
139b
strengths, identification, 144b
Client-centered model, 136
Client instructional needs, 2–3
Clinical behavior guidelines, 119t–121t
Clinical bias (reduction), stereotypes
(identification), 152b
Clinical competence, stages (Benner),
320t
Clinical decision-making, 56–57, 56f
enhancement of, 373
process, critical thinking (application),
52–57, 52t
Clinical decision support systems
(CDSSs), 356
computerized, 376–377
concerns in, 381–382, 382b
usage, 381–382, 382b
Clinical encounters, 189

Clinical judgment, 1–2, 43–58
case example, 44b
concepts, 43
clarification, 53
definitions, 44
evidence-based practice, 50b
Clinical nurse colleagues, 318
Clinical nurse leader, 316
Clinical practice
guidelines, 377
three C's of, 15
Clinical preceptors, 318–319
Clinical simulations, 317
Closed-ended questions, 69
Closed therapeutic groups, 108
CMS. *See* Centers for Medicare and
Medicaid Services
Code of Ethics for Nurses
American Nurses Association, 31–33,
33b, 52
International Code of Ethics adoption,
31–33
Coding, 367
in healthcare, 368–369
Cognition, 125
Cognitive, resilience and, 392
Cognitive abilities, 153t
Cognitive behavioral model, 121
nursing strategies, 125
Cognitive behavioral therapy (CBT), 232
Cognitive development, 250
case study, 250b
stages of, 251t
Cognitive dissonance, 49
Cognitive distortions, 125b
Cognitive impairment, symptoms of, 277
Cognitive processing
deficits
assistance, strategies, 244b
impairment, 238–239
children, 239
etiology, 239
incidence, 238–239
older adults, 239
Cognitive processing deficits, 213
Cognitive reappraisal, 129f
Cognitive restructuring, 232
Cohesion, 104, 104b
Cohesiveness, 107
facilitation of, 104b
therapeutic factors, 111t
Co-leadership, 109
Collaboration, 31, 176, 329
barriers to, 331b
characteristics of, 350, 350f
conflict into, 336b
decision-making, 351b

Collaboration (Continued)
  definition, 328, 332
  dynamic process, 329, 332–333
  effective, 336–337
  practice, 328
  in relational continuity, 350
  resolution process, 339
  shared common goals, 329
  team, 324
  theoretical model concepts, 328
Collaborative characteristics, relational
    continuity on, 350
Collaborative communication, 60
Collaborative culture, creating, 332–333
Collaborative partnership, 138–139
Collaborative patient-centered relation-
    ships, 135–137
Collegiality, 329–330, 330b
COMFORT communication model, 305b
"Command" hallucinations, 293
Commendations, 167
Communicating medical orders, in HIT
    system, 365–366
Communication, 135
  abilities, assessment of, 241
  addressing, barriers, 2, 100b
  American Nurses Association stan-
      dards for, 61b
  applications, 9–10, 18–19, 35
  barriers to, 14–15, 331b
    strategies to remove, 337–341
  clarity and safety in, 1, 12–27, 337–339
  collaborative, 60
  computer-mediated, in community,
      375–376
  concepts, 59–60
  continuity of care, 345–355, 354b
  deficits, 348
  definition, 1–2, 59
  developing education skills, 317–318
  difficulties, symptoms, 277
  effective, 29, 328
    barriers to, 331–332
  empathy, usage, 189
  environment, 6
  environmental awareness, 63–64
  environmental factors, 65
  errors, addressing in-hospital patient
      transfers, 1
  evidence-based practice, 82b
  factors influencing, 61–64, 64b
    barriers, 61–62
  fatigue and, 15
  fragmentation in, 14
  functions of, within healthcare sys-
      tems, 8
  gender differences, 82–83, 250

Communication (Continued)
  guidelines for, 30–31
  hands-free, 374
  health, 6–7
  healthcare system, 4
  in health teaching and coaching, 2–3,
      206–217
  humor, usage, 73
  improve, during handoffs, 23, 23b
  intercultural communication, 88–101
  interdisciplinary, opportunities, 342
  interprofessional, 328–344, 339b
    improved, 335t
  interprofessional education and
      practice, 9
  lack of, 246
    case example of, 246b
  metacommunication, 75
  metaphors, usage, 73
  miscommunication, 14, 348
  models, 4, 4f, 62
    linear, 4
    transactional, 4
  nonpunitive culture in, creation of,
      15–17
  nurse self-awareness, 63
  nursing, 5
    efforts for, 24–26
    professional guides for, 28–42
  nursing's metaparadigm, 5
  older adults
    assessment interviews, guidelines
        for, 272–274, 272b
    healthcare and, 268
    nurse and, 269t
    promoting wellness, 274
    strategies, assess and care for,
        271–272
  open communication, 324, 329, 329b
  other suggestions, 72–73
    avoid overload, 72
    focus, 72–73
  patient and family, 60, 60f
  patient-centered care, 4–5
  with peers, 321
  person, 6
  personal factors, 64
  professional nursing, 7–8, 7b
  as promoter of continuity, 350
  promotion, healthy work environ-
      ment, 341b
  as QSEN's six competencies, 31
  role relationship within nursing, 3
  safety, problems and recommended
      best practices in, 16t
  schizophrenia communication simula-
      tion, 245b

Communication (Continued)
  sensory disabilities, 247t
  shared partnership, 65
    developing, 67
  skills, 62t, 188–189
  sociocultural factors, effects, 81–83
  standardization, 17–18
  standardized tools, 12, 19–22
    and lists, 340–341
  strategies, 241
  in stressful situations, 218–234,
      233b
  styles
    applications, 83, 83b–84b
    concepts, 75–76, 76b
    factors, 75–76
    improvement, 85b
    quick profile, 84b
    variation in, 75–87, 87b
  with supervisors, 321
  team training, outcomes of, 333
  teamwork and, 330, 331b
  technology, 371–385, 384b
    applications of, 379–384
    for assisting patients, in self-
        management, 378
    clinical practice guidelines
        in, 377
    computerized clinical decision
        support systems in,
        376–377
    computer-mediated, in community,
        375–376
    decentralized access in, 372–373
    facilitation, 371–372
    issues in, 383–384
    patient engagement in, 377, 377b
    for patient health self-management,
        377–378
    patient-nurse communication
        outcomes in, 379
    for personal health records, 378
    usage, 73
  theoretical concepts, 2–3
    interpersonal communication, 2
    message barriers, 2
    process, 2–3
  theories. See Communication theories
  therapeutic, 63
  touch, 148f
  treatment-related communication
      disabilities, 246b
  unclear, reframing, 338t
  verbal styles, 77–78, 78b
  voice-activated, 374
Communication accommodation theory,
    81

Communication deficit
  applications of, 241–247
  associated with mental disorders, 239–240
  case example of, 236b
  communicating with patients, 235–248, 246b
  concepts of, 235–237
  early recognition of, 241
  evidence-based practice, development of, 240b
  goal in, 236
  hearing loss, 237, 237f
  incidence, 236
  legal mandates, 236–237
  patient advocacy, 247
  referrals, 246
  types of, 237–240
  vision loss, 237–238
Communication silos, 333
Communication theories, 1–11
  components, 3
    environment, 3
    feedback, 3
    meaning, 3
    messages, 3
    process, 3
    receiver, 3
    sender, 3
    symbols, 3
    transmission, 3
  concepts, 1–5
  self-disclosure, 3
  systems theory, 3
Communicators, role relationship, 86
Community
  anticipatory guidance, 265
  children, nurse advocacy, 265–266
  community-based education, 191
  computer-mediated communication, 375–376
  definition, 201
  empowerment, 201–202
    health promotion models, 202–203
  engagement, guiding principles, 201b
  family-centered relationships, 169
  resources, 289
    mobilization, 291
  support groups, 265
Community support, stress, 229
Compassion fatigue, 311
Competence stage, 320
Competition, 176
Complicated grief, 302
Comprehensive discharges, nursing actions in, 348b
Compromise, 176

Computerized charting, 366–367
Computerized clinical decision support systems, 376–377
  outcomes of, 377
Computerized health information technology systems, 356–359
  electronic records in, 359–360
    ease of access in, 360
    interoperability in, 359–360, 360b
    portability in, 360
  usage, 358–359, 358t, 359f
Computerized provider order entry (CPOE) systems, 356
  usage, 363
Computer literacy, in HIT system, 365
Computer-mediated communication, in community, 375–376
Confidentiality, 39
  in electronic longitudinal plans of care, 364
  HIPAA requirements, 287
Conflict
  accommodation, 176
  antecedents, 331
  applications, 180–182
  avoidance, 176
  case example, 185b
  causes, 173
  clear statements, usage, 188
  collaboration, 176
  communication skills, 188–189
  competition, 176
  compromise, 176
  concepts, 172–179
  containment, 188
  context, understanding, 175–176
  definition, 172
  defusing, home healthcare (provision), 189
  encounter
    evaluation/debriefing, 188
    preparation, 182–183
    timing, 182
  escalation, prevention, 189
  evidence-based practice, 179b
  hostility, defusing, 189
  interpersonal sources of, 331b
  issues, defining, 181b
  I statements, usage, 177, 188
  moderate pitch, usage, 178
  nature, 173
  nursing communication interventions, 183t
  organizational policies and practices, 174
  outcomes, 175
    dysfunction, 178
    positive growth, 178

Conflict (Continued)
  personal responses, 176b
    understanding, 175–178
  pitch/tone, usage, 188
  presence, assessment, 180–181
    case example, 180b–181b
  prevention, 180
    organizational strategies for, 342
  resolving, 172–190
  respect, demonstration, 188
  response
    structure, 177
    styles, 176
  safety, 179
  self-control, maintenance, 185
  situation, perspective, 182
  sources of, 335
  staff management, 174–175
  statements, clarity (usage), 188
  style, development, 176
  talk, usage, 186
  techniques, 181–182
  tension-reducing actions, usage, 186–188
  therapeutic communication skills, usage, 182, 186–188
  vocal tone, usage, 178
  workplace, individual strategies to deal with, 337
Conflict resolution, 175, 333
  applying, process, 182–185
  barriers, avoidance, 336
  case example, 181b–182b
  encounter, preparation, 182–183
    focus on issue, 183
    goal, 182–183
    manage feelings, 182–183
    own contribution, 182
  goal, 175
  information, organization, 183–184
  options, generation, 184
  physician–nurse conflict resolution, 336–337
  possibilities, 184
  principles, 175, 175f
  steps, 334–336
    promotion, 340b
  strategies, 339, 340b
  techniques, 181–182
Confusion, 239f
Congruent nonverbal behaviors, usage, 79
Connect Appreciate Respond Empower (C.A.R.E.), 156
Connotation, 76–77
Consciousness level, communication (absence), 246
  case example of, 246b

Consent, informed, 39–40, 40b
  duration of, 40
  surrogates and, 40
Constructive confrontations, 144
Constructive criticism, 333
  example, 341b
Constructive feedback, 144
Consumer-driven healthcare, electronic
    health information technology
    system in, 358t
Containment, 188
Content problem issue, 173
Context, changes (factors), 56
Continuing education, 320–321
Continuity of care (COC),
    communicating for, 345–355,
    354b
  applications, 350–354
  barriers to, 347
  case management, 347
    advocacy, 353
    chronic conditions, management
      of, 353
    communication, 352, 352b
    national guidelines, 352
    strategies, 352–353
  case study, 346b
  characteristics, 346, 347f
  collaboration, 350, 350f
  concepts, 345–349
  coordination, 350
  definitions, 345
  discharge planning, 351
  evidence-based practice, 349b
  family caregivers, 353–354
  incidence, 345
  informational continuity, 351
  large data sets/big data, 353
  management continuity,
    351–354
  miscommunication, 348
  organization problems, 348–349
  patient-centered care, dimensions,
    347f
  patient system navigation, 351–352
  planning care transitions, key elements
    in, 347, 348t
  promoters, 349
  relational continuity, 350–351
  relational or personal characteristics,
    349
  theory-based conceptual frameworks,
    346–347
  transition and discharge planning, 347,
    348t, 351, 352b
Convergence, 81
Coordination, in COC, 350

Coping, 222–225
  abilities, 153t
  case example of, 223b
  defensive coping strategies, 223–225
  emotion-focused coping strategies, 223
  maladaptive, 225
  mechanisms, 231
  older adults, 296
  personal coping strategies, examina-
    tion, 223b
  problem-focused, 223
  protective, 308
  strategies, 222–223
    children, 252
    crisis, relationship, 289
    parents, 252–253
  types of, 223
Corrective recapitulation, of primary
    family, 111t
COVID-19 pandemic, 44, 93, 301, 363,
    387
  loss during, 301
Crew resource management, 22
  briefing in, 22
  debriefing in, 22
  patient safety outcomes for, 22
  tools for, 22
Criminal law, 35
Crisis, 218, 284–298, 297b
  action plan, implementing, 290
  alternative options, 289
  applications for, 286–296
  behavioral emergencies and, 285
  community resources, 289
  concepts of, 284–286
  coping strategies, incorporate, 289
  definition, 284–285
  developmental crisis, 285
  disaster management, 295–296
  encouragement, providing, 290
  evidence-based practice for, 286b
  explicit information, providing,
    288–289
  family support, 290
  follow-up protocol, 291
  goal of, 286
  goals, establishment, 289–290
  intervention, 285
    communication, 287–288
    initial family responses to,
      290b–291b
    strategies, structuring, 286–291
  lethality and mental status, 287, 287b
  mental health emergencies, 291–295
    types of, 292–293
  nature, understanding, 287b
  nursing model for, 286

Crisis (Continued)
  occurrence, 284
  partial solutions for, 289
  personal strengths, affirming, 288
  personal support systems, 289b
  problems, identifying, 288–289
  problem-solving, 285
  psychosis, 293–295
  rapport, establishment, 287–288
  recoil, 285
  response pattern, 285
  restoration or reconstruction, 285
  sexual assault (mental health
    emergencies), 293
  shock, 285
  situation, reflective response in, 288b
  situational crisis, 251, 285
  state, 284
  strategies, crisis, intervention, 290
  structure, providing, 290
  support system, 289
  tasks, designing, 290
  termination, 291
  theoretical frameworks of, 285
  types, 285
  violence (mental health emergencies),
    292–293, 292t
Crisis intervention teams (CIT), 295
Criteria, application, 55–56
Critical life events, 221–222
Critical thinker, characteristics of, 48–49,
    48t
Critical thinking, 1–2, 43–58
  affective component, 49
  application, 50, 52t
  barriers, 49
  cognitive process, 49
  decision support system in, 376–377,
    376b
  enhancement of, 373
  learning process, summarization, 57
Cross-cultural awareness, 95
Cross-cultural communication, 154
Cues, 63–64
Cultural assessment, domains (Purnell),
    92t
Cultural authenticity, 90b
Cultural competence, 97
  Purnell's model of, 90
Cultural determinants of healthcare,
    93–94
Cultural differences, incorporating,
    308–309
Cultural diversity, 91, 93b
  lack in healthcare providers, 91
  points of, 90b
  professional health education and, 91

Cultural humility, 99
Culturally competent care, improving, 97, 98f
Culturally competent nurse
  characteristics, 98–99
    attitude, 99
    cultural humility, 99
    knowledge, 98
    skills, 98–99
    time orientation, 99
    use of interpreters, 99
Culturally diverse patient, care of, 96–97
Cultural needs, addressing, 308–309
Cultural nursing care, Madeleine Leininger's theory of, 90–91
Cultural patterns, 89
Cultural relativism, 94
  case example, 94b
  definition of, 94
Cultural sensitivity, 99
Culture
  authenticity, 90b
  competence, 97
  definitions, 88
  diversity, 90b, 91, 93b
  expectations, 80
  in healthcare, 91–95
    access, 92
    beliefs, 91–92
    economics, 92
    genetic *versus* cultural determinants of health status, 92
    health disparity, 92–94
    outcomes, 92
  impact, 203
  importance, 95–96
  learning, 89–90
  patterns, 89
  perceptions, 99b
  relativism, 94
  sensitivity, 99
Cumulative Index to Nursing and Allied Health (CINAHL), 252b, 261
Cyber health education, for health promotion, 382–383

D
Data
  integration, 54
  missing, identification, 54
  new, obtaining, 54–55
Data entry errors, 366–367
Death
  acceptance and, 302
  anger and, 301
  bargaining and, 301–302

Death (*Continued*)
  care providers at, 310–311, 310f, 311b
  childhood, 309–310
  denial and, 301
  depression and, 302
  final loss, 301
  good death, 310–311, 311b
  immanent death, guidelines for communicating with patients, 309b
  imminent death, family communication needs, 308b
  Kübler-Ross's stages of, 301–302
Debriefing, 22, 291, 342
Decentralized remote access, 371
Decision-making
  collaborative, 351b
  decision support system in, 376–377, 376b
  shared decision-making, 143–144, 143b
Decision talk, 144
Deep breathing, 232, 392
Defensive coping strategies, 223–225
Deficits, types, 237–240
Delegation, principles, 322b
Delirium, 278t
Dementia, 240, 240b, 277, 278t
  advanced dementia, client care, 280
  advocacy, 280
  clients, communication, 279b
  early cognitive changes, signs, 279b
  symptoms, behavioral communication interventions, 281t–282t
Democratic group leader, 109
Denial, loss stage, 301
Denotation, 76–77
Deontologic model, 45
Deprescribing, care transition model, 349
Depression, 278t
  loss stage, 302
Destructive criticisms, 339
Developing awareness, phases of grief, 302
Developmental crisis, 285
Developmental factors, patient's, 212–213
Difficult discussions, 145–146
Digital devices, 373
Direct patient care nurses, 315–316
Disability-related needs, 272–273
Disaster
  definition, 295
  situations, 295
Disaster management, 295–296
  in healthcare settings, 296
  planning for, 295–296
Disbelief, in phases of grief, 302

Discharge checklist, care transition model, 349
Discharge planning, 347, 348t, 352b
  in continuity of care, 351
Discussion groups, 111, 112t
Disease
  prevention, 197–198
    immunizations, 192b
    primary prevention, 195
    secondary prevention, 195
    tertiary prevention, 195
Disease-specific apps, 373–374
Disengagement, 137–138
Disruptive behaviors, 331–332
  definition, 331
  document and report, 341
  elimination, collaborative culture, 332–333
  incidence of incivility, 332
  nurse outcomes, 332
  organization outcomes, 332
  patient outcomes, 332
  process, 332
Distortions, cognitive, 125b
Distress, 220
  moral, 36–37
  symptoms, stabilization of, 286
Distributive justice, 47
Divergence, 81
Diversity
  cultural diversity, 90b, 91, 93b
  existence, 91
  in nursing profession, 93b
Doctor of Nursing Practice, 316–317
  terminal practice degree, 316–317
Documentation, 356, 357f
  clarity in, 361
  efficiency in, 361
  legal record, 35
  nursing
    essentials of, 361–362
    improved completeness of, 359f, 362
    other formats for, 363
  partnering with patients in, 360–361
  on patient's health record, 366
  standards of, 364–365
Domains of cultural assessment (Purnell), 92t
Do not resuscitate (DNR) directives, 307
Drug abuse, pain in older adults, 273
Duty-based model, 45
Dysfunction, 178

E
Eastern mind-body programs, 391
EBP. *See* Evidence-based practice
Economics, 92

e-Documentation, in health information technology systems, 356–370
Effective communication, 328
　barriers to, 331–332
　case example of, 30b
　concepts of, 29
　defined, 29
　outcomes of, 8
Effective feedback, 71
Efficient care, enhancement of, 373
Ego defense mechanisms, 223, 224t
Ego despair, 269–270
Ego development model (Erikson), 269–270
Ego identity, 119
Ego integrity, 269–270
eHealth. *See* Telehealth
Elder abuse, 270
Electronic health information technology system, in consumer-driven healthcare, 358t
Electronic health record (EHR), 359–360
　in culture of patient safety, 367t
　data entry errors, 366–367
　documenting patient information in, 360–361
　ease of access in, 360
　efficiency of, 361
　information flow in, 360, 360b
　interoperability in, 359–360, 360b
　nursing action problems, 366, 366b
　patient access, 361
　portability in, 360
　safety of patient care, 17
Electronic longitudinal plans of care, 363–364
Electronic nursing competencies, 380
Email, 377
　guidelines for, 380
e-Mobile nurse-patient healthcare communication, 377
Emotional attitude, 392
Emotional meanings, communication, 85f
Emotional value, 125
Emotion-focused coping strategies, 223
Emotions, validating and normalizing, 169
Empathy, 61, 150
　absence, 150
　applications, 156–157
　usage, 189
Empowerment, 149
　absence, 149
　method, 156
　social support, impact, 200–201
　strategies, 156, 200
　　case example, 200b
　structural, 323

End-of-life, 168
End-of-life (EOL) care, 304, 311b
　for children, 264
　communication in, 307–308
　　guidelines for, 309b
　cultural differences, incorporating, 308–309
　cultural needs, addressing, 308–309
　decision-making, 306–307
　　principles guiding, 307b
　ethical and legal issues, 307
　family and team conferences for, 307
　family education, 307–308
　issues and approaches in, 306–307
　patient-centered care relationships, 145b
　patients, 308
　spiritual needs attending, 309
End-of-Life Nursing Education Consortium (ELNEC), 304
Engel, George, 302
Environment, 3, 6
Environmental awareness, communication, 63–64
Environmental deprivation, impact, 238f
Environmental hazards, orientation to, 243–244
EOL. *See* End-of-life (EOL) care
Epidemiologic data, in HIT system, 363
Erikson, Erik
　ego development model, 269–270
　theory of psychosocial development, 119, 119t–121t
Error databases, 14
Errors
　as system problems, 14
　underreporting of, in punitive climate, 14–15
Ethical codes, 31–34, 33f, 33b
Ethical decision-making, 1–2, 43–58
　case example, 48b, 53b
　concepts, 43
　models, 45–47
　steps in, 47–48
Ethical dilemma, 45
　case example, 45b, 57b
　communication, 11b
　　family, 170b
　　strategies for health promotion, 204b
　health teaching, 217b
　intrapersonal communication, 393b
　patient-centered therapeutic relationships, 146b
　resolving conflict, 190b
　self-concept, 130b
　solving, 50–52
　therapeutic relationship bridges, 158b

Ethical reasoning, 44–48
　barriers, 49
　personal knowledge, 44–45
Ethical standards, codes containing, 31–34, 33f
Ethical support, of patient's right of autonomy, 1–2, 57b
Ethical theories, 45–47
Ethnicity, and related concepts, 94–95
Ethnocentrism, 94
　case example, 94b
Eustress, 220
Evidence-based practice (EBP), 18b, 138b
　development of, 8b–9b, 17, 36b, 349b, 367t
　effective communication, 66b
　in patient care, 10t
　use of, 10
E-visits, 375–376
Examination, skepticism, 55
Exemplary nurse leaders, 324b
Exercise, 390
Exercise therapy, 111
Existential factors, 111t
Experiential learning, 317
Expert stage, 320
Expressive aphasia, 238, 244
External stressors, 218
Eye contact, 79
　attention, 80–81

F
Facial expression, 79
　attention, 80
Facilitative body language, usage, 79
Family
　anxiety, decrease (nursing interventions), 230t
　applications, 163–170
　assessing coping strategies, 167b
　bedside rounds, 165–166
　care options, 307, 308b
　case example, 160b
　communicating with, 160–171
　composition, 161
　with critically ill patient, 161t, 167–169
　　breaking bad news, 168
　　commendations, 167
　　evaluation, 168–169
　　incorporating family strengths, 167
　　informational support, 167–168
　definition, 160–161
　evidence-based practice, 163b
　family-centered care, 251–253, 252b
　helping cope, 168b
　improve numeracy, 207, 208f
　legacies, 162

Family (Continued)
    meetings, 165
    needs in intensive care unit, 167b
    relationships, impact (assessment), 229
    strengths, incorporating, 167
    theoretical frameworks, 161–162
Family caregivers
    ability of, 349
    continuity for, 353–354
Family-centered care, 163–167
    assessment, 164, 164b
    implementation, 166–167
    intervention, 164–165
        interventive questioning, 165
        problem identification, 164
    nursing care plan, 166b
    orientation, 163–164
    planning, 165–166
    positive and negative family responses,
        165b
    therapeutic questions, 164b
Family-centered relationships in commu-
    nity, 169
Family communication
    concepts, 160–171
    using technology to enhance, 170
Family involvement, 213
Family members, teaching, 168
Fatigue
    communication and, 15
    compassion fatigue, 311
FAX, guidelines for, 380
Federal Emergency Management Agency
    (FEMA), 295–296
Federation of European Countries, ethi-
    cal codes, 44
Feedback, 3, 71–72, 215, 216b
    loops, 62–63
Feelings, 184
    focus on, 288
    identification, 288
        reflective listening responses for, 288
    processing strong, 228
FEMA. See Federal Emergency
    Management Agency
"Fight-or-flight" patterns, 220
Figure-ground phenomenon, 117f
Flexner's criteria, role and, 314b
Flow sheets, in documenting nursing
    care, 363
Focused questions, 68–69
Forming phase
    groups, 106
    therapeutic groups, 112–113
Fragmentation, 14
Fully integrated computerized systems,
    371

Functional capabilities, restoration of, 286
Functional similarity, 104, 104b
Functional status
    assessment of, 272–273
    definition of, 272–273

G
Gaze aversion, 80–81
Gaze-controlled communication com-
    puter programs, 246
Gender, 82–83
    bias, 84b
    differences
        communication, 250
        impact, 82–83, 155
    nurse behavior and, 333
    self-concept, 118
General adaptation syndrome, 220–221
General systems theory, 161, 162f
Generational diversity, 81–82, 333
Genetic versus cultural determinants of
    health status, 92
Gestures, 79
    attention, 79
Global aphasia, 238, 244
Global health promotion agendas, 196
Goal-based model, 45
God, belief in, 229
Good death, 310–311, 311b
Grief, 303
    acute grief, 302
    anticipatory grief, 302, 302b
    case study on, 302b
    in children, 264, 310
    complicated, 302
    concepts, 301–303
    developing awareness in, 302
    disbelief phase of, 302
    Engel's constructs, 302
    Lindenmann's construct, 302
    patterns of, 302
    reactions, psychiatric management,
        285
    restitution phase of, 302
    shock phase of, 302
Group presentations, 215
Groups
    activity, 111
    adjourning phase, 107
    applications, 109–114
    artistic, 111
    closed therapeutic groups, 108
    co-leadership, 109
    communication in, 102–114
        concepts, 102–103
        healthcare, relationship, 103
    definition, 102

Groups (Continued)
    discussion, 111, 112t
    dynamics, 105
        task and maintenance functions in,
            107b
    environment, safety (creation), 108
    forming phase, 106
    goals, 103–104
    health education, 111
    health-related groups, applications,
        108
    heterogeneous groups, 108
    homogeneous groups, 108
    leadership, 108–109
        case example, 109b
    member composition, 104–105
    membership, 108
    norming phase, 107
    norms, 104–105
    open groups, 108
    performing phase, 107
    primary groups, 102–103
    process, 105–107
    professional work, 111–112
    purpose, 103
    role
        expectations, 106b
        functions, 107–108
        positions, 105
    secondary groups, 103
    size, 104–105
    small group communication therapy,
        characteristics, 103–108
    specific norms, 105
    storming phase, 106
    support, 110–111
    therapeutic factors, 111t
    therapeutic groups, 109–110
        type and purpose, 103t
    think, 113
Guided imagery, 232

H
Habits, 49
Hallucinations, 293
Handheld devices, usage, 382b
Handheld internet devices, 371
Hands-free communication, 374
Hardiness, 225
Health, 6–7
    definitions, 191
    disparities, 196–197, 204
        causes, 197
        nurse role, 197
    disruptions, impact, 143
    health-related support groups, 201
    maintenance, critical elements, 192f

Health *(Continued)*
  professionals, core competencies, 315f
  profile, development, 197b
  promotion, activities, areas, 276b
  teaching, 276–277
Health and lifestyle monitoring apps, 382
Healthcare
  coding systems in, 368–369
  cultural diversity, points, 90b
  durable power of attorney for, 307
  home-based, 237
  interpreters, usage, 99
  laws in
    classifications of, 34–35
    statutory, 34
  partnerships, formation with, 264–265
  self-concept, significance, 116
  settings
    communication, gender, differences,
      82–83
    disaster management in, 296
  stress, sources, 227
  workers, violence (increase), 173–174
Healthcare communication
  aging and, 268
  culture, importance, 95–96
Healthcare delivery
  paradigm shift in, 6–7
  trends in, 9–10
Healthcare system, 4, 5f
  functions of communication within, 8
Healthcare team
  conflict resolution among, 340b
  transitional sending/receiving, core
    functions, 352b
Health disparity, 92–94
  cultural determinants of healthcare,
    93–94
  etiology, 93
  incidence, 93
  social determinants of health, 93
Health education groups, 111
Health information technology (HIT)
    systems, e-documentation in,
    356–370, 373f
  applications of, 365–369
  concepts, 356–365
  electronic longitudinal plans of care,
    363–364
  electronic records, documenting
    patient information, 360–361
  health outcome through large data
    sets, 362–363
  nursing documentation, improved
    completeness, 362
  partnering with patients, 360–361
  quality of care, 362

Health information technology (HIT)
    systems, e-documentation
    in *(Continued)*
  work-arounds, 366
  workload, 366
Health Insurance Portability and
    Accountability Act (HIPAA), regula-
    tory compliance to, 38, 38b
Health literacy
  case examples, 203b
  core constructs of, 211, 211t
Health organization imperative, stress,
    225
Health professionals, 351b
Health promotion, 269, 270b
  activities, 191
  agendas, 196
  applications, 198–204
  case example, 197b
  communication strategies,
    191–205
  concepts, 191–198
  culture, impact, 203
  definitions, 191
  developmental level, 203–204
  evidence-based practice, 197b
  health education, 198–199
  model, 202–203
    Pender's, 192, 193b
    revision, 193f
  nursing goals on, 271–272
  population concept, 201–202
  protective factors, 195–196
  social determinants, 196
  strategies, 198
  theoretical concepts in, 192–195
    Bandura's social learning theory,
      194–195, 195b
    Prochaska's transtheoretical model
      for change, 194
Health teaching
  applications, 209–215
  concepts, 206–209
  definition, 206–209
  evaluation and documentation,
    214–215
  evidence-based practice, 209b
  feedback, 215, 216b
  group presentations, 215
  theory, 206–208
Healthy habits, 389, 390f
Healthy People 2030
  goals of, 236
  older adults, 269
Healthy work environment, standards
  for, 329, 329b
Hearing, sensory loss, 242b

Hearing loss, 237, 237f
  children, 237
  communication strategies, 241
    case example of, 241b–242b
  etiology, 237
  incidence, 237
  older adults, 237
"Helper" group member, 105
Helping relationships, social relationships
    (differences), 134t
Heterogeneous groups, 108
Hierarchy of needs (Maslow). *See*
    Maslow's hierarchy of needs
Higher power, belief in, 229
High-esteem, behaviors, 126t
Hildegard Peplau's interpersonal nursing
    theory, 136
HIPAA. *See* Health Insurance Portability
    and Accountability Act
Hobbies, as communication strategy, 260
  case example of, 260b
Holmes and Rahe scale, 222
Home-based healthcare, 237
Home health nurse, 276f, 353f
Homeostasis, 220
Homogeneous groups, 108
Hope, installation of, 111t
Hospice care, definition, 300
Hospital
  physically ill children, communication,
    257
  prehospitalization preparation, 251
Hospital situations, personal space
    (respect), 158
Hostility, 228–229
  defusing, 189
Huddle, 23
Human rights-based model, 45
Humor, 73, 392
  usage, 86
Hyperactive disorders, 263

I
Ideal self, 118
Identifying claims, 53
Identity, 123
  diffusion, 119
  personal, 123–125
    case example, 124b
    cognition, 124b, 125
    cognitive reappraisal, 129f
    enhancement, patient-centered
      interventions (usage),
      124b
    exercise, 126b
    nursing strategies, 125
    perception, 124–125, 124b–125b

Identity (Continued)
    spiritual aspects, 128–129
    supportive nursing strategies, 125
    therapeutic strategies, 129
Illness
    environmental deprivation, impact, 238f
    information, understanding (overesti-
        mating), 257
I lose, You lose situation, 176
I lose, You win situation, 176
Imitative behavior, 111t
Immanent death, guidelines for commu-
    nicating with patients, 309b
Imminent death, family communication
    needs, 308b
Improved communication, 14
Indirect feedback, 215
Individualized care, 134
Individualized teaching plans, 211–214
    adaptations for cognitive processing
        deficits, 213
    components of patient education,
        211–212
    creating successful teaching plan, 214
    developing measurable objectives, 214
    developmental factors, 212–213
    family involvement, 213
    shared decision-making, 211
Infants
    communication with, 255b–257b, 257
    verbal communication skills, absence,
        157f
Infection control, device use for, 380
Inferences, 55
Informatics, 365
Information
    collection, 53
    confidential, professional sharing of,
        39–40
    flow in electronic health records, 360,
        360b
    imparting, 111t
    organization, 183–184
        background information, 183–184
    provision, 78, 229–230
    real-time interactive communication
        for, 371
Informational continuity, 351
    definition of, 346
Informational support, 167–168
Informed consent, 39–40, 40b
    duration of, 40
    surrogates and, 40
In-hospital biomedical monitoring, 374
Inquiry, 43
Instant messaging, personal use guide-
    lines, 380–381, 380t

Instrumental activities of daily livings
    (IADLs), 272
Intensive care unit (ICU), treatment-
    related communication deficits,
    246b
Intercultural communication, 2, 88–101
    application, 95–99
    case example, 94b
    concepts, 88–91
    cultural variation, 89
    definitions, 94
    evidence-based practice, 95b
    incidence, 89
    Szalay's process model, 90
    theoretical frameworks, 90–91
Interdisciplinary communication, oppor-
    tunities for, 342
Interdisciplinary courses, 317–318, 317b
Interdisciplinary rounds
    callouts and time-outs, 23–24
    huddle, 23
    team meetings and, 23–24
Interdisciplinary team
    palliative care, 304
    role clarity, 350
Internal stressors, 218
International Code of Ethics, 31–33
International Council of Nurses (ICN),
    30–31
Interoperability, in electronic records,
    359–360, 360b
Interpersonal boundaries, defined, 61
Interpersonal communication, 2
Interpersonal competence, 83–84
Interpersonal learning, 111t
Interpersonal relationship, self-concept
    in, 115–130
Interpreters, usage, 99
Interprofessional communication,
    328–344, 339b, 343b
    applications, 333–342
    improved, 335t
Interprofessional education, 9
Intervention, 97, 184
    evaluation, 56
    feelings, 184
    metacommunication, 184
    name conflict issue, 184
    request behavior change, 184
Interviews, guidelines for effective initial
    assessment, 135b
Intrapersonal communication, 386–394
    applications, 389–393
    burnout, 387–389
    concepts, 386–389
    definition, 386
    evidence-based practice, 389b

Intrapersonal communication (Continued)
    goals, 387
    interventions, 390–392
    self-talk, 387
    theory, 387
    types, 390–392
Involvement, term (usage), 137–138
I PASS the BATON TeamSTEPPS Model
    with, 22, 23t
I statements
    case example, 177b–178b
    effectiveness, 188
    usage usage, 177, 188
I win now, but then lose, You lose
    situation, 176

J
Jargon, usage, 85–86
Johns Hopkins Mobile Integrated
    Healthcare Model, 347
Just culture system, 15
Justice, 47
    case example, 47b
    exercise, 51b
    social worth, 47
    unnecessary treatment, 47
    veracity, 47

K
Kant, Immanuel, 45
Kinesthetic learners, 209–210
Knowledge, 98
    technology and, 379
Kolesar v. Jeffries, 364
Kübler-Ross, Elisabeth, 301

L
Laissez-faire group leaders, 109
Language, 94–95
    deficits, verbal communication impair-
        ment, 238
    difficulties, assistance (strategies), 244b
    facilitative body language, usage, 79
    paralanguage, 77–78
Laptop computers, 373
Large data sets, 353
Laughter, 73
Laws, in healthcare
    civil, 34–35
    classifications of, 34–35
    criminal, 35
    statutory, 34
Leader communication, 113
Leadership, 108–109
    case example, 109b
    of work groups, 111

Learning
    delays, 244–245
    experiential, 317
    questions to assess, 212, 212b
LEARN model, 97
Legal liability, in nurse-patient relation-
        ships, 35
Legal mandates, 236–237
Legal record, documentation as, 35
Legal standards, 34–35
Leininger, Madeleine, 90–91
Lethality, assessing, 287, 287b
Licensed nurses, 322, 322b
Life
    quality of, 270
    review, 274
Lifestyle
    healthy diet, exercise, 196f
    management, technology, 378
    promotion, 231–232
Limit-setting plan, development guide-
        lines, 263b
Lindemann, Eric, 302
Lindemann's grief construct, 302
Linear communication models, 4
Linear model, of communication, 62
Listening
    active, 67–68
        simulation exercise, 68b
    responses, negative, 71t
Location, impact, 83
Loss
    acceptance, 302
    anger, 301
    applications, 304–311
    bargaining, 301–302
    concepts, 301
    death final loss, 301
    denial, 301
    depression, 302
    meaning of, 301b
    multiple losses, 301
    theoretical frameworks for,
        301–302
Love and belonging needs, 136–137
Low self-esteem, behaviors, 126t

M
Madeleine Leininger's theory of cultural
        nursing care, 90–91
Magnet culture, characteristics, 324
Magnet hospital, 323–324
Magnet model components, 325f
Magnet Recognition Program, 324
Maladaptive coping, 225
Malpractice, in nurse-patient relation-
        ships, 35

Manageable workload, work environ-
        ment and, 324
Management continuity, 351–354
    definition of, 346
Mandatory reporting, 39
Manifest behaviors, 153t
Maslow's hierarchy of needs, 36,
        136–137, 137f, 270
Mass trauma situations, 295
    elements of, 296t
MCI. See Mild cognitive impairment
Meaning, 3, 76–77
Meaningful use, 358–359
Medical home, 249, 350
Medical jargon, 85–86
Medical orders, 365–366
Medical paternalism, autonomy versus,
        46
Medication
    process, 17b
    self-management of, 275
    teaching, 275b
Meditation, 232, 391, 391b
    techniques, 233b
Member responsibilities, 112
Members, 113
Mental disorders, communication
        deficits associated with,
        244–245
Mental health emergencies,
        291–295
    communication deescalation tips for,
        292b
    psychosis, 293–295
    sexual assault, 293
    suicide, 293–295
    types of, 292–293
    violence, 292–293, 292t
Mental health problems, 263
Mental illness, 239
Mental incompetence, 280
Mental processing deficits,
        communication, 244–245
Mental status
    assessment, 287, 287b
    testing, 273b
Mentor, 319
Message, 3
    barriers, 2
    clarity, 332
    competency, 84
    context, 86
    nonverbal message, 78
Metacommunication, 75, 184
    case example, 76b
    term, usage, 75
Metaphors, 73

m-Health, 371–385, 384b
    applications, 379–384
    concepts, 371–379
    devices, 373
        biomedical sensors, 374
        cellular phones, 373
        mobile biomedical sensors, 374, 374f
        smart phones, 373
        tablets and laptop computers, 373,
            374b
        usage, 382b
    outcomes, 378–379, 382–384
    patient engagement, 382–384
Microaggressions, 118
Microassaults, 118
Mild cognitive impairment (MCI), 277
Mind-body therapies, 232
Mindfulness, 390–391, 391b
Mini-meditation, 393, 393b
Mini-Mental State Examination
        (MMSE), 273b
    measures, 272
Miscommunication, 14, 348
    errors, 1
    problems, 29
Missing data, identification, 54
Mistrust, 94, 149–150
MMSE. See Mini-Mental State
        Examination
Mnemonics, 43
Mobile biomedical sensors, 374, 374f
Mobile health monitoring systems,
        373–374
    apps
        for communication with nurse or
            physician, 374
        for healthcare providers, 373
        for individuals in community,
            373–374
Model behaviors, that convey respect, 337
Moderate pitch, usage, 178
Monopolizing phase, 113
Moral distress, 36–37, 51
Moral problem, 46
Moral uncertainty, 50–51
Motivation, 199
Motivational interviewing (MI), 193b,
        199–200, 212
    case example, 199b
Multiple losses, 301
Mutuality, 150–151
    in decision-making, 260
    evaluation, 151b
Mutual respect, 332
Mutual storytelling technique, usage,
        259b
Mutual trust, 350–351

N

National Center for Interprofessional Practice and Education, 328
National culturally and linguistically appropriate services (CLAS) standards, 97–98
National health promotion agendas, 196
National Prevention Strategy, 196f
Near miss incidents, reporting, 14–15
Negative attributions, 118
Negative listening responses, 71t
Networking, 324
New data, obtaining, 54–55
Noise, 65
Nonassertive behavior, 179
Nonmaleficence, 46–47
Nonpain symptom control, approaches in end-of-life care, 306
Nonpunitive culture, creation of, 15–17
Nonspecific physiologic responses, 220–221
Nonverbal behaviors
    anxiety, association, 153b
    body cues, attention, 80–81
    congruent nonverbal behaviors, usage, 79
    gestures and expressions, 75
    interpretation of, 81
Nonverbal clues, 185
Nonverbal communication, 1, 78–81
Nonverbal messages, 78–79
Nonverbal style
    components, 76
    factors, 78–81
        case example, 81b
Norming phase
    group, 107
    therapeutic groups, 113
Novice stage, 319
Nurse-family relationships, 163–164
Nurse-patient communication, 2–3
Nurse-patient relationships
    barriers, reduction, 157–158
    conflict, presence (assessment), 180–181
    introductions, usage, 138b
    involvement in, 86
    malpractice and legal liability in, 35
    model of patient centeredness, 133f
    professional communication
        nonverbal style factors, 78–81
        styles (impact), 77t
        verbal style factors, 77–78, 78b
Nurses
    barriers, 132
    behavior, factors that affect, 333
    direct patient care, 315–316
    disengagement, 137–138

Nurses (Continued)
    managers, 316
    new, mentoring, 337
    obstacles to effective communication within, 64
    and older adult communication, 269t
    overinvolvement, warning signs, 137
    PhD-prepared researcher, 317
    presence, 140–142
    rights of, 323
    role, nurse–patient role relationships, 325–326
    scientist, 317
    self-disclosure, 132
    social media and, 37t
    stress issues for, in palliative care setting, 311, 311b
    suicide and, 295
Nurse self-awareness, communication, 63
Nurse-specific initiatives, 17, 17b
Nursing, 5
    actions
        empathy, application, 156–157
        levels, 157t
    behaviors
        usage, 186t–187t
    communication in, standards as guides to, 28
    concepts, 1–11, 13–14
    culturally competent communication, 96
    defining. See Professional nursing
    diagnoses, identification, 49
    ethical dilemmas, solving, 50–52
    intervention classification finding, application of, 368b
    knowledge, 96
    language, 96
    mentorship, 3
    nonverbal cultural differences, 96
    professional
        diversity, presence, 93b
        evolution of, 13
    role in supporting patients, 212, 214f
    roles (Peplau), 136b
    skills, 96–97
    standardized language terminology in, 368
    teamwork, 23
Nursing care communication, competencies, 10
Nursing communication
    professional guides for, 28–42
    concepts of, 28–31
Nursing documentation
    essentials of, 361–362
    improved completeness of, 359f, 362
    other formats for, 363

Nursing practice, coding in, 368f
Nursing process, 35–36
    prioritize, 36, 37b
    values clarification and, 49–50
Nursing's metaparadigm, 5
Nursing support, 133

O

Objectives, 208, 214, 214b–215b
Observe hand movements, 79
Occupational therapy, 111
Older adults
    assessment
        for cognitive changes, 272, 273b
        of functional status, 272–273
        interviews, communication guidelines for, 272, 272b
        level of social support, 273–274
        mental health, 273
        pain, 273
    cognitive impairment
        processing, 239
        relationships, 277–280
    cognitively intact, 276f
    communicating with, 267–283, 282b
    dementia
        definition, 277
        delirium, depression, contrast, 278t
        symptoms (behavioral communication interventions), 281t–282t
    disability-related needs in, 272–273
    elder abuse, 270
    fundamental rights, 268b, 271
    health promotion for, 269, 270b, 276
        teaching, 277b
    Healthy People 2030, 269
    hearing loss, 237
    integrated health promotion, 276
    mental health issues, 270–271, 271b
    mental status testing with, 273b
    nurses and communication, 269t
    pain range in, estimates of, 305
    promoting wellness, 274
    short-term memory, 279
    strategies, assess and care for, 271–272
    stress issues for, 229
    term, usage of, 267
    trauma, coping, 296
    verbal cues, 279
    vision loss, 238
Online information, access to, 377
Open communication, 324, 329, 329b
    usage, 340–341
Open dialogue, commitment to, 337
Open-ended questions, 68, 200
    asking, 68b

Option talk, 144
Orem's self-care deficit nursing theory of nursing, 387
Organizational climate, 342
  in work environment, 323
Organizational policies and practices, 174
Organizational system, understanding, 342
Organizations, safety communication guidelines, 14
Orientation, 319
Orientation/assessment phase, 136, 145
  patient-centered care, 134
  therapeutic relationships, 142–143
Orientation, family-centered care, 163–164
Ottawa Charter for Health Promotion, 196
Outcomes, effective communication and, 29–30

P

Pain, 304–306
  assessment of, 305, 306f
  assessment scale, 261
  "breakthrough," 305–306
  care problem, 261–262
  management, 261–262
    narcotic medication for, 305–306
    nonpharmacologic strategies, 306
  nonverbal indicators of, 305
  in older adults
    alternative methods, 273
    chronic pain, definition, 273
    drug abuse, 273
    medications, 273
  symptoms of, 261
  treatment of, 262
  types of, 305
  Wong–Baker FACES Pain Rating Scale, 305, 306f
Palliative care, 304–306
  aspects of, 304, 304b
  case study, 299b
  children, 309–310
  definitions, 300
  dimensions of, 300b
  evidence-based practice, 303b
  goal, 300
  healthcare provider role, 300
  incidence, 300
  location, 304
  nursing initiatives, 304
  nursing role, 308, 310f
  process, 304
  situations, 300–301
    barriers to communication, 301

Palliative care (Continued)
    professional readiness, 300–301
    stress issues for nurses, 311, 311b
    team approaches, 304–306
Panning care and discharges (Ray Bolton), 353b
Paradigm shift in healthcare delivery, 6–7
Paralanguage, 77–78
Paraphrasing, 69
  exercise, 70b
Parents
  communication guidelines, 265b
  coping strategies, 252–253
  healthcare partnership formation, 264–265
  of special healthcare needs children communication, 265–266
  stress, sources of, 253
Parkinson's disease, 219b
Participants
  observation, 141–142
  responsiveness, 86
  roles, 86
Paternalism, medical, autonomy *versus*, 46
Patient, 308
  advocacy, 78
    roles, 324–326, 325b
  after death, care, 311
  assessment, 52–53
  behavioral reaction, 288
  best practices standards, access, 55
  body language, 292–293
  cognitive processing deficits, assistance (strategies), 244b
  communication
    engaging in, 66
    guidelines, 309b
    obstacles to effective, 64
    strategies, 246b
  culturally diverse, care, 96–97
  emotional response, 288
  engaging, 287–288
  health record, documentation, 366
  with hearing loss, 241
    case example, 241b–242b
  improve numeracy, 207, 208f
  involvement, encouragement, 78
  level of health literacy, 25–26
  literacy and education, 208–209
  as members of the health team, 25
  mental processing deficits, communication with, 244–245
  misidentification, prevention, 24
  nonverbal body cues, attention, 80–81
  preferences, assessment, 96t
  privacy, protection, 37–39

Patient (Continued)
    confidentiality, 39
    ethical responsibility, 38–39
    HIPAA regulatory compliance, 38, 38b
    The Joint Commission privacy regulations, 38
  responsiveness, 86
  role, 325–326
  safety outcomes, 17
  with sensory loss, 243b
  strengths, identification, 127–128
  transfers of care, 14
  treatment-related communication disabilities, 245–246
  values, 49
  violent behavior, 292
  with vision loss, 242–243
    case example, 243b
  worth, validation, 78
Patient-centered care, 4–5, 5b, 31
  in continuity of care, 347f
  model, 332
  team collaboration, 335f
Patient-centered care process
  orientation/assessment phase, 134
  termination phase, 135
  working phase, 135
Patient-centered care relationships, 131–132
  characteristics of, 132–134
    individualized care, 134
    nursing support, 133
    patient, 132
    respect, 133
  elements of, 134–135
Patient-centered communication
  applications, 65–67
  characteristics of, 61–63
    content, 61
    goals, 61
  developing, 59–74
Patient-centered education, 211–212
Patient-centered verbal communication skills, 210b
Patient disease management, 378
Patient diversity, 2
Patient education, definition, 206
Patient focus, 10
Patient health self-management, technology, 377–378
Patient identifier number, lack of, 14
Patient-nurse communication, outcomes, 379
Patient-provider collaborations, 25
Patient Self-Determination Act of 1991, 46, 307

Patient system navigation, 351–352
Pediatric nursing procedures, 262b
Peers, communication with, 321
Pender's health promotion model, 192, 193f
Peplau, Hildegard
    interpersonal nursing theory, 136
    nursing roles, 136b
Performing phase
    group, 107
    therapeutic groups, 113
Person, 6
Personal coping strategies, examination, 223b
Personal health literacy, definition, 206
Personal health records (PHRs), 378
Personal identity, 123–125
    case example, 124b
    cognition, 124b, 125
    cognitive reappraisal, 129f
    enhancement, patient-centered interventions (usage), 124b
    exercise, 126b
    nursing strategies, 125
    perception, 124–125, 124b–125b
    spiritual aspects, 128–129
        case example, 129b
        nursing strategies, 129
    supportive nursing strategies, 125
    therapeutic strategies, 129
Personality theory, 118–119
Personal medical identification number, 364
Personal resources, strengthening, 285
Personal space
    respect, 158
        hospital situations, 158
    violation, impact, 154
Personal strengths, affirming, 288
Personal support systems, 289b
Personal value
    professional value versus, 49
    system, development, 49
Physical activity, usage, 188
Physical appearance, 115
Physically ill children, communication with, 257
Physical motivators, 195
Physical space, in work environment, 323
Physical therapist, 276f
Physician–nurse conflict resolution, 336–337
Piaget cognitive development stages, 251t
Pitch
    moderation, 77–78
    usage, 188
Plain language, 210

Planning care transitions, key elements in, 347, 348t
Play, communication strategy, 258–259
Point of care, 361
    applications, 380
    capability, 371
    technology for communicating at, 372–373, 373f
Policies, 342
Portal technology, 378, 378b
Positive reinforcement, 342
Positivity, 390
Possible selves, term (usage), 116
Posttraumatic stress disorder (PTSD), 220
Posture, 79
    attention, 80
Poverty, 93–94
Practice discipline, nursing, 7
Practice prevention, 390
PRECEDE-PROCEED model, 202
    definitions, 203t
    PRECEDE diagnostic behavioral factors, example, 202t
Precipitating event, 288
Prehospitalization preparation, 251
Presbycusis, 237
Presbyopia, 238
Preschoolers, child communication in, 258–259
Presence, 140–142
Primary groups, 102–103
Pre-interaction phase, therapeutic relationships, 142
Prioritize self-care, 389
Privacy, 63
    in electronic longitudinal plans of care, 364
    protection, 37–39
        confidentiality, 39
        ethical responsibility, 38–39
        HIPAA regulatory compliance, 38, 38b
        The Joint Commission privacy regulations, 38
Private space, ensuring (actions), 158
Problem-focused coping strategies, 223
Problem, identification, 55
Problem-solving, 50
Process, 3
Process issue, 173
Prochaska's transtheoretical model for change, 194
Professional caring, 7–8
Professional communication
    definition, 59
    functions of, 60
    skills, 63
    styles (impact), 77t

Professional health education, and cultural diversity, 91
Professionalism, 313–318
    in nursing, 314
Professional nursing, 7–8, 7b
    art, 7
    caring, 7–8
    core value of, 7–8
    practice discipline, 7
Professional nursing, roles, 314–315, 314b, 315f, 316b
    scope of practice, 314–315
    socialization, 318–319
Professional skill acquisition, 319–320
Professional standards for scope of nursing, 30–31
Professional value
    acquisition, 52
    five core values of, 49b
    personal value versus, 49
    system, 49
Professional work groups, 111–112
Profession's culture, 318
Proficiency stage, 320
Progressive relaxation, 232
Protective coping, 308
Protective factors, 195–196
Proxemics, 65, 80, 85, 153–154
Proximity to patient, 168
Psychological behavioral problems, child communication, 255–257
Psychological first aid (PFA), core actions for, 293
Psychosis, mental health emergencies, 293–295
Psychosocial development theory (Erikson), 119, 119t–121t, 122b
Punitive climate, underreporting of errors in, 14–15
Purnell, Larry, 90
    domains of cultural assessment, 92t
Purnell's model of cultural competence, 90

Q

Quality and Safety Education for Nurses (QSEN), 12, 31
    attitude, 180
    competency, 32t, 148
    mastering, 249
Quality assurance, in HIT system, 362
Quality, care, communicating clearly for, 17
Quality discharge planning, 347
Quality of care, HIT system, 362
Quality of life, 6
    functionality framework, 270

Questions
    circular questions, 69
    closed-ended questions, 69
    focused questions, 68–69
    open-ended questions, 68, 68b, 200
    three wishes, 261
Quick self-stress assessment, 389, 389t

R

Racism, 94
Radiofrequency identification (RFID), 24, 374–375
Radio frequency identification chips, 375
Rape, interpersonal victimization, 293
Rapport, building, 66–67, 96–97
Readiness assessment, Prochaska model (usage), 195b
Reality, presentation, 73
Reality orientation groups, 110
Real-time interactive communication, 371
Reasoning process, 52t
Receiver, 3
Reception failures, 29
Receptive aphasia, 238
Recognition, 389
Recoil, 285
Re-Engineered Discharge Toolkit (RED), 352
Referrals, 169
Reflection, 69–70
    exercise, 70b
Reflection and analysis, 393
Reflective listening response, usage, 288
Reflective responses, usage, 288b
Registered nurses, Bill of Rights, 323b
Relational continuity, 350–351
    collaborative and, characteristics of, 350
    definition of, 346
Relationships. See also Nurse-patient relationships
    barriers, reduction, 157b
    helping relationships, social relationships (differences), 134t
    style factors, impact, 85
Relaxation routines, 393, 393b
Relaxation techniques, 188
Reminiscence groups, 110
Remote site monitoring, 374
Remotivation groups, 110
Reporting, mandatory, 39
Resilience, 224–225, 386, 389–390
    training, 392–393
Resolution. See Conflict resolution

Respect, 61, 86, 133, 147–148, 333
    absence, 147
    convey, child communication, 264
    demonstration, 188
    model behaviors, 337
    mutual respect, 332
    personal space, 158
        hospital situations, 158
Responses
    assertive responses, 180b
    listening, negative, 71t
    structure, 177
    styles, 176
    verbal, 64–65
Restatement, 69
Restitution phase, 302
RFID. See Radiofrequency identification
Rights, of nurses, 323
Robert Wood Johnson Foundation, 328
Roles, 326b
    advanced practice nurses, 316
    application of, 318–326
    of case manager, 349
    clarity, 315, 332, 339, 350
    competencies, 316
    concepts of, 313–318
    developmental stages of, 319
    evidence-based practice, 318b
    expectations and, 313
    Flexner's criteria and, 314b
    funding, 349
    networking, 324
    nurse practice roles, 315–317
    of other health professionals, 351b
    patient advocacy, 324–326, 325b
    performance, 128
        case example, 128b
    professionalism and, 313–318
    professional nursing role competencies, 314–315, 314b, 315f, 316b
    relationships, 86, 128b
        nurse–patient, 325–326
        within nursing, 321–322
    socialization, steps in, 319–323
    technology and, 315
    theoretical constructs, 313–314
    theory, 314
    work environment and, 313–318

S

Safety, 179
    communication guidelines for, 14
    culture of, 13, 15–17
    definition of, 13
    goals of, 13
    HIT systems, 361–362
    incidences of, 13, 13b

Safety (Continued)
    case example, 13b
    innovations that foster, 15–18
    policies for, 24–25
    technology-oriented solutions create a climate of, 24
SANE program. See Sexual Assault Nurse Examiner
Schizophrenia, communication simulation, 245b
School age children, communication, 259–260
Science of teaching, 207
Scientific method, 43
Scope of practice, 30
Secondary groups, 103
Secure instant messaging, 377
Self
    actual self, 118
    definition, 118
    ideal self, 118
    management strategies, 139
    presence, 140–142
    therapeutic use, 137
Self-awareness, 137, 139, 322–323
    approaches in end-of-life care, 306
    communication and, 65
Self-clarity, 116
Self-concept
    application, 121–129
    body image, 115
    case example, 118b
    characteristics, 116f, 121–129
    clarity, 116
    concepts, 115–121
    definition, 115–118
    development, 116–117
    evidence-based practice, 122b
    features and functions, 116
    frameworks, 118–119
    gender, 118
    interpersonal relationships, 117–118
    microassaults, 118
    negative attributions, 118
    nursing strategies, 123–124
    patterns and nursing diagnosis, 122–123
    personality theory, 118–119
    physical appearance, 115
    self-clarity, 116
    spiritual aspects, 128–129
    theoretical frameworks, 118–119
    therapeutic strategies, 129
Self-control, maintenance, 185
Self-disclosure, 3, 132
Self-efficacy, 127–129, 192
    role performance, 128

Self-esteem, 115, 125–127
  behaviors, association, 126t
  case example, 116b
  definition of, 115
  development of, 116–117
  therapeutic strategies, 127
Self-fulfilling prophecies, 116
Self-identification (exercise), 117b
Self-management, strategies, 143
Self-reflection, 339
Selye, Hans, 220, 387
Sender, 3
Sensory function, loss of, 242b
Sensory loss, hearing/vision, 242b
Sensory perceptions, degree, 153t
Sentinel event, 293–294
Set boundaries, 390
Sexual assault, mental health emergencies, 293
Sexual Assault Nurse Examiner (SANE) program, 293
Shared decision-making, 143–144, 143b, 211, 332
  definition, 206
  process, steps, 144
Shared goals, 350
Shared mental model, 329
  value of, 329
Shock, 285
  in phases of grief, 302
Short-term memory, impact, 279
Short-term therapeutic relationships
  adaptation, 145–146
  orientation phase, 145
  termination phase, 144–145
  working phase, 145
Silence, 70–71, 71t
  allowance, 79
Simulations
  skills acquisition through, 19
  usage, 57
Situational crisis, 251, 285
Situation, background, assessment, recommendation (SBAR), 20, 334
  advantage of, 21
  example of, 20b
  on mobile communications, 374b
  patient safety outcomes of, 20–22
  simulation exercise for, 21b
  structured communication format, 20t
  usage, 20–22
Skills, 98–99
Slang, usage, 85–86
Sleep, 391–392
Small group communication therapy, characteristics, 103–108

Smartphones, 373
  apps, 244
  guidelines for, 380
Social cognitive competency, 84
Social determinants
  importance, 197
  of health, 93
Social isolation, 271
Socialization, 111t, 274
Socializing agents, 318
Social justice, 47
Social learning theory (Bandura), 194–195, 314
  case example, 195b
Social media
  advances in, 40
  case example in, 40b
  online guidelines for nurses using, 37t
  privacy cautions in, 40–41
  usage, 40–41, 381
Social relationships, helping relationships (differences), 134t
Social support, 229
  aging, relationship, 274–275
  assessment, 229
  description, 201
  level, dependence, 275
Social worth, 47
Solution
  agree, 185
  restate, 185
Speech
  deficits, verbal communication impairment, 238, 244
  difficulties, client assistance (strategies), 244b
  speech-generating devices, 244
Spiritual distress, 128
  issues, 129b
Spirituality, 128
Spiritual needs
  assessment, 128
  attending, 309
Spiritual support
  aging (relationship), 274–275
  stress, 229
Staff-focused consultation, 188
Staff management, 174–175
  active interventions, 174
  outcomes, 175
  postevent, 174
  preventive interventions, 174
Staff, supervision of, 321–322
Standardized handoff tools, 24
  patient safety outcomes in, 24
Standardized language terminology, in nursing, 368

Standardized tools, for communication, 12, 17–18
  patient safety outcome in, 17
  usage, introduction to, 19–22
Standards of care, 307
State Boards of Nursing, 31
Statutory laws, 34
Stereotypes
  identification, 152b
  impact, 152
  learning, 152
  negative stereotypes (valuation), emotions (impact), 152
STOPP (Screening Tool of Older Person's Inappropriate Prescriptions), 349
Storming phase
  group, 106
  therapeutic groups, 113
Storytelling
  as communication strategy, 259
  mutual technique, usage, 259b
Stranger anxiety, 257
"Stranger" role, 140
Strategic career planning, 321
Stress, 386
  acute, 220
  allostasis model of, 221f
  anger, 228–229
  applications of, 225–233
  assessment of, 225–228
    tool, 228b
  behavioral observations, 227–228
  case example, 387b
  chronic, 220
  cognitive behavioral approaches, 232
  community support, 229
  concept/definition of, 218
  coping, 222
  critical incident, 221–222
  distress, 220–221
  education for, reduction, 229–230
  etiology, 219
  eustress, 220
  feelings, processing, 228
  gender, 220
  general adaptation syndrome, 220–221
  goals, development, 230–231
    case example of, 231b
  guided imagery, impact, 232
  health organization imperative, 225
    nurses, 225
    organizations, 225
  hormones, 221
  hospital-related sources, 227
  hostility, 228–229
  impact

Stress *(Continued)*
    assessment of, 229
    factors, 226b
  incidence of, 218–219, 386
  intervention, 229
    tool, 228b
  issues
    addressing, 226
    for children, 229
  levels, 220
  meditation, 232
    techniques, 233b
  mind-body therapies, 232
  models, 220–222
  patient-centered approach, 227
  personal sources of, 219b
  prevention, 227
  primary appraisal, 222
  priority setting of, 231
  progressive relaxation, usage, 232
  psychosocial frameworks, 221–222
  reactions, primary/secondary appraisal
    in, 222f
  reduction, 390
  reduction measures, 339–340
  resilience, 224–225
  responses, 220, 386
  secondary appraisal, 222
  social support, 229
    assessment, 231
  spiritual support, 229
  support groups, 229
  support network, 229
  symptoms, 219–220
  systemic physiologic response, 220
  transactional model of, 222
Stressors, 119t–121t
  definition of, 218
  response, 221
Structural empowerment, 323
Style factors, impact, 85
Suffering, client understanding (desire), 148
Suicide, 388
  American Nurses Credentialing Center
    Competencies, 294–295
  assisted, 307
  behavior, 293–294
  definition, 293, 293f
  incidence, 293
  interventions, 294
    crisis team, 295
    safety planning, 295
  nurses and, 295
  passive suicidal wishes and actions, 294
  prevention, 295
  risk factors, 294, 294b
  screening and assessment, 294

Summarization, 70
Sundowning, 280
Supervisors, communication with, 321
Support groups, 110–111
Support network, stress, 229
Support system, 341–342
Surgical unit, conflict on, 330b
Surrogates, informed consent and, 40
Symbols, 3
System failures, 29
Systemic physiologic response, 220
System problems, 349
Systems theory, 3
Szalay's process model of intercultural
    communication, 90

T
Tablets, 373
Talk
  choice talk, 144
  decision talk, 144
  option talk, 144
  usage, 186
Talking down, avoidance, 86
Taxonomy, definition, 368
TCAB. *See* Transforming Care at the Bedside
Teach-back method, 214–215, 215b
Teaching
  care plans, 214, 214b
  strategies at different development
    levels, 212, 213t
Team care, 10
Team meetings, interdisciplinary rounds
    and, 23–24
Teams
  communication, improves, 330t
  members, nurse behavior toward, 333
TeamSTEPPS. *See* Team Strategies and
    Tools to Enhance Performance and
    Patient Safety
TeamSTEPPS training, 330, 330t
Team Strategies and Tools to Enhance
    Performance and Patient Safety
    (TeamSTEPPS), 22–23, 330t,
    333–334, 334b, 335f
  with I PASS the BATON, 22, 23t
Team training
  in communication, outcomes of, 333
  models for, 22–23
  patient safety outcomes of, 23–24
  program, 330t
Teamwork, 31, 334
  communication and, 330, 331b
Technology
  application programs (apps), 372
  in patient-centered relationships, 73
  use, 379–380

Technology-oriented solutions, climate
    of patient safety, 24
  patient safety outcomes in, 24
Telehealth, 374f, 375
Tension-reducing actions, usage, 186–188
Termination phase, 136
  short-term therapeutic relationships,
    144–145
  therapeutic relationships, 135
Termination phase, patient-centered
    care, 135
Texting
  personal use guidelines, 380–381
  secure instant messaging, 377
The Joint Commission, privacy
    regulations, 38
Theory of Culture Care (Leininger), 90–91
Therapeutic communication
  characteristics of, 63f
  definition of, 63
  dynamic interactive process, 63
  skills, usage, 182, 186–188
Therapeutic groups, 109–110
  adjourning phase, 113
  applications, 109–114
  forming phase, 112–113
  monopolizing phase, 113
  norming phase, 113
  performing phase, 113
  purpose, 103t
  storming phase, 113
  types, 103t
Therapeutic relationship bridges, 147–159
  acceptance, impact, 151–152
  anxiety, impact, 152–153
  applications, 156–158
  barriers, 147–159
  caring, 148
    process, steps, 156
  case study, 148b
  concepts, 147–151
  cultural barriers, 154–155
  empathy, 150
  empowerment, 149
    strategies, 156
  evidence-based practice, 155b
  gender differences, 155
  mutuality, 150–151
  nurse-client relationships, barriers
    (reduction), 157–158
  nursing actions, empathy (applica-
    tion), 156–157
  personal space, violation (impact), 154
  respect, 147–148
  stereotyping, impact, 152
  trust, 149–150
  veracity, 151

Therapeutic relationships
  applications, 137–146
  collaborative partnership, 135–139
  concepts, 131–137
  definitions, 131
  goals, 139
  involvement, level, 137–138
    maintenance, 138
  orientation phase, 142–143
  participant observation, 141–142
  patient-centered, 131–146
    characteristics of, 132–134
    collaborative, 135–137
    elements of, 134–135
    phases of, 142–145
    self-management, 139
  preinteraction phase, 142
  short-term relationships
    adaptation, 145–146
    orientation phase, 145
    termination phase, 144–145
    working phase, 145
  termination phase, 135
  theoretical frameworks, 136–137
  working (exploitation/active intervention) phase, 143–144
Thinking
  critical thinking, 48–50
  errors, 125
  types of, 43, 44f
"Three wishes question," 261
Time, 63
Timely follow-up, care transition model, 349
Time orientation, 99
Time-outs, 23–24
Timing, 65
TJC. See The Joint Commission
Toddlers (child communication), 257–258
Tone
  moderation, 77–78
  usage, 188
  vocal, usage, 178
Touch, 79–80
  aging, 280
Transactional communication models, 4
Transactional models, of communication, 62–63
Transformational leadership, 323
Transforming Care at the Bedside (TCAB), 25
  patient safety outcomes, 25
Transition and discharge planning, 347, 348t, 351, 352b
Transition Care Model, 346
Transition healthcare model, 269

Transmission, 3
Transmission failures, 29
Trauma
  children, cope with, 296
  older adults, cope with, 296
Treatment
  pain, 262
  procedures, child preparation, 262b
  related communication deficits, 246b
Trust, 149–150
  definition, 141
  establishment, 141
  mistrust, 149–150
  promotion, techniques, 149b
  truthfulness, impact, 47

U
Unit checklists, usage, 19
Universality, 111t
Universal norms, 105
Unlicensed assistive personnel, 321
Unnecessary treatment, 47
Unresolved conflict, 178
Unwarranted put-downs, 339–340
Utilitarian-based model, 45

V
Validation, 72, 98–99
Values
  clarification, 49–50
  emotional value, 125
  identification, 53–54
Veracity, 151
  of child communication, 264
  trust, relationship, 47
Verbal behaviors, anxiety (association), 153b
Verbal communication, 1, 76–77
  case example, 76b
  impairment, 238, 244
  skills, absence, 157f
Verbalization, usage, 186
Verbal responses, 64–65
Verbal style
  components, 76
  factors, 77–78, 77f, 78b, 85–86
Veterans Administration Clinical Team Training Program, 23
Video recording, self-analysis, 84b
Violence
  avoidance, nursing behaviors, 186t–187t
  behavioral indicators of, 292t
  case example, 173b–174b
  mental health emergencies, 292–293, 292t
  risk, incidence statistics, 174

Vision, sensory loss, 242b
Vision loss, 237–238
  children, 238
  communication strategies, 242–243
    case example of, 243b
  etiology, 238
  incidence, 237–238
  older adults, 238
Visual learners, 209–210
Vocalics, 85
Vocalization
  pitch/tone, moderation, 77–78
  variation, 78
Vocera, 374
Voice-activated communication, 374
von Bertalanffy, Kurt, 161–162

W
Walking meditation, 393b
Wearable biomedical sensors, 374
  uses, 381
Well-being, 191
  maintenance, critical elements, 192f
Wellness, aging and, 274
Wellness Initiative for Senior Education (WISE), 274
Wireless devices, usage, 382b
Wireless technology, 372
Wisdom, 270
Wong–Baker FACES Pain Rating Scale, 305, 306f
Words, meaning (interpretation), 76
Workable relationships (establishment), trust (impact), 149
Work-arounds, 25, 366
Work environment, 313–318
  creating safe, supportive, 323–324
Work flow, enhancement, 371, 374–375
Work groups
  effective and ineffective, 112t
  leadership, 111
  professional, 111–112
Working phase, brief therapeutic relationship, 136, 145
  applications, 143–144
Working phase, patient-centered care, 135
Workload, HIT system, 366
World Health Organization (WHO), 31
World view, 94
Written communication, 1
  strategies for, 210, 210b
Written materials, usage, 25
Written orders, 365–366

Z
Zoom, 331b